ANNALS OF
THE NEW YORK ACADEMY
OF SCIENCES

Volume 713

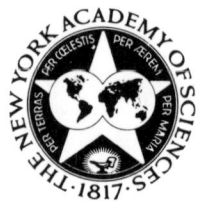

EDITORIAL STAFF

Executive Editor
BILL BOLAND

Managing Editor
JUSTINE CULLINAN

Associate Editor
ANGELA C. FINK

The New York Academy of Sciences
2 East 63rd Street
New York, New York 10021

THE NEW YORK ACADEMY OF SCIENCES
(Founded in 1817)
BOARD OF GOVERNORS, July 1993–June 1994

CYRIL M. HARRIS, *Chairman of the Board*
JOSHUA LEDERBERG, *President*
HENRY M. GREENBERG, *President-Elect*

Honorary Life Governor
WILLIAM T. GOLDEN

Vice-Presidents
EDWARD COHEN   JERROLD WILLIAM MABEN   MARTIN L. LEIBOWITZ

Secretary-Treasurer
HENRY A. LICHSTEIN

Elected Governors-at-Large
BARRY R. BLOOM   RONALD BRESLOW   SUSANNA CUNNINGHAM-RUNDLES
MARTHA R. MATTEO   DOROTHY NELKIN   RICHARD A. RIFKIND
DAVID E. SHAW   WILLIAM C. STEERE, JR.   SHMUEL WINOGRAD

CHARLES A. SANDERS, *Past Chairman*   HELENE L. KAPLAN, *General Counsel* [ex officio]
RODNEY W. NICHOLS, *Chief Executive Officer* [ex officio]

CHOLECYSTOKININ

ANNALS OF THE NEW YORK ACADEMY OF SCIENCES
Volume 713

CHOLECYSTOKININ

*Edited by Joseph R. Reeve Jr., Viktor Eysselein,
Travis E. Solomon, and Vay Liang W. Go*

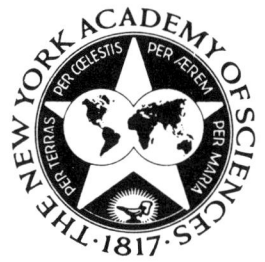

*The New York Academy of Sciences
New York, New York
1994*

Copyright © 1994 by the New York Academy of Sciences. All rights reserved. Under the provisions of the United States Copyright Act of 1976, individual readers of the Annals are permitted to make fair use of the material in them for teaching and research. Permission is granted to quote from the Annals provided that the customary acknowledgment is made of the source. Material in the Annals may be republished only by permission of the Academy. Address inquiries to the Executive Editor at the New York Academy of Sciences.

Copying fees: For each copy of an article made beyond the free copying permitted under Section 107 or 108 of the 1976 Copyright Act, a fee should be paid through the Copyright Clearance Center, Inc., 222 Rosewood Drive, Danvers, MA 01923. For articles of more than 3 pages, the copying fee is $1.75.

∞ The paper used in this publication meets the minimum requirements of American National Standard for Information Sciences—Permanence of Paper for Printed Library Materials, ANSI Z39.48-1984.

Library of Congress Cataloging-in-Publication Data

Cholecystokinin / edited by Joseph R. Reeve, Jr., . . . [et al.].
    p. cm. — (Annals of the New York Academy of Sciences, ISSN 0077-8923 ; v. 713)
    ISBN 0-89766-857-X (cloth : alk. paper). — ISBN 0-89766-858-8 (paper : alk. paper)
    1. Cholecystokinin—Physiological effect—Congresses. I. Reeve, Joseph R. II. Series.
    [DNLM: 1. Cholecystokinin—congresses. 2. Receptors, Cholecystokinin—congresses. W1 ANA626YL 1994]
Q11.N5 vol. 713
[QP572.C5]
500 s—dc20
[612.3'2]
DNLM/DLC   94-4554
for Library of Congress   CIP

SP
Printed in the United States of America
ISBN 0-89766-857-X (cloth)
ISBN 0-89766-858-8 (paper)
ISSN 0077-8923

ANNALS OF THE NEW YORK ACADEMY OF SCIENCES
Volume 713
March 23, 1994

CHOLECYSTOKININ[a]

Editors
JOSEPH R. REEVE JR., VIKTOR EYSSELEIN,
TRAVIS E. SOLOMON, AND VAY LIANG W. GO

Conference Organizers
JOSEPH R. REEVE JR., VIKTOR EYSSELEIN, JOYCE FRIED,
TRAVIS E. SOLOMON, AND VAY LIANG W. GO

CONTENTS

A Tribute to Viktor Mutt. *By* THE EDITORS.......... xiii

Preface and Introduction. *By* JOSEPH REEVE JR., JOYCE FRIED, VIKTOR EYSSELEIN, TRAVIS SOLOMON, and VAY LIANG W. GO.......... xv

Opening Lecture

Historical Perspectives on Cholecystokinin Research. *By* VIKTOR MUTT.......... 1

Part I. The Biochemistry and Molecular Biology of Cholecystokinin

Natural and Synthetic CCK-58. Novel Reagents for Studying Cholecystokinin Physiology. *By* JOSEPH R. REEVE JR., VIKTOR E. EYSSELEIN, F. J. HO, P. CHEW, STEVEN R. VIGNA, RODGER A. LIDDLE, and CHRIS EVANS.......... 11

Regulation of Cholecystokinin Gene Expression in Rat Intestine. *By* RODGER A. LIDDLE.......... 22

Peptides Related to Cholecystokinin in Nonmammalian Vertebrates. *By* GÜNTHER KREIL and CHRISTIAN WECHSELBERGER.......... 32

Is Invertebrate CCK-Like Immunoreactivity Caused by Asp-Phe-Amides Similar to the lymnaDFamides (a New Family of Molluscan Neuropeptides)? *By* ANDERS H. JOHNSEN and JENS F. REHFELD.......... 39

Part II. The Biochemistry and Molecular Biology of Cholecystokinin Receptors

Cellular Mechanisms Mediating Agonist-Stimulated Calcium Influx in the Pancreatic Acinar Cell. *By* STEPHEN J. PANDOL, ANNA GUKOVSKAYA, TRISTRAM D. BAHNSON, and VINCENT E. DIONNE.......... 41

Cholecystokinin Receptor Family. Molecular Cloning, Structure, and Functional Expression in Rat, Guinea Pig, and Human. *By* STEPHEN A. WANK, JOSEPH R. PISEGNA, and ANDREAS DE WEERTH.......... 49

[a]This volume is the result of a conference entitled **CCK 1993: International Symposium** held in Chatham (Cape Cod), Massachusetts on May 19–22, 1993.

The CCK-B/Gastrin Receptor. Identification of Amino Acids That Determine Nonpeptide Antagonist Affinity. *By* A. S. KOPIN, M. BEINBORN, Y.-M. LEE, E. W. MCBRIDE, and S. M. QUINN 67

Part III. Pharmacology of Cholecystokinin and Its Antagonists

Biological Evaluation of JMV180 Cholecystokinin Analogs. *By* M. AMBLARD, M. F. LIGNON, N. BERNAD, A. M. NOEL-ARTIS, L. HAUAD, J. LAUR, M. RODRIGUEZ, M. C. GALAS, D. FOURMY, and J. MARTINEZ 79

Distinguishing Multiple CCK Receptor Subtypes. Studies with Guinea Pig Chief Cells and Transfected Human CCK Receptors. *By* ROBERT T. JENSEN, JIA-MING QIAN, JAW-TOWN LIN, SAMUEL A. MANTEY, JOSEPH R. PISEGNA, and STEPHEN A. WANK 88

Novel CCK Analogs for Studying CCK-B Receptor. *By* CHIZUKO YANAIHARA, ATSUKAZU KUWAHARA, MUTSUAKI SUZUKI, MINORU HOSHINO, MIN LI, LI QIN ZHENG, KAZUHISA KASHIMOTO, YASUO TAKEDA, KAZUAKI IGUCHI, TOHORU MOCHIZUKI, and NOBORU YANAIHARA 107

The Ureidoacetamides, a Novel Family of Non-peptide CCK-B/Gastrin Antagonists. *By* G. A. BÖHME, P. BERTRAND, C. GUYON, M. CAPET, C. PENDLEY, J. M. STUTZMANN, A. DOBLE, M. C. DUBROEUCQ, G. MARTIN, and J. C. BLANCHARD 118

Part IV. Neurophysiology of Cholecystokinin

CCK Elicits and Modulates Vagal Afferent Activity Arising from Gastric and Duodenal Sites. *By* GARY J. SCHWARTZ and TIMOTHY H. MORAN 121

Ionic Mechanisms Underlying Cholecystokinin Action in Rat Brain. *By* P. BODEN and G. N. WOODRUFF 129

Cholecystokinin Modulates Dopamine-Mediated Behaviors. Differential Actions in Medial Posterior *versus* Anterior Nucleus Accumbens. *By* JACQUELINE N. CRAWLEY 138

Integration of Postprandial Function in the Proximal Gastrointestinal Tract. Role of CCK and Sensory Pathways. *By* HELEN E. RAYBOULD and K. C. KENT LLOYD 143

CCK in Cerebral Cortex and at the Spinal Level. *By* T. HÖKFELT, P. MORINO, V. VERGE, M.-N. CASTEL, C. BROBERGER, X. ZHANG, M. HERRERA-MARSCHITZ, J. J. MEANA, U. UNGERSTEDT, X.-J. XU, J.-X. HAO, M. J. C. PUKE, ZS. WIESENFELD-HALLIN, Å. SEIGER, J. HUGHES, A. VARRO, and G. DOCKRAY 157

Gastric Distention Induces c-Fos Immunoreactivity in the Rat Brain Stem. *By* KATHLEEN A. FRASER and JOSEPH S. DAVISON 164

Part V. Gastrointestinal Physiology of Cholecystokinin

Feedback Inhibition of Cholecystokinin Secretion by Bile Acids and Pancreatic Proteases. *By* GARY M. GREEN 167

Effects of CCK on Pancreatic Function and Morphology. *By* CLAUS NIEDERAU, REINHARD LÜTHEN, and TOBIAS HEINTGES 180

Acid-Base Interactions during Exocrine Pancreatic Secretion. Primary Role for Ductal Bicarbonate in Acinar Lumen Function. *By* STEVEN D. FREEDMAN and GEORGE A. SCHEELE 199

Role of CCK in Gallbladder Function. *By* BIRGIT TER-BORCH GRAM SCHJOLDAGER 207

Effect of Cholecystokinin on Gastric Motility in Humans. *By* CHRISTOPH BEGLINGER 219

Effects of Dietary Fat on Postprandial Gastrointestinal Motility Are Inhibited by a Cholecystokinin Type A Receptor Antagonist. *By* R. DE GIORGIO, V. STANGHELLINI, M. RICCI MACCARINI, A. M. MORSELLI-LABATE, G. BARBARA, L. FRANZOSO, L. C. ROVATI, R. CORINALDESI, L. BARBARA, AND V. L. W. GO 226

Part VI. Satiety

Cholecystokinin and Satiety: A Time Line. *By* GREGORY N. ERVIN 232

Satiating Effect of Cholecystokinin. *By* G. P. SMITH and J. GIBBS 236

Brain Regions Where Cholecystokinin Exerts Its Effect on Satiety. *By* RAFAEL R. SCHICK, VOLKER SCHUSDZIARRA, TONY L. YAKSH, and VAY LIANG W. GO 242

Endogenous CCK and the Peripheral Neural Substrates of Intestinal Satiety. *By* ROBERT C. RITTER, LYNNE A. BRENNER, and CONNIE S. TAMURA 255

Role of Cholecystokinin in the Regulation of Satiation and Satiety in Humans. *By* R. J. LIEVERSE, J. B. M. J. JANSEN, A. A. M. MASCLEE, and C. B. H. W. LAMERS 268

Part VII. The Role of Cholecystokinin in Disease

The Cholecystokinin Hypothesis of Anxiety and Panic Disorder. *By* JACQUES BRADWEJN and DIANA KOSZYCKI 273

Cholecystokinin Stimulates Ca^{2+} Mobilization and Clonal Growth in Small Cell Lung Cancer through CCK_A and CCK_B/Gastrin Receptors. *By* THOMAS HERGET, TARIQ SETHI, S. VINCENT WU, JOHN H. WALSH, and ENRIQUE ROZENGURT 283

Cholecystokinin Hyperresponsiveness in Dysmotility-Type Nonulcer Dyspepsia. *By* A. S. B. CHUA, T. G. DINAN, L. C. ROVATI, and P. W. N. KEELING 298

CCK, Schizophrenia, and Anxiety. CCK-B Antagonists Inhibit the Activity of Brain Dopamine Neurons. *By* KURT RASMUSSEN 300

A Second Generation of Non-Peptide Cholecystokinin Receptor Antagonists and Their Possible Therapeutic Potential. *By* S. B. FREEDMAN, S. PATEL, A. J. SMITH, K. CHAPMAN, A. FLETCHER, J. A. KEMP, G. R. MARSHALL, R. J. HARGREAVES, K. SCHOLEY, E. C. MELLIN, R. M. DIPARDO, M. G. BOCK, and R. M. FREIDINGER 312

Poster Papers

A Processing-Independent Analysis (PIA) for Human Procholecystokinin and Its Products. *By* LEA I. PALOHEIMO and JENS F. REHFELD 319

Regulation of the Human Cholecystokinin Gene. *By* KARIN PEDERSEN, FINN CILIUS NIELSEN, and JENS F. REHFELD 321

cDNA Deduced Procionin. Structure and Expression Pattern in Protochordates Resembles that of Procholecystokinin in Mammals. *By* J. U. THORUP, H.-J. MONSTEIN, A. H. JOHNSEN, and J. F. REHFELD 324

Evidence for a Helix-Turn-Helix in the NH_2-Terminus of CCK-58. *By* ANDREW K. S. LEE, HUGH B. NICHOLAS, JR., and GRACE L. ROSENQUIST. 328

Characterization of Cholecystokinin Receptors in Rat Pancreas. Evidence for Expression of CCK-A Receptors But Not CCK-B (Gastrin) Receptors. *By* WEIGONG ZHOU, STEPHEN P. POVOSKI, NANCY A. ROSEN, DANIEL S. LONGNECKER, and RICHARD H. BELL, JR. 331

Cholecystokinin Receptors in Cells of the Immune System. *By* MARIE-FRANCOISE LIGNON, NICOLE BERNAD, and JEAN MARTINEZ.......... 334

Molecular Cloning, Functional Expression, and Chromosomal Localization of the Human Cholecystokinin Type A Receptor. *By* JOSEPH R. PISEGNA, ANDREAS DE WEERTH, KONRAD HUPPI, and STEPHEN A. WANK............. 338

CCK_8-Evoked Ca^{2+} Mobilization in Pancreatic Acinar Cells. Evidence for a Regulatory Role of Protein Kinase C by Phosphorylation-Dependent Inhibition of Signaling through the High-Affinity CCK Receptor. *By* P. H. G. M. WILLEMS, H. J. M. VAN HOOF, M. G. H. VAN MACKELENBERGH, J. G. J. HOENDEROP, S. E. VAN EMST–DE VRIES, and J. J. H. H. M. DE PONT.. 343

$Gastrin_{13}$ Binds to CCK_B Brain Membrane Receptors Coupled to G Protein in Guinea Pig Brain Membranes. *By* J. C. LALLEMENT, J. C. GALLEYRAND, A. C. LIMA-LEITE, P. FULCRAND, and J. MARTINEZ............ 346

Rat Pancreatic Nucleoside Diphosphate Kinase, a Novel Regulator of Cholecystokinin Receptor Affinity. Cloning and Expression. *By* GEORGE T. BLEVINS, JR., ELS M. A. VAN DE WESTERLO, PAULETTE M. BLEVINS, and JOHN A. WILLIAMS 350

Combined Dose-Ratio Analysis for the CCK-B Antagonist Virginiamycin in Guinea Pig Ileum. *By* M. CORSI, G. DAL FORNO, B. OLIOSI, C. PIETRA, F. TH. M. VAN AMSTERDAM, and D. G. TRIST.. 353

CCK-B Antagonists Exhibit Antidepressant-Like Effects and Potentiate Endogenous Enkephalin Analgesia. Correlation with *in Vivo* Binding Affinities and Brain Penetration. *By* C. DURIEUX, M. DERRIEN, R. MALDONADO, O. VALVERDE, A. BLOMMAERT, M.-C. FOURNIÉ-ZALUSKI, and B. P. ROQUES 355

Effect of Hypothalamic Microinjection and Ventricular Perfusion of CCK Receptor Antagonists on Gut Myoelectrical Activity. *By* S. NITECKI, G. J. HARTY, and J. H. SZURSZEWSKI 358

Use of *Ex Vivo* Binding to Estimate Brain Penetration and Central Activity of CCK-B Antagonists. *By* SMITA PATEL, KERRY L. CHAPMAN, ALISON J. SMITH, ANNE HEALD, and STEPHEN B. FREEDMAN 360

The CCK_A Receptor Antagonist SR 27897 Differentially Influences the Activity of A_9 and A_{10} Dopaminergic Neurons in the Rat. *By* V. SANTUCCI, C. GUEUDET, O. THURNEYSSEN, D. GULLY, P. SOUBRIE, and G. LE FUR 364

Comparison of the Effects of the CCK-Receptor Antagonist Loxiglumide and the M_1-Receptor Antagonist Telenzepine on the Pancreatic Protein Response to Intraduodenal Tryptophan in Dogs. First Results. *By* STEPHAN TEYSSEN and MANFRED V. SINGER.. 368

Effects of CCK-A Antagonist Devazepide on Inhibition of Feeding by Duodenal Infusion of Oleic Acid in Rats. *By* TODD A. WOLTMAN and ROGER D. REIDELBERGER.. 372

The CCK-B Antagonist LY288513 Blocks Diazepam-Withdrawal-Induced Increases in Auditory Startle Response. *By* KURT RASMUSSEN, DAVID R. HELTON, JAMES E. BERGER, and ELIZABETH SCEARCE............................... 374

Evaluation of Brain Penetration of CCK-B Antagonists. *By* M. C. DUBROEUCQ, C. GUYON, F. MANFRE, M. CAPET, M. BARREAU, P. BERTRAND, B. JEANTAUD, A. DOBLE, and J.-C. BLANCHARD.................. 377

[^{3}H]SNF 8702 Autoradiography of CCK-B Receptors in Guinea Pig Brain and Studies with a Cloned Rat CCK-B Receptor. *By* RICHARD J. KNAPP, EWA MALATYNSKA, SHINICHI HASHIMOTO, SUNAN FANG, MARY HUNT, JAMES K. WAMSLEY, PAM PETERSON, TERESA ZALEWSKA, VICTOR J. HRUBY, and HENRY I. YAMAMURA.. 380

Effects of Cholecystokinin Octapeptide on Potassium Currents in Cultured Sympathetic Neurons. *By* HU XIAN and DAVID L. KREULEN 384

Cholecystokinin Receptor Subtypes Regulate Dopamine D_2 Receptors in Rat Neostriatal Membranes. Involvement of D_1 Receptors. *By* XI-MING LI, PETER B. HEDLUND, and KJELL FUXE 386

Intraduodenal Acid Augments Oleic Acid (C18)-Induced Cholecystokinin Release. *By* R. J. BRODISH, B. W. KUVSHINOFF, A. S. FINK, J. TURKELSON, D. W. MCFADDEN, and T. E. SOLOMON............................. 388

Potentiation of Acid-Induced Pancreatic Bicarbonate Output by Amino Acid Is Mediated by Neural Elements, but Not by Circulating Cholecystokinin. *By* R. J. BRODISH, B. W. KUVSHINOFF, A. S. FINK, D. W. MCFADDEN, J. TURKELSON, and T. E. SOLOMON 391

Role of CCK in the Regulation of Dynamic and Tonic Mechanical Response of the Human Gastric Fundus to Lipids. *By* M. A. MESQUITA, D. G. THOMPSON, N. K. AHLUWALIA, L. E. A. TRONCON, M. D'AMATO, and L. C. ROVATI.. 393

Selectivity and Potency of New Basic CCK-B Antagonists. *By* L. C. ROVATI, M. D'AMATO, W. PERIS, L. REVEL, and F. MAKOVEC................................ 395

Differential Effects of CCK on Longitudinal and Circular Smooth Muscle of Chicken Ileum. Mechanisms Involved. *By* E. FERNÁNDEZ, M. T. MARTÍN, A. G. FERNÁNDEZ, and E. GOÑALONS 398

CCK-8 Contracts the Gallbladder and Colon through Different Mechanisms in the Ferret. *By* S. MITAN and BEVERLEY GREENWOOD 401

Stimulation by the Ancestral Member of the CCK/Gastrin Family, Cionin, of Trout Gallbladder Contraction. *By* ANDERS H. JOHNSEN, BIRGIT SCHJOLDAGER, and JØRGEN JØRGENSEN 404

Inhibitory Action of CCK-OP on Rat Proximal Colon. *By* S. KISHIMOTO, H. MACHINO, H. KOBAYASHI, K. HARUMA, G. KAJIYAMA, A. MIYOSHI, and K. FUJII.. 407

Gastrin-Releasing Peptide and CCK after Intraduodenal Inhibition of Proteases. *By* H. KÖHLER, R. NUSTEDE, R. STREICH, and F.-E. LÜDTKE.... 410

Role of CCK in the Physiological Control of Gastroduodenal and Intestinal Motility in Chickens. *By* V. MARTINEZ, M. JIMENEZ, E. FERNANDEZ, E. GOÑALONS, and P. VERGARA... 413

Cholecystokinin in Human Stomach. Immunohistochemical Investigations on the Distribution and the Effects on Gastric Motility *in Vitro. By* S. MICHALSKI, H. HERKEN, K. GOLENHOFEN, G. LEPSIEN, R. NUSTEDE, H. KÖHLER, and F. E. LÜDTKE 417

Role of Substance P in the Regulation of Ion Transport of CCK_A and CCK_B Receptors in Mouse Ileum. *By* R. K. RAO, S. LEVENSON, S.-N. FANG, V. J. HRUBY, H. I. YAMAMURA, and F. PORRECA................................ 420

Cholecystokinin-Induced Pancreatic Growth Involves the High-Affinity CCK Receptor and Concomitant Activation of Tyrosine Kinase and Phospholipase D. *By* N. RIVARD, G. RYDZEWSKA, and J. MORISSET 422

Role of Intraluminal Nutrients in Feedback Regulation of Pancreatic Enzyme Secretion. *By* ALAN W. SPANNAGEL and GARY M. GREEN 424

On the Influence of CCK Receptor Blockade on GRP-Mediated Pancreatic Secretion. *By* F. STÖCKMANN, R. NUSTEDE, R. SCHLEMMINGER, H. KÖHLER, G. RAMADORI, and H.-J. PEIPER.. 427

Diurnal Variation in the Effects of Type A CCK Receptor Antagonist Devazepide on Meal Patterns in Rats. *By* DANIEL A. CASTELLANOS and ROGER D. REIDELBERGER.. 429

Cholecystokinin Inhibits Food Intake at a Peripheral Extragastric Site. *By* T. T. ZITTEL, B. V. ELM, R. K. TEICHMANN, H. D. BECKER, and H. E. RAYBOULD 431

Expression of CCK-A and CCK-B/Gastrin Receptors in Enterochromaffin-Like Cell Carcinoids of *Mastomys natalensis*. *By* OLA NILSSON, LARS KÖLBY, BO WÄNGBERG, STEPHEN A. WANK, and HÅKAN AHLMAN 435

Growth of Azaserine-Induced Putative Preneoplastic Nodules in the Rat Pancreas Is Mediated Specifically by Way of Cholecystokinin-A Receptors. *By* STEPHEN P. POVOSKI, WEIGONG ZHOU, DANIEL S. LONGNECKER, BILL D. ROEBUCK, and RICHARD H. BELL, JR. 439

Endogenous CCK in the Control of Gastric Secretory Response to Meal in Normal Subjects and Duodenal Ulcer Patients. *By* J. W. KONTUREK, R. STOLL, W. DOMSCHKE, and S. J. KONTUREK 442

Second Messenger Activators Regulate CCK mRNA in the Human Neuroepithelioma Cell Line SK-N-MCIXC. *By* B. L. MANIA-FARNELL, B. J. MERRILL, H. I. YAMAMURA, and T. P. DAVIS.. 446

Loxiglumide, a CCK-A Antagonist, in Irritable Bowel Syndrome. A Pilot Multicenter Clinical Study. *By* P. A. CANN, L. C. ROVATI, H. L. SMART, R. C. SPILLER, and P. J. WHORWELL 449

Clinical Efficacy and Prokinetic Effect of the CCK-A Antagonist Loxiglumide in Nonulcer Dyspepsia. *By* A. S. B. CHUA, M. BEKKERING, L. C. ROVATI, and P. W. N. KEELING 451

Cholecystokinin in the Hormonal Stimulation of Amino Acid Uptake and Pancreatic Enzyme Secretion. *By* J. W. KONTUREK, A. GABRYELEWICZ, R. STOLL, and W. DOMSCHKE 454

Concluding Remarks

Summary and Conclusions. *By* VAY LIANG W. GO... 457

Subject Index 459
Index of Contributors 465

Financial assistance was received from:

- AMERICAN GASTROENTEROLOGICAL ASSOCIATION
- A/M GROUP, MERCK INC.
- BECKMAN INSTRUMENTS, INC.
- DU PONT, NEN RESEARCH PRODUCTS (BOSTON, MASSACHUSETTS)
- GLAXO INC.
- JANSSEN PHARMACEUTICA RESEARCH FOUNDATION
- MARION MERRELL DOW
- MERCK & CO., INC.
- MERCK RESEARCH LABORATORIES
- NATIONAL INSTITUTES OF HEALTH (NATIONAL INSTITUTE OF DIABETES AND DIGESTIVE AND KIDNEY DISEASES GRANT R13 DK-46628-01)
- NATIONAL SCIENCE FOUNDATION (AWARD NUMBER IBN-9223310)
- PACKARD INSTRUMENT COMPANY
- RHÔNE-POULENC RORER
- WARNER-LAMBERT/PARKE DAVIS

The New York Academy of Sciences believes it has a responsibility to provide an open forum for discussion of scientific questions. The positions taken by the participants in the reported conferences are their own and not necessarily those of the Academy. The Academy has no intent to influence legislation by providing such forums.

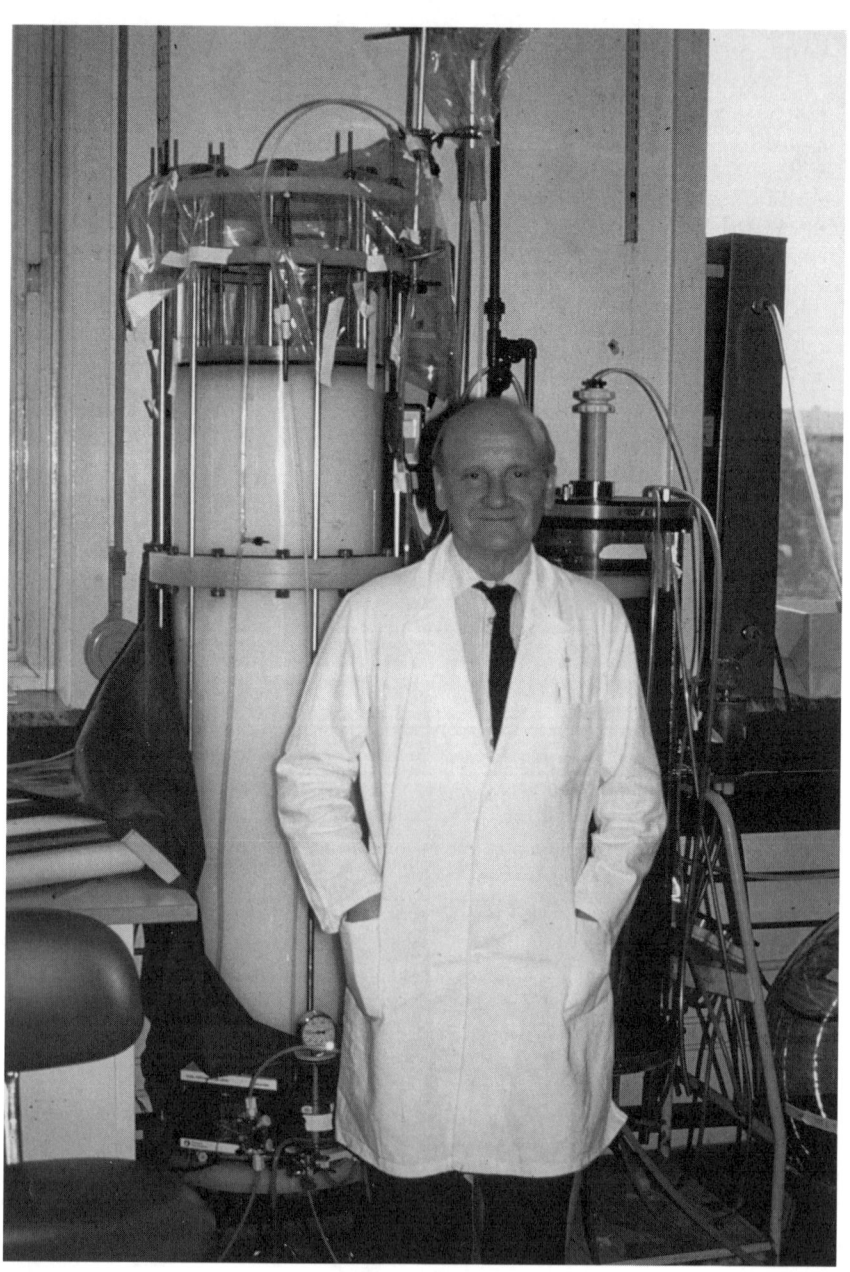

Viktor Mutt

A Tribute to Viktor Mutt

In recognition of his pioneering research on the chemistry and physiology of cholecystokinin, this volume is in honor of Professor Viktor Mutt.

It was more than 60 years after Bayliss and Starling in 1902 posed the question of whether the "substance exciting the liver is the same as that exciting the pancreas" that Professor Mutt answered it by purifying and chemically characterizing a peptide that contained 33 amino acids and both cholecystokinetic and pancreozyminic activities — CCK_{33}.

Professor Mutt has since then generously provided CCK_{33} to investigators throughout the world. Scientists from across the globe owe a great debt of gratitude to this considerate gentleman who has provided them with the means to study the physiology of cholecystokinin and who has supplied the basis for molecular biological studies of cholecystokinin and its receptor.

Those who know him also know that this brilliant, creative scientist long associated with the Karolinska Institute in Stockholm could not do otherwise than be generous. He is a genuinely warm, unpretentious, caring family man who must have one of the world's longest Christmas card lists. He has—and keeps—friendships that number in the hundreds.

And despite the high status in which this man, Viktor Mutt, is held by the world's scientific community, he is quite modest: so self-effacing that when presented with an award at the banquet given in his honor at the same Chatham symposium that yielded this volume, he said that the award would be especially dear to him because it came from his peers. The truth is that there were indeed many of Dr. Mutt's colleagues at the banquet that night, but few, if any, peers.

Those who have visited the professor can also tell you how difficult it is to keep up with this energetic man. No matter what he is working on, he always has time—or makes time—to talk with a visitor, to personally conduct the visitor on a guided tour of his laboratories (assuming that his guest can match his pace), no matter if that visitor is, like Professor Mutt, another scientist of great international renown or simply an undergraduate who is researching careers in bioscience. Included among the many attendees of the Chatham conference who benefitted from such hospitality were every single one of the symposium's organizers.

For many years, even though Dr. Mutt was our only source of cholecystokinin, his unselfish distribution of the peptide led to the development of immunological assays that have been used to purify other molecular forms of cholecystokinin from several species. It also led to the development of biological assays used in further studies on:

- The specificity of cholecystokinin receptors,
- The function of high and low affinity states of cholecystokinin receptors,
- Second messengers that communicate binding of cholecystokinin to other regions of the cell, and
- Cellular responses to these second messengers.

The magnitude of his contribution is made all the more impressive by the fact that cholecystokinin is but one of many biologically active peptides that have been purified and chemically characterized in Professor Mutt's laboratory. His generosity with his purified peptide or, in many cases, rather crude purification fractions has provided the basis for the careers of a great many investigators.

All of us who study biologically active peptides are indebted to Professor Mutt for his dedication to science, his kind generosity, and his drive for excellence. He is truly a model that all of us can look up to in our pursuit of knowledge.

—THE EDITORS

Preface and Introduction

JOSEPH REEVE JR.,[a] JOYCE FRIED,[b]
VIKTOR EYSSELEIN,[c] TRAVIS SOLOMON,[d]
AND VAY LIANG W. GO[e]

[a]CURE: VA/UCLA Gastroenteric Biology Center
UCLA School of Medicine and
West Los Angeles Veterans Administration Center
Los Angeles, California 90073

[b]University of California School of Medicine
Los Angeles, California 90024-1722

[c]Harbor-UCLA Medical Center
Division of Gastroenterology
Torrance, California 90509

[d]VA Medical Center
Kansas City, Missouri 64128

[e]The Brain Research Institute
University of California School of Medicine
Los Angeles, California 90024-1761

Pancreatic secretion and contraction of the gallbladder were among the first recognized physiological activities of substances stored in the small intestine. Viktor Mutt of Sweden, the man whom this volume is honoring, helped demonstrate that both of these physiological phenomena were mediated by the same peptide, cholecystokinin (CCK).

A peptide found in endocrine and neural cells in the periphery as well as in central neurons, cholecystokinin's role in normal and pathological physiology is being studied widely. Continuing interest in cholecystokinin is evidenced by the large number of publications on CCK, its receptors, and its receptors' agonists and antagonists.

The vague concept of a symposium on cholecystokinin first took form at the 1992 meeting of the American Gastroenterological Association when we, the organizers of the symposium, began planning the scientific program, fund-raising strategies, and the administrative organization of the symposium.

It had been 8 years since the first international conference on neuronal cholecystokinin in Brussels, Belgium, in July 1984. Sponsored by the Queen Elizabeth Medical Foundation of Belgium and the New York Academy of Sciences, it was organized by Jean-Jacques Vanderhaeghen and Jacqueline N. Crawley and was reported in the *Annals of the New York Academy of Sciences,* Vol. 448.

It had been 4 years since the most recent international meeting on cholecystokinin, held in the United Kingdom at Robinson College, Cambridge, in September 1988 and organized by John Hughes, Graham Dockray, and Geoffrey Woodruff. The proceedings of that meeting were published in a book entitled "The Neuropeptide Cholecystokinin (CCK)," edited by the three organizers.

Since the Cambridge meeting, landmark advances have been made in cholecystokinin research, advances that had been no more than hopeful wishes in 1988, as can readily be seen by comparing that volume to this one. Since then, for example, the structure of CCK_A and CCK_B receptors has been determined, and it is now accepted that the CCK_B and gastrin receptor are the same; this is a giant step that will help investigators unravel the puzzle of structure-function relationships. At the Cambridge meeting, antagonists that have since become the backbone of cholecystokinin physiology were first described; this volume looks at the utility of those antagonists. As a final example, several additional specific receptor agonists and antagonists have been developed since 1988 that will further our understanding of cholecystokinin physiology.

The purpose of our symposium, we decided, would be twofold: (1) to provide for an exchange of information among investigators from several specialty areas and (2) to recognize, through such activities as a banquet in his honor, the contributions that Professor Viktor Mutt has made in the study of cholecystokinin. (Dr. Mutt's written perspective on the history of cholecystokinin research is included in this volume.) Our hope was that participants would leave the symposium with insights that would enhance their own research and that some fruitful collaborations might result from the informal, yet exciting, atmosphere of the meeting. We hope that this volume might achieve more of those same results.

It was Joyce Fried who set up the administrative organization and, among other tasks, selected the site for the conference: Chatham Bars Inn on Cape Cod, Massachusetts, a truly inspired choice. Her organization also handled the appropriate logistics involved in arranging transportation, setting up scientific programs, distributing publicity, sending out invitations, following through on fund raising, and all the other myriad activities that go into creating a successful meeting—and profoundly successful it *was*!

The chairs of the various sessions (Jens Rehfeld, Viktor Eysselein, Laurence Miller, John Williams, Jerry Gardner, Noboru Yanaihara, Helen Raybould, John Walsh, Travis Solomon, Graham Dockray, Gregory Ervin, and Guido Adler) gave the organizers valuable input from the very beginning. Graham Dockray gave us particularly valuable advice on practical aspects of the meeting as well as helping us select speakers to invite. He also presented to Professor Mutt the award honoring his achievements.

The quality of the papers contributed to this book is but one indication of the value of the session chairs' participation in the intellectual organization of the symposium. The conference sessions were organized into seven major sections, a structure that is reflected in the chapter headings for this volume. Covered in these seven sections are:

I. Structure and processing of procholecystokinin in various species and the regulation of its mRNA.
II. Recent data on the structure of the cholecystokinin receptor, effects of its site-directed mutagenesis, and cellular responses of binding agonist to cholecystokinin receptors.
III. The use of synthetic agonists and antagonists specific for subtypes of the cholecystokinin receptor.
IV. Central actions of cholecystokinin and how stimulation of central neurons can have peripheral effects.
V. The role of cholecystokinin as an endocrine peptide, including how it is released and how it acts on pancreas, gallbladder, and gastric motility.
VI. Central/peripheral cholecystokinin: does it act as a satiety factor or not?
VII. Evidence that cholecystokinin plays a role in both central and peripheral disease states.

Each paper in this volume states the scientific opinions of its author(s). The editors have made no substantive changes. Each reflects many of the recent advances in the biochemistry, molecular biology, physiology, and cell biology of cholecystokinin and its receptors. Many indicate paths that will be followed in future research. Such new reagents as specific agonists and antagonists, expressed receptors, and synthetic molecular forms of cholecystokinin will allow future investigators to make new breakthroughs in how this important peptide, cholecystokinin, expresses its actions.

For enabling us to hold this enormously helpful symposium and produce this volume, we, the organizers, gratefully acknowledge the contributions of the American Gastroenterological Association (which enriched the symposium by funding travel scholarships for 23 young investigators), the National Institutes of Health (National Institute of Diabetes and Digestive and Kidney Diseases Grant Number R13 DK-46628-01), and the National Science Foundation (Award Number IBN-9223310), which provided funding for travel scholarships, as well as the many industry contributors listed in the Table of Contents.

We also acknowledge and express our appreciation to Martin Dodge for his help in gathering the manuscripts for this volume, nagging authors to get their papers submitted by the deadline, organizing the table of contents, and interacting with the publisher.

Finally, we wish to thank the participants who contributed significant time, knowledge, ideas, and excitement. Ultimately, it was they who made the meeting a great success. Among them are not only the speakers, but also those investigators who submitted abstracts and came to the meeting at their own expense to make valuable contributions to our understanding of cholecystokinin. The abstracts submitted by many of these investigators were of such quality and significance that we, the organizers, decided to invite all of them to submit extended abstracts for this volume—which almost all did. The organizers are proud to be associated with this excellent group of participants who made the meeting such a stimulating and enjoyable experience, one that made it well worth the effort to bring it together.

Historical Perspectives on Cholecystokinin Research[a]

VIKTOR MUTT

Department of Biochemistry II
Karolinska Institute
171 77 Stockholm, Sweden

In a preliminary report to the Royal Society on January 23, 1902, Bayliss and Starling[1] described the discovery of a substance in extracts of the mucosa of the upper intestine, which on intravenous administration caused the pancreas to secrete and suggested the name secretin. Later the same year, they[2] investigated if secretin had any effect on other organs and found that its only other effect was the stimulation of bile flow from the liver. They pointed out that the French workers Henri and Portier had also described this latter effect of secretin, but inasmuch as the secretin preparation they used presumably was contaminated by bile acids and as these were known to stimulate biliary secretion, their findings were inconclusive. The secretin preparation used by Bayliss and Starling was free of bile. Bayliss and Starling concluded that: "The question arises whether the substance exciting the liver is the same as that exciting the pancreas. It would be appropriate that the same body should perform both functions, but we must leave the question at present undecided." The question remained undecided for 62 years until it was shown that secretin, which we had isolated in an essentially pure form, had a weak but distinct choleretic action in the dog[3] or perhaps until Bodanszky and coworkers[4] synthesized a polypeptide with the amino acid sequence that we had found for natural secretin and the synthetic material too was found to have choleretic activity.

Meanwhile, Okada from Tokyo, working at the Institute of Physiology at University College, carried out extensive investigation of the different effects of feeding various types of food on biliary secretion and also confirmed that intravenously administered secretin stimulated biliary secretion. University College was evidently a good place for a visiting scientist. Okada[5] wrote: "All the experiments recorded in this paper were carried out on dogs, and the operations of them were performed for me by Professor Starling."

Okada, however, did not confine himself to investigating only the hepatic secretion of bile. He studied the contractibility of the gallbladder and found that contractions increased during digestion compared with food deprivation, but he did not mention any effect of intravenously administered secretin on gallbladder contractibility.[6]

In 1919 Braga and Campos[7] in Brazil found that a preparation of secretin caused emptying of the gallbladder. During the 1920s physiologists and clinicians became increasingly interested in the regulation of gallbladder function. Boyden found in cats that the gallbladder emptied after a meal of egg yolk and cream,[8,9] and on this basis clinical tests were started.[10] Whitaker demonstrated in dogs that physiological emptying of the gallbladder was caused by the contractile activity of the smooth muscle, as suggested by the work of Doyon[11] in 1893, and not, as assumed by many

---

[a] Investigations from the author's laboratory were supported by grants from the Swedish Medical Research Council and funds of the Karolinska Institute.

physiologists, by pressure from its neighboring organs during digestion.[12] Whitaker further showed that nervous mechanisms did not play an essential role in the regulation of gallbladder activity. He also investigated a preparation of secretin and found no definite effect on the gallbladder.

The picture was clarified substantially by the work of Ivy and Oldberg. In 1927 they[13] described experiments showing that in anesthetized cats or dogs the intravenous administration of a purified preparation of secretin resulted in a rise in intragallbladder pressure which was not inhibited by atropine. They also showed in dogs that emptying of the gallbladder prefilled with radiopaque material could be visualized roentgenographically. Their findings were also reported in greater detail in the February 11, 1928 issue of *JAMA,*[14] where they concluded that: "These observations, we believe, prove not only that the gall-bladder of the cat and dog 'contracts,' but also that a highly purified extract of the intestinal mucosa causes the gallbladder to evacuate, and that it is highly probable that the evacuation of the gall-bladder is brought about partially, if not completely, by a hormone identical with 'secretin', or a new hormone which controls the tonus of the gall-bladder." Subsequently, they[15] stated that since the previous report, ". . . Kloster, Lueth and Ivy have made preparations for us, the use of which indicate that 'secretin' does not cause the gall-bladder to contract but that it is some substance closely associated with 'secretin' because it is possible to prepare a solution of 'secretin' which is free of the gall-bladder excitant."

Moreover, Ivy and Oldberg performed cross-circulation experiments in which introduction of dilute HCl into the duodenum of the donor dog resulted in gallbladder contraction in the donor as well as the recipient dog. They concluded that: "These observations, if they do not prove, certainly show that a hormone mechanism must be considered, at least, as one of the mechanisms concerned in the normal evacuation of the gall-bladder. We propose the term 'cholecystokinin' to designate the active principle which causes the gall-bladder to contract." In describing these experiments, Ivy and Oldberg wrote: "After some consideration, we have decided to name the substance in intestinal extracts which causes the gall bladder to contract, 'cholecystokinin' (that which excites or moves the gall bladder).[16] Some evidence will be presented in a later paper which leads us to believe that the gall-bladder contracting principle is different from secretin." Various observations soon accumulated to suggest that cholecystokinin was a rather remarkable substance. If its physiological function was to contract the gallbladder, what then did it do in species, like the horse, which did not have a gallbladder? Although it stimulated the smooth muscle of the gallbladder to contract, it relaxed another smooth muscle, that of the sphincter of Oddi.[17]

The discovery of secretin had been followed by intense attempts in many laboratories to isolate it. In view of the obvious potentialities of CCK for practical clinical work, it is surprising that for many years, except for a solitary attempt by Ågren,[18] work on its purification remained confined to the laboratory in which CCK had been discovered. We too did not intentionally start to purify it. Instead, having isolated secretin in an essentially pure form,[19,20] we decided also to purify pancreozymin. Pavlov[21] and his coworkers had shown that the pancreatic juice secreted in response to acidification of the upper intestine had a low concentration of protein, whereas the juice secreted in response to stimulation of the vagus was rich in protein. Mellanby[22] had concluded that secretin stimulated the pancreas to secrete water and inorganic electrolytes, mainly sodium bicarbonate, and that the vagus stimulated it to secrete enzymes. However, Harper and Raper,[23] following up observations made by Harper and Vass, showed that extracts of the mucosa of the upper intestine contained a substance that on intravenous administration stimulated the pancreas to secrete enzymes; they named this substance pancreozymin.[23]

The existence of pancreozymin as a substance distinct from secretin was soon confirmed by Ivy and coworkers.[24] Thereafter, using dogs with subcutaneously transplanted pancreatic glands, Wang and Grossman[25] carried out their well known study of the effects of various substances, introduced into the intestine, on the release of secretin and pancreozymin. In this paper they noted that substances that were effective in releasing pancreozymin had earlier been found to be active in releasing cholecystokinin.

As reported elsewhere,[26,27] to isolate secretin we had worked out a method for the preparation of a concentrate of thermostable intestinal peptides, CTIP, which contained a large subgroup of peptides present in the tissues of the upper intestine. In brief, the method entails short boiling of the intestine to denature proteolytic enzymes, followed immediately by freezing of the boiled tissue material. The frozen material is minced and peptides are extracted from it with dilute acetic acid at low temperature. After filtering, peptides are adsorbed from the filtrate to alginic acid, eluted with 0.2 M HCl, and precipitated from the eluate, following adjustment of its pH to about 3 with sodium acetate, by saturation with NaCl. This precipitate is CTIP.

We had located pancreozymin activity to a certain "methanol-insoluble" side fraction from the preparation of secretin from CTIP. The purification of pancreozymin from this side fraction proceeded over a number of steps of size-exclusion and ion-exchange chromatography of a type that had become routine for the purification of peptides. An uncommon step, important from a practical point of view, was the precipitation of pancreozymin from solution in aqueous ethanol with butanol. This removed highly toxic impurities and enabled the pancreozymin preparation to be used in humans. As expected, the intravenous administration of our pancreozymin preparations stimulated the secretion of pancreatic enzymes but, unexpectedly, also the expulsion of bile from the gallbladder.[28-30] Similar observations were made in England by Howat and coworkers.[31]

To both groups of investigators the obvious explanation was that the pancreozymin preparations were contaminated by CCK. However, further purification of pancreozymin in our laboratory led to parallel increases in the pancreozyminic and cholecystokinetic activities of the preparations,[32] and we began to suspect that pancreozymin and cholecystokinin were one and the same substance.[33,34] The suspicion was strengthened by the finding that the two activities could be abolished by mild oxidation, under conditions in which the activity of secretin remained unaffected, and could be recovered by reduction of the oxidized material.[35] Such behavior was known earlier for several peptide hormones and, in the case of ACTH, was shown to be due to the reversible oxidation of a residue of methionine to one of methionine sulfoxide.[36] Considerably later, in the case of the vasoactive intestinal peptide VIP, we found that oxidation of a methionine residue in a hormonal peptide to the corresponding sulfoxide does not necessarily affect the activity of the peptide, although it changes its chromatographic behavior.[37] Because cholecystokinin-pancreozymin (CCK-PZ), as we now called it, contained residues of methionine, we decided to cleave it with cyanogen bromide according to a technique described by Gross and Witkop.[38] Among the cleavage products we identified aspartyl-phenylalanine amide,[39] which suggested that CCK-PZ had the COOH-terminal sequence -Met-Asp-Phe-NH$_2$. Completely unexpectedly this was found to be identical to the corresponding part of the sequence of gastrin.

Gastrin had been isolated by 1962 by Gregory and Tracy[40] from porcine antral tissue in the form of two heptadecapeptides, the acid hydrolysates of which had the same amino acid compositions.[41] When their amino acid sequences were determined, they were identical except that the phenolic group of the single tyrosine residue was free in one case (gastrin I) but esterified with sulfuric acid in the other (gastrin II).[42] It was also evident that CCK-PZ belonged to the group of naturally occurring peptides that instead of having a free COOH-terminal carboxyl group had a COOH-terminal alpha amide structure. This structural feature was first described for oxytocin[43,44] and vasopressin.[45,46] Subsequently it was found in a large number of hormonal and toxic peptides, and the enzymatic mechanism for its formation, from glycine-extended precursors, was clarified.[47,48] When the COOH-terminally amidated decapeptide caerulein was discovered in the skin of the frog Hyla caerulea, isolated and sequenced by Erspamer and coworkers,[49] it was evident that CCK-PZ, gastrin, and caerulein had an identical COOH-terminal pentapeptide amide sequence, which in gastrin was linked directly to a preceding residue of tyrosine but displaced from such a residue by an intervening residue of methionine in CCK, and one of threonine in caerulein. The phenolic group of the tyrosine residue was found to be esterified with sulfuric acid in CCK-PZ and caerulein, as in gastrin II. Elucidation of structure activity relationships for CCK-PZ has been interwoven with, and influenced by, similar studies on gastrin and caerulein.[49–51]

From such studies it was evident that sulfation of the tyrosine residue was essential for strong cholecystokinetic and pancreozyminic activity. However, one study showed that it was the strong acidic charge as such, and its position with respect to the peptide backbone, rather than specifically the tyrosine-O-sulfate that was necessary for activity. Substitution of the residue of tyrosine-O-sulfate by a residue of serine-O-sulfate in the COOH-terminal heptapeptide of CCK-PZ produced a peptide with very weak activity, whereas substitution with a residue of epsilon-hydroxynorleucine sulfate resulted in a peptide with strong activity.[52] The CCK-PZ that we had isolated proved to be a tritriacontapeptide, the complete amino acid sequence of which was elucidated in two publications, one in 1968[53] and the other in 1971.[54] It is: Lys-Ala-Pro-Ser-Gly-Arg-Val-Ser-Met-Ile-Lys-Asn-Leu-Gln-Ser-Leu-Asp-Pro-Ser-His-Arg-Ile-Ser-Asp-Arg-Asp-Tyr-(SO_3)-Met-Gly-Trp-Met-Asp-Phe-NH_2.

During this work it was found that the COOH-terminal octapeptide, which could be released, albeit sluggishly, by degradation of the tritriacontapeptide with trypsin, exhibited the complete cholecystokinetic and pancreozyminic activities of the whole molecule. Later the sequence of CCK-39, a form of CCK in which the sequence of the first isolated tritriacontapeptide was extended from its NH_2-terminus by the hexapeptide Tyr-Ile-Gln-Gln-Ala-Arg, was disclosed.[55] Remarkably, conversion of CCK-39 to CCK-33 entails a cleavage between two basic amino acid residues in a pair, rather than C-terminally to them. The isolation of CCK-33 and CCK-39 brought to a conclusion the main part of our work with CCK. Others, however, went on. Forms of CCK both longer than CCK-39 and shorter than CCK-33 have been isolated from the intestine of various species. Thus, CCK-58 was isolated, first from dog intestine[57] and subsequently from that of several other mammalian species, including man.[58] Recently, CCK-83 was isolated from human intestine, giving insight into the order in which the various biosynthetic steps leading from preprocholecystokinin to the different forms of the mature hormone occur.[59] As to forms shorter than CCK-33, from dog intestine CCK-25, CCK-18, CCK-8, CCK-7, and CCK-5 were isolated,[60] and CCK-22 together with CCK-8 from rat[61] and guinea pig[62] intestines. Isolation and sequence determination of these various forms of CCK were substantially facilitated by the availability of the amino acid sequence of preprocholecystokinin, which had been deduced from the experimentally determined nucleotide sequences for the rat,[63,64] pig,[65] mouse,[66,67] and human[68] forms of it.

An article of great importance in the understanding of CCK was published by

Vanderhaeghen and coworkers[69] in 1975. They described a "brain gastrin immunoreactive peptide, BGP," in the CNS of vertebrates. Dockray[70] found that the immunochemical properties of BGP were more CCK-like than gastrin-like and that on size-exclusion chromatography, BGP resembled CCK-8.

Soon thereafter, Straus et al.[71] described immunohistochemical experiments suggesting the presence of CCK-8 in rabbit cerebrocortical neurons, and Muller et al.,[72] using a combination of immunochemistry with electrophoretic and chromatographic methods, provided evidence for the presence of CCK-8 together with a larger form of CCK in pig brain. The presence of immunoreactive CCK in brain extracts from cats, rats, rabbits, and guinea pigs was reported by del Mazo.[73]

Rehfeld, using sequence-specific radioimmunoassays in combination with size-exclusion chromatography, concluded that CCK was present in the brain in both humans and pig and that it was heterogeneous in the brain as well as the small intestine.[74]

Vanderhaeghen together with Robberecht and Deschodt-Lanckman[75] found that BGP in extracts of a 100,000 × g pellet of postmortem human cerebral grey matter had a charge and size resembling that of CCK-8, and that it, like CCK-8, released amylase from rat pancreatic fragments and stimulated adenylate cyclase activity in rat pancreatic plasma membranes. Nevertheless, they also found that the amount of BGP in the extracts was much higher if determined by bioassay rather than radioimmunoassay.

Any doubts as to the presence of CCK in the CNS were definitely dispelled by the isolation of CCK-8 from sheep brain by Dockray et al.[76] An enormous amount of work in different laboratories on the possible physiological or pharmacological importance of CCK in the nervous system has followed these initial observations and continues without any signs of abating. Many developments until about 1985 were discussed at an international conference on neuronal CCK.[77] Although CCK-8 was the first form of CCK to actually be isolated from brain and has since been isolated from the brains of a substantial number of other mammalian species, including the human,[78] CCK-58 too has been isolated from dog,[79] pig,[80] and ox[81] brain. However, neither CCK-33 nor CCK-39 has been isolated from brain.

In our work on the amino acid sequence of CCK we found that selective cleavage of the peptide chain at certain amino acid residues is of value. Thus, besides the already mentioned nonenzymatic cleavage of CCK-33 with CNBr at methionyl residues, complete cleavage of it with trypsin released CCK-8, whereas on limited cleavage a substantial amount of CCK-8 remained attached to the tryptic tetrapeptide that preceded it in the intact peptide chain, giving CCK-12. Thrombin cleaved only one of the four bonds cleaved by trypsin, that between the NH_2-terminal hexapeptide and the following pentapeptide. Consequently, limited cleavage by trypsin and cleavage by thrombin sufficed to establish the order in which the five tryptic peptides occurred in intact CCK-33. Incidentally, we had earlier found thrombin useful in a similar situation, when determining the amino acid sequence of secretin.[82] We also found that enterokinase, in contrast to trypsin, releases CCK-8 swiftly from CCK-33 and CCK39.[83] An endoprotease, apparently very different from enterokinase, was recently purified from a rat brain synaptosome preparation and found to release CCK-8 from CCK-33.[84]

Today, when sophisticated machinery is available with which the amino acid sequences of peptides the size of CCK-58 may be determined using only a few nanomols of peptide, it may appear antiquated to be interested in enzymes that cleave peptide chains at specific residues. However, there are many naturally occurring peptides with, in various ways, blocked NH_2-terminal amino groups. In these cases, direct sequencing is not possible, at least not from the amino end, and the usual way to proceed is to produce fragments of the peptide by enzymatic degradation.

Therefore, until mass spectroscopists so refine their techniques that determination of amino acid sequences by any technique other than mass spectroscopy is obsolete, cleavage of peptides with enzymes of high specificity will continue to be useful. A welcome addition to this set of tools is an endopeptidase cleaving specifically at asparaginyl residues, recently discovered.[85] Also, the indication that the chicken may have an enzyme cleaving specifically at phenylalanyl bonds[86] is promising.

The isolation of CCK has had many interesting spin-off effects. For example, using a preparation of highly purified pancreozymin (CCK) which they had obtained from our laboratory, Hokin and Hokin[87] found that the stimulation of amylase secretion from pancreas slices *in vitro* was accompanied by what they termed a phospholipid effect, that is, increased incorporation of phosphate into a phospholipid fraction of tissue, an effect that they had observed earlier after stimulation of the pancreas with acetylcholine.[88] Largely through the work of Michell[89] and Berridge,[90] this effect was later understood to be due to the widely distributed diacylglycerol-phosphoinositide second messenger system.

A striking feature of current investigations of signal transmission by hormonal peptides is the search for nonpeptidal receptor agonists and antagonists. The first instance of success with this type of work was the discovery by Gardner and coworkers[91] that dibutyryl guanosine 3',5'-cyclic monophosphate was a competitive antagonist of the action of CCK on pancreatic acinar cells.

Unexpected and of far reaching nutritional and economic consequences[92] was the discovery by Schlatter *et al.*[93] that the alpha methyl ester of the COOH-terminal dipeptide of gastrin, and therefore of CCK and of caerulein, was more than 100 times sweeter than cane sugar.

The question may be asked if by now all major properties of CCK have been disclosed or if surprises can still be expected. Recent findings suggest that there might. It has long been known that the cholecystokinetic and pancreozyminic activities of CCK are exerted by its COOH-terminal part. Recently, however, Richter and Schwandt[94] found that a synthetic peptide with a sequence identical to the 1-21 sequence of CCK-33 had a lipolytic activity on human adipose tissue, an effect that CCK-8 did not have.

The finding of CCK in brain was unexpected. Likewise unexpected was the recent finding by Persson and coworkers[95] that in several mammalian species, CCK-like immunoreactivity and mRNA for preproCCK are present in male germ cells, suggesting that CCK may play a role in fertilization.

Friedman *et al.*[96] recently found that expression of the gene for preproCCK occurs in certain pediatric tumors and suggested that this could be useful for differential diagnosis of tumor types. The group of peptides to which CCK belongs was recently expanded by the discovery, in the protochordate *Ciona intestinalis,* of cionin with its two adjacent residues of tyrosine-O-sulfate and its possible implications in the understanding of the evolution of gastrin and CCK.[97] In mammals, however, the CCK-gastrin group of hormonal peptides still comprises only these two individual peptides. However, there is some reason to believe that additional ones may remain to be discovered.[98]

Finally, it should be realized that CCK could not have been discovered by way of any genome project. The amino acid sequence of preproCCK could have been deduced from the nucleotide sequence of the DNA corresponding to it, and peptides representing sequences of it, flanked by pairs of basic amino acids, synthesized. These synthetic peptides would have been practically inactive, however, because the two important posttranslational modifications, amidation of the COOH-terminal phenylalanine and esterification of the phenolic group of the tyrosine residue in position 7 from the COOH-terminus with sulfuric acid, would not have been evident from the deduced sequence. Today, the signals specifying for these two types of modifications are known, so now additional peptide hormones requiring just these two modifications for activity need not be missed on deduction from nucleotide sequences. But there are other types of posttranslational modifications for which no signal is known. For instance, in 1981 Erspamer and coworkers[99] had already isolated the opioid peptide dermorphin from the skin of a South American frog and found that it contained a residue of D-alanine in position 2. However, Kreil and coworkers[100] showed that the precursor protein to dermorphin has L-alanine in the corresponding position. Subsequently, several peptides with either D-alanine or L-methionine in position 2 but with exclusively L-amino acids in their precursors were discovered in frog skin.[101,102] Also, in several species of mollusc, peptides with different D-amino acids in their positions 2 were discovered.[103–105] Although precursor proteins to these molluscan peptides have not yet been described, it is reasonable to assume that in analogy with those for the amphibian peptides, they too contain L-amino acids exclusively. In no case is either the mechanism of conversion of the L-residue to a D-residue or the signal stating that such a conversion should take place known. It may be of interest to note that recently high concentrations of D-serine were found in rat brain.[106]

The foregoing is a rather sketchy outline of the history of CCK. More thorough treatment of various aspects of CCK are to be found in earlier reviews.[77,107–110]

REFERENCES

1. BAYLISS, W. M. & E. H. STARLING. 1902. Proc. Roy. Soc. **69:** 352–353.
2. BAYLISS, W. M. & E. H. STARLING. 1902. J. Physiol. (Lond.) **28:** 325–353.
3. JONSSON, G., L. SUNDMAN & L. THULIN. 1964. Acta Physiol. Scand. **62:** 287–290.
4. VAGNE, M., G. F. STENING, F. P. BROOKS & M. I. GROSSMAN. 1968. Gastroenterology **55:** 260–267.
5. OKADA, S. 1914/15. J. Physiol. (Lond.) **49:** 457–482.
6. OKADA, S. 1915/16. J. Physiol. (Lond.) **50:** 42–46.
7. BRAGA, J. G. & C. M. CAMPOS. 1919. Gazeta Clinica (Brazil) **17:** 65–69.
8. BOYDEN, E. A. 1923. Anat. Rec. **24:** 388–426.
9. BOYDEN, E. A. 1925. Anat. Rec. **30:** 333–356.
10. BOYDEN, E. A. 1926. Anat. Rec. **33:** 201–239.
11. DOYON, M. 1893. Arch. Physiol. Normal et Patologique **25:** 710–719.
12. WHITAKER, L. R. 1926. Am. J. Physiol. **78:** 411–436.
13. IVY, A. C. & E. OLDBERG. 1927. Proc. Soc. Exp. Biol. Med. **25:** 113–115.
14. IVY, A. C. & E. OLDBERG. 1928. J. Am. Med. Assoc. **90:** 445–446.
15. IVY, A. C. & E. OLDBERG. 1928. Proc. Soc. Exp. Biol. Med. **25:** 251–252.
16. IVY, A. C. & E. OLDBERG. 1928. Am. J. Physiol. **86:** 599–613.
17. SANDBLOM, P., W. L. VOEGTLIN & A. C. IVY. 1935. Am. J. Physiol. **113:** 175–180.
18. ÅGREN, G. 1939. Scand. Arch. Physiol. **81:** 234–243.
19. JORPES, J. E. & V. MUTT. 1961. Acta Chem. Scand. **15:** 1790–1791.
20. JORPES, J. E., V. MUTT, S. MAGNUSSON & B. B. STEELE. 1962. Biochem. Biophys. Res. Comm. **9:** 275–279.
21. PAVLOV, J. P. 1900. Ein Vortrag. Das Experiment als zeitgemässe und einheitliche Methoden medizinischer Forschung.: 1–48. Bergmann. Wiesbaden.
22. MELLANBY, J. 1925. J. Physiol. **60:** 85–91.
23. HARPER, A. A. & H. S. RAPER. 1943. J. Physiol. **102:** 115–125.
24. GREENGARD, H., M. I. GROSSMAN, J. R. WOOLLEY & A. C. IVY. 1944. Science **99:** 350–351.

25. WANG, C. C. & M. I. GROSSMAN. 1951. Am. J. Physiol. **164:** 527–545.
26. MUTT, V. 1978. *In* Gut Hormones. (S. R. Bloom, ed.: 21–27. Churchill Livingstone. Edinburgh, London.
27. MUTT, V. 1980. *In* Gastrointestinal Hormones. G. B. J. Glass, ed.: 85–126. Raven Press. NY.
28. WERNER, B. & V. MUTT. 1954. Scand. J. Clin. & Lab. Invest. **6:** 228–236.
29. BRODÉN, B. 1958. Acta Radiol. **49:** 25–29.
30. EDHOLM, P. 1960. Acta Radiol. **53:** 257–265.
31. DUNCAN, P. R., A. A. HARPER, H. T. HOWAT, S. OLEESKY & H. VARLEY. 1952. Gastroenterologia **78:** 349–353.
32. JORPES, J. E., V. MUTT & K. TOCZKO. 1964. Acta Chem. Scand. **18:** 2408–2410.
33. JORPES, J. E. & V. MUTT. 1961. Ann. Int. Med. **55:** 395–405.
34. JORPES, J. E. & V. MUTT. 1966. Acta Physiol. Scand. **66:** 196–202.
35. MUTT, V. 1964. Acta Chem. Scand. **18:** 2185–2186.
36. DEDMAN, M. L., T. H. FARMER & C. J. O. R. MORRIS. 1961. Biochem. J. **78:** 348–352.
37. MUTT, V. 1981. Peptides 2(suppl. 2): 209–214.
38. GROSS, E. & B. WITKOP. 1961. J. Am. Chem. Soc. **83:** 1510.
39. MUTT, V. & J. E. JORPES. 1967. Biochem. Biophys. Res. Comm. **26:** 392–397.
40. GREGORY, R. A. 1962. *In* Surgical Physiology of the Gastro-Intestinal Tract, Symposium. A. N. Smith, ed.: 57–70. Edinburgh Royal College. Edinburgh.
41. GREGORY, R. A. & H. J. TRACY. 1972. Gut **5:** 103–114.
42. GREGORY, H., P. M. HARDY, D. S. JONES, G. W. KENNER & R. C. SHEPPARD. 1964. Nature (Lond.) **204:** 931–933.
43. DU VIGNEAUD, V., C. RESSLER & S. TRIPPET. 1953. J. Biol. Chem. **205:** 949–957.
44. TUPPY, H. 1953. Biochim. Biophys. Acta **11:** 449–450.
45. DU VIGNEAUD, V., H. C. LAWLER & E. A. POPENOE. 1953. J. Am. Chem. Soc. **75:** 4880–4881.
46. ACHER, R. & J. CHAUVET. 1953. Biochim. Biophys. Acta **12:** 487–488.
47. BRADBURY, A. F., M. D. A. FINNIE & D. G. SMYTH. 1982. Nature **298:** 686–688.
48. KATOPODIS, A. G., D. PING, C. E. SMITH & S. W. MAY. 1991. Biochemistry **30:** 6189–6194.
49. ANASTASI, A., V. ERSPAMER & R. ENDEAN. 1967. Experientia **23:** 699–700.
50. YANAIHARA, N., N. SUGIURA, K. KASHIMOTO, T. NARUSE, C. YANAIHARA & T. SOLOMON. 1984. *In* Peptides. Proceedings of the 18th European Peptide Symposium, Djurönäset, Sweden, June 10–15. U. Ragnarsson, ed.: 373–378. Almqvist and Wiksell, Uppsala, Sweden
51. VINAYEK, R., R. T. JENSEN & J. D. GARDNER. 1987. Am. J. Physiol. **252:** G178–G181.
52. BODANZSKY, M., J. MARTINEZ, G. P. PRIESTLEY, J. D. GARDNER & V. MUTT. 1978. J. Med. Chem. **21:** 1030–1035.
53. MUTT, V. & J. E. JORPES. 1968. Eur. J. Biochem. **6:** 156–162.
54. MUTT, V. & J. E. JORPES. 1971. Biochem. J. **125:** 57–58p.
55. MUTT, V. 1976. Clin. Endocrinol. 5(Suppl.): 175s–183s.
56. GROSSMAN, M. I. 1970. Gastroenterology **58:** 128.
57. EYSSELEIN, V. E., J. R. REEVE, JR., J. E. SHIVELY, D. HAWKE & J. H. WALSH. 1982. Peptides **3:** 687–691.
58. EYSSELEIN, V. A., G. A. EBERLEIN, M. SCHAEFFER, D. GRANDT, H. GOEBELL, W. NIEBEL, G. L. ROSENQUIST, H. E. MEYER & J. R. REEVE, JR. 1990. Am. J. Physiol. **258:** G253–G260.
59. EBERLEIN, G. A., V. E. EYSSELEIN, M. T. DAVIS, T. D. LEE, J. E. SHIVELY, D. GRANDT, W. NIEBEL, R. WILLIAMS, J. MOESSNER, J. ZEEH, H. E. MEYER, H. GOEBELL & J. R. REEVE, JR. 1992. J. Biol. Chem. **267:** 1517–1521.
60. REEVE, J. R., JR., V. E. EYSSELEIN, J. H. WALSH, C. M. BEN-AVRAM & J. E. SHIVELY. 1986. J. Biol. Chem. **261:** 16392–16397.
61. ENG, J. H., B.-H. DU, Y.-C. E. PAN, M. CHANG, J. D. HULMES & R. S. YALOW. 1984. Peptides **5:** 1203–1206.
62. ZHOU, Z.-Z., J. ENG, Y.-C. E. PAN, M. CHANG, J. D. HULMES, J.-P. RAUFMAN & R. S. YALOW. 1985. Peptides **6:** 337–341.

63. DESCHENES, R. J., L. J. LORENZ, R. S. HAUN, B. A. ROOS, K. L. COLLIER & J. E. DIXON. 1984. Proc. Natl. Acad. Sci. USA **81**: 726–730.
64. DESCHENES, R. J., R. S. HAUN, C. L. FUNCKES & J. E. DIXON. 1985. J. Biol. Chem. **260**: 1280–1286.
65. GUBLER, U., A. O. CHUA, B. J. HOFFMAN, K. J. COLLIER & J. ENG. 1984. Proc. Natl. Acad. Sci. USA **81**: 4307–4310.
66. FRIEDMAN, J., B. S. SCHNEIDER & D. POWELL. 1985. Proc. Natl. Acad. Sci. USA **82**: 5593–5597.
67. VITALE, M., A. VASHISHTHA, D. J. POWELL & J. M. FRIEDMAN. 1990. Nucleic Acids Res. **19**: 169.
68. TAKAHASHI, Y., K. KATO, Y. HAYASHIZAKI, T. WAKABAYASHI, E. OHTSUKA, S. MATSUKI, M. IKEHARA & K. MATSUBARA. 1985. Proc. Natl. Acad. Sci. USA **82**: 1931–1935.
69. VANDERHAEGHEN, J.-J., J. C. SIGNEAU & W. GEPTS. 1975. Nature **257**: 604–605.
70. DOCKRAY, G. J. 1976. Nature **264**: 568–570.
71. STRAUS, E., J. E. MULLER, H.-S. CHOI, F. PARONETTO & R. S. YALOW. 1977. Proc. Natl. Acad. Sci. USA **74**: 3033–3034.
72. MULLER, J. E., E. STRAUS & R. S. YALOW. 1977. Proc. Natl. Acad. Sci. USA **74**: 3035–3037.
73. DELMAZO, J. 1977. Gastroenterology **72**(abstr.): A24/1047.
74. REHFELD, J. F. 1978. J. Biol. Chem. **253**: 4022–4030.
75. ROBBERECHT, P., M. DESCHODT-LANCKMAN & J. J. VANDERHAEGHEN. 1978. Proc. Natl. Acad. Sci. USA **75**: 524–528.
76. DOCKRAY, G. J., R. A. GREGORY & J. B. HUTCHISON. 1978. Nature **274**: 711–713.
77. VANDERHAEGHEN, J.-J. & J. N. CRAWLEY, EDS. 1985. Neuronal Cholecystokinin. Ann. N.Y. Acad. Sci. **448**: 1–697.
78. MILLER, L. J., I. JARDINE, E. WEISSMAN, V. L. W. GO & D. SPEICHER. 1984. J. Neurochem. **43**: 835–840.
79. EYSSELEIN, V. E., J. R. REEVE, JR., J. E. SHIVELY, C. MILLER & J. H. WALSH. 1984. Proc. Natl. Acad. Sci. USA **81**: 6565–6568.
80. TATEMOTO, K., H. JÖRNVALL, S. SIIMESMAA, G. HALLDÉN & V. MUTT. 1984. FEBS **174**: 289–293.
81. ENG, J., H.-R. LI & R. S. YALOW. 1990. Regul. Peptides **30**: 15–19.
82. MUTT, V., S. MAGNUSSON, J. E. JORPES & E. DAHL. 1965. Biochemistry **4**: 2358–2362.
83. MUTT, V., K. TATEMOTO, M. CARLQUIST & A. LIGHT. 1981. Biosci. Rep. **1**: 651–659.
84. VIERECK, J. C. & M. C. BEINFELD. 1992. J. Biol. Chem. **267**: 19475–19481.
85. ABE, Y., K. SHIRANE, H. YOKOSAWA, H. MATSUSHITA, M. MITA, I. KATO & S-I. ISHII. 1993. J. Biol. Chem. **268**: 3525–3529.
86. BJÖRNSKOV, I., J. F. REHFELD & A. H. JOHNSEN. 1992. Peptides **13**: 595–601.
87. HOKIN, L. E. & M. R. HOKIN. 1956. J. Physiol. **132**: 442–453.
88. HOKIN, M. R. & L. E. HOKIN. 1953. J. Biol. Chem. **203**: 967–977.
89. MICHELL, R. H. 1975. Biochim. Biophys. Acta **215**: 81–147.
90. BERRIDGE, M. J. 1983. Biochem. J. **212**: 849–858.
91. PEIKIN, S. R., C. L. COSTENBADER & J. D. GARDNER. 1979. J. Biol. Chem. **254**: 5321–5327.
92. SMITH, V. J., R. A. GREEN & T. R. HOPKINS. 1989. J. Assoc. Off. Anal. Chem. **72**: 30–33.
93. MAZUR, R. H., J. M. SCHLATTER & A. H. GOLDKAMP. 1969. J. Am. Chem. Soc. **91**: 2684–2691.
94. RICHTER, W. O. & P. SCHWANDT. 1989. Horm. Metab. Res. **21**: 216–217.
95. PERSSON, H., J. F. REHFELD, A. ERICSSON, M. SCHALLING, M. PELTO-HUIKKO & T. HÖKFELT. 1989. Proc. Natl. Acad. Sci. USA **86**: 6166–6170.
96. FRIEDMAN, J. M., M. VITALE, J. MAIMON, M. A. ISRAEL, M. E. HOROWITZ & B. S. SCHNEIDER. 1992. Proc. Natl. Acad. Sci. USA **89**: 5819–5823.
97. JOHNSEN, A. H. & J. F. REHFELD. 1990. J. Biol. Chem. **265**: 3054–3058.
98. VARRO, A. 1989. Neurochem. Int. **14**: 505–510.
99. MONTECUCCHI, P. C., R. DECASTIGLIONE, S. PIANI, L. GOZZINI & V. ERSPAMER. 1981. Int. J. Peptide Protein Res. **17**: 275–283.
100. RICHTER, C., R. EGGER & G. KREIL. 1987. Science **238**: 1200.

101. Mor, A., A. Delfour, S. Sagan, M. Amiche, P. Pradelles, J. Rossier & P. Nicolas. 1989. FEBS. **255:** 269–274.
102. Richter, K., R. Egger, L. Negri, R. Corsi, C. Severini & G. Kreil. 1990. Proc. Natl. Acad. Sci. USA **87:** 4836–4839.
103. Fujimoto, K., I. Kubota, Y. Yasuda-Kamatani, H. Minakata, K. Nomoto, M. Yoshida, A. Harada, Y. Muneoka & M. Kobayashi. 1991. Biochem. & Biophys. Res. Comm. **177:** 847–853.
104. Ohta, N., I. Kubota, T. Takao, Y. Shimonishi, Y. Yasuda-Kamatani, H. Minakata, K. Nomoto, Y. Muneoka & M. Kobayashi. 1991. Biochem. Biophys. Res. Comm. **178:** 486–493.
105. Fujisawa, Y., T. Ikeda, K. Nomoto, Y. Yasuda-Kamatani, H. Minakata, P. T. M. Kenny, I. Kubota & Y. Muneoka. 1992. Comp. Biochem. Physiol. **102C:** 91–92.
106. Hashimoto, A., T. Nishikawa, T. Hayashi, N. Fujii, K. Harada, T. Oka & K. Takahashi. 1992. FEBS. **296:** 33–36.
107. Jorpes, J. E. & V. Mutt. 1973. *In* Handb. Exp. Pharm. J. E. Jorpes & V. Mutt, eds.: **34:** 1–2. Springer Verlag. Berlin.
108. Mutt, V. 1980. *In* Gastrointestinal Hormones, G. B. J. Glass, ed.: 169–222. Raven Press. New York.
109. Mutt, V. 1988. *In* Adv. Metab. Dis. Vol. II. V. Mutt, ed.: 251–320. Academic Press. San Diego.
110. Rehfeld, J. F. 1989. *In* Handb. Physiol. G. M. Makhlouf & S. G. Schultz, eds. Vol. II: 337–354. American Physiological Society. Bethesda, Maryland.

Natural and Synthetic CCK-58

Novel Reagents for Studying Cholecystokinin Physiology[a]

JOSEPH R. REEVE JR.,[b,c] VIKTOR E. EYSSELEIN,[d]
F. J. HO,[b] P. CHEW,[b] STEVEN R. VIGNA,[e]
RODGER A. LIDDLE,[e] AND CHRIS EVANS[b]

[b]CURE: VA/UCLA Gastroenteric Biology Center
UCLA School of Medicine and
West Los Angeles Veterans Administration Center
Los Angeles, California 90073

[d]Harbor-UCLA Medical Center
Torrance, California 90509

[e]Departments of Cell Biology and Medicine
Duke University Medical Center
Box 3709
Durham, North Carolina 27710

For CCK-58 to be of sufficient relevance to continue studying its physiology, several criteria should be fulfilled: (1) It should be a major stored form in the tissue where it is synthesized. (2) It should be a major molecular form released from the cell. (3) It should be found in several species. (4) It should have a different physiology from other molecular forms of cholecystokinin. (5) CCK-58 should be available in sufficient amounts for biological and chemical characterization. All of these criteria have been fulfilled for CCK-58, and significant insight into the physiology of cholecystokinin should result from further studies of its biology.

This paper reviews some of the initial experiments with natural and synthetic CCK-58 that indicate that the activity expressed by its carboxyl terminus is influenced by other regions of the peptide. It is postulated that the influence comes from a stable tertiary structure. The small amounts of natural CCK-58 that have been purified have not been sufficient for determination of tertiary structure by chemical means such as nuclear magnetic resonance. Fortunately, receptors are very sensitive biological probes for structure-function relationships. Therefore, CCK-58 is an important tool for evaluating how tertiary structure can alter expression of biological activity. The structures of CCK-58 and CCK-8 are shown in FIGURE 1. This figure depicts how the 50 additional amino acids, on the amino terminus of CCK-58, may influence expression of its carboxyl terminal eight amino acids.

I. CCK-58 IS A MAJOR STORED FORM OF CHOLECYSTOKININ

CCK-58 is a major molecular form of cholecystokinin in many but not all species.[1] Cholecystokinin-like immunoreactivity eluting from HPLC columns in the region of

---

[a]This work was supported by NIH RO1 grants DK 33850 and DK 38626, by NSF grant IBN-9118986 by the Veterans Administration Research Service, and by NIH Center Grant DK 41301. Support by the Peptide Biochemistry and Molecular Probes Core of the CURE: VA/UCLA Gastroenteric Biology Center is gratefully acknowledged.

[c]Address for correspondence: Joseph R. Reeve, Jr., Building 115, Room 115, CURE, VA Wadsworth, Los Angeles, CA 90073.

CCK-58 is over 80% of the total immunoreactivity in some species. To detect CCK-58 with minimal degradation analytical amounts of extracts must be processed quickly and HPLC separation of the various molecular forms completed within 1 hour of the start of extraction.[1]

The proportion of CCK-58 stored in tissues may be higher than previously reported for two reasons: (1) CCK-58 may be degraded into smaller forms during processing of tissue extracts. (2) CCK-58 may not be as cross-reactive as other molecular forms of cholecystokinin.

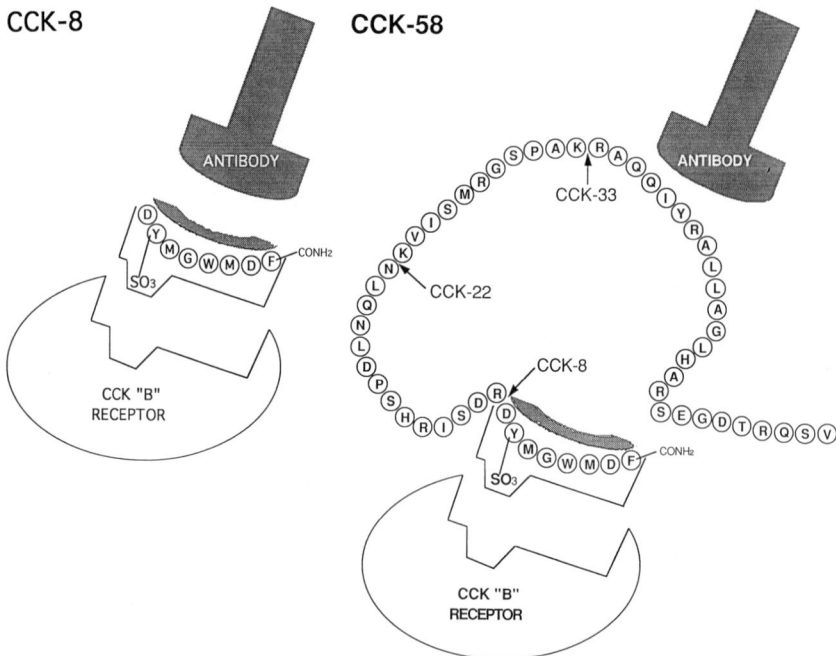

FIGURE 1. The structures of CCK-8 and CCK-58 as well as how the amino terminal 50 amino acids in CCK-58 may influence the activity of its carboxyl terminus are shown. It can be seen that antibodies and receptors alike have no steric hindrance for binding to CCK-8. However, antibody is sterically hindered from binding to the carboxyl terminus of CCK-58, whereas the CCK "B" receptor is not hindered at all. This could possibly be due to a difference in binding orientations. Not shown is the possibility that the amino terminus may actually stabilize a preferred binding conformation to the carboxyl terminus of CCK-58 with the CCK "A" receptor.

CCK-58 can be cleaved into smaller molecular forms in intestinal extracts during analytical or preparative chromatography. Cholecystokinin immunoreactivity eluting in the same position as CCK-58 routinely comprises over 70% of the total immunoreactivity in intestinal extracts.[2] However after several purifications, using the same reverse phase HPLC column, the proportion of CCK-58 dropped to less than 20% (unpublished observation). As soon as this column was replaced by another step, CCK-58 again became the most abundant molecular form of cholecystokinin detected in intestinal extracts. The loss of CCK-58 must be due to its conversion into smaller molecular forms by enzymes. This conversion can be inhibited by reduction of pH, time, temperature, and contamination by enzymes left on columns from earlier extracts. The lability of CCK-58 in extracts or even on columns in 0.1% trifluoroacetate means that estimates of its prevalence are likely to be low. The use of exogenous CCK-58 identical in structure to the endogenous peptide will allow investigators to evaluate recovery and cross-reactivity of CCK-58 in intestinal extracts.

CCK-8 has been considered the only molecular form of cholecystokinin in the brain. However, CCK-58 has been purified and sequenced from brain in several species.[3–5] In canine brain, if the diminished cross-reactivity with antibody 5135 is accounted for, CCK-58 would be in nearly the same abundance as CCK-8.[3] As in the intestine, no exogenous peptide has been used to study degradation in extracts. A major question in all research on stored forms is how much of the processing is done in the cell of synthesis *versus* how much occurs after cell disruption by tissue extraction procedures. It is possible that conversion of CCK-58 into smaller forms occurs during the extraction and initial purification steps. It is reasonable to assume that CCK-58 is a major molecular form of cholecystokinin in the brain and that our understanding of its abundance will change when exogenous CCK-58 is used to validate both the degradation and the cross-reactivity of the endogenous peptides.

II. CCK-58 IS A MAJOR RELEASED FORM OF CHOLECYSTOKININ

Not only is CCK-58 a major molecular form of cholecystokinin stored in intestine and brain, but it is also a major endocrine form of cholecystokinin. Immunoreactivity eluting in the same place as CCK-58 is the predominant cholecystokinin immunoreactivity in plasma from dog[6] and one of the major forms in human postprandial plasma.[7] The relative abundance of CCK-58 detected in blood may be higher than reported for two reasons: (1) CCK-58 is degraded in plasma. CCK-58 can only be detected in plasma if its degradation is inhibited by the addition of acid to blood and plasma.[7] It is possible that acidification of plasma does not entirely stop the enzymatic cleavage and that some of the detected forms are still products of degradation. (2) CCK-58 is less immunoreactive than are other forms of cholecystokinin. This has been demonstrated using human, canine, and porcine CCK-58 which are 30–50% as reactive as synthetic CCK-8 with several carboxyl terminal antibodies.[2,8–10] The detected relative abundance of CCK-58 in the circulation may increase if degradation is inhibited more fully or if an assay is developed that detects CCK-58 as well as other molecular forms of cholecystokinin.

The relative amounts of various cholecystokinin molecular forms in stimulated canine plasma are shown in TABLE 1 (adapted from ref. 6). CCK-58 immunoreactivity was 64% of the total cholecystokinin immunoreactivity. If the known cross-reactivity of CCK-58 is used to correct the relative amounts, CCK-58 accounts for over 80% of the circulating forms of cholecystokinin. Recently, another laboratory has confirmed that CCK-58 is a major form in dog blood.[11] Thus CCK-58 is the predominant endocrine form of cholecystokinin in dog. Others have not observed such a high abundance of CCK-58 in the circulation of another species, pig.[12] The availability of synthetic CCK-58 for cross-reactivity and recovery studies will allow future investigators to determine if species differences are due to real dissimilarities in circulating proportions or to variations in cross-reactivity or recovery.

TABLE 1. Molecular Forms of Cholecystokinin in Plasma after Stimulation of its Release

Molecular Form	Uncorrected Immunoreactivity[a] (fmol/ml plasma)	Percentage of Total
Early[b]	0.1	1
CCK-8	0.5	8
CCK-33,-39	0.9	14
Intermediate[b]	0.6	9
CCK-58	4.2	64
Late[b]	0.3	4

[a]Values expressed are the means for nine experiments with seven dogs.

[b]Early, intermediate, and late forms refer to their position on HPLC. No standards eluted in these regions, so their chemical structures are unknown. The intermediate form eluted differently on various columns. The early form could be oxidized CCK-8 and the late form could be unsulfated CCK-58.

III. CCK-58 IS FOUND IN SEVERAL SPECIES

CCK-58 has been purified and characterized from intestinal or brain extracts of dog,[2,3,13] pig,[4,14] human,[8] rat,[15] cow,[5] rabbit (Reeve et al., unpublished observations), and cat (Rosenquist et al., unpublished observations). Its presence in multiple species and in different tissues indicates that the processing that forms CCK-58 from procholecystokinin is widespread. The proportion of CCK-58 to other molecular forms has not been adequately studied, because no CCK-58 standards have been available for bioassay or radioimmunoassay measurements. The concentrations of purified CCK-58 and synthetic CCK-8 have been compared by amino acid analysis and radioimmunoassay. Human and dog CCK-58 were approximately 30–50% as immunoreactive as synthetic CCK-8 with a carboxyl terminal antibody.[2,8]

IV. CCK-58 IS DIFFERENT IN SEVERAL BIOLOGICAL SYSTEMS THAT REGULATE THE EXPRESSION OF CHOLECYSTOKININ BIOACTIVITY

Several biological systems regulate the expression of cholecystokinin bioactivity after secretion from its cell of synthesis. These systems include metabolism in the circulation, cleavage in interstitial fluid, binding to the receptor, activation of the receptor, inactivation at the receptor, and recycling of the receptor. The bioactivity of various molecular forms of cholecystokinin involves all these systems. If CCK-58 is very different at any one of these systems, its physiology could greatly differ from other, more often studied forms of cholecystokinin.

Receptor Binding of CCK-8 and Canine CCK-58 at CCK "B" Receptors

Brain and stomach contain the CCK "B"/gastrin receptor.[16,17] Previous studies have shown little difference in the potency of CCK-8 and CCK-33 at this receptor as long as they were sulfated in the seventh position from the carboxyl terminus.[18] The desulfated forms had about one tenth the potency of the sulfated forms.[18] Mouse brain (CCK "B") receptors were prepared as previously described.[18] The ability of chemically characterized CCK-8 and canine CCK-58 to inhibit the saturable binding of a radiolabeled analog of cholecystokinin, ^{125}I-dTyr-Gly-Asp-Tyr(SO$_3$H)-Nle-Gly-Trp-Nle-Asp-Phe-NH$_2$, was compared. The peptides were equipotent at the CCK "B" receptor (FIG. 2). This finding suggests that CCK-58 has all the necessary components for biological activity and confirms that the natural CCK-58 did not contain modifications in its carboxyl terminus that diminished its activity.

Receptor Binding of CCK-8 and Canine CCK-58 at Low Affinity CCK "A" Receptors

CCK-33 is reported to be less potent than CCK-8 on the low affinity CCK "A" receptors on rat pancreatic acinar membranes.[19,20] However, the CCK-33 used was from natural sources and was not chemically characterized.

Mouse pancreatic acini membrane (CCK "A") receptors were prepared as previously described.[19] The same CCK-8 and canine CCK-58 preparations were used to displace label from the CCK "B" receptors as were used for the pancreatic acini membranes. CCK-58 was more potent than CCK-8 at these low affinity CCK "A" receptors. These data strongly suggest that the amino terminus of CCK-58 stabilizes its carboxyl terminus in a confirmation that enhances its ability to bind CCK "A" receptors.

Canine CCK-58 Is Less Potent Than Synthetic CCK-8 for Release of Amylase from Pancreatic Acini

Release of amylase is a validated method of comparing the potency of various molecular forms of cholecystokinin.[21] It was first felt that CCK-33 was less potent

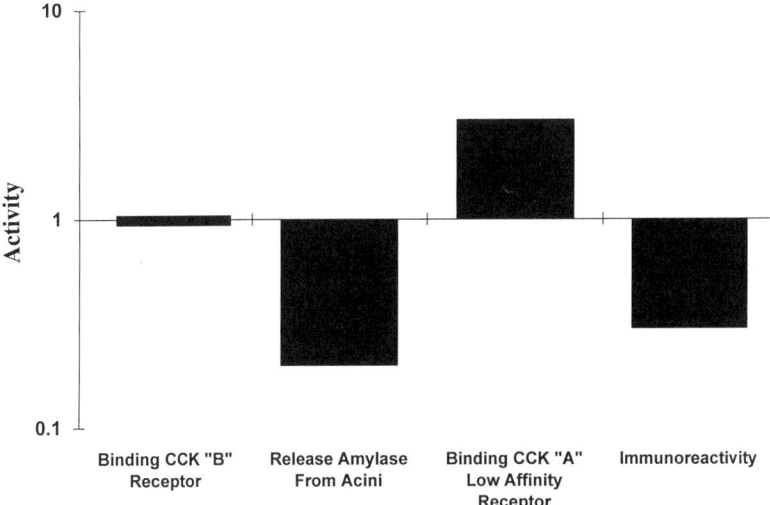

FIGURE 2. Comparison of the activities of CCK-8 and CCK-58. Both peptides bind equally at the CCK "B" receptor. CCK-58 is less potent for amylase release from isolated pancreatic acini and for reaction with carboxyl terminal antibody 5135. CCK-58 is more potent for displacement of label from low affinity CCK "A" receptors.

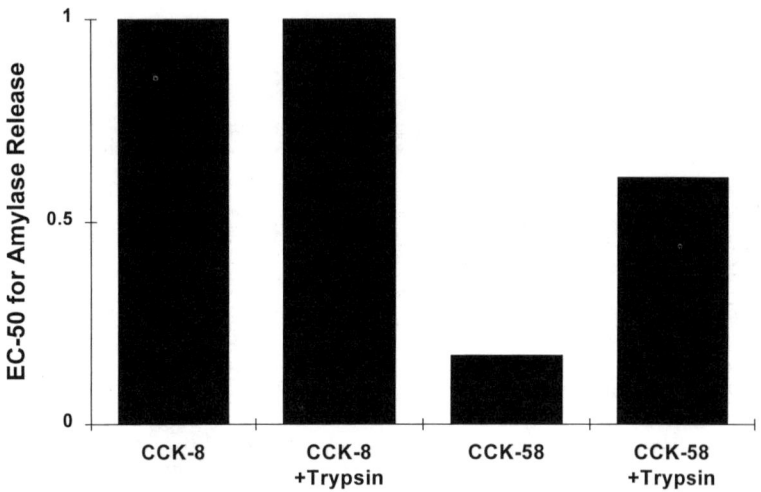

FIGURE 3. The EC_{50} for the release of amylase from isolated pancreatic acini of CCK-8 and CCK-58 with and without trypsin digestion. Trypsin did not change the activity of CCK-8, but it greatly increased the activity of CCK-58.

than CCK-8 for release of amylase from isolated pancreatic acini.[22] Subsequent experiments that used chemically characterized CCK-33 and CCK-8 showed that the two peptides had equal activity.[23] This observation confirmed earlier studies that postulated that the reduced activity of CCK-33 was caused by its loss onto container surfaces.[24] The discrepancy of the results demonstrates the need for careful chemical characterization of stock solutions before attempting to compare the potency of various molecular forms of cholecystokinin.

It was already reported that CCK-58 is less potent than CCK-8 for release of amylase from pancreatic acini.[25] These results were confirmed with the same purified CCK-58 used for the receptor binding studies just described (FIG. 2). It appears that the decrease in activity was due to shielding of the carboxyl terminus by some region of the amino terminus. This shielding is a good indication that CCK-58, unlike other molecular forms of cholecystokinin, has a stable tertiary structure.

Canine CCK-58 Has the Same Bioactivity As CCK-8 When Its Amino Terminus Is Cleaved Away

The concentrations of highly purified canine CCK-58 and synthetic CCK-8 were determined by amino acid analysis. These stock solutions were diluted with 0.05 M acetic acid containing 0.1% albumin before the final dilution into assay buffer[25] or tryptic digestion buffer. The bioactivities of CCK-58, CCK-8, and trypsin-treated CCK-58 and CCK-8 were compared. A separate portion of each peptide was chromatographed on a reverse phase HPLC column (chromatography data are summarized below, but not shown). FIGURE 3 shows the EC_{50} for each of the digested and undigested peptides compared to untreated CCK-8. Trypsin treatment did not change the position or bioactivity of CCK-8. Trypsin treatment of CCK-58 caused all cholecystokinin immunoreactivity to elute earlier than CCK-58 (in the region from the position of CCK-8 to that of CCK-33) and increased the bioactivity to nearly that of CCK-8.

SYNTHETIC CANINE CCK-58

As pointed out, all of the foregoing results were obtained using natural CCK-58. There is always the possibility that it was purified with a contaminant that could influence the results. A further test of the hypothesis that CCK-58 has a structure that influences its activity would be to show similar results with synthetic CCK-58.

Synthesis of CCK-58

The chemical synthesis of CCK-58 is the object of a more detailed report, but a brief summary can be given. Canine CCK-58 was synthesized in a filter flask connected to nitrogen and vacuum using FMOC strategies. The PAL resin was used so that a peptide amide was formed after cleavage from the resin. FMOC amino acids were coupled to the growing peptide chain using a carbodiimide reagent. The coupling and the deprotection reactions were monitored by ninhydrin, and the synthesis did not proceed until these reactions were judged to be more than 98% complete. In preliminary experiments more than 40% of the crude synthetic peptide eluted in the region of CCK-58. However, the yield was less than 5% of the expected amount of peptide. Experiments are underway to improve this yield. However, sufficient CCK-58 has been purified to allow its chemical and biological characterization. It should be pointed out that even though only 2% of the resin was used in these preliminary experiments and less than 5% of the expected amount was recovered (0.1% of the CCK-58 synthesized), nevertheless 100 nmol of pure synthetic CCK-58 was obtained. This is more CCK-58 than can be obtained by extraction from 1 kg of canine intestine. Synthetic peptide was sufficient to do all the chemical and biological studies described below.

Chemical Characterization of Synthetic CCK-58

Amino Acid Analysis. Purified synthetic CCK-8 and CCK-58 were stored in the same HPLC buffers in which they were purified. Three aliquots of each peptide (10, 10, and 20 µl) were put into hydrolysis tubes, the TFA and acetonitrile were removed by vacuum, and the peptides were hydrolyzed. Compositions were as expected from the structures of CCK-58 and CCK-8. Concentrations of stock solutions of peptides determined before and after the bioassay experiments were essentially the same.

HPLC Coelution of Natural and Synthetic CCK-58. Synthetic CCK-58 and purified natural CCK-58 were injected separately and together for comparison on gradient and isocratic (FIG. 4) reverse phase HPLC. Under both types of reverse phase chromatographies the coinjected peptides eluted as single peaks.

Mass Spectral Analysis. The masses of synthetic and natural CCK-58 were the same within the limits of the mass spectrometer. The only chemical change not detected by mass spectrometry that would change the activity of the peptides is deamidation of the carboxyl phenylalanine. Both peptides had the same bioactivity on isolated acini and the same immunoreactivity, demonstrating that the phenylalanine was amidated.

Mass Spectral Analysis of Tryptic Peptides. Synthetic and natural CCK-58 were digested by trypsin, and the digestion products were separated on a microbore

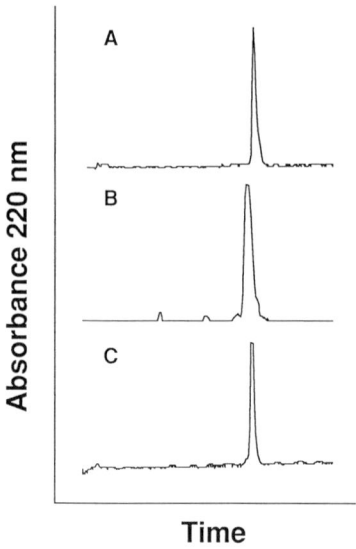

FIGURE 4. Isocratic analysis of synthetic and natural CCK-58: (**A**) natural canine CCK-58 purified from dog intestines; (**B**) synthetic canine CCK-58; and (**C**) coinjection of natural and synthetic CCK-58.

HPLC. Each peak in the effluent had its mass analyzed by an on-line mass spectrometer. All the tryptic peaks for natural and synthetic CCK-58 had the same mass, further confirming the identity of their structures.

Microsequence Analysis of CCK-58. The sequence of synthetic CCK-58 was determined by microsequence analysis and is the same as the structure for natural CCK-58.[2]

BIOACTIVITY OF SYNTHETIC CCK-58

The release of amylase stimulated by synthetic CCK-58 was compared to that of synthetic CCK-8. As with the natural peptide, CCK-58 was about one third as potent as CCK-8. This confirms that the natural CCK-58 was purified in a fully bioactive form, and it provides convincing evidence that it was the shielding of the amino terminus, and not modifications of the carboxyl terminus, that caused the decrease in activity compared to that of CCK-8.

Now that the importance of the tertiary structure of CCK-58 in the expression of biological activity for pancreatic acini has been demonstrated, it is imperative that other aspects of expression of biological activity be evaluated. Other elements in the regulation of biological activity include metabolism in the circulation, interstitial fluid, and at the receptor, binding at the receptor, and activation of the receptor.

SIGNIFICANCE OF CCK-58 IN UNDERSTANDING THE PHYSIOLOGY OF CHOLECYSTOKININ

Circulating Levels of Cholecystokinin

If CCK-58 is the major circulating form of cholecystokinin, and bioassay and radioimmunoassay do not detect it as well as they do other molecular forms of cholecystokinin, then the circulating levels of cholecystokinin have been underestimated. It must be stressed that the lack of cross-reactivity of CCK-58 is well documented only in man and dog. Further studies are needed to determine if CCK-58 in other species is less bioactive or immunoreactive.

A question that arises is, why is the proportion of CCK-58 lower in the circulation than in stored tissue? Three possible answers come to mind: (1) CCK-8 is preferentially released from the intestine; (2) CCK-58 is cleared more rapidly from the circulation than are other molecular forms; and (3) CCK-58 is degraded into smaller forms in the plasma. It is unlikely that there is a mechanism for selectively releasing CCK-8 from the intestine. It is known that CCK-58 has a much longer circulation half-life than does CCK-8.[26] It is therefore very possible that CCK-58 is being degraded in plasma after it is withdrawn from the body. If it is still degraded in acidified plasma, it may be present in even higher proportions than reported.[6,8]

Physiological Relevance of the CCK "A" Receptor Low Affinity States

The relevance of the low affinity state of the CCK "A" has been questioned because the affinity is lower than the highest apparent blood concentrations of cholecystokinin. This concept needs to be reevaluated in light of our findings that (1) both radioimmunoassay and bioassay have underestimated the chemical concentrations of circulating cholecystokinin; and (2) CCK-58 has a higher potency than do other molecular forms of cholecystokinin at the low affinity CCK "A" receptor. Therefore, it is likely that the low affinity state of the CCK "A" receptor is of physiological significance.

Potential Relevance of CCK-58 at the CCK "B"/Gastrin Receptor

Gastrin circulates in blood at 10 times higher concentrations than does cholecystokinin. Gastrin and cholecystokinin bind equally to the gastrin/CCK "B" receptor, so it has been assumed that cholecystokinin would have little influence on this receptor. However, inasmuch as all measurements of cholecystokinin may be underestimated, CCK-58 could possibly have some effect at the gastrin receptor even in the presence of gastrin.

CONCLUSIONS

The present data strongly suggest that CCK-58 has a stable tertiary structure that influences its biological activity. This structure enhances the binding of CCK-58 to low affinity CCK "A" receptors, inasmuch as CCK-58 is about three times more potent than CCK-8 for binding to pancreatic membranes. This tertiary structure does not influence binding to CCK "B" receptors, yet it diminishes the immunoreactivity and bioactivity of CCK-58 at high affinity CCK "A" receptors. In addition, something in the structure of CCK-58 slows its clearance from the circulation. Since CCK-58 differs from other molecular forms of cholecystokinin in most biological systems that govern the expression of cholecystokinin bioactivity, it is a novel tool for studying cholecystokinin physiology.

SUMMARY

CCK-58 is a unique reagent for testing how segments of a peptide far removed from its active site can influence the expression of its biological activity. Indications of tertiary structure have come from studies with natural peptide purified from canine small intestine. These studies gave clear indications that tertiary structure affects CCK-58 bioactivity, but the small quantities of CCK-58 available made it impossible to characterize completely how tertiary structure influenced bioactivity. Canine CCK-58 was synthesized manually using a solid support and was purified by reverse phase high pressure liquid chromatography (HPLC). Synthetic CCK-58 was characterized by isocratic reverse phase and gradient HPLC, amino acid analysis, mass spectral analysis, sequence analysis, and three bioassays. Synthetic and natural canine CCK-58 had the same elution profiles, amino acid composition, sequence, and mass. The two peptides were equipotent for the stimulation of pancreatic secretion. Natural canine CCK-58 was equipotent to CCK-8 for CCK "B" receptor binding, a further indication of the purity of the natural peptide. However, natural CCK-58 was more potent than CCK-8 for CCK "A" receptor binding and less potent than CCK-8 for stimulation of pancreatic secretion. These data support the concept that CCK-58 has a stable tertiary structure. This structure does not affect its binding to CCK "B" receptors, enhances its binding to low affinity CCK "A" receptors, and decreases its activity expressed through binding to high affinity CCK "A" receptors. The concept of a stable tertiary structure is also supported by the fact that many antibodies directed towards the carboxyl terminus of cholecystokinin react better with CCK-8 than CCK-58. The availability of synthetic CCK-58 will allow analysis of its tertiary structure by physical and chemical methods as well as studies on how peptide tertiary structure can affect receptor binding, receptor activation, metabolism in blood, degradation in interstitial fluid, and inactivation at the receptor. Evaluating all of these systems will help investigators understand the regulation of cholecystokinin activity by its major endocrine form, CCK-58.

ACKNOWLEDGMENT

Help in manuscript preparation was provided by Ziv Termeforoosh.

REFERENCES

1. EBERLEIN, G. A., V. E. EYSSELEIN & H. GOEBELL. 1988. Cholecystokinin-58 is the major molecular form in man, dog and cat but not in pig, beef and rat intestine. Peptides **9:** 993–998.
2. REEVE, J. R., JR., V. E. EYSSELEIN, J. H. WALSH, C. M. BEN-AVRAM & J. E. SHIVELY. 1986. New molecular forms of cholecystokinin. Microsequence analysis of forms previously characterized by chromatographic methods. J. Biol. Chem. **261:** 16392–16397.
3. EYSSELEIN, V. E., J. R. REEVE, JR., J. E. SHIVELY, C. MILLER & J. H. WALSH. 1984. Isolation of a large cholecystokinin precursor from canine brain. Proc. Natl. Acad. Sci. USA **81:** 6565–6568.
4. TATEMOTO, K., H. JORNVALL, S. SIIMESMAA, G. HALLDEN & V. MUTT. 1984. Isolation and characterization of cholecystokinin-58 (CCK-58) from porcine brain. FEBS Lett. **174:** 289–293.
5. ENG, J., H. R. LI & R. S. YALOW. 1990. Purification of bovine cholecystokinin-58 and sequencing of its N-terminus. Regul. Pept. **30:** 15–19.
6. EYSSELEIN, V. E., G. A. EBERLEIN, W. H. HESSE, M. V. SINGER, H. GOEBELL & J. R. REEVE, JR. 1987. Cholecystokinin-58 is the major circulating form of cholecystokinin in canine blood. J. Biol. Chem. **262:** 214–217.

7. EBERLEIN, G. A., V. E. EYSSELEIN, W. H. HESSE, H. GOEBELL, M. SCHAEFER & J. R. REEVE, JR. 1987. Detection of cholecystokinin-58 in human blood by inhibition of degradation. Am. J. Physiol. **253:** G477–G482.
8. EYSSELEIN, V. E., G. A. EBERLEIN, M. SCHAEFFER, D. GRANDT, H. GOEBELL, W. NIEBEL, G. L. ROSENQUIST, H. E. MEYER & J. R. REEVE, JR. 1990. Characterization of the major form of cholecystokinin in human intestine: CCK-58. Am. J. Physiol. **258:** G253–G260.
9. TURKELSON, C. M., J. R. REEVE, JR. & T. E. SOLOMON. 1990. Low immunoreactivity of canine cholecystokinin-58. Gastroenterology **99:** 646–651.
10. HOCKER, M., W. E. SCHMIDT, H. M. WILMS, F. LEHNHOFF, R. NUSTEDE, A. SCHAFMAYER & U. R. FOLSCH. 1990. Measurement of tissue cholecystokinin (CCK) concentrations by bioassay and specific radioimmunoassay: Characterization of the bioactivity of CCK-58 before and after tryptic cleavage. Eur. J. Clin. Invest. **20:** S45–S50.
11. SUN, G., T.-M. CHANG, W. XUE, J. F. Y. WEY, K. Y. LEE & W. Y. CHEY. 1992. Release of cholecystokinin and secretin by sodium oleate in dogs: Molecular form and bioactivity. Am. J. Physiol. **262:** G35–G43.
12. CANTOR, P. & J. F. REHFELD. 1989. Cholecystokinin in pig plasma: Release of components devoid of a bioactive COOH-terminus. Am. J. Physiol. **256:** G53–G61.
13. EYSSELEIN, V. E., J. R. REEVE, JR., J. E. SHIVELY, D. HAWKE & J. H. WALSH. 1982. Partial structure of a large canine cholecystokinin (CCK58): amino acid sequence. Peptides **3:** 687–691.
14. MCINTOSH, C. H., M. A. DAHL, Y. N. KWOK, V. MUTT, N. SPRUSTON & J. C. BROWN. 1988. Isolation from porcine intestinal extracts of a cholecystokinin-like peptide and a peptide with homology to cytochrome oxidase polypeptide VII and chymodenin. Can. J. Physiol. Pharmacol. **66:** 1407–1414.
15. TURKELSON, C. M., T. E. SOLOMON, L. BUSSJAEGER, J. TURKELSON, M. RONK, J. E. SHIVELY, F. J. HO & J. R. REEVE, JR. 1988. Chemical characterization of rat cholecystokinin-58. Peptides **9:** 1255–1260.
16. KOPIN, A. S., Y. M. LEE, E. W. MCBRIDE, L. J. MILLER, M. LU, H. Y. LIN, L. F. KOLAKOWSKI, JR. & M. BEINBORN. 1992. Expression cloning and characterization of the canine parietal cell gastrin receptor. Proc. Natl. Acad. Sci. USA **89:** 3605–3609.
17. WANK, S. A., J. R. PISEGNA & A. DE WEERTH. 1992. Brain and gastrointestinal cholecystokinin receptor family: Structure and functional expression. Proc. Natl. Acad. Sci. USA **89:** 8691–8695.
18. SAITO, A., I. D. GOLDFINE & J. A. WILLIAMS. 1981. Characterization of receptors for cholecystokinin and related peptides in mouse cerebral cortex. J. Neurochem. **37:** 483–490.
19. SAKAMOTO, C., J. A. WILLIAMS, K. Y. WONG & I. D. GOLDFINE. 1983. The CCK receptor on pancreatic plasma membranes: Binding characteristics and covalent cross-linking. FEBS Lett. **151:** 63–66.
20. JENSEN, R. T., G. F. LEMP & J. D. GARDNER. 1980. Interaction of cholecystokinin with specific membrane receptors on pancreatic acinar cells. Proc. Natl. Acad. Sci. USA **77:** 2079–2083.
21. LIDDLE, R. A., I. D. GOLDFINE, M. S. ROSEN, R. A. TAPLITZ & J. A. WILLIAMS. 1985. Cholecystokinin bioactivity in human plasma. Molecular forms, responses to feeding, and relationship to gallbladder contraction. J. Clin. Invest. **75:** 1144–1152.
22. VILLANUEVA, M. L., S. M. COLLINS, R. T. JENSEN & J. D. GARDNER. 1982. Structural requirements for action of cholecystokinin on enzyme secretion from pancreatic acini. Am. J. Physiol. **242:** G416–G422.
23. LIDDLE, R. A., J. ELASHOFF & J. R. REEVE, JR. 1986. Relative bioactivities of cholecystokinins-8 and -33 on rat pancreatic acini. Peptides **7:** 723–727.
24. SOLOMON, T. E., T. YAMADA, J. ELASHOFF, J. WOOD & C. BEGLINGER. 1984. Bioactivity of cholecystokinin analogues: CCK-8 is not more potent than CCK-33. Am. J. Physiol. **247:** 1)-P G105–1.
25. REEVE, J. R., JR., V. EYSSELEIN, G. A. EBERLEIN, P. CHEW, F. J. HO, V. D. HUEBNER, J. E. SHIVELY, T. D. LEE & R. A. LIDDLE. 1991. Characterization of canine intestinal cholecystokinin-58 lacking its carboxyl-terminal nonapeptide. Evidence for similar post-translational processing in brain and gut. J. Biol. Chem. **266:** 13770–13776.
26. HOFFMANN, P., G. A. EBERLEIN, J. R. REEVE, JR., R. H. BÜNTEL, D. GRANDT, H. GOEBELL & V. E. EYSSELEIN. 1993. Comparison of clearance and metabolism of infused CCK-8 and CCK-58 in dog. Gastroenterology, in press.

Regulation of Cholecystokinin Gene Expression in Rat Intestine[a]

RODGER A. LIDDLE[b]

Department of Medicine
Duke University Medical Center and
Durham VA Medical Center
Durham, North Carolina 27710

Intestinal cholecystokinin (CCK) is produced by discrete endocrine cells within the mucosa of the proximal small intestine.[1] CCK secretion is regulated by ingested foods and involves a negative feedback system in which active proteases in the lumen of the proximal small intestine inhibit CCK release.[2,3] Conversely, elimination of protease activity in the intestine stimulates CCK secretion.[4] Accordingly, in the rat, protein, by virtue of its ability to serve as a substrate for proteases but not amino acids, stimulates CCK secretion.[5] These observations served as the basis for a model to determine if stimulation of CCK secretion is associated with regulation of CCK gene expression. Additional studies examined the manner in which intestinal CCK hormone content, CCK mRNA levels, and CCK secretion are regulated by (1) food deprivation, (2) inhibitory influences of somatostatin, and (3) stimulation by bombesin. These studies were designed to elucidate the complex interactions that enable the intestine to adapt to changing demands for hormone synthesis and secretion.

DIETARY REGULATION OF CCK GENE EXPRESSION

All studies were performed on male Sprague-Dawley rats weighing 250–350 g. Where appropriate, rats were prepared with indwelling intraduodenal and intravenous or intraperitoneal cannulas and maintained in modified Bollman cages.[6] Rats were fed an elemental diet of 3.5 ml/h Vivonex (Norwich Eaton Pharmaceuticals, Norwich, NY) by continuous duodenal perfusion and had free access to water. After 72 hours, animals were perfused intraduodenally with soybean trypsin inhibitor (SBTI, 50 mg/h for 24 hours). The effects of these dietary manipulations on plasma CCK levels are shown in FIGURE 1. The Vivonex diet consists primarily of free amino acids and carbohydrate and contains little fat. Consequently this elemental diet did not cause an increase in plasma CCK. However, with instillation of trypsin inhibitor intraduodenally, there was a significant and sustained elevation in CCK levels to over five times basal levels. To examine the relation between CCK secretion and CCK mRNA levels, intestine from the same animals was harvested for preparation of RNA. Poly A⁺ RNA was prepared as described[7] and northern analysis performed using cDNA probes for either CCK[8] or β-actin[9] (FIG. 2). Only a single band of ~ 750 bases was identified on northern blot and indicated that CCK mRNA was more abundant in the proximal than in the distal small intestine. Equivalent amounts of

---

[a]This work was supported by NIH grant DK 38626, the Stedman Center for Clinical Nutrition, and the Department of Veterans Affairs.
[b]Address correspondence to: Rodger A. Liddle, MD, Department of Medicine, Box 3913, Duke University Medical Center, Durham, NC 27710.

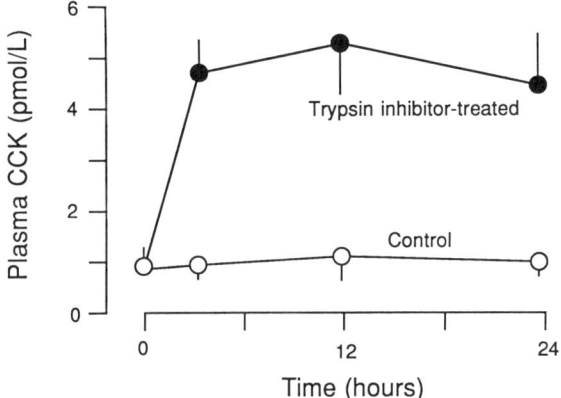

FIGURE 1. Effect of trypsin inhibitor administration on plasma CCK levels. Rats were fed by continuous intraduodenal perfusion either an elemental diet alone (○) or an elemental diet plus trypsin inhibitor (●). At the times indicated, blood was collected for measurements of CCK. Each point is the mean ± SEM of four animals. A statistically significant increase in plasma CCK levels was noted in animals treated with trypsin inhibitor ($p < 0.05$). (From Liddle et al.[6] with permission.)

β-actin mRNA were present in both tissues. In animals fed the elemental diet, CCK mRNA levels were relatively low (FIG. 3). However, by 4 hours, significant increases in steady-state CCK mRNA levels in the intestine were observed in trypsin inhibitor-treated rats than in control animals, and mRNA levels remained elevated for the duration of trypsin inhibitor perfusion. No changes were found in β-actin mRNA levels. To determine if these observed changes in CCK RNA levels were transcriptional, nuclear run-on assays were performed. In this assay, transcripts that are initiated in the whole cell are elongated in isolated nuclei and reflect the ongoing rate of transcription.[10] Five micrograms of CCK cDNA, plasmid pBR322, and β-actin were immobilized onto nitrocellulose filters and hybridized with nuclear

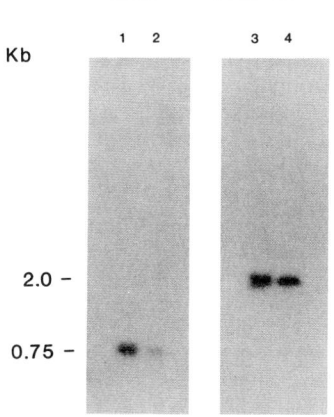

FIGURE 2. Northern analysis of poly A$^+$ RNA from rat proximal (*lanes 1 and 3*) and distal (*lanes 2 and 4*) intestine using CCK or β-actin cDNA probes. (From Liddle et al.[6] with permission.)

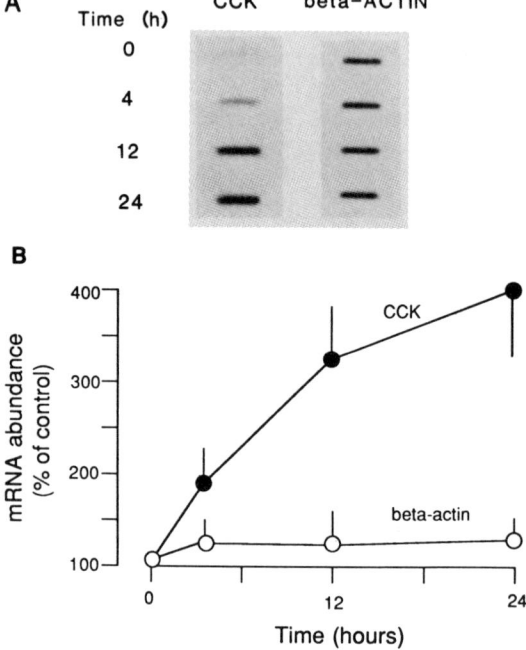

FIGURE 3. Effect of trypsin inhibitor feeding on CCK mRNA levels. Coincident with measurements of plasma CCK shown in FIGURE 1, RNA was slotted onto nitrocellulose filters and hybridized with CCK or β-actin cDNA probes. Densitometry scanning of slot blots is shown in relation to duration of trypsin inhibitor administration ($n = 4$). (From Liddle et al.[6] with permission.)

transcription run-on products (FIG. 4). Nuclei from trypsin inhibitor-treated intestine at 4 hours increased the CCK hybridization signal 300% over the corresponding unstimulated control signal. In comparison, there was no change in the β-actin signal. The addition of 2 μg/ml of α-amanitin (a concentration that preferentially inhibits RNA polymerase II)[10] markedly reduced the signal obtained. This finding demonstrated that CCK gene transcription was increased under conditions of trypsin inhibitor perfusion, indicating that the elevation in steady-state mRNA levels was due, at least in part, to regulation of the CCK gene at the transcriptional level.

In contrast to dietary stimulation of gastrointestinal function, food deprivation produces a variety of metabolic and endocrine effects. In the gastrointestinal tract, starvation reduces duodenal CCK levels[11] but not somatostatin levels.[12,13] Increases in tissue content of other gastrointestinal hormones such as glucose-dependent insulinotropic peptide (GIP) have also been associated with prolonged fasting.[13] However, little is known about how food deprivation alters synthesis and secretion of these hormones, which may be important for the restoration of hormone function after periods of fasting.

To determine if fasting alters CCK gene expression, CCK mRNA levels were quantified in rat intestine. Within 1 day, fasting specifically reduced CCK mRNA levels (relative to β-actin mRNA) in the small intestine (FIG. 5). This effect was reversed by refeeding as CCK mRNA levels were restored to control values after 1 day of refeeding a normal chow diet. In contrast to the effects on CCK mRNA, no change was noted in somatostatin mRNA levels with either fasting or refeeding. The decrease in CCK mRNA relative to β-actin and somatostatin mRNA levels indicates that dietary stimulation is necessary for maintaining high levels of CCK gene expression.

REGULATION OF CCK GENE EXPRESSION BY SOMATOSTATIN

It is likely that endocrine cells of the gastrointestinal tract are under the influence of both stimulatory and inhibitory influences. In experimental animals, somatostatin has previously been demonstrated to inhibit the secretion of many hormones including CCK.[14] The observation that somatostatin levels remained high in rats despite food deprivation at a time when CCK mRNA levels declined raised the possibility that somatostatin might influence CCK gene expression. To test this hypothesis, somatostatin-14 was infused intravenously into rats that were simultaneously treated with intraduodenal trypsin inhibitor. As expected, in the absence of somatostatin, trypsin inhibitor treatment stimulated CCK release as reflected by an elevation in plasma CCK levels (FIG. 6). Somatostatin infusion (1 μg/kg · h) not only reduced trypsin inhibitor-stimulated plasma CCK levels but also significantly lowered CCK mRNA levels in the intestine. No effect on intestinal CCK hormone content was noted. These observations suggest that somatostatin exerts an inhibitory effect on CCK gene expression.

NEUROHORMONAL STIMULATION OF CCK GENE EXPRESSION

Intestinal hormones appear to be regulated by a complex of stimulatory and inhibitory factors. Important among these are neural and paracrine influences. In particular, the neuropeptide bombesin (or its mammalian counterpart, gastrin releasing peptide) has been shown to stimulate CCK release in animals, intestinal segments, and isolated cell preparations.[15–18] However, it is not known if stimulation

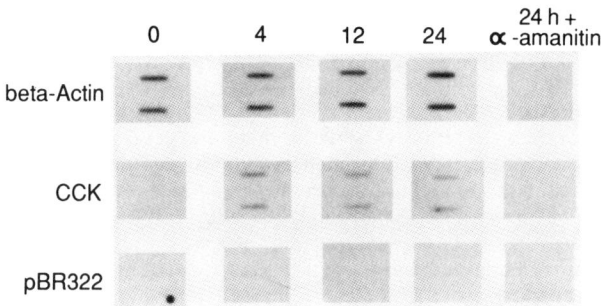

FIGURE 4. Effect of trypsin inhibitor feeding on CCK gene transcription. Nuclear run-on assays were performed from the proximal small intestinal mucosa of animals treated with trypsin inhibitor administered intraduodenally. The duration of treatment is shown ranging from 0–24 hours. The radioactive signal seen with both β-actin and CCK was inhibited by the addition of α-amanitin. (From Liddle et al.[6] with permission.)

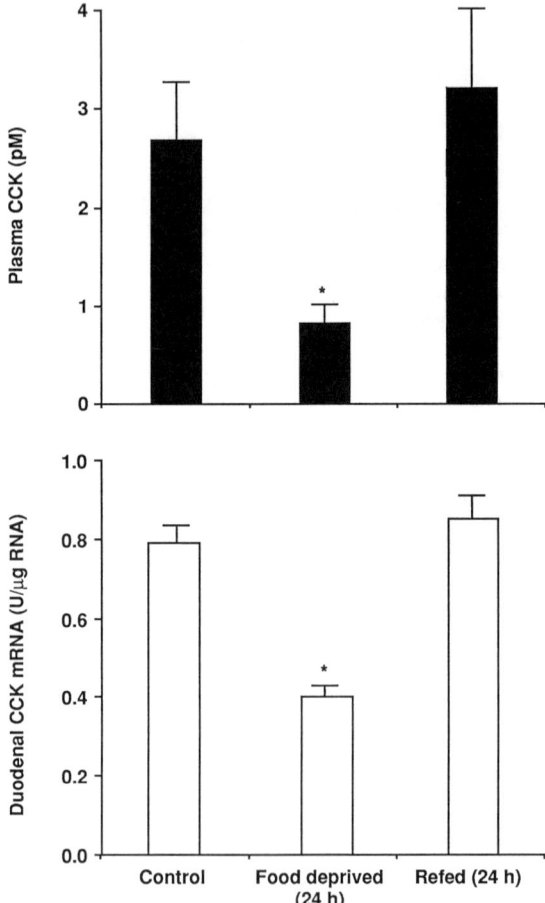

FIGURE 5. Effect of food deprivation and refeeding on plasma and intestinal CCK. Plasma CCK concentrations (**a**) and duodenal CCK mRNA levels (**b**) are shown relative to the duration of food deprivation. Each point is the mean ± SEM of five animals. (* = $p < 0.05$). (Modified from Kanayama and Liddle.[28])

of hormone secretion is also responsible for increased gene expression as suggested by dietary feeding experiments. Inasmuch as bombesin stimulates CCK secretion by a neurohormonal pathway and not by virtue of luminal stimulation, it was proposed that treatment of rats with bombesin would provide a mechanism for determining if secretion was instrumental in stimulation of CCK gene expression. For these studies, rats received intravenous infusions of bombesin ranging from 0.25–16 μg/kg · h. Concentrations of 4 μg/kg · h and greater significantly increased plasma CCK levels (FIG. 7). However, despite continuous bombesin administration, CCK levels returned to basal within 4 hours, consistent with the development of tachyphylaxis to bombesin.[19] Furthermore, despite stimulating CCK release, bombesin had no effect on CCK mRNA levels. Together, these findings indicate that stimulation of CCK secretion alone is not sufficient to increase gene expression.

DISCUSSION

The complementary DNA encoding cholecystokinin was originally isolated from a rat medullary thyroid carcinoma cell line.[8] Not only has this clone been used as the probe for quantifying CCK mRNAs, but it also led to the identification of the rat CCK gene and characterization of its promoter region.[20,21] These studies have identified several *cis*- and *trans*-acting elements that are responsible for expression of the CCK gene.[21] In particular, regions homologous to cAMP- and 12-O-tetradecoanoylphorbol-13-acetate (TPA)-responsive elements described in other genes are present in the 5' upstream region of the CCK gene. These regions imply that CCK gene expression may be regulated by intracellular cAMP and activation of protein kinase C. It follows then that factors that modify cAMP or protein kinase C within the CCK cell might regulate CCK gene expression.

In the current studies, CCK mRNA levels were affected by diet and neurohormonal regulators. Dietary stimulation of CCK secretion produced by intraduodenal administration of trypsin inhibitor significantly increased CCK mRNA relative to nonregulated genes such as β-actin. Nuclear run-on studies demonstrated that this increase was due, at least in part, to an increase in gene transcription rates. In

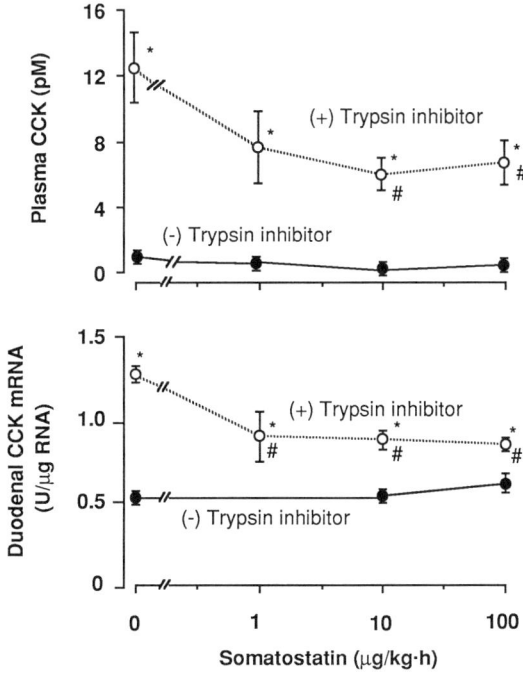

FIGURE 6. Effect of somatostatin infusion on plasma CCK concentrations and duodenal CCK mRNA levels. Somatostatin-14 was infused at the doses indicated simultaneously with (●) or without (○) intraduodenal perfusion of trypsin inhibitor for 24 hours. Each point is the mean ± SEM of 4–8 animals. #Values statistically different from trypsin inhibitor treatment in the absence of somatostatin infusion; *values statistically different from control ($p < 0.05$). (Modified from Kanayama and Liddle[29] with permission.)

contrast to the stimulatory effects of diet, fasting reduced CCK mRNA levels. This decrease was rapidly reversed by refeeding. The mechanisms by which diet stimulates the CCK cell are incompletely understood. Studies demonstrating negative feedback regulation of CCK secretion by diet recently provided evidence for regulation of CCK release by two CCK-releasing factors.[22-24] One of these factors, monitor peptide, stimulates CCK release directly through a calcium-dependent and possibly receptor-mediated mechanism.[25,26] It is hypothesized that monitor peptide

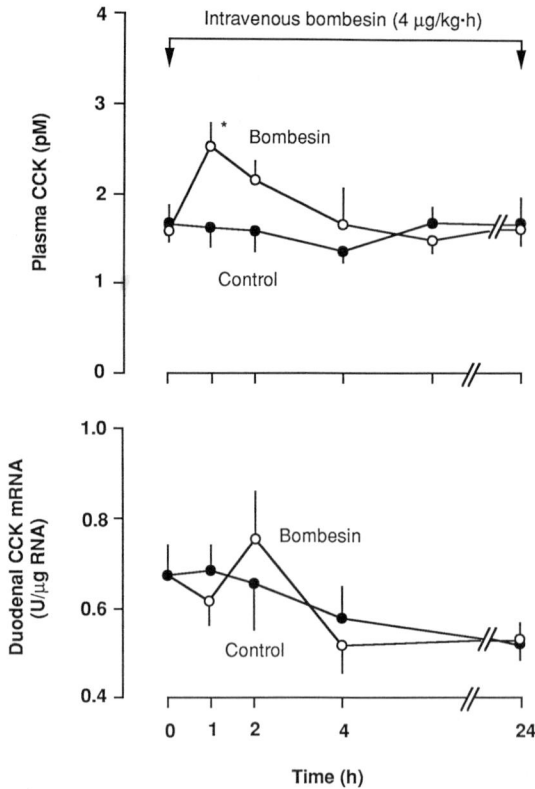

FIGURE 7. Effect of bombesin infusion on plasma CCK concentrations and duodenal CCK mRNA levels. Bombesin was infused intravenously at a rate of 4 μg/kg · h for 24 hours. Each point is the mean ± SEM of 4–8 animals. *Values statistically different from time 0 ($p < 0.05$). (From Kanayama and Liddle[30] with permission.)

increases intracellular calcium ion concentration in CCK cells through activation of the phosphoinositide cascade. In this scheme, ligand binding to its receptor would activate phospholipase C which would, in turn, liberate inositol trisphosphate (IP_3) and diacylglycerol from PIP_2. IP_3 would then cause the release of calcium ion from intracellular stores, whereas the generation of diacylglycerol would be expected to activate protein kinase C. It is interesting to speculate that elevation in protein kinase C activity through this pathway might provide a signal for CCK gene regulation through appropriate promoter regions such as the TPA-responsive element.

In contrast, many of the inhibitory effects of somatostatin are believed to be mediated by effects on intracellular cAMP. Identification of a cAMP-responsive element in the CCK gene lends credence to the hypothesis that the effect of somatostatin in reducing CCK gene expression, as was observed in the present studies, might be through effects on gene transcription. In other endocrine cells, somatostatin receptors have been identified on the cell membrane.[27] Although it is unknown whether similar receptors exist on the CCK cell, the potent effects of somatostatin on CCK release make this an attractive possibility and are consistent with the foregoing hypothesis for regulation of gene expression.

It was previously unknown if the increase in CCK mRNA levels observed with dietary stimulation was unique to luminal stimulation of CCK release or if other factors that would stimulate CCK secretion, such as neurohormonal stimulation, also affected CCK gene expression. The present study demonstrated that bombesin stimulated CCK secretion but did not affect steady-state CCK mRNA levels in the intestine. Therefore, it appears that neurohormonal stimulation of CCK release differs from dietary stimulation of CCK secretion and that secretion of CCK is not obligatorily linked to CCK gene expression. The several possible explanations for this difference may be related to: (1) possible differences in the intracellular signals generated by dietary stimulation *versus* bombesin stimulation and their effects on gene transcription; (2) the magnitude of stimulated secretion as reflected by the lower plasma CCK levels with bombesin infusion *versus* luminal stimulation; or (3) the duration of stimulation, because tachyphylaxis was seen within 4 hours of bombesin treatment but did not occur with chronic dietary stimulation. Therefore, the ability to stimulate CCK gene expression may be related to the magnitude or duration of cellular stimulation.

CCK, like most other gastrointestinal hormones, increases in the blood in response to ingestion of food; therefore, dietary stimulation appears to be the most important factor regulating CCK under physiological conditions. However, other gut hormones such as somatostatin and bombesin which are also modified by diet also affect CCK. Although we have examined only a few factors that modify intestinal CCK, the regulatory pathways are undoubtedly more complex. Future studies will attempt to dissect this multitude of interrelationships. At present it is clear that both CCK secretion and gene expression are regulated at multiple levels by dietary and neurohormonal factors.

ACKNOWLEDGMENTS

The author thanks Shuji Kanayama, Alex McDonald, and Jackie Carter for their essential contributions to these studies.

REFERENCES

1. BUCHAN, A., J. POLAK, E. SOLCIA, C. CAPELLA, D. HUDSON & A. PEARSE. 1978. Electron immunohistochemical evidence for the human intestinal I cell as the source of CCK. Gut **19:** 403–407.
2. GREEN, G. M. & R. L. LYMAN. 1972. Feedback regulation of pancreatic enzyme secretion as a mechanism for trypsin inhibitor-induced hypersecretion in rats. Proc. Soc. Exp. Biol. Med. **140:** 6–12.

3. OWYANG, C., D. S. LOUIE & D. TATUM. 1986. Feedback regulation of pancreatic enzyme secretion–suppression of cholecystokinin release by trypsin. J. Clin. Invest. **77:** 2042–2047.
4. LIDDLE, R. A., I. D. GOLDFINE & J. A. WILLIAMS. 1984. Bioassay of plasma cholecystokinin in rats: Effects of food, trypsin inhibitor, and alcohol. Gastroenterology **87:** 542–549.
5. LIDDLE, R. A., G. M. GREEN, C. K. CONRAD & J. A. WILLIAMS. 1986. Proteins but not amino acids, carbohydrates, or fats stimulate cholecystokinin secretion in the rat. Am. J. Physiol. **251:** G243–G248.
6. LIDDLE, R. A., J. D. CARTER & A. R. MCDONALD. 1988. Dietary regulation of rat intestinal cholecystokinin gene expression. J. Clin. Invest. **81:** 2015–2019.
7. AVIV, H. & P. LEDER. 1972. Purification of biologically active globin messenger RNA by chromatography on oligothymidylic acid-cellulose. Proc. Natl. Acad. Sci. USA **69:** 1408–1412.
8. DESCHENES, R. J., L. J. LORENZ, R. S. HAUN, B. A. ROOS, K. J. COLLIER & J. E. DIXON. 1984. Cloning and sequence analysis of a cDNA encoding rat preprocholecystokinin. Proc. Natl. Acad. Sci. USA **81:** 726–730.
9. CLEVELAND, D. W., M. A. LOPATA, R. J. MACDONALD, N. J. COWAN, W. J. RUTTER & M. W. KIRSCHNER. 1980. Number and evolutionary conservation of alpha- and beta-tubulin and cytoplasmic beta- and gamma-actin genes using specific cloned cDNA probes. Cell **20:** 95–105.
10. MCKNIGHT, G. S. & R. D. PALMITER. 1979. Transcriptional regulation of the ovalbumin and conalbumin genes by steroid hormones in the chick oviduct. J. Biol. Chem. **254:** 9050–9058.
11. KOOP, I., T. KIMMICH, H. KOOP & R. ARNOLD. 1987. Effect of food deprivation on the function of the intestinal cholecystokinin-producing cell in the rat. Digestion **38:** 114–123.
12. TANNENBAUM, G. S., O. RORSTAD & P. BRAZEAU. 1979. Effect of prolonged food deprivation on the ultradian growth hormone rhythm and immunoreactive somatostatin tissue levels in the rat. Endocrinology **104:** 1733–1738.
13. SHULKES, A., Y. CAUSSIGNAC, C. B. LAMERS, T. E. SOLOMON, T. YAMADA & J. H. WALSH. 1983. Starvation in the rat: Effect on peptides of the gut and brain. Aust. J. Exp. Biol. Med. Sci. **61:** 581–587.
14. WALSH, J. H. 1987. Gastrointestinal hormones. *In* Physiology of the Gastrointestinal Tract. L. R. Johnson, ed.: 181–253. Raven Press. New York.
15. GHATEI, M. A., R. T. JUNG, J. C. STEVENSON, C. J. HILLYARD, T. E. ADRIAN, Y. C. LEE, N. D. CHRISTOFIDES, D. L. SARSON, K. MASHITER, I. MACINTYRE & S. R. BLOOM. 1982. Bombesin: Action on gut hormones and calcium in man. J. Clin. Endocrinol. & Metab. **54:** 980–985.
16. JANSEN, J. B. M. J. & C. B. H. W. LAMERS. 1984. Effect of bombesin on plasma cholecystokinin in normal persons and gastrectomized patients measured by sequence-specific radioimmunoassays. Surgery **96:** 55–60.
17. CUBER, J. C., F. VILAS, N. CHARLES, C. BERNARD & J. A. CHAYVIALLE. 1989. Bombesin and nutrients stimulate release of CCK through distinct pathways in the rat. Am. J. Physiol. **256:** G989–G996.
18. SHARARA, A. I., E. P. BOURAS, M. A. MISUKONIS & R. A. LIDDLE. 1993. Evidence for indirect dietary regulation of cholecystokinin release in rats. Am. J. Physiol. **265:** G107–G112.
19. PANDOL, S. J., R. T. JENSEN & J. D. GARDNER. 1982. Mechanism of [Tyr^4] Bombesin-induced desensitization in dispersed acini from guinea pig pancreas. J. Biol. Chem. **257:** 12024–12029.
20. DESCHENES, R. J., R. S. HAUN, C. L. FUNCKES & J. E. DIXON. 1985. A gene encoding rat cholecystokinin. J. Biol. Chem. **260:** 1280–1286.
21. HAUN, R. S. & J. E. DIXON. 1990. A transcriptional enhancer essential for the expression of the rat cholecystokinin gene contains a sequence identical to the −296 element of the human c-fos gene. J. Biol. Chem. **265:** 15455–15463.

22. Lu, L., D. Louie & C. Owyang. 1989. A cholecystokinin releasing peptide mediates feedback regulation of pancreatic secretion. Am. J. Physiol. **256:** G430–G435.
23. Miyasaka, K., D. Guan, R. A. Liddle & G. M. Green. 1989. Feedback regulation by trypsin: Evidence for intraluminal CCK-releasing peptide. Am. J. Physiol. **257:** G175–G181.
24. Iwai, K., S. I. Fukuoka, T. Fushiki, M. Tsujikawa, M. Hirose, S. Tsunasawa & F. Sakiyama. 1987. Purification and sequencing of a trypsin-sensitive cholecystokinin-releasing peptide from rat pancreatic juice. J. Biol. Chem. **262:** 8956–8959.
25. Bouras, E. P., M. A. Misukonis & R. A. Liddle. 1992. Role of calcium in monitor peptide-stimulated cholecystokinin release from perifused intestinal cells. Am. J. Physiol. **262:** G791–G796.
26. Liddle, R. A., M. A. Misukonis, L. Pacy & A. E. Balber. 1992. Cholecystokinin cells purified by fluorescence-activated cell sorting respond to monitor peptide with an increase in intracellular calcium. Proc. Natl. Acad. Sci. USA **89:** 5147–5151.
27. Yamada, T. & T. Chiba. 1989. Somatostatin. *In* The Gastrointestinal System. Volume II. Neural and Endocrine Biology. G. M. Makhlouf, ed.: 431–454. Oxford University Press. New York.
28. Kanayama, S. & R. A. Liddle. 1991. Influence of food deprivation on intestinal cholecystokinin and somatostatin. Gastroenterology **100:** 909–915.
29. Kanayama, S. & R. A. Liddle. 1990. Somatostatin regulates duodenal cholecystokinin and somatostatin messenger RNA. Am. J. Physiol. **258:** G358–G364.
30. Kanayama, S. & R. A. Liddle. 1991. Regulation of intestinal cholecystokinin and somatostatin mRNA by bombesin in rats. Am. J. Physiol. **261:** G71–G77.

Peptides Related to Cholecystokinin in Nonmammalian Vertebrates

GÜNTHER KREIL AND CHRISTIAN WECHSELBERGER

Institute of Molecular Biology
Austrian Academy of Sciences
A-5020 Salzburg, Austria

The hormones gastrin and cholecystokinin (CCK) belong to the same family of mammalian peptides. Both were originally isolated from the gastrointestinal tract and subsequently shown to be present also in brain.[1-3] Different forms of these peptides varying in size exist in these tissues, but these are liberated from their precursors by differential proteolysis (to be described). The two hormones have the same COOH-terminal pentapeptide sequence. The main difference is that gastrin contains a tyrosine residue six amino acids from the carboxyl end, whereas in CCK tyrosine is the seventh residue (FIG. 1). The tyrosine residues are invariably sulfated in the various forms of CCK, but they are only partially sulfated in gastrins.

From amphibian skin, three peptides, termed caeruleins, have been isolated which belong to the same family,[4,5] and from the position of the sulfated tyrosine residue, these skin peptides are of the CCK type.

It has been assumed that gastrin, CCK, and caerulein are derived from a common ancestor that was present early in the evolution of vertebrates. This review summarizes our current knowledge of nonmammalian members of this family, and their possible phylogeny is discussed.

GASTRIN-LIKE PEPTIDES FROM DIFFERENT SPECIES

A peptide with the carboxy-terminal sequence Trp-Met-Asp-Phe-amide was isolated from chicken antrum by Dimaline *et al.*[6] From the position of the tyrosine, this would appear to be a CCK-like hormone (FIG. 1). Outside this region, the chicken peptide which contains 36 amino acids shows very little similarity to either mammalian gastrin-34 or CCK-33. The presence of this peptide in a region considered to be the counterpart of the mammalian pyloric antrum suggests that the chicken peptide is an avian gastrin. In line with this possibility, it was shown that this peptide stimulates secretion of gastric acid but has no effect on pancreatic secretion.

Similar findings for a reptilian and an amphibian species were recently presented (FIG. 1). Peptides were isolated from the antrum of a turtle and a frog[7] which are clearly related to the chicken peptide just mentioned. The homology is about 50% between both the chicken and turtle and the turtle and frog peptides, respectively. Again, similarity to the mammalian counterparts is low, albeit somewhat higher in the case of CCK.

CCK-LIKE PEPTIDES IN DIFFERENT VERTEBRATES

Different forms of CCK (CCK-83, CCK-58, CCK-39, CCK-33, CCK-22, CCK-8, and CCK-5) were isolated from several mammalian species. CCK-8 is the predominant form in brain, whereas the larger peptides are more abundant in intestine.

Peptides closely related or even identical to mammalian CCK-8 are also present in chicken[8] and frog brain.[7,9] The caeruleins mentioned earlier, which are present in skin secretion of frogs from several different families, are also CCK-like peptides. These data then indicate that peptides containing the common sequence Tyr-Xaa-

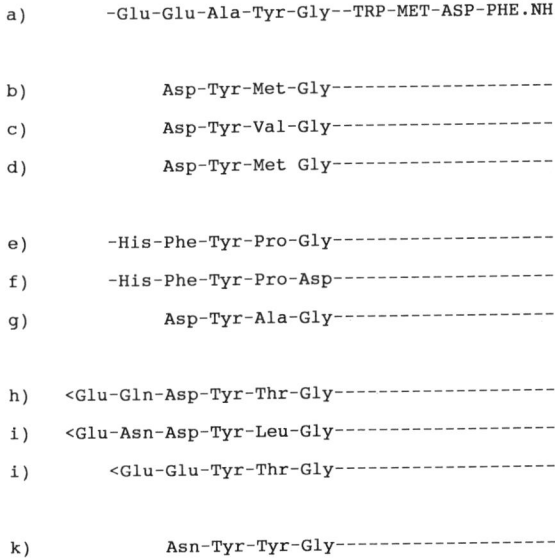

FIGURE 1. Comparison of peptides of the CCK/gastrin family from different vertebrates. (a) Mammalian gastrin; (b) typical mammalian and chicken brain CCK-8; (c) guinea pig and chinchilla CCK-8; (d) CCK from brain of *X. laevis* (as predicted from the sequence of cDNA clones); (e) antral peptide from turtle; (f) antral peptide from chicken; (g) antral peptide from a frog; (h–j) caeruleins from amphibian skin; and (k) cionin from *Ciona intestinalis* (see text for relevant references). <Glu = pyroglutamic acid.

Yaa-Trp-Met-Asp-Phe-amide are present in brain and intestine of amphibia, reptilia, and birds. In contrast, peptides related to gastrin which contain tyrosine as the sixth residue from the carboxyl end have so far only been found in mammals.

CIONIN

As reported by Johnsen and Rehfeld,[10] the neural ganglion of the protochordate *Ciona intestinalis* contains a peptide belonging to the gastrin-CCK family (FIG. 1).

Interestingly, this octapeptide, termed cionin, contains two sulfated tyrosine residues in positions six and seven from the carboxyl end, and thus combines the characteristic features of mammalian gastrin and CCK. On this basis, it is likely that cionin represents an ancestral form of these peptide hormones. By point mutations, either of the two tyrosines could be changed to other residues, thus giving rise to CCK or gastrin.

PRECURSORS FOR PEPTIDES OF THE CCK-GASTRIN FAMILY AS DEDUCED FROM CLONED cDNAs

With the advent of recombinant DNA techniques, the cDNAs encoding the precursors of gastrin,[11-13] CCK,[14,15] and caerulein[16,17] were investigated. In fact, the gastrin precursor was the first in which partial sequence of the corresponding cDNA was obtained by a degenerate oligonucleotide predicted from the amino acid sequence to screen a cDNA library.[11] This later became a standard technique for the isolation of cDNAs.

Both mammalian gastrin and CCK are derived from simple precursors of similar size, each containing a single copy of the corresponding hormone. The different forms of these hormones arise through proteolytic cleavage at single arginine residues present in the respective precursor polypeptides. After the COOH-terminal phenylalanine, the typical processing sequence Gly-Arg-Arg is present, followed by a short extension peptide. Cholecystokinin and gastrin peptides of different length terminating with Phe-Gly rather than the Phe-amide were isolated from different tissues,[18-20] indicating that endoproteolytic cleavage can precede the formation of the terminal amide. The COOH-terminal flanking peptide of the CCK precursor contains two tyrosines that are both sulfated.[21,22] Conversely, in the corresponding peptide of the gastrin precursor the serine residue is partially phosphorylated.[23]

As expected from the known amino acid sequences of the longer forms of gastrin and CCK, the sequence of the precursors of these hormones shows no discernible homology in the corresponding pre- and pro-segments. However, the similarity in the parts encoding the common carboxy-terminal structure of the mature hormones extends beyond the ensuing processing sites into the COOH-terminal extension peptides (FIG. 2). The homology in this region is striking. This is also evident at the

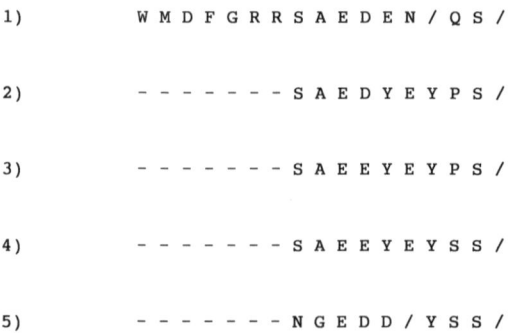

```
1)        W M D F G R R S A E D E N / Q S /

2)        - - - - - - - S A E D Y E Y P S /

3)        - - - - - - - S A E E Y E Y P S /

4)        - - - - - - - S A E E Y E Y S S /

5)        - - - - - - - N G E D D / Y S S /
```

FIGURE 2. Comparison of the COOH-terminal sequences of CCK and gastrin precursors of different species. (1) Human gastrin; (2) rat and mouse CCK; (3) human CCK; (4) *X. laevis* CCK; and (5) *X. laevis* caerulein. Stop codons are marked (/).

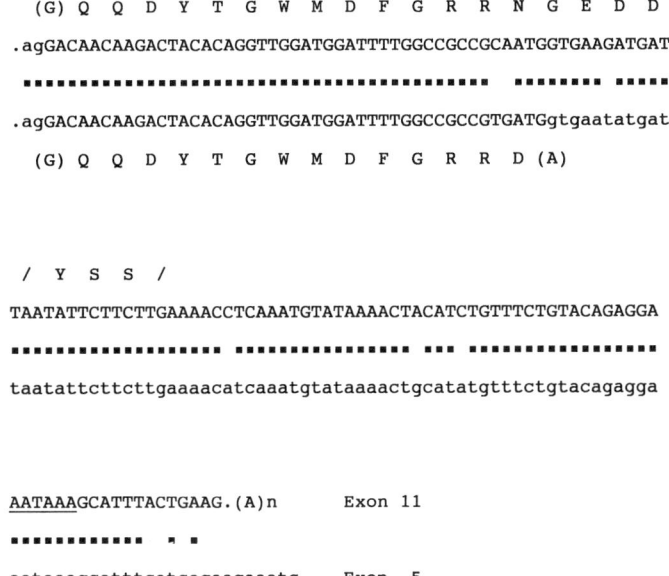

FIGURE 3. Comparison of the nucleotide sequence of exon 11 (*upper lines*) and exon 5 (*lower lines*) of the gene for the type III caerulein precursors (modified from ref. 28). Intron sequences are written in *small letters*. Stop codons are marked (/); the polyadenylation signal is *underlined*.

nucleotide level where, for example, the Gly-Arg-Arg-Ser sequence is in all instances encoded by GGC-CGC/T-CGC-AGT. Moreover, the genes for these hormone precursors[24,25] contain an intron located at about the same site in the coding region, namely, after the first base of the 71st and 72nd codon of prepro-gastrin and prepro-CCK, respectively. This indicates that a distant evolutionary relationship may exist between these two genes.

The precursors of caerulein have also been analyzed via cDNA cloning. From cDNA libraries prepared from skin of *Xenopus laevis,* clones encoding four different caerulein precursors were analyzed.[16,17] The deduced precursor polypeptides contained one, three, or four copies of the mature product. Moreover, processing of these precursors also yielded several copies of antibacterial peptides which can form an amphipathic helix.[26,27] The caerulein precursors are thus much more complex than the precursors of mammalian gastrin and CCK. However, these contain also a COOH-terminal extension that is clearly related to the corresponding mammalian counterparts (FIG. 2).

In addition to cDNAs, genes encoding the caerulein precursors of type I and III were also investigated.[28] Exons encoding the additional caerulein copies have clearly been generated by exon duplication. By the introduction of a new splice site at the 3'-end, these exons are smaller than the putative original exon encoding the last copy and the 3'-untranslated part of the respective mRNAs. However, sequences of the introns following this new splice site are still highly homologous to the corresponding part of the larger exon (FIG. 3). In the course of this work, an additional exon was found which could potentially encode a new peptide only distantly related to CCK.[28] It is currently not known if this exon is expressed in cells of *X. laevis*.

Recently, cDNAs encoding a precursor of CCK were isolated from a library prepared from brain of *X. laevis*.[29] This simple precursor is similar to the CCK precursors of mammalian origin; it contains a single copy of the mature hormone close to the COOH-end. In this case, the similarity of the carboxy-terminal extension peptide to those of mammalian CCK precursors is striking. Data confirm earlier results indicating that CCK-like rather than caerulein-like peptides are present in the brain of amphibia.[7] In addition, there is a high degree of homology between the 3'-parts of the cDNAs encoding the brain CCK and the skin caerulein precursors of *X. laevis* (FIG. 4); however, no similarity could be detected in other regions of the cDNA and the deduced amino acid sequences.[29]

CONCLUDING REMARKS

The data of Johnsen and Rehfeld[10] demonstrate that genes encoding peptides of the CCK-gastrin family were already present in protochordates. Early in the evolu-

```
         N  D  R  D  Y  M  G  W  M  D  F  G  R  R  S  A  E  E  Y  E
.ATGACAGAGACTACATGGGTTGGATGGATTTTGGCCGTCGCAGTGCTGAAGAATATGAA
 ■  ■ ■■■■■■■■ ■■■■■■■■■■■■■■■■■■■■ ■■■■ ■■ ■■■■■■  ■■ ■■
.GACAACAAGACTACACAGGTTGGATGGATTTTGGCCGCCGCAATGGTGAAGATGATTAA
 G  Q  Q  D  Y  T  G  W  M  D  F  G  R  R  N  G  E  D  D  /

 Y  S  S  /
TATTCCTCGTGAAAACTCAAAATATATCAAATGTTCCCCTGTTTCTGTACAGATGAAATAA
■■■■■ ■■ ■■■■■■■■  ■■■■ ■■■ ■■■  ■ ■ ■■■■■■■■■■■■■■■ ■■■■■■■
TATTCTTCTTGAAAACCTCAAATGTATAAAA-CTACATCTGTTTCTGTACAGAGGAAATAA
 Y  S  S  /

AGTAATTTGCTGTCTTT.(A)n          CCK-PRECURSOR
■■ ■ ■■■ ■■■
AGCA-TTTACTGAAG.(A)n            CAERULEIN (exon 11)
```

FIGURE 4. Comparison of the 3'-end of the cDNA encoding the CCK precursor from amphibian brain (*upper line*) and the last exon of the gene for the type III caerulein precursor (*lower line*). The polyadenylation signals are *underlined;* stop codons are marked (/). (A)n stands for the poly-A tail of the mRNAs.

tion of vertebrates, genes for CCK precursors found in mammals were apparently present. This is indicated by our recent analysis of a cDNA encoding such a precursor in the brain of a frog.[29] Starting with the putative ancestor, the cionin precursor, the codon for tyrosine in position 6 from the COOH-terminus, TAT or TAC, was already mutated to ATG coding for methionine in amphibia. Furthermore, additional peptides with the structural characteristics of CCK are present in antrum and in skin of amphibia.

Data currently available make it likely that the phylogenetic tree of CCK-like peptides has at least three branches. According to this view, the first branch involves genes for the typical CCK precursors found in mammalian brain and intestine and, more recently, in amphibian brain. The second branch is represented by the genes encoding the caerulein precursors present in amphibian skin. These complex genes could have arisen early in amphibian evolution through duplication of the 3'-terminal exon of the gene for a CCK precursor. Additional duplications of this exon and mutations leading to a new 3'-splice site would have yielded the additional caerulein copies. These exons were combined with exons encoding antibacterial peptides to yield the complex genes for the caerulein precursors as found in *X. laevis*. The third branch is represented by the genes encoding the precursors of the CCK-like peptides from the antrum of a frog, a reptile, and a bird. Again, these genes may have evolved by duplication of the 3'-exon of the gene of an ancestral CCK precursor.

This leaves open to question the evolutionary history of the genes encoding mammalian gastrin. Peptides of this type have so far been detected only in mammals. The simplest assumption is that gastrin originated from antrum peptides of other vertebrates by deletion of the codon for the sixth amino acid from the COOH-end. Clearly, additional data on peptide and cDNA sequences from different species are needed to test whether the evolution of the CCK-gastrin family can be described by this simple phylogenetic tree.

ACKNOWLEDGMENTS

We thank Prof. J. F. Rehfeld (University of Copenhagen) for helpful suggestions.

REFERENCES

1. BELLEROCHE, J. DE & G. J. DOCKRAY, EDS. 1984. Cholecystokinin in the Nervous System. Verlag Chemie. Basel.
2. REHFELD, J. F. 1989. Cholecystokinin. *In* Handbook of Physiology. The Gastrointestinal System, vol. II: Neural and Endocrine Biology. G. M. Maklouf & S. G. Schultz, eds.: 337–358. American Physiological Society. Bethesda, MD.
3. REHFELD, J. F. 1991. Progastrin and its products in the cerebellum. Neuropeptides **20:** 239–245.
4. ERSPAMER, V. & P. MELCHIORRI. 1980. Active polypeptides: From amphibian skin to gastrointestinal tract and brain of mammals. Trends Pharmacol. Sci. **1:** 391–395.
5. ERSPAMER, V., P. MELCHIORRI, G. FALCONIERI ERSPAMER, P. C. MONTECUCCHI & R. DE CASTIGLIONE. 1985. *Phyllomedusa* skin: A huge factory and store-house of a variety of active peptides. Peptides **6**(Suppl. 3): 7–12.
6. DIMALINE, R., J. YOUNG & H. GREGORY. 1986. Isolation from chicken antrum, and primary amino acid sequence of a novel 36-residue peptide of the gastrin/CCK family. FEBS Lett. **205:** 318–322.
7. JOHNSEN, A. H. & J. F. REHFELD. 1992. Identification of cholecystokinin/gastrin peptides in frog and turtle. Evidence that cholecystokinin is phylogenetically older than gastrin. Eur. J. Biochem. **207:** 419–428.
8. FAN, Z. W., J. ENG, M. MIEDEL, J. D. HOLMES, Y.-C. E. PAN & R. S. YALOW. 1987. Cholecystokinin octapeptides purified from chinchilla and chicken brains. Brain Res. Bull. **18:** 757–780.
9. DIMALINE, R. 1983. Is caerulein amphibian CCK? Peptides **4:** 457–462.
10. JOHNSEN, A. H. & J. F. REHFELD. 1990. Cionin: A disulfotyrosyl hybrid of cholecystokinin and gastrin from the neural ganglion of the protochordate *Ciona intestinalis*. J. Biol. Chem. **265:** 3054–3058.
11. AGARWAL, K. L. & B. E. NOYES. 1980. Studies on gastrin mRNA structure using an oligonucleotide probe. Ann. N.Y. Acad. Sci. **343:** 433–442.
12. YOO, O. J., T. POWELL & K. L. AGARWAL. 1982. Molecular cloning and nucleotide sequence of full-length cDNA coding for porcine gastrin. Proc. Natl. Acad. Sci. USA **79:** 1049–1053.
13. BOEL, E., J. VUUST, F. NORRIS, K. NORRIS, A. WIND, J. F. REHFELD & K. A. MARCKER. 1983. Molecular cloning of human gastrin cDNA: Evidence for evolution of gastrin by gene duplication. Proc. Natl. Acad. Sci. USA **80:** 2866–2869.
14. DESCHENES, R. J., L. J. LORENZ, R. S. HAUN, B. A. ROOS, K. J. COLLIER & J. E. DIXON.

1984. Cloning and sequence analysis of a cDNA encoding rat preprocholecystokinin. Proc. Natl. Acad. Sci. USA **81:** 726–730.
15. GUBLER, U., A. O. CHUA, B. J. HOFFMAN, K. J. COLLIER & J. ENG. 1984. Cloned cDNA to cholecystokinin mRNA predicts an identical prepro-cholecystokinin in pig brain and gut. Proc. Natl. Acad. Sci USA **81:** 4307–4310.
16. HOFFMANN, W., T. C. BACH, H. SELIGER & G. KREIL. 1983. Biosynthesis of caerulein in the skin of *Xenopus laevis:* Partial sequence of precursors as deduced from cDNA clones. EMBO J. **2:** 111–114.
17. RICHTER, K., R. EGGER & G. KREIL. 1986. Sequence of prepro-caerulein cDNAs cloned from skin of *Xenopus laevis:* A small family of precursors containing one, three, or four copies of the final product. J. Biol. Chem. **261:** 3676–3680.
18. SUGANO, K., G. W. APONTE & T. YAMADA. 1985. Identification and characterization of glycine-extended post-translational processing intermediates of pro-gastrin in porcine stomach. J. Biol. Chem. **260:** 11724–11729.
19. REHFELD, J. F. & H. F. HANSEN. 1986. Characterization of prepro-cholecystokinin products in the porcine cerebral cortex: Evidence of different processing pathways. J. Biol. Chem. **261:** 5832–5840.
20. REHFELD, J. F. 1986. Accumulation of nonamidated prepro-gastrin and preprocholecystokinin products in porcine pituitary corticotrophs: Evidence of post-translational control of cell differentiation. J. Biol. Chem. **261:** 5841–5847.
21. ADRIAN, T. E., J. DOMIN, A. J. BACARESE-HAMILTON & S. R. BLOOM. 1986. Is the C-terminal flanking peptide of rat cholecystokinin double sulphated? FEBS Lett. **196:** 5–9.
22. VARRO, A., J. YOUNG, H. GREGORY, J. CSEH & G. J. DOCKRAY. 1986. Isolation, structure and properties of the C-terminal flanking peptides of preprocholecystokinin from rat brain. FEBS Lett. **204:** 386–390.
23. DOCKRAY, G. J., A. VARRO, H. DESMOND, J. YOUNG, H. GREGORY & R. A. GREGORY. 1987. Post-translational processing of the porcine gastrin precursor by phosphorylation of the COOH-terminal fragment. J. Biol. Chem. **262:** 8643–8647.
24. WIBORG, O., L. BERGLUND, E. BOEL, F. NORRIS, K. NORRIS, J. F. REHFELD, K. A. MARCKER & J. VUUST. 1984. Structure of a human gastrin gene. Proc. Natl. Acad. Sci. USA **81:** 1067–1069.
25. TAKAHASHI, Y., K. KATO, Y. HAYASHIZAKI, T. WAKABAYASHI, E. OHTSUKA, S. MATSUKI, M. IKEHARA & K. MATSUBARA. 1985. Molecular cloning of the human cholecystokinin gene by use of a synthetic probe containing deoxyinosine. Proc. Natl. Acad. Sci. USA **82:** 1931–1935.
26. GIBSON, B. W., L. POULTER, D. H. WILLIAMS & J. E. MAGGIO. 1986. Novel peptide fragments originating from PGLa and the caerulein and xenopsin precursors from *Xenopus laevis.* J. Biol. Chem. **261:** 5341–5349.
27. RICHTER, K., H. ASCHAUER & G. KREIL. 1985. Biosynthesis of peptides in the skin of *Xenopus laevis:* Isolation of novel peptides predicted from the sequence of cloned cDNAs. Peptides **6**(suppl. 3): 17–21.
28. VLASAK, R., O. WIBORG, K. RICHTER, S. BURGSCHWAIGER, J. VUUST & G. KREIL. 1987. Conserved exon-intron organization in two different caerulein precursor genes of *Xenopus laevis.* Additional detection of an exon potentially coding for a new peptide. Eur. J. Biochem. **169:** 53–58.
29. WECHSELBERGER, C. & G. KREIL. 1993. The cholecystokinin precursor from brain of *Xenopus laevis* is homologous to its mammalian counterpart. In preparation.

Is Invertebrate CCK-Like Immunoreactivity Caused by Asp-Phe-Amides Similar to the lymnaDFamides (a New Family of Molluscan Neuropeptides)?

ANDERS H. JOHNSEN AND JENS F. REHFELD

Department of Clinical Biochemistry
KB 3011, Rigshospitalet
University of Copenhagen
Blegdamsvej 9, DK-2100 Copenhagen, Denmark

Cholecystokinin (CCK) and gastrin constitute a peptide family that is characterized by the common amidated COOH-terminus Trp-Met-Asp-Phe · NH_2. The structures of CCK and gastrin have been identified in several mammalian and nonmammalian vertebrates. Recently, we identified a putative ancestral member of the CCK/gastrin family, cionin, from the protochordate *Ciona intestinalis*.[1] Invertebrate CCK/gastrin-like peptides have not yet been identified, but comprehensive immunochemical evidence indicates the existence of such peptides. (For a review see ref. 2.) However, exact structural information is impossible to obtain by immunochemical methods. Thus, great care is warranted in the interpretation, especially of the results obtained by immunocytochemistry. Several reports have described CCK/gastrin-like immunoreactivity in nervous tissue of molluscs. The aim of the present work was to disclose the nature of peptides responsible for CCK/gastrin-like immunoreactivity in invertebrates. The pond snail, *Lymnaea stagnalis*, was chosen, because it is well characterized, especially with respect to its nervous system,[3] and because it was within reach for obtaining sufficient material.

The CCK-like immunoreactivity was extracted from the central nervous system of 6,000 animals. The peptides were purified in 5–6 HPLC steps monitored by an antiserum that recognizes the biologically active COOH-terminus of cholecystokinin and gastrin. Five trideca-peptides were isolated.[4] They were identified by sequence analysis and plasma-desorption mass spectrometry (FIG. 1).

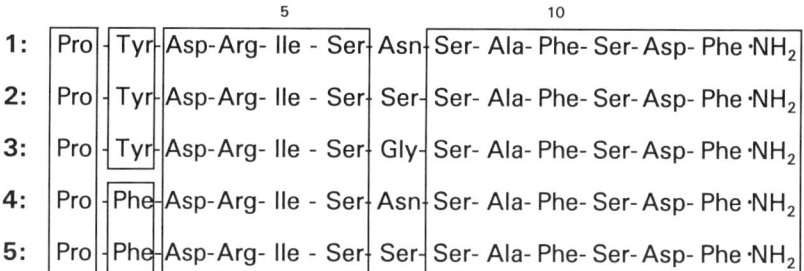

FIGURE 1. Sequences of lymnaDFamide 1–5.

lymnaDFamide-1	Pro -Tyr-Asp-Arg- Ile - Ser-Asn-Ser- Ala- Phe- Ser-	Asp- Phe ·NH₂
CCK	-Arg -Ile - Ser-Asp-Arg-Asp-Tyr-Met-Gly- Trp-Met-	Asp- Phe ·NH₂
gastrin	-Leu -Glu- Glu- Glu- Glu- Glu- Ala- Tyr- Gly- Trp-Met-	Asp- Phe ·NH₂

FIGURE 2. Alignment of lymnaDFamide-1 with the last 13 residues of human CCK and gastrin.

The peptides are named lymnaDFamides to acknowledge the identity with the COOH-terminal dipeptide of the mammalian neuroendocrine peptides CCK and gastrin (FIG. 2). LymnaDFamide-1 was tested on trout gallbladder, which responds equally to CCK and gastrin. It had no effect in concentrations up to 2 μM, whereas 0.1 μM CCK-8-s induced a maximal contractile response. We propose that the lymnaDFamides belong to an Asp-Phe-amide superfamily including CCK and gastrin. The lymnaDFamides and related peptides are likely to cross-react with many antisera directed against the COOH-terminal part of CCK/gastrin. Thus, we suggest that the widespread CCK/gastrin immunoreactivity in invertebrates is due to peptides belonging to such an Asp-Phe-amide superfamily rather than to genuine CCK/gastrin peptides.

REFERENCES

1. JOHNSEN, A. H. & J. F. REHFELD. 1990. Cionin: A disulfotyrosyl hybrid of cholecystokinin and gastrin from the neural ganglion of the protochordate *Ciona intestinalis*. J. Biol. Chem. **265:** 3054–3058.
2. JOHNSEN, A. H. & J. F. REHFELD. 1993. Phylogeny of gastrin. *In* Gastrin. J. H. Walsh, ed.:15–27. Raven Press. New York.
3. GERAERTS, W. P. M., A. B. SMIT, K. W. LI & P. L. HORDIJK. 1992. The light green cells of *Lymnaea*: A neuroendocrine model system for stimulus-induced expression of multiple peptide genes in a single cell type. Experientia **48:** 464–473.
4. JOHNSEN, A. H. & J. F. REHFELD. 1993. LymnaDFamides, a new family of neuropeptides from the pond snail, *Lymnaea stagnalis*. Clue to cholecystokinin immunoreactivity in invertebrates? Eur. J. Biochem. **213:** 875–879.

Cellular Mechanisms Mediating Agonist-Stimulated Calcium Influx in the Pancreatic Acinar Cell

STEPHEN J. PANDOL,[a] ANNA GUKOVSKAYA,
TRISTRAM D. BAHNSON, AND VINCENT E. DIONNE

*Departments of Medicine and Pharmacology
University of California and
Department of Medicine
Veterans Affairs Medical Center
San Diego, California 92161*

The function of the pancreatic acinar cell is to synthesize, store, and secrete digestive enzymes.[1] Historically, the pancreatic acinar cell has been an important model in providing the initial observations about the phosphoinositide/calcium signaling pathway. The initial observation that phosphatidylinositol turnover occurred during hormonal stimulation was made by Hokin and Hokin[2] in 1953 using pigeon pancreatic slices. Inositol 1,4,5-trisphosphate (IP_3) was first demonstrated to mobilize intracellular calcium stores by Streb *et al.*[3] in 1983 using permeabilized pancreatic acinar cells.

Hormones and neurotransmitters regulate pancreatic secretion by way of two separate intracellular signal transduction systems. Some agonists such as vasoactive intestinal peptide and secretin cause secretion by activating adenylyl cyclase which increases intracellular cyclic adenosine monophosphate (cAMP).[4,5] Other agonists such as cholecystokinin (CCK), acetylcholine analogs, and bombesin stimulate digestive enzyme secretion in these cells by causing changes in cellular phosphoinositides and calcium.[4–7] The present article focuses on the signal transduction system used by these agonists.

Cholecystokinin, cholinergic agents, and bombesin peptides cause a phospholipase C-mediated hydrolysis of phosphatidylinositol-4,5-bisphosphate to IP_3 and 1,2-diacylglycerol.[4,8,12] IP_3 mobilizes calcium from intracellular stores,[3] whereas 1,2-diacylglycerol activates protein kinase C.[8–12] The release of Ca^{2+} from internal stores by the agonist is both rapid and transient. Ca^{2+} release occurs within one to a few seconds depending on the concentration of agonist.[13–17] The release results in a rapid rise in free intracellular Ca^{2+} concentration ($[Ca^{2+}]_i$).[13–17] The increase in $[Ca^{2+}]_i$ causes activation of a plasma membrane Ca^{2+} ATPase, resulting in Ca^{2+} efflux from the cell and a return of $[Ca^{2+}]_i$ towards resting levels.[18] Return of $[Ca^{2+}]_i$ towards resting levels takes place in 3–5 minutes.[13–17] After release of the intracellular pool of Ca^{2+}, there is activation of Ca^{2+} entry across the plasma membrane.[2,19] This Ca^{2+} entry results in a sustained increase in $[Ca^{2+}]_i$ during stimulation, and this increased $[Ca^{2+}]_i$ is dependent on the presence of extracellular $CaCl_2$.[20]

Both internal Ca^{2+} release and Ca^{2+} entry have essential roles in mediating enzyme secretion. The release of intracellular Ca^{2+} by agonists or Ca^{2+} ionophores causes a burst in enzyme secretion lasting about as long as the transient increase in

---

[a]Address for correspondence: Stephen J. Pandol, MD, Veterans Affairs Medical Center (111D), 3350 La Jolla Village Dr., San Diego, CA 92161.

$[Ca^{2+}]_i$.[8,13,20] Thus, intracellular Ca^{2+} release is sufficient to cause secretion in the absence of extracellular Ca^{2+}.[8,13,20] However, during sustained agonist stimulation, continued enzyme secretion is dependent on extracellular Ca^{2+}.[2,20-22] That is, in the absence of extracellular Ca^{2+}, enzyme secretory rates return to resting levels after the initial transient increase in $[Ca^{2+}]_i$.

Calcium oscillations have also been observed in pancreatic acinar cells. Low concentrations of CCK and acetylcholine analogs as well as maximally effective concentrations of the CCK analog JMV-180 can cause sustained oscillations of $[Ca^{2+}]_i$.[23-25] Although the mechanisms of $[Ca^{2+}]_i$ oscillations and the role of oscillations in enzyme secretion are controversial, each oscillatory increase in $[Ca^{2+}]_i$ would be expected to stimulate a burst in enzyme secretion.

MECHANISMS MEDIATING CALCIUM ENTRY

Relationship to Internal Calcium Stores

Although the mechanisms of agonist-induced intracellular Ca^{2+} release have been described, the mechanisms regulating Ca^{2+} entry have been difficult to establish. It is now generally accepted that this Ca^{2+} entry is activated by depletion of intracellular Ca^{2+} stores, a mechanism referred to as the "Capacitative Model" by Putney.[26,27] This model was proposed to account for the observed coupling between intracellular Ca^{2+} release and Ca^{2+} entry in a variety of tissues. In the first version of the model,[26] it was proposed that depletion of the pool activated the pathway for Ca^{2+} entry because the pool and the plasma membrane Ca^{2+} influx mechanism were in a close anatomic relationship. The Ca^{2+} entered the pool directly after crossing the plasma membrane. The depletion-activated Ca^{2+} entry would provide Ca^{2+} for refilling the intracellular stores. In addition, during continued stimulation, Ca^{2+} release from the stores would provide a source of Ca^{2+} to be released into the cytoplasm. This release into the cytoplasm would result in increased $[Ca^{2+}]_i$ during continued stimulation.

Observations since this first version of the Capacitative Model indicate that Ca^{2+} probably does not enter the pool directly after crossing the plasma membrane. Experiments in both pancreatic acinar cells and parietal cells demonstrated that the intracellular Ca^{2+} storage organelles could take up Ca^{2+} from the entire cytoplasm, not just from specialized regions between the storage organelles and the plasma membrane.[28,29] In these studies the cells were stimulated with carbachol; atropine was then added immediately after release of Ca^{2+} from internal stores and before significant Ca^{2+} efflux from the cells occurred. With the addition of atropine, all of the cytoplasmic Ca^{2+} returned to the stores. In a variation of this experiment, Muallem et al.[30] demonstrated that cytosolic Ca^{2+} chelators prevented refilling of intracellular Ca^{2+} stores, suggesting that Ca^{2+} must traverse the cytoplasm before it could enter the stores.

Another approach to demonstrating the relationship between intracellular stores and plasma membrane Ca^{2+} influx made use of the tumor promoter drug thapsigargin. This agent depletes the intracellular stores by inhibiting the Ca^{2+} ATPase of the stores without raising levels of inositol phosphates.[31,32] Depletion of Ca^{2+} from intracellular stores with thapsigargin resulted in activation of the Ca^{2+} entry mechanism.[33] These results indicated that Ca^{2+} entry is activated as a result of Ca^{2+} depletion. In addition, they indicated that inositol phosphates are not necessary for this activation. Because of the experimental results just described, Putney[27] revised the Capacitative Model of Ca^{2+} entry to include the provision for a soluble messenger system coupling Ca^{2+} pool depletion to activation of Ca^{2+} entry.

Role of Cyclic GMP As a Soluble Messenger Mediating Ca^{2+} Entry

The most challenging issue at present is the elucidation of the messenger system linking intracellular Ca^{2+} pool depletion to activation of plasma membrane Ca^{2+} entry. Irvine has proposed that the phosphorylated metabolite of IP_3, inositol 1,3,4,5-tetrakisphosphate (IP_4), has a role in mediating Ca^{2+} entry.[34-36] This proposal came initially from findings in sea urchin eggs where the full fertilization response could be elicited with a combination of IP_3 and IP_4, but not with IP_3 alone, in the presence of external Ca^{2+}.[34] Subsequently, cell perfusion and electrophysiologic measurements of Ca^{2+}-activated K^+ channels in lacrimal cells demonstrated that perfusion of cells with IP_3 alone caused only transient activation of the Ca^{2+}-activated K^+ channels.[35,36] The addition of IP_4 to the intracellular perfusate and Ca^{2+} to the extracellular media was necessary for sustained channel activation. Although these results suggest a possible role for IP_4 in mediating Ca^{2+} entry, as discussed earlier, the finding that thapsigargin can activate Ca^{2+} entry in the absence of inositol phosphates suggests that IP_4 is not required. Furthermore, as described in more detail below, we have been unable to demonstrate a direct effect of IP_4 on Ca^{2+} entry using the patch-clamp recording method.[37]

Our laboratory has presented evidence that cyclic guanosine monophosphate (cGMP) may be a mediator that activates Ca^{2+} entry in pancreatic acinar cells.[38] It has been known for several years that agonists that mobilize intracellular Ca^{2+} stores also increase cellular cGMP levels in pancreatic acinar cells as well as a variety of other tissues.[39,40] However, the role of cGMP in these tissues has not been determined. In a survey of the relationships between cGMP and Ca^{2+} metabolism in the pancreatic acinar cell, we found that cGMP was necessary for carbachol-induced activation of the Ca^{2+} entry pathway.[38] For these experiments, we used the pharmacologic agent LY83583, which is known to inhibit cGMP formation in a variety of tissues.[38,56] Using fura-2 loaded acini and measurements of $[Ca^{2+}]_i$, we found that this agent had no effect on the ability of carbachol to release Ca^{2+} from internal stores. However, LY83583 inhibited Ca^{2+} entry both during and after carbachol stimulation when refilling of the intracellular Ca^{2+} stores occurs. Previous experiments have demonstrated that activation of Ca^{2+} entry is necessary for refilling the stores at termination of the stimulation.[41-43] Thus, these results indicated that cGMP formation coincident with agonist stimulation was necessary for activation of Ca^{2+} entry.

In a recent series of experiments,[37] we identified an inward current corresponding to Ca^{2+} entry in pancreatic acinar cells using an approach similar to the one that Hoth and Penner[44] used to demonstrate Ca^{2+} entry in mast cells. This approach included measurements of whole cell currents using patch clamp recordings made under various conditions of intracellular Ca^{2+} depletion. Recording conditions included an excess of extracellular Ca^{2+} (10 mM) and the inclusion of the Ca^{2+} chelator BAPTA in the perfusing intracellular saline to buffer $[Ca^{2+}]_i$ to low levels (1–75 nM). Under these conditions, intracellular application of IP_3, which caused Ca^{2+} depletion in the presence of BAPTA, activated an inward current with a reversal potential of approximately +45 mV. When substitutions for extracellular Ca^{2+} were made with Mn^{2+}, N-methyl-D-glucamine$^+$, Ni^{2+}, or Cd^{2+}, the current was partially reversed. These results indicated that Ca^{2+} store depletion resulted in a measurable inward current that, at least in part, was carried by Ca^{2+}.

We found that a similar current could be activated by extracellular application of carbachol or intracellular application of cGMP (but not cAMP) under conditions when $[Ca^{2+}]_i$ was clamped at 74 nM to prevent low $[Ca^{2+}]_i$ from depleting intracellular Ca^{2+} stores. Finally, the inward current was not activated by the intracellular application of IP_4. These results suggested that cGMP is sufficient to activate Ca^{2+} entry and may mediate the effect of agonists on Ca^{2+} entry in pancreatic acinar cells.

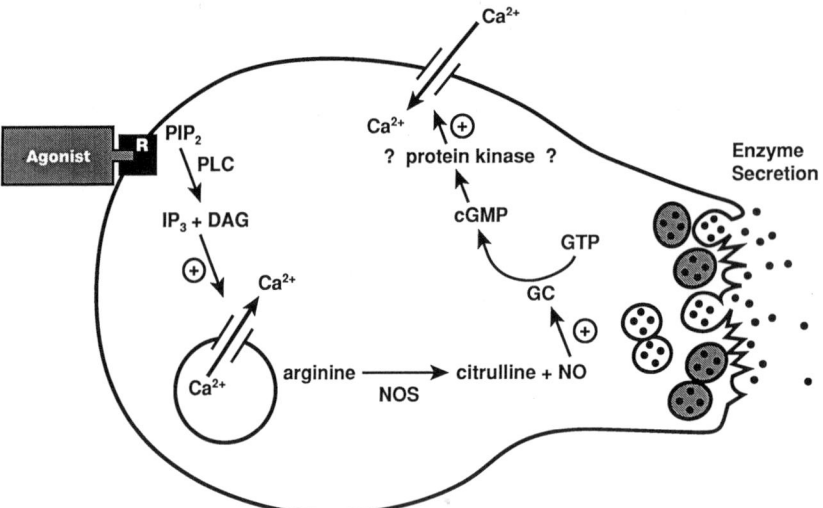

FIGURE 1. Proposed pathway of agonist-mediated Ca^{2+} entry in the pancreatic acinar cell. The agonist represents either CCK, acetylcholine, or bombesin. The agonist stimulates an increase in IP_3 by a phospholipase C-mediated breakdown of phosphatidylinositol 4,5-bisphosphate. The IP_3, in turn, activates the IP_3 receptor/Ca^{2+} channel on the internal stores to release Ca^{2+} into the cytoplasm. This release results in both an increase in $[Ca^{2+}]_i$ and a depletion of intracellular Ca^{2+} stores. By mechanisms that are not yet well defined, depletion of Ca^{2+} stores results in activation of nitric oxide (NO) synthase which converts arginine to citrulline and NO. The NO, in turn, activates soluble guanylyl cyclase resulting in an increase in cGMP. Finally, the cGMP mediates Ca^{2+} entry by either a direct action on some cGMP-modulated membrane conductance or indirectly by a cGMP-dependent process (e.g., kinase or phosphodiesterase).

Unresolved Issues

Although the results just described suggest that Ca^{2+} store depletion or cGMP can regulate Ca^{2+} entry, the relationships between Ca^{2+} release from the stores and the observed increase in cGMP are not known. Further investigations of this pathway should determine the mechanisms regulating cGMP formation in the cell. A number of messengers have been suggested to regulate cGMP formation in eukaryotic cells. These include arachidonic acid and/or its oxidative metabolites,[45] nitric oxide (NO) and different NO-derived compounds,[45–47] and carbon monoxide.[48,49] We have developed preliminary evidence that NO is produced by agonists in pancreatic acini and that this NO is responsible for mediating the increase in cGMP caused by the agonists under some conditions.[50] Further experiments will be required to determine how Ca^{2+} depletion of the intracellular stores causes activation of NO synthase.

The finding that cGMP can activate Ca^{2+} entry suggests that the pathway involves either a cGMP-dependent enzymatic step or a direct interaction of cGMP with a membrane conductance (e.g., ion channel or ion transporter). Examples of cyclic nucleotide-gated channels are found in cardiac myocytes,[51] neurons,[52] photoreceptors,[53,54] and olfactory tissue.[55]

SUMMARY

FIGURE 1 summarizes our current concept of a signaling mechanism to explain agonist-induced Ca^{2+} entry in the pancreatic acinar cell. We propose that cGMP can modulate Ca^{2+} entry under conditions of internal Ca^{2+} store depletion and that the NO signaling system may be involved in coupling Ca^{2+} depletion to cGMP formation. The finding that Ca^{2+} entry after Ca^{2+} store depletion can occur with no elevation in $[Ca^{2+}]_i$[37] raises the possibility that alternative signaling pathways may converge to stimulate cGMP formation or that additional messengers may activate plasmalemmal Ca^{2+} entry mechanisms in parallel.

REFERENCES

1. PALADE, G. 1975. Intracellular aspects of the process of protein synthesis. Science **189:** 347–358.
2. HOKIN, M. R. & L. E. HOKIN. 1953. Enzyme secretion and incorporation of P^{32} into phospholipids of pancreas slides. J. Biol. Chem. **203:** 967–977.
3. STREB, H., R. F. IRVINE, M. J. BERRIDGE & I. SCHULZ. 1983. Release of Ca^{2+} from a nonmitochondrial intracellular store in pancreatic acinar cells by inositol-1,4,5-trisphosphate. Nature Lond. **306:** 67–69.
4. HOOTMAN, S. R. & J. A. WILLIAMS. 1987. Stimulus-secretion coupling in the pancreatic acinar cells. *In* Physiology of the Gastrointestinal Tract. 2nd Ed. L. R. Johnson: 1129–1146. Raven Press. New York.
5. GARDNER, J. P. & R. T. JENSEN. 1987. Secretagogue receptors on pancreatic acinar cells. *In* Physiology of the Gastrointestinal Tract. 2nd Ed. L. R. Johnson, ed.: 1109–1128. Raven Press. New York.
6. WILLIAMS, J. A. 1980. Regulation of pancreatic acinar cell function by intracellular calcium. Am. J. Physiol. **238:** G269–G279.
7. SCHULZ, I. 1980. Messenger role of calcium in function of pancreatic acinar cells. Am. J. Physiol. **239:** G335–G347.
8. BRUZZONE, R. 1990. The molecular basis of enzyme secretion. Gastroenterology **99:** 1157–1176.
9. PANDOL, S. J. & M. S. SCHOEFFIELD. 1986. 1,2-diacylglycerol, protein kinase C and pancreatic enzyme secretion. J. Biol. Chem. **261:** 4439–4444.
10. MATOZAKI, T. & J. A. WILLIAMS. 1989. Multiple sources of 1,2-diacylglycerol in isolated rat pancreatic acini stimulated by cholecystokinin. Involvement of phosphatidylinositol biophosphate and phosphatidylcholine hydrolysis. J. Biol. Chem. **264:** 14729–12734.
11. STREB, H., J. P. HESLOP, R. F. IRVINE, I. SCHULZ & J. J. BERRIDGE. 1985. Relationships between secretagogue-induced Ca^{2+} release and inositol phosphate production in permeabilized pancreatic acinar cell. J. Biol. Chem. **260:** 7309–7315.
12. BERRIDGE, M. J. & R. F. IRVINE. 1989. Inositol phosphates and cell signalling. Nature (Lond.) **341:** 197–205.
13. PANDOL, S. J., M. S. SCHOEFFIELD, G. SACHS & S. MUALLEM. 1985. Role of free cytosolic calcium in secretagogue-stimulated amylase release from dispersed acini from guinea pig pancreas. J. Biol. Chem. **260:** 10081–10086.

14. POWERS, R. W., P. C. JOHNSON, M. J. HOULIHAN, A. K. SALUJA & M. L. STEER. 1985. Intracellular Ca^{2+} levels and amylase secretion in quin-2-loaded mouse pancreatic acini. Am. J. Physiol. **248:** C535–C541.
15. OCHS, D. L., J. I. KORENBROT & J. A. WILLIAMS. 1985. Relationship between agonist-induced changes in the concentration of free intracellular calcium and secretion of amylase by pancreatic acini. Am. J. Physiol. **249:** G389–G398.
16. MERRITT, J. E. & R. P. RUBIN. 1985. Pancreatic enzyme secretion and cytosolic free calcium. Effects of ionomycin, phorbol dibutyrate and diacylglycerol alone and in combination. Biochem. J. **230:** 151–159.
17. BRUZZONE, R., T. POZZAN & C. B. WOLLHEIM. 1986. Caerulein and carbamoylcholine stimulate pancreatic amylase release at resting cytosolic free Ca^{2+}. Biochem. J. **235:** 139–143.
18. MUALLEM, S., T. G. BEEKER & S. J. PANDOL. 1988. Role of Na^+/Ca^{2+} exchange and the plasma membrane Ca^{2+} pump in hormone-mediated Ca^{2+} efflux from pancreatic acini. J. Membrane Biol. **102:** 153–162.
19. PANDOL, S. J., M. S. SCHOEFFIELD, C. J. FIMMEL & S. MUALLEM. 1987. The agonist-sensitive calcium pool in the pancreatic acinar cell. Activation of plasma membrane Ca^{2+} influx mechanism. J. Biol. Chem. **262:** 16963–16968.
20. KRIMS, P. E. & S. J. PANDOL. 1988. Free cytosolic calcium and secretagogue-stimulated initial pancreatic exocrine secretion. Pancreas **3:** 383–390.
21. SCHEELE, G. & A. HAYMOVITS. 1979. Cholinergic and peptide-stimulated discharge of secretory protein in guinea pig pancreatic lobules. J. Biol. Chem. **254:** 10364–10370.
22. GARDNER, J. D. & R. T. JENSEN. 1981. Regulation of pancreatic enzyme secretion in vitro. In Physiology of the Gastrointestinal Tract. L. R. Johnson, ed.: 831–871. Raven Press. New York.
23. MATOZAKI, T., B. GOKE, Y. TSUNODA, M. RODRIGUEZ, J. MARTINEZ & J. A. WILLIAMS. 1990. Two functionally distinct cholecystokinin receptors show different modes of action on Ca^{2+} mobilization and phospholipid hydrolysis in isolated rat pancreatic acini studies using a new cholecystokinin analog. JMV-180. J. Biol. Chem. **265:** 6247–6254.
24. OSIPCHUK, Y. V., M. WAKUI, D. I. YULE, D. U. GALLACHER & O. H. PETERSON. 1990. Cytoplasmic Ca^{2+} oscillations evoked by receptor stimulation, G-protein activation, internal application of inositol trisphosphate or Ca^{2+}: Simultaneous microfluorimetry and Ca^{2+} dependent Cl^- current recording in single pancreatic acinar cells. Embo J. **9:** 697–704.
25. PETERSEN, C. C., E. C. TOESCU & O. H. PETERSEN. 1991. Different patterns of receptor-activated cytoplasmic Ca^{2+} oscillations in single pancreatic acinar cells: Dependence on receptor types, agonist concentration and intracellular Ca^{2+} buffering. Embo J. **10:** 527–533.
26. PUTNEY, J. W., JR. 1986. A model for receptor-regulated calcium entry. Cell Calcium **7:** 1–12.
27. PUTNEY, J. W., JR. 1990. Capacitative calcium entry revisited. Review article. Cell Calcium **11:** 611–624.
28. MACHEN, T. E. & P. A. NEGULESCU. 1988. Release and reloading of intracellular Ca^{2+} stores after cholinergic stimulation of the parietal cell. Am. J. Physiol. **254:** C498–C504.
29. MUALLEM, S., M. S. SCHOEFFIELD, C. J. FIMMEL & S. J. PANDOL. 1988. Agonist-sensitive calcium pool in the pancreatic acinar cell. II. Characterization of reloading. Am. J. Physiol. **255:** G229–G235.
30. MUALLEM, S., M. KHADEMAZAD & G. SACHS. 1990. The route of Ca^{2+} entry during reloading of the intracellular Ca^{2+} pool in pancreatic acini. J. Biol. Chem. **265:** 2011–2016.
31. THASTRUP, O., P. J. CULLEN, D. K. DROBAK, M. R. HANLEY & A. P. DAWSON. 1990. Thapsigargin, a tumor promoter discharges intracellular Ca^{2+} stores by specific inhibition of endoplasmic reticulum Ca^{2+} ATPase. Proc. Natl. Acad. Sci. USA **87:** 2466–2470.
32. JACKSON, T. R., S. I. PATTERSON, O. THASTRUP & M. R. HANLEY. 1988. A novel tumor promotor, thapsigargin, transiently increases cytoplasmic free Ca^{2+} without generation of inositol phosphates in NG115-40IL neuronal cells. Biochem. J. **253:** 81–86.
33. TAKEMURA, H., A. R. HUGHES, O. THASTRUP & J. W. PUTNEY, JR. 1989. Activation of

calcium entry by the tumor promotor, thapsigargin, in parotid acinar cells. Evidence that an intracellular calcium pool, and not an inositol phosphate, regulates calcium fluxes at the plasma membrane. J. Biol. Chem. **264:** 12266–12272.

34. IRVINE, R. F. & R. M. MOOR. 1986. Micro-injection of inositol 1,3,4,5-tetrakisphosphate activates sea urchin eggs by a mechanism dependent on external Ca^{2+}. Biochem. J. **240:** 917–920.
35. MORRIS, A. P., D. V. GALLACHER, R. F. IRVINE & O. H. PETERSEN. 1987. Synergism of inositol trisphosphate and tetrakisphosphate in activating Ca^{2+}-dependent K^+ channels. Nature **330:** 653–655.
36. CHANYGA, L., D. V. GALLACHER, R. F. IRVINE, B. V. L. POTTER & O. H. PETERSON. 1989. Inositol 1,3,4,5-trisphosphate is essential for sustained activation of the Ca^{2+}-dependent K^+ current in single internally perfused lacrimal cells. J. Membrane Biol. **109:** 85–93.
37. BAHNSON, T. D., S. J. PANDOL & V. E. DIONNE. 1993. Cyclic GMP modulates depletion-activated Ca^{2+} entry in pancreatic acinar cells. J. Biol. Chem. **268:** 10808–10812.
38. PANDOL, S. J. & M. S. SCHOEFFIELD-PAYNE. 1990. Cyclic GMP mediates the agonist-stimulated increase in plasma membrane calcium entry in the pancreatic acinar cell. J. Biol. Chem. **265:** 12846–12853.
39. DEMEYTS, P. & J. HANOUNE. 1982. Plasma membrane receptors and function. *In* The Liver: Biology and Pathobiology. I. Arias, H. Popper, D. Schacter & D. A. Shafritz, eds.: 551–580. Raven Press. New York.
40. YOUNG, J. A., D. I. COOK, E. W. VAN LENNEP & M. ROBERTS. 1987. Secretion of the major salivary glands. *In* Physiology of the Gastrointestinal Tract. 2nd Ed. L. R. Johnson, ed.: 773–816. Raven Press. New York.
41. PANDOL, S. J., M. S. SCHOEFFIELD, C. J. FIMMEL & S. MUALLEM. 1987. The agonist-sensitive calcium pool in the pancreatic acinar cell: Activation of plasma membrane calcium influx mechanism. J. Biol. Chem. **262:** 16963–16968.
42. MUALLEM, S., M. S. SCHOEFFIELD, C. J. FIMMEL & S. J. PANDOL. 1988. Agonist-sensitive calcium pool in the pancreatic acinar cell. I. Permeability properties. Am. J. Physiol. **255:** G221–G228.
43. MUALLEM, S., M. S. SCHOEFFIELD, C. J. FIMMEL & S. J. PANDOL. 1988. Agonist-sensitive calcium pool in the pancreatic acinar cell. II. Characterization of reloading. Am. J. Physiol. **255:** G229–G235.
44. HOTH, H. & R. PENNER. 1992. Depletion of intracellular calcium stores activates a calcium current in mast cells. Nature **355:** 353–356.
45. WALDMAN, S. A. & F. MURAD. 1987. Cyclic GMP synthesis and function. Pharmacol. Rev. **39:** 163–196.
46. MURAD, F., C. K. MITTAL, W. P. ARNOLD, S. KATSUKI & H. KIMURA. 1978. Guanylate cyclase: Activation by azide, nitro compounds, nitric oxide, and hydroxyl radical and inhibition by hemoglobin and myoblobin. Adv. Cyclic Nucleotide Res. **9:** 145–158.
47. FEELISCH, M. & E. A. NOACK. 1987. Correlation between nitric oxide formation during degradation of organic nitrates and activation of guanylate cyclase. Eur. J. Pharmacol. **139:** 19–30.
48. PALMER, R. M. J., D. S. ASHTON & S. MONCADA. 1988. Vascular endothelial cells synthesize nitric oxide from L-arginine. Nature (Lond.) **333:** 664–666.
49. TAYEH, M. A. & M. A. MARLETTA. 1989. Macrophage oxidation of L-arginine to nitric oxide, nitrite, and nitrate. Tetrahydrobiopterin is required as a cofactor. J. Biol Chem. **264:** 19654–19658.
50. GUKOVSKAYA, A. S. & S. J. PANDOL. 1993. Nitric oxide regulates neurotransmitter induced cGMP rise and Ca^{2+} influx in pancreatic acinar cells. Gastroenterology (Abstr.) **104:** A306.
51. DIFRANCESCO, D. & P. TORTORA. 1991. Direct activation of cardiac pacemaker channels by intracellular cyclic AMP. Nature **351:** 145–147.
52. PAPE, H. C. & D. A. MCCORMICK. 1989. Noradrenaline and serotonin selectively modulate thalamic burst firing by enhancing a hyperpolarization-activated cation currents. **340:** 715–718.
53. FESENKO, E. E., S. S. KOLESNIKOV & A. L. LYUBARVSKY. 1985. Induction by cyclic GMP of

cationic conductance in plasma membrane of retinal rod outer segment. Nature **313:** 310–313.
54. KAUPP, U. B. & K. W. KOCH. 1992. Role of cGMP and Ca^{2+} in vertebrate photoreceptor excitation and adaptation. Ann. Rev. Physiol. **54:** 153–175.
55. NAKAMURA, T. & G. H. GOLD. 1987. A cyclic nucleotide-gated conductance in olfactory receptor cilia. Nature **325:** 442–444.
56. MULSCH, A., R. BUSSE, S. LIEBAU & U. FORSTERMANN. 1988. LY 83583 interferes with the release of endothelium-derived relaxing factor and inhibits soluble guanylate cyclase. J. Pharmacol. Exp. Ther. **247:** 283–288.

Cholecystokinin Receptor Family

Molecular Cloning, Structure, and Functional Expression in Rat, Guinea Pig, and Human

STEPHEN A. WANK,[a] JOSEPH R. PISEGNA,
AND ANDREAS DE WEERTH

Digestive Diseases Branch
National Institute of Diabetes and Digestive and Kidney Diseases, and
National Institutes of Health
Bethesda, Maryland 20892

The cholecystokinin (CCK) and gastrin family of peptides share a common COOH-terminal pentapeptide-amide amino sequence and can be found throughout the gastrointestinal, central (CNS), and peripheral nervous systems.[1,2] Receptors for CCK have been biologically and pharmacologically classified on the basis of their relative affinity for sulfated and nonsulfated CCK agonists and selective antagonists into as many as four receptor types, CCK_A, CCK_B, gastrin, and receptors preferring the COOH-terminal tetrapeptide common to CCK and gastrin, CG-4.[3] The CCK_A type receptor (CCK_AR) has high affinity only for sulfated CCK and the antagonist L-364,718[4] and has been described on pancreatic acinar cells,[5] gallbladder smooth muscle,[6] chief,[7] and D^8 cells of gastric mucosa, select areas of the central and peripheral nervous systems,[9] and tumoral cell lines such as the pancreatic acinar carcinoma cell line AR4-2J[10] and the human neuroblastoma cell line CHP 212.[11] Some pharmacological and biochemical data suggest that two subtypes of CCK_ARs exist: one in the pancreas and another in the gallbladder.[12-15] Furthermore, multiple studies of the stoichiometry of CCK_AR binding indicate the presence of at least two receptors on pancreatic acinar cells, a high affinity receptor with low capacity and a low affinity receptor with high capacity;[16,17] however, kinetic studies indicate the presence of a single CCK_AR existing in two affinity states, high and low.[18] The CCK_B receptor subtype (CCK_BR) has a 3–10-fold higher affinity for sulfated CCK-8 than does gastrin and prefers the antagonist L-365,260.[19] CCK_BRs have been found on cells throughout the central nervous system,[20,21] immune cells such as monocytes[22] and T lymphocytes,[23] and tumoral cell lines such as the AR4-2J cell line[24] and human leiomyosarcoma cells.[25] Gastrin type receptors have an equal affinity for CCK-8 and gastrin and also prefer the antagonist L-365,260 with the exception of the canine gastrin receptor.[19] Gastrin receptors have been described in gastric mucosa on parietal,[26] chief,[7] and ECL[27] cells, gallbladder[28] and stomach smooth muscle[29] cells, neoplastic cells such as small cell lung carcinoma,[30] and gastric and colonic carcinoma,[31] and on pancreatic acinar cells of the guinea pig,[32] dog,[33] and calf.[34] CG-4 type receptors have 500–1,000-fold higher affinity for CG-4 than for CCK-8 and gastrin and have been described on isolated perfused hog pancreatic islet cells in biological assays where they mediate the release of insulin, glucagon, somatostatin, and pancreatic polypeptide.[35]

---

[a] To whom correspondence should be addressed.

STRUCTURE OF RAT CCK_A AND CCK_B RECEPTORS

We recently cloned and functionally expressed both the CCK_AR[36] and CCK_BR[37] from rat pancreas and brain cDNA libraries, respectively. Analysis of their deduced amino acid sequences indicates that these receptors are highly homologous (48% amino acid identity) and contain seven regions of hydrophobic residues corresponding to transmembrane domains (FIG. 1). This finding suggests their membership in the guanine nucleotide-binding regulatory protein-coupled superfamily of receptors[38] and is consistent with their reported modulation by guanine nucleotides.[39] Both sequences contain at least three consensus sites for N-linked glycosylation, consistent with the heavy and variable degree of glycosylation reported using ligand affinity cross-linking techniques[40] and consensus sites for protein kinase C phosphorylation[41] consistent with studies of CCK-8 and TPA-stimulated phosphorylation of serine and threonine residues on pancreatic CCK_ARs[42] (FIG. 1). For both the CCK_AR and CCK_BR, there are conserved cysteines in the first and second extracellular loops that may form a disulfide bridge required for stabilization of the tertiary structure as demonstrated for rhodopsin,[43] β-adrenergic,[44] and muscarinic receptors[45] (FIG. 1). A cysteine in the carboxy-terminus may be a membrane-anchoring palmitoylation site similar to rhodopsin and the β-adrenergic receptors[46,47] (FIG. 1).

RAT PANCREATIC ACINI EXPRESS A SINGLE CLASS OF CCK_A RECEPTORS

To address an old and persistent question of whether the broad dose-inhibition curve for radiolabeled CCK binding to pancreatic acini is the result of interaction with two distinct classes of receptors, high and low affinity classes of receptors, or interaction with a single class of receptors capable of existing in high and low affinity states, we performed radioligand binding dose inhibition studies in COS-7 cells transfected with the cloned rat CCK_AR cDNA inserted in the mammalian expression vector pCDL-SRα.[48] Similar to the native receptor,[49] the recombinant receptor has a 1,000-fold greater affinity for CCK-8 than for gastrin-17-1 and more than a 100-fold greater affinity for CCK_AR-specific antagonist L-364,718 than for the CCK_BR-specific antagonist L-365,260[37] (FIG. 2). For both the cloned and native receptors, the dose-inhibition curve with the agonist CCK-8 was broad (FIG. 2) and best fit[50] by a two-site model with high (0.7 ± 0.1 nM) and low (53 ± 7 nM) affinity binding sites (TABLE 1).[15] In contrast, the antagonist dose inhibition curve with L-364,718 was narrow with equal affinity for both high (0.8 ± 0.8 nM) and low (0.7 ± 0.7 nM) affinity binding sites (TABLE 1).[51] These results demonstrate that high and low affinity CCK receptor binding sites previously attributed to two distinct receptors can now be attributed to a single receptor existing in two different affinity states.

GALLBLADDER AND PANCREAS EXPRESS IDENTICAL CCK_A RECEPTORS

Pharmacological and functional studies demonstrate a CCK_A receptor subtype in both pancreas and gallbladder.[5,6] However, some pharmacological[12-15] and affinity cross-linking studies[52-54] of CCK receptors from pancreas and gallbladder suggest that these two tissues possess two different subtypes of CCK_ARs. To determine the identity of CCK_ARs between gallbladder and pancreas, we cloned the CCK_AR from each tissue.[55] Using a rat CCK_AR cDNA probe,[18] we cloned guinea pig gallbladder

Rat CCK_A Receptor

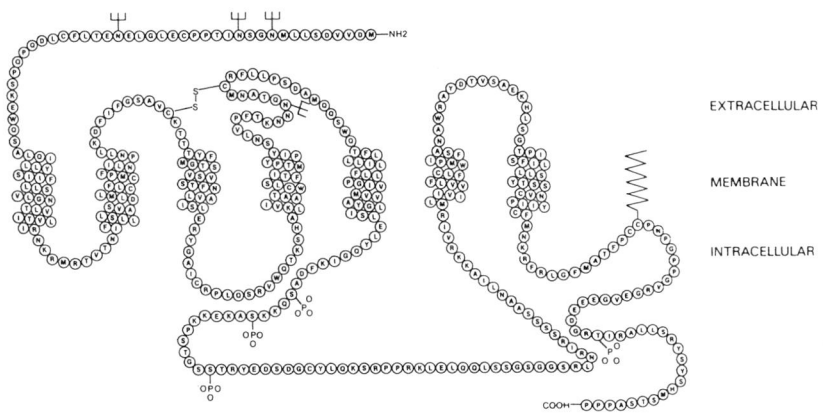

Rat CCK_B Receptor

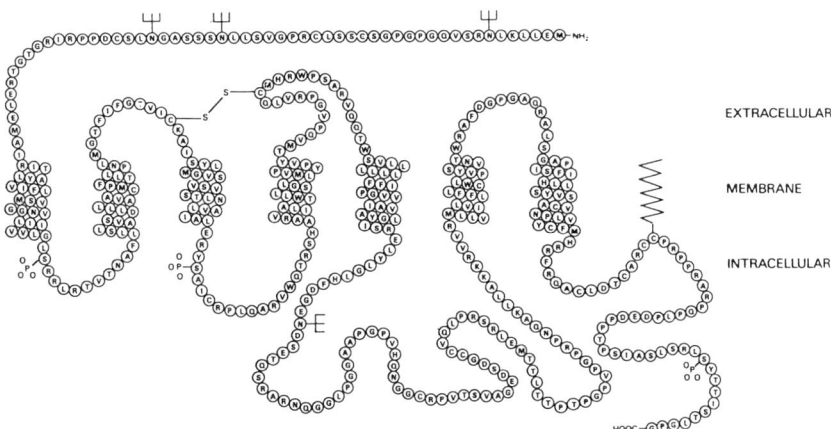

FIGURE 1. Schematic models of rat CCK_A and CCK_B receptors. Deduced amino acid sequences (using amino acid letter symbols) of rat CCK_A (*top*)[36] and CCK_B (*bottom*)[37] receptors showing putative transmembrane helices, consensus sites for putative *N*-linked glycosylation (tridents), serine and threonine phosphorylation by protein kinase C and A ($-PO_3$), and conserved cysteines in the first and second extracellular loops possibly forming a disulfide bridge ($-S-S-$)[33–35] and a conserved cysteine in the cytoplasmic tail possibly palmitoylated (jagged line extending into the membrane).[36,37] ($-NH_2$, amino terminus; $-COOH$, carboxy terminus).

CCK_AR by hybridization screening of a gallbladder cDNA library. Guinea pig pancreas CCK_AR cDNA was cloned via the polymerase chain reaction (PCR) using primers from the guinea pig gallbladder CCK_AR 5' and 3' noncoding regions. CCK_AR clones from guinea pig gallbladder and pancreas had identical nucleotide sequences.[55] The deduced amino acid sequences are 89% homologous to those of the rat CCK_A receptor (FIG. 3). Radioligand binding dose inhibition studies of transiently expressed receptors in COS-7 cells exhibited a CCK_AR pharmacologically similar to the native[49] and cloned rat CCK_AR[37,55] (FIG. 3). These studies indicate that the CCK_ARs in guinea pig gallbladder and pancreas are identical and do not support

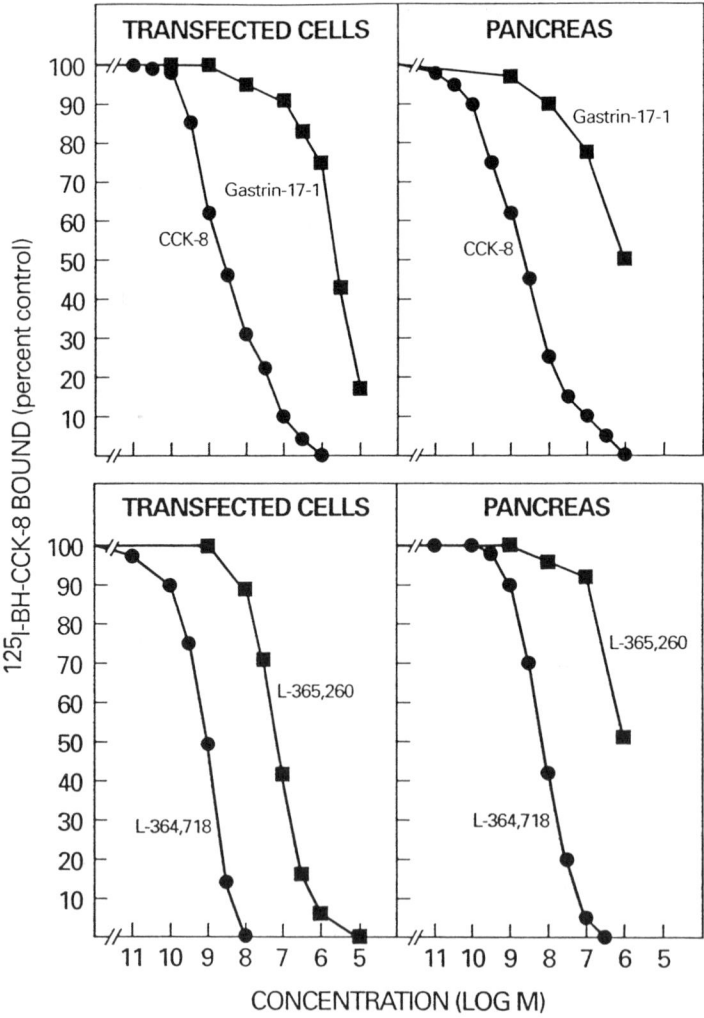

FIGURE 2. Comparison of the ability of CCK receptor agonists and antagonists to inhibit binding of [^{125}I]BH-CCK-8 to COS-7 cells expressing the recombinant rat CCK_A receptor and pancreatic acini expressing native CCK receptors. COS-7 cells were transfected with the mammalian expression vector pCDL-SRα containing the human CCK_A receptor cDNA. Transfected COS-7 cells or pancreatic acini were incubated with either the tracer alone or increasing concentrations of agonists CCK-8 or gastrin-17-I (*top panel*) or antagonists L-365,260 and L-364,718 (*bottom panel*). Data are presented as percent saturable binding (total binding in the presence of labeled hormone alone minus binding in the presence of 1 μM CCK-8).

TABLE 1. Comparison of the Affinities of CCK-8 and L-364,718 for CCK_A Receptors on Transfected COS-7 Cells and Pancreatic Acini[a]

	Affinity (nM)	
Ligand	Transfected COS-7 Cells	Pancreatic Acini
CCK-8		
K_d High	0.70 ± 0.1	0.46 ± 0.2
K_d Low	53 ± 7	47 ± 13
L-364,718		
K_d High	0.8 ± 0.8	3.0 ± 0.8
K_d Low	0.7 ± 0.7	4.0 ± 1.2

[a]Data in Figure 1 were analyzed using the nonlinear least-squares, curve-fitting program, LIGAND.[50] Values given are means ± SD.

previous studies, suggesting that gallbladder and pancreas possess different $CCK_A R$ subtypes.[55]

STRUCTURE AND FUNCTIONAL EXPRESSION OF HUMAN CCK_A RECEPTORS

Little is known about the structure, pharmacology, and cell biology of human $CCK_A Rs$ because of the difficulty in obtaining either fresh human tissue or long-term cultures in nontransformed cells expressing the $CCK_A R$. Human gallbladders in patients undergoing cholecystectomy possess a single CCK_A binding site that is functionally and biochemically intact in diseased specimens.[53] Therefore, we elected to PCR clone the human $CCK_A R$ cDNA from a surgical gallbladder specimen using 5' and 3' noncoding sequences obtained from screening a human genomic library with the recently cloned rat $CCK_A R$ cDNA.[36] The cloned receptor encodes a unique 428 amino acid protein having >90% homology to the rat and guinea pig $CCK_A R$ (FIG. 3).[55] To demonstrate, for the first time, the precise pharmacology of a pure human $CCK_A R$, the cloned $CCK_A R$ was expressed in COS-7 cells, and ligand binding dose-inhibition studies were performed[55] (FIG. 4). [^{125}I]-BH-CCK-8 binding inhibition by CCK-8 ($IC_{50} = 3 \times 10^{-9}$ nM) was 600-fold more potent than gastrin-17-I ($IC_{50} = 1.8 \times 10^{-6}$ nM), and inhibition by the CCK_A receptor antagonist L-364,718 ($IC_{50} = 0.8 \times 10^{-9}$ nM) was 25-fold more potent than the $CCK_B R$-specific antagonist L-365,260 ($IC_{50} = 2 \times 10^{-8}$ nM) (FIG. 4). These findings are characteristic of a $CCK_A R$ subtype pharmacology and are similar to that reported previously for $CCK_A R$ on CHP 212 human neuroblastoma cells[11] as well as for native[2] and transfected[37] rat and guinea pig[49,55] $CCK_A Rs$.

To demonstrate that the human $CCK_A R$ cDNA encodes a functional CCK_A receptor capable of activating phospholipase C, we measured the increase of phosphoinositides stimulated by CCK-8 in COS-7 cells expressing the transfected receptor. CCK-8 caused a 6.8-fold dose-dependent increase in total inositol phosphates with a detectable increase at 0.1 nM, a half-maximal increase at 3.0 nM and a maximal increase at 100 nM (FIG. 5). This response was nearly completely inhibited by the $CCK_A R$-specific antagonist L-364,718 at 0.1 μM (FIG. 5). These results are in close agreement with previous studies of $CCK_A Rs$ on the human neuroblastoma cell line CHP212.[11]

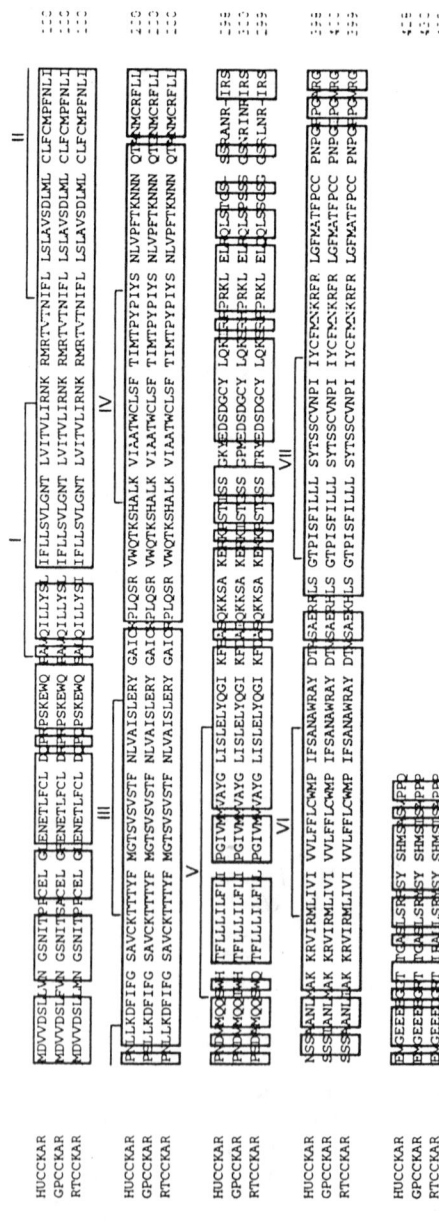

FIGURE 3. Alignment of the human CCK$_A$ receptor (HUCCKAR), guinea pig CCK$_A$ receptor (GPCCKAR), and rat CCK$_A$ receptor (RATCCKAR) deduced protein sequences. Using the "Pileup" program sequence analysis package of the Genetics Computer Group,[56] the human CCK$_A$ receptor[53] was aligned for maximal homology with the rat[36] and guinea pig CCK$_A$[55] receptors. Shown here using amino acid letter symbols is the result of this alignment with *solid lines* indicating putative transmembrane domains and *boxed letters* indicating amino acids from guinea pig and rat not conserved in the human receptor sequence.

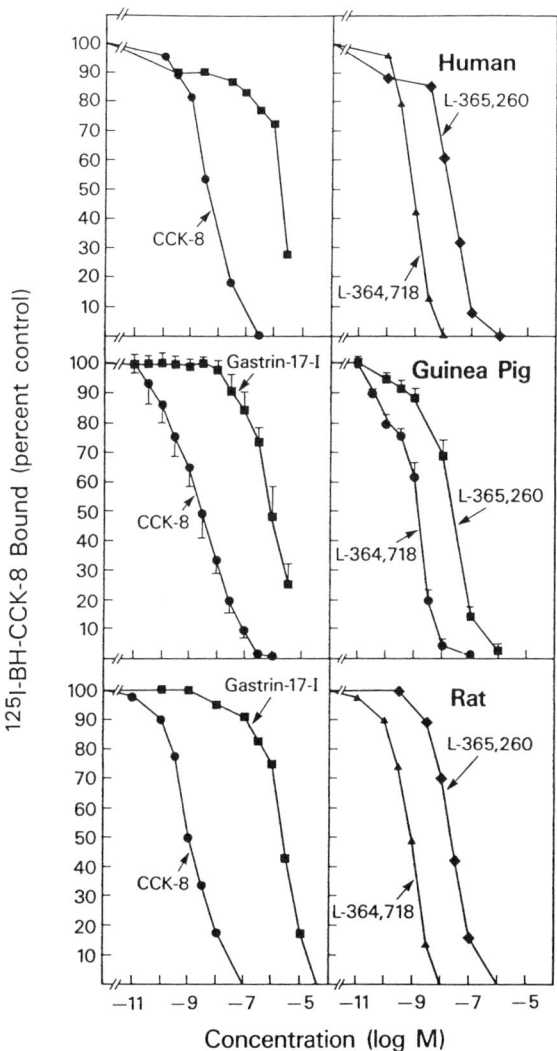

FIGURE 4. Ability of CCK receptor agonists and antagonists to inhibit binding of ^{125}I-BH-CCK-8 to COS-7 cells expressing either the human, guinea pig, or rat CCK_A receptors. COS-7 cells were transfected with the expression vector pCDL-SRα[48] containing either human (*top panel*), guinea pig (*middle panel*), or rat (*bottom panel*) CCK_A receptor DNA sequences. [^{125}I]-BH-CCK8 (50 pM) was incubated either alone or with increasing concentrations of agonists (CCK-8 and gastrin-17-I) (*left panel*) or antagonists (L-364,718 and L-365,260) (*right panel*). Data are presented as percent saturable binding (total binding in the presence of radiolabeled hormone alone minus binding in the presence of 1 μM CCK-8). Each experiment was performed in duplicate, and the results given are the means from at least two separate experiments.

GALLBLADDER EXPRESSES TYPICAL CCK$_B$ RECEPTORS

Although in vivo[57] and gallbladder muscle strip[58] studies suggest that CCK$_A$Rs mediate gallbladder contraction, studies of isolated smooth muscle cells suggest that two types of receptors mediate contraction.[29] One type is consistent with a CCK$_A$R interacting preferentially with CCK-8 and L-364,718. The other type is a novel receptor interacting preferentially with gastrin unlike the CCK$_B$R which interacts nearly equally with CCK-8 and gastrin.[29] However, like the CCK$_B$R, this novel receptor interacts preferentially with L-365,260.[29] To determine if the novel gastrin-preferring receptor on gallbladder smooth muscle cells is a new member of the CCK

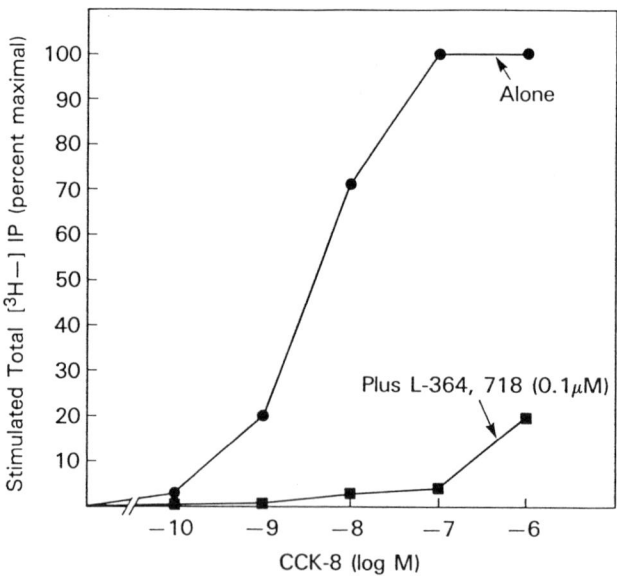

FIGURE 5. Ability of CCK-8 alone or CCK-8 plus L-364,718 to stimulate total [^{3}H]inositol phosphate generation in COS-7 cells transfected with the human CCK$_A$ receptor. Data are expressed as the percentage of maximal increase obtained using 1 uM CCK-8. CCK-8 (1 uM) increased [^{3}H]inositol phosphates from a basal level of 4,235 ± 808 dpm to 28,676 ± 1,495 dpm (mean ± SEM).

receptor family, we used the CCK$_A$R cDNA from guinea pig gallbladder[55] to screen a guinea pig gallbladder cDNA library under high and low stringency conditions.[28] The clones, identified only under low stringency conditions, had a 90% identity with rat CCK$_B$R (FIG. 6).[28] This degree of sequence homology is in the range expected for a species-dependent variation of the same receptor and suggests that the newly cloned gallbladder cDNA encodes a CCK$_B$R subtype. To determine the subtype pharmacology of the cloned receptor, dose-inhibition binding studies of transiently expressed receptors in COS-7 cells were performed. The recombinant guinea pig gallbladder receptor had an approximately threefold greater affinity for CCK-8 than gastrin-17-1 and a 100-fold greater affinity for the CCK$_B$R-specific antagonist L-365,260, than for

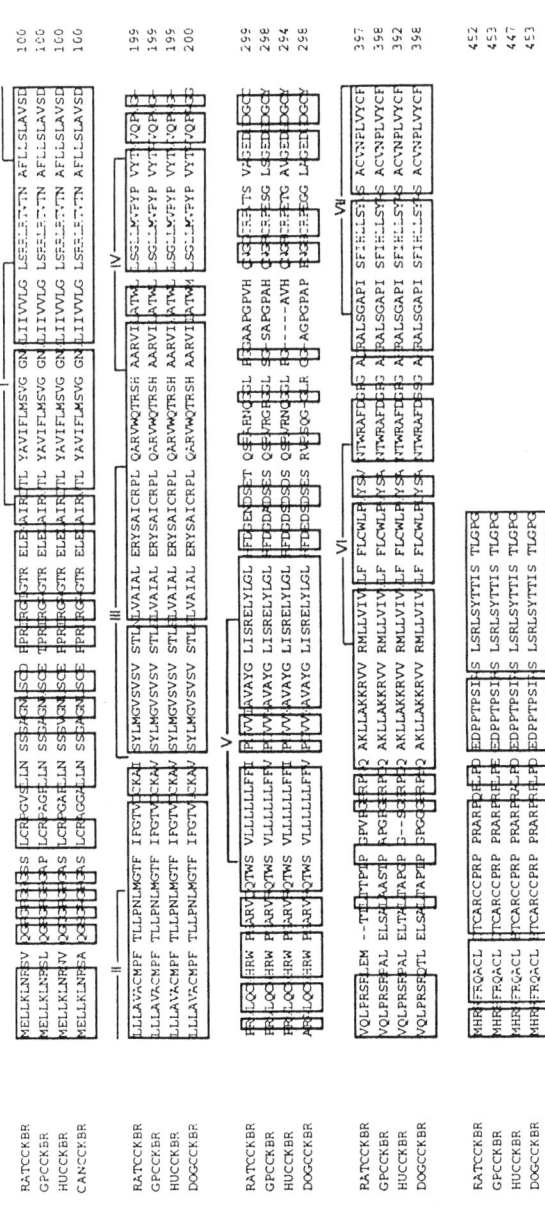

FIGURE 6. Alignment of the rat CCK$_B$ receptor (RATCCKBR), guinea pig CCK$_B$ receptor (GPCCKBR), human CCK$_B$ receptor (HUCCKBR), and canine CCK$_B$ receptor (CANCCKBR) deduced protein sequences. Using the "Pileup" program sequence analysis package of the Genetics Computer Group,[56] the rat,[36] guinea pig,[28] human CCK$_B$,[60] and canine[61] CCK$_B$ receptors were aligned for maximal homology. Shown here using amino acid letter symbols is the result of this alignment with *solid lines* indicating putative transmembrane domains and *boxed letters* indicating amino acids from guinea pig and rat not conserved in the human receptor sequence.

the CCK_AR-specific antagonist L-364,718 (FIG. 7).[28] These results are in close agreement with the pharmacological profile of the native[49] and recombinant rat CCK_BR (FIG. 7) and further support that the cDNA clone from guinea pig gallbladder is a typical CCK_BR subtype.

STRUCTURE AND FUNCTIONAL EXPRESSION OF HUMAN CCK_B RECEPTORS

Similar to the human CCK_AR, little is known about the human CCK_BR structure, pharmacology, and cell biology. Therefore, we used the rat CCK_BR cDNA to isolate a clone from a human brain cDNA library by hybridization screening.[60] This clone lacked the 5' terminal 82 nucleotides necessary to complete the coding sequence. These last nucleotides were obtained from human stomach cDNA by the polymerization chain reaction using a degenerate 5' noncoding sequence primer derived from rat and guinea pig.[60] The nucleotide sequence obtained from stomach and brain were identical and encoded a 447 amino acid protein that was 90% and 91% identical to the rat and guinea pig CCK_BRs, respectively (FIG. 6). To confirm that the CCK_BR clones isolated from both human brain and stomach encode a functional CCK_BR and to demonstrate for the first time the precise pharmacology of a pure human CCK_BR, radioligand-binding dose-inhibition studies were performed. [^{125}I]-BH-CCK-8 binding inhibition by CCK-8 ($EC_{50} = 3 \times 10^{-9}$ nM) was twofold more potent than gastrin-17-I ($EC_{50} = 6.4 \times 10^{-9}$ nM) and inhibition by the CCK_BR antagonist L-365,260 ($EC_{50} = 1 \times 10^{-8}$ nM) was 50-fold more potent than that of the CCK_AR-specific antagonist L-364,718 ($EC_{50} = 5 \times 10^{-7}$ nM) (FIG. 7).[59] These findings are similar to those reported previously for native[49] and recombinant rat CCK_BRs[37] (FIG. 7) and native CCK_ARs in the transformed human T-lymphocyte, JURKAT cells,[22] and in a human small cell carcinoma cell line.[30]

To demonstrate that the human CCK_BR cDNA encodes a functional CCK_BR capable of activating phospholipase C, we measured the increase of phosphoinositides stimulated by CCK-8 in COS-7 cells expressing the transfected receptor. CCK-8 caused a 4.6-fold[60] dose-dependent increase in total inositol phosphates with a detectable increase at 0.1 nM, a half-maximal increase at 3.0 nM, and a maximal increase at 100 nM (FIG. 8). This response was nearly completely inhibited by the CCK_BR-specific antagonist L-365,260 at 0.1 μM (FIG. 8). These results are in close agreement with previous studies of CCK_BRs on guinea pig chief cells[7] and rabbit[62] and canine parietal cells.[63]

NORTHERN AND SOUTHERN BLOT HYBRIDIZATIONS IDENTIFY ONLY TWO MEMBERS OF THE CCK RECEPTOR FAMILY: CCK_A AND CCK_B RECEPTORS

The heterogeneity in the reported pharmacology and biochemical cross-linking data detailed earlier in this chapter and the examples set by other receptor families (e.g., receptors for dopamine, serotonin, somatostatin as well as numerous other hormone receptors) would suggest that there may be other members of the CCK receptor family. Hybridization screening of cDNA libraries from human brain and gallbladder, guinea pig gallbladder, stomach, a 90% pure chief cell preparation and rat brain, pancreas and AR4-2J cells, and a genomic library from human placenta identified only CCK_A and CCK_B receptors. To discover potential new members of

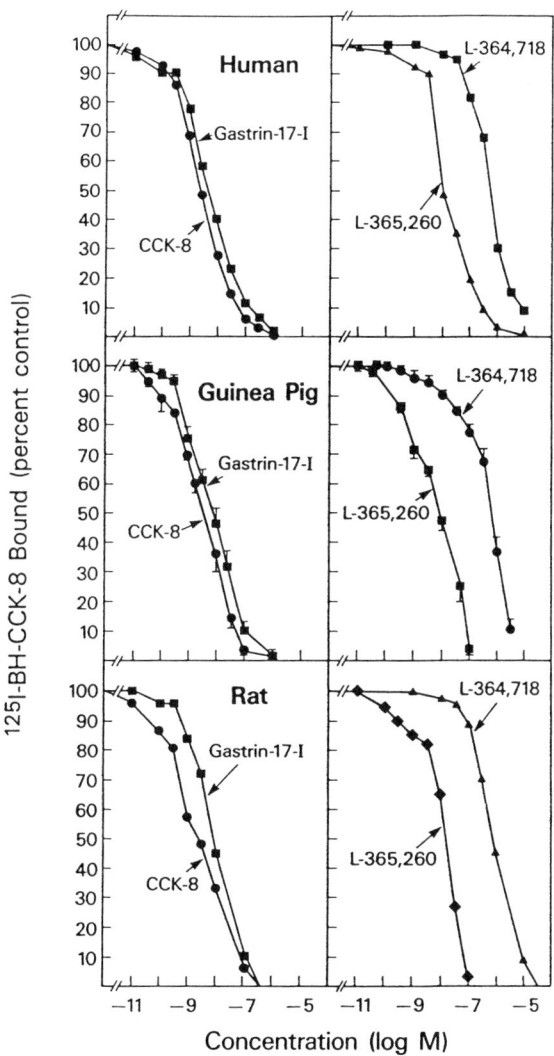

FIGURE 7. Ability of CCK receptor agonists and antagonists to inhibit binding of ^{125}I-BH-CCK-8 to COS-7 cells expressing either human, guinea pig, or rat CCK$_B$ receptors. COS-7 cells were transfected with the expression vector pCDL-SRα[48] containing either the human (*top panel*), guinea pig (*middle panel*), or rat (*bottom panel*) CCK$_B$ receptor cDNA sequences. ^{125}[I]-BH-CCK8 (50 pM) was incubated either alone or with increasing concentrations of agonists (CCK-8 and gastrin-17-I) (*left panel*) or antagonists (L-364,718 and L-365,260) (*right panel*). Data are presented as percent saturable binding (total binding in the presence of radiolabeled hormone alone minus binding in the presence of 1 μM CCK-8). Each experiment was performed in duplicate, and the results given are the means from at least two separate experiments.

the CCK receptor family in addition to the CCK_A and CCK_B receptors, we performed Northern and Southern blot hybridization for human, guinea pig, and rat tissues using species-specific radiolabeled full-length coding sequence cDNA probes for both the CCK_AR and CCK_BR on the respective blots from each species. Northern blot hybridization was performed under both high and low stringency conditions using 2 μg of poly (A)+ mRNA from each tissue. The same blot for each species was hybridized with either the CCK_AR or the CCK_BR species-specific probe.[28,36,37,55,59,60] Northern hybridization resulted in species-specific heterogeneity in transcript size and distribution in some tissues for both the CCK_AR (human, 6 kb in gallbladder; guinea pig, 4.4 kb in 60% pure parietal cell preparation, 90% pure chief cell

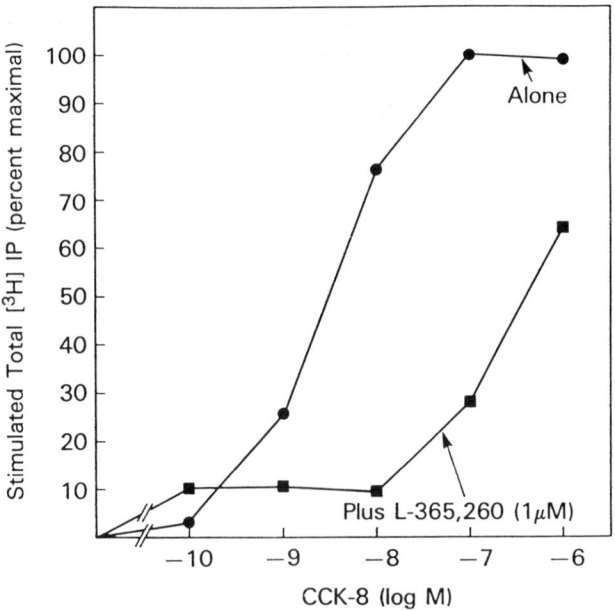

FIGURE 8. Ability of CCK-8 alone or CCK-8 plus L-365,260 to stimulate total [^{3}H]inositol phosphate generation in COS-7 cells transfected with the human CCK_B receptor. Data are expressed as the percentage of maximal increase obtained using 1 μM CCK-8. CCK-8 (1 μM) increased [^{3}H]inositol phosphates from a basal level of 4,896 ± 496 dpm to 22,289 ± 615 dpm (mean ± SEM).

preparation, gastric glands, brain, and pancreas; rat, 2.7 kb in pancreas and AR4-2J cell; FIG. 6) and the CCK_BR (human, variably spliced 2.8 and 3.3 kb transcripts in brain, stomach, pancreas, liver, lung, and gallbladder; guinea pig, variably spliced 2.2 and 2.4 kb transcripts in a 60% pure parietal cell preparation, 90% pure chief cell preparation, gastric glands, and brain; rat, 2.7 kb in brain cortex and pancreas; FIG. 9). No new hybridizing transcripts suggestive of potential new members of the CCK receptor family were found even under low stringency hybridizing conditions (data not shown).

Southern blot hybridization was performed using 10 μg of restriction enzyme digested genomic DNA from each species that was hybridized with either CCK_AR or

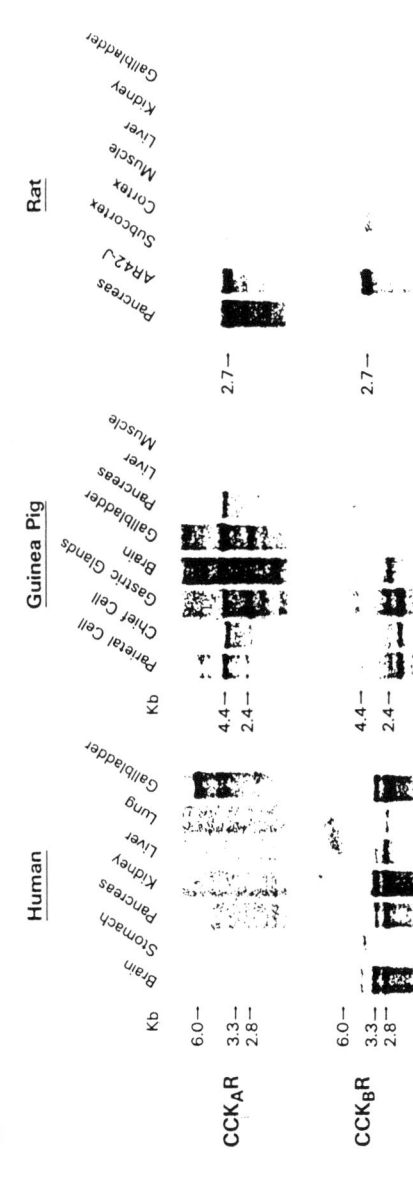

FIGURE 9. Northern blot analysis of poly (A)+ RNA from human, guinea pig, and rat tissues. Two micrograms of poly (A)⁺, RNA from each of the tissues indicated were separated on a 1.5% denaturing/formaldehyde agarose gel, probed with the full coding region of the species-specific CCK$_A$ (*upper panel*) or CCK$_B$ (*lower panel*) [^{32}P] random prime labeled receptor cDNA. The blot was then washed under high stringency conditions (3 × 20' washes with 0.1 × SSC/0.1% SDS @ 42°C), exposed for 48 hours, and scanned with a phosphorimager (Molecular Dynamics). The size and migration of standard RNA are indicated on the left in kb.

CCK$_A$ RECEPTOR

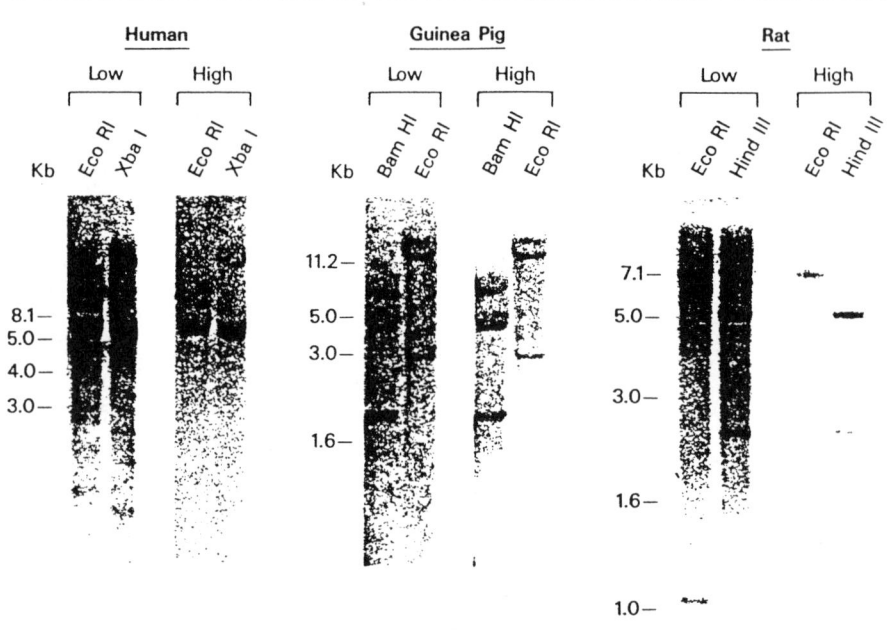

CCK$_B$ RECEPTOR

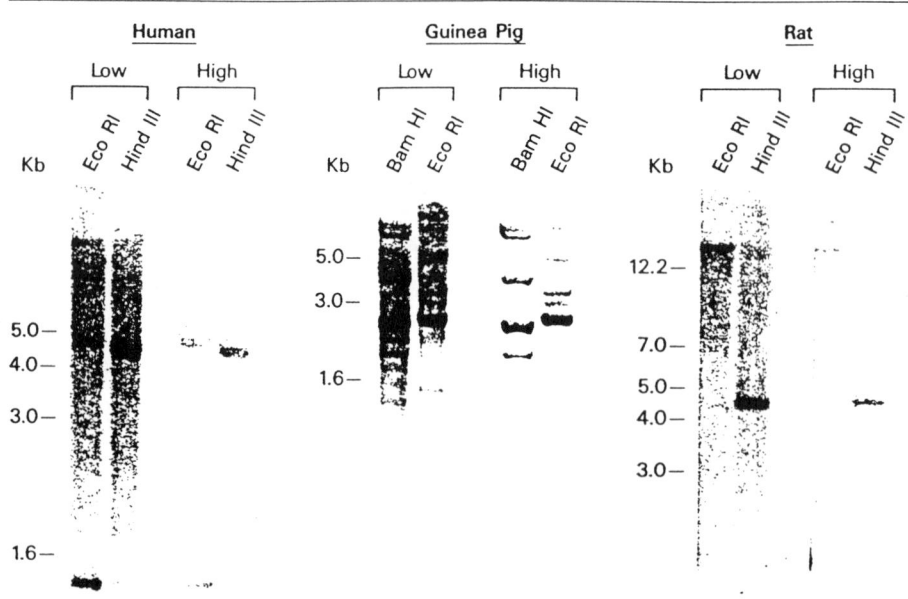

FIGURE 10. See legend on facing page.

CCK_BR species-specific probes under both high and low stringency conditions (ref. 59 and unpublished data; FIG. 10). No hybridizing restriction fragments were identified under low stringency conditions that did not also remain under high stringency conditions and, therefore, no new members of the CCK receptor family could be identified. The presence of multiple hybridizing restriction fragments under both high and low stringency conditions seen with guinea pig DNA probably represents fragments of the same receptor cut within the multiple introns known to exist in these receptors (ref. 64 and unpublished data).

GASTRIN RECEPTORS ARE CCK_B RECEPTORS ON PARIETAL CELLS

The affinity of rat, guinea pig, and human CCK_BRs for antagonists L-364,718 and L365,260 (FIG. 7) differ significantly from the canine gastrin receptor.[19] The canine parietal cell gastrin receptor has almost a sevenfold greater affinity for the CCK_A receptor antagonist L-364,718 than for the gastrin receptor antagonist L-365,260.[61] This divergence in canine gastrin receptor reversal in affinity for antagonists L-364,718 and L-365,260 is due to a single nucleotide change leading to a single amino acid change (human nucleotide #349, V to L, FIG. 6) in the sixth transmembrane domain.[62] Similar to the human brain and stomach CCK_BR,[60] PCR cloning of the CCK_BR from canine brain (unpublished data) results in the identical cDNA nucleotide sequence reported for the canine parietal gastrin receptor.[61] Furthermore, the identification of only a single CCK_BR by low and high stringency cDNA library, Northern and Southern blot hybridization suggests that gastrin receptors are simply CCK_BRs on parietal cells and do not represent a third type of CCK receptor.

SUMMARY

A review of the literature encompassing numerous pharmacological, physiological, and biochemical studies indicates the presence of at least four CCK receptor types, CCK_A, CCK_B, gastrin, and CG-4 receptors. Multiple subtypes of the CCK_AR have been postulated to account for the differences in pharmacology or affinity cross-linking of CCK_ARs between pancreas and gallbladder and the presence of high and low affinity CCK_ARs on pancreatic acini. Multiple subtypes of the CCK_BR have been postulated to explain the differences in pharmacology and physiology between gastric and gallbladder smooth muscle CCK_BRs. We recently cloned and functionally expressed both the CCK_AR and the CCK_BR from rat, guinea pig, and human. The CCK_AR and CCK_BR are 48% homologous and constitute a family of receptors within the guanine nucleotide-binding regulatory protein-coupled superfamily of receptors. Each receptor is highly conserved between species. A single cDNA encoding a single

←

FIGURE 10. Southern blot analysis. Ten micrograms of human, guinea pig, and rat genomic DNA was digested with the indicated restriction endonucleases, blotted onto Nytran, and the same blot hybridized with either the [^{32}P] random prime labeled, species-specific CCK_A (*upper panel*) or CCK_B (*lower panel*) receptor, full coding region, cDNA probe. The blot was exposed for 48 hours and processed using a phosphorimager (Molecular Dynamics) following each of the low ($3 \times 20'$ washes with $2.0 \times SSC/0.1\%$ SDS @ 37°C) and high ($3 \times 20'$ washes with $0.1 \times SSC/0.1\%$ SDS @ 42°C) stringency washes. The size and migration of standard DNA are indicated on the left in kb.

protein is present in both pancreas and gallbladder and can account for both high and low affinity CCK_ARs found on pancreatic acini when transfected into COS-7 cells. A single cDNA encoding a single CCK_BR protein is present in both the central nervous system and the periphery including the gastrointestinal system. Therefore, the gastrin receptor is actually a CCK_BR present on parietal cells. Genomic and cDNA library hybridization as well as Northern and Southern hybridization studies among rat, guinea pig, and human species identifies only two members of the CCK receptor family, CCK_AR and CCK_BR. Although these studies do not identify other closely related members of the CCK receptor family, they do not rule out the existence of other less closely related members. Furthermore, differences in tissue and species-specific posttranslational processing, receptor coupling, and associated membrane protein and lipid heterogeneity may be among some of the other factors that may account for the phenotypic expression of more receptor subtypes than molecular studies would predict.

REFERENCES

1. HILL, D. R., N. J. CAMPBELL, T. M. SHAW & G. N. WOODRUFF. 1987. J. Neurosci. **7:** 2967–2976.
2. JENSEN, R. T., S. A. WANK, W. H. ROWLEY, S. SATO & J. D. GARDNER. 1989. Trends Pharmacol. Sci. **10:** 418–423.
3. MENOZZI, D., J. D. GARDNER & P. N. MATON. 1989. Am. J. Physiol. **257:** G73–G79.
4. CHANG, R. S. L. & V. J. LOTTI. 1986. Proc. Natl. Acad. Sci. USA **83:** 4923–4926.
5. SANKARAN, H., I. D. GOLDFINE, C. W. DEVENEY, K.-Y. WONG & J. A. WILLIAMS. 1980. J. Biol. Chem. **255:** 1849–1853.
6. BITAR, K. N. & G. M. MAKHOULF. 1982. Am. J. Physiol. **242:** G400–407.
7. QIAN, J.-M., W. H. ROWLEY & R. T. JENSEN. 1993. Am. J. Physiol. **264:** G718–G728.
8. SOLL, A. H., D. A. AMIRIAN, K. P. THOMAS, J. PARK, J. D. ELASHOFF, M. A. BEAVEN & T. YAMADA. 1984. Am. J. Physiol. **247:** G714–G723.
9. MORAN, T. H., P. H. ROBINSON, M. S. GOLDRICH & P. R. MCHUGH. 1975. Brain Res. **362:** 986–989.
10. LOGSDON, C. D. 1986. J. Biol. Chem. **261:** 2096–2101.
11. KLUEPPELBERG, U. G., X. MOLERO, R. W. BARRETT & L. J. MILLER. 1990. Mol. Pharmacol. **38:** 159–163.
12. JENSEN, R. T., Z.-H. ZHOU, R. B. MURPHY, S. W. JONES, I. SETNIKAR, L. A. ROVATI & J. D. GARDNER. 1986. Am. J. Physiol. **251:** G839–G846.
13. MACOVEC, F., R. CHRISTE, M. BANI, L. REVEL, I. SETNICAR & A. L. ROVATI. 1986. Eur. J. Med. Chem. **21:** 9–20.
14. MACOVEC, F., R. CHRISTIE, M. BANI, M. PACINI, I. SETNIKAR & L. A. ROVATI. 1985. Arzneim-Forsch. **36:** 1048–1051.
15. YANAIHARA, C., N. SIGURA, K. KASHIMOTO, M. KONDO, M. KAWAMURA, S. NARUSE, A. YASUI & N. YANAIHARA. 1985. Biomed. Res. **6:** 111–115.
16. SANKARAN, H., I. D. GOLDFINE, A. BAILEY, V. LICKO & J. A. WILLIAMS. 1982. Am. J. Physiol. **242:** G250–G257.
17. MENOZZI, D., R. VINAYEK, R. T. JENSEN & J. D. GARDNER. 1991. J. Biol. Chem. **266:** 10385–10391.
18. WANK, S. A., R. T. JENSEN & J. D. GARDNER. 1988. Am. J. Physiol. **255:** G106–G112.
19. LOTTI, V. J. & R. S. L. CHANG. 1989. Eur. J. Pharmacol. **162:** 273–280.
20. INNIS, R. B. & S. H. SNYDER. 1980. Proc. Natl. Acad. Sci. USA **77:** 6917–6921.
21. SAITO, A., H. SANKARAN, I. D. GOLDFINE & J. A. WILLIAMS. 1980. Science **208:** 1155–1156.
22. LIGNON, M., N. BERNAD & J. MARTINEZ. 1991. Mol. Pharmacol. **39:** 615–620.
23. SACERDOTE, P., C. J. WIEDERMANN, L. M. WAHL, C. B. PERT & M. R. RUFF. 1991. Peptides **12:** 167–176.
24. LAMBERT, M., N. D. BUI & J. CHRISTOPHE. 1991. Reg. Peptides **322:** 151–167.
25. PEARSON, R. K., E. M. HADAC & L. J. MILLER. 1989. Am. J. Physiol. **256:** 1005–1010.

26. SOLL, A. H., D. A. AMIRIAN, K. P. THOMAS, L. P. REEDY & J. D. ELASHOFF. 1984. J. Clin. Invest. **73:** 1434–1447.
27. TIELEMANS, Y., J. AXELSON, F. SUNDLER, G. WILLEMS & R. HAKANSON. 1990. Gut **31:** 274–278.
28. DEWEERTH, A., J. R. PISEGNA & S. A. WANK. 1993. Gastroenterology **104:** A497.
29. GRIDER, J. R. & G. M. MAKHLOUF. 1990. Am. J. Physiol. **259:** G184–G190.
30. YODER, D. B. & T. W. MOODY. 1987. Peptides **8:** 151–167.
31. SINGH, P., B. RAE-VENTER, C. M. TOWNSEND, T. KHALIL & J. C. THOMPSON. 1985. Am. J. Physiol. **249:** G761–G769.
32. YU, D.-H., M. NOGUCHI, Z. C. ZHOU, M. L. VILLANUEVA, J. D. GARDNER & R. T. JENSEN. 1987. Am. J. Physiol. **253:** G793–G801.
33. FOURMY, D., A. ZAHEDI, R. FABRE, M. GUIDET, L. PRADAYROL & A. RIBET. 1987. Eur. J. Biochem. **165:** 683–692.
34. LE MEUTH, V., V. PHILOUZE, M. FORMAL, I. LE HUEROU-LURON, N. VAYSSE, C. GESPACH, N. GUILLOTEAU & D. FOURMY. 1992. Regul. Peptides. **40:** 209.
35. REHFIELD, J. F., L.-I. LARSSON, N. R. GOTTERMANN, T. W. SCHWARTZ, J. J. HOLST, S. L. JENSEN & J. S. MORLEY. 1980. Nature **284:** 33–38.
36. WANK, S. A., R. HARKINS, R. T. JENSEN, H. SHAPIRA, A. DE WEERTH & T. SLATTERY. 1992. Proc. Natl. Acad. Sci. USA **89:** 3125–3129.
37. WANK, S. A., J. R. PISEGNA, P. & A. DEWEERTH. 1992. Proc. Natl. Acad. Sci. USA **89:** 8691–8695.
38. DOHLMAN, H. G., M. G. CARON & R. J. LEFKOWITZ. 1987. Biochemistry **26:** 2657–2663.
39. MERRIT, J. E., C. W. TAYLOR, R. P. RUBIN & J. W. PUTNEY. 1986. Biochem. J. **236:** 337–343.
40. PEARSON, R. K., L. J. MILLER, E. M. HADAC & S. P. POWERS. 1987. J. Biol. Chem. **262:** 13850–13856.
41. GRAFF, J. M., D. J. STUMPO & P. J. BLACKSHEAR. 1989. J. Biol. Chem. **264:** 11912–11919.
42. KLUEPPELBERG, U. G., L. K. GATES, F. S. GORELICH & L. J. MILLER. 1991. J. Biol. Chem. **266:** 2403–2408.
43. KARNIK, S. S., J. P. SAKMANN, H. A. CHEN & G. KHORANA. 1988. Proc. Natl. Acad. Sci. USA **85:** 8459–8463.
44. DIXON, R. A., I. S. SIGAL, M. R. CANDELORE, R. B. REGISTER, E. RANDS & C. D. STRADER. 1987. EMBO. J. **6:** 3269–3275.
45. HULME, E. C., N. J. BIRDSALL & N. J. BUCKLEY. 1990. Ann. Rev. Pharmacol. Toxicol. **30:** 633–673.
46. O'DOWD, B., M. HNATOWICH, M. B. CARON, R. J. LEFKOWITZ & M. BOUVIER. 1989. J. Biol. Chem. **264:** 7564–7569.
47. OVCHINIKOV, Y. A., N. G. ABDULAEV & A. S. BOGACHUK. 1988. FEBS Lett. **230:** 1–5.
48. TAKEBE, Y., M. SEIKI, J.-I. FUJISAWA, P. HOY, K. YOKOTA, K.-I. ARAI, M. YOSHIDA & N. ARAI. 1988. Mol. & Cell. Biol. **8:** 466–472.
49. JENSEN, R. T., S. C. HUANG, T. VON SCHRENCK, S. A. WANK & J. D. GARDNER. 1990. In GI Endocrinology: Receptors and Post-Receptor Mechanisms. J. T. Thompson, C. M. Townsend, G. A. Greely, Jr., P. L. Rayford, Jr., C. W. Cooper, P. O. Singh & N. Rubin, eds.: 95–113. Academic Press, Inc. New York, NY.
50. MUNSON, P. J. & D. RODBARD. 1980. Anal. Biochem. **107:** 220–229.
51. WANK, S. A. 1992. Gastroenterology **102:** A297.
52. PEARSON, R. K., L. J. MILLER, E. M. HADAC & S. P. POWERS. 1987. J. Biol. Chem. **262:** 13850–13856.
53. SCHJOLDAGER, B., X. MOLERO & L. J. MILLER. 1989. Gastroenterology **96:** 1119–1125.
54. SCHJOLDAGER, B., M. J. SHAW, S. P. POWERS, P. H. SCHMALZ, J. SZURSZEWSKI & L. J. MILLER. 1988. Am. J. Physiol. **254:** G294–G299.
55. DEWEERTH, A., J. R. PISEGNA & S. A. WANK. 1993. Am. J. Physiol. **265:** G1116–G1121.
56. DEVEREAUX, J., P. HAEBRLI & O. SMITHIES. 1984. Nucleic Acids Res. **12:** 387–395.
57. LIDDLE, R. A., B. J. GERTZ, S. KANAYAMA, L. BECCARIA, L. D. COKER, T. A. TURNBULL & E. T. MORITA. 1989. J. Clin. Invest. **84:** 1220–1225.
58. GRIDER, J. R. & G. M. MAKHLOUF. 1990. Gastroenterology **92:** 175–189.

59. DEWEERTH, A., J. R. PISEGNA & S. A. WANK. 1993. Biochem. Biophys. Res. Commun. **194:** 811–818.
60. PISEGNA, J. R., A. DEWEERTH, K. HUPPI & S. A. WANK. 1992. Biochem. Biophys. Res. Comm. **189:** 296–303.
61. KOPIN, A. S., Y.-M. LEE, E. W. MCBRIDE, L. J. MILLER, M. LU, H. Y. LIN, L. F. KOLAKOWSKI & M. BEINBORN. 1992. Proc. Natl. Acad. Sci. USA **89:** 3605–3609.
62. BEINBORN, M., Y.-M. LEE, E. MCBRIDE, S. M. QUINN & A. S. KOPIN. 1993. Nature **362:** 348–350.
63. ROCHE, S., J.-P. BALI, J.-C. GALLEYRAND & R. MAGOUS. 1991. Am. J. Physiol. **260:** G182–G188.
64. CHIBA, T., S. K. FISHER, J. PARK, E. B. SEGUIN, B. W. AGRANOFF & T. YAMADA. 1988. Am. J. Physiol. **255:** GG99–G105.
65. SONG, I., D. R. BROWN, R. N. WILTSHIRE, J. M. TRENT & T. YAMADA. 1993. Gastroenterology **104:** A856.

The CCK-B/Gastrin Receptor

Identification of Amino Acids That Determine Nonpeptide Antagonist Affinity[a]

A. S. KOPIN,[b] M. BEINBORN, Y.-M. LEE, E. W. McBRIDE, AND S. M. QUINN

*Division of Gastroenterology and
GRASP Digestive Disease Center
New England Medical Center
Tufts University School of Medicine
Boston, Massachusetts 02111*

Gastrin and cholecystokinin (CCK) share an identical carboxy-terminal pentapeptide amide, a domain critical for receptor binding. Based on the binding of agonists as well as antagonists, receptors within the gastrin/CCK family have traditionally been divided into two major subtypes: CCK-A and CCK-B/gastrin.[1]

The CCK-A receptor is found in pancreas, gallbladder, and isolated brain nuclei. CCK-B/gastrin receptors are present on smooth muscle cells and parietal cells ("gastrin" receptors) and are the predominant brain CCK receptor ("CCK-B"). Although CCK-A and CCK-B/gastrin receptors can easily be distinguished on the basis of both agonist and antagonist binding, small differences in agonist binding have created controversy regarding the existence of distinct "CCK-B" and "gastrin" receptor subtypes. Our data suggest that the CCK-B and gastrin receptors represent a single subtype[2] and that species differences underlie part of the heterogeneity in ligand binding reported within the CCK-B/gastrin receptor subclass.[3]

As a first step towards understanding receptor function at a molecular level, we used a COS-7 cell expression cloning system to isolate a cDNA encoding the parietal cell gastrin receptor (FIG. 1). The first requirement in this cloning strategy was to isolate mRNA from cells with abundant gastrin receptors. On the basis of A. H. Soll's earlier observations,[4] we used an enriched (95%) preparation of canine parietal cells as starting material. From these cells, size selected (>1.5 kb) mRNA was isolated and used to make a cDNA expression library in the vector pcDNA1 (Invitrogen).

Pools of library DNA, representing 3,000–10,000 primary recombinants, were transfected into COS-7 cells. Forty-eight hours after transfection, cells were incubated with ^{125}I CCK-8 as well as with ^{125}I D-Tyr-Gly-[(Nle^{28,31})-CCK-26-33], a CCK analog that includes a free amino group available for chemical cross-linking.[5] Inasmuch as COS-7 cells do not normally have gastrin or CCK receptors, only cells expressing the recombinant gastrin receptor bound the radioligand. Following the binding assay, excess radioligand was washed away, and the cells were fixed in glutaraldehyde. Slides were then dipped in photoemulsion, exposed in the dark for 72 hours, developed, and examined under the microscope.

After two million primary recombinants were screened, a pool expressing the

---

[a]This work was supported by National Institutes of Health Grants DK01934, DK46767, and the Digestive Disease Research Center P30-DK34928.
[b]To whom correspondence should be addressed.

Parietal cell mRNA
↓
Plasmid expression library: DNA Pools
↓
Transfect COS-7 cells
↓

125I CCK-8 Binding
Fixation

↓

Emulsion: 72 hrs
Develop

↓

Enrich positive pool

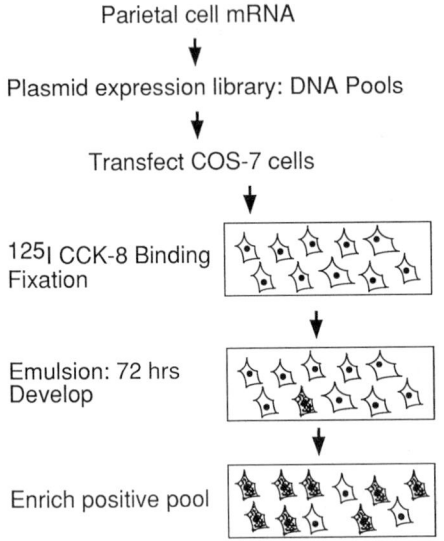

FIGURE 1. Strategy for cloning the parietal cell "gastrin" receptor. Construction of a canine parietal cell cDNA expression library and radioligand autoradiography screening for a COS-7 cell expressing the gastrin receptor (see text for details). Adapted from ref. 20.

gastrin receptor cDNA, GR-1, was identified. FIGURE 2 shows a phase contrast view of the first positive COS-7 cell expressing the gastrin receptor. The positive pool was subdivided and enriched until a single clone was isolated. This cDNA was sequenced on both strands.

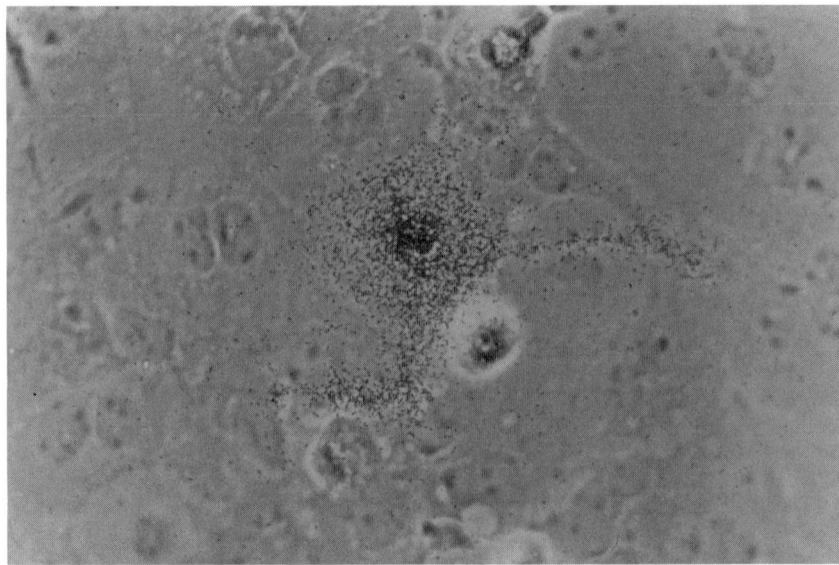

FIGURE 2. Phase contrast photomicrograph shows silver grains clustered over the first COS-7 cell expressing the recombinant gastrin receptor.

The canine CCK-B/gastrin receptor cDNA has an open reading frame encoding a 453 amino acid protein.[6] Hydropathy analysis suggests seven transmembrane domains characteristic of other G-protein coupled receptors. Examination of the deduced amino acid sequence reveals many features typical of the β-adrenergic receptor superfamily. There are two cysteine residues, one in the first extracellular loop and one in the second which may be involved in a disulfide bond similar to that found in rhodopsin.[7] The third cytoplasmic loop and the carboxy terminus are rich in threonine and serine residues which may serve as potential sites of phosphorylation analogous to those found in rhodopsin and in the β$_2$-adrenergic receptor.[8] The amino terminus of the cloned receptor includes three potential asparagine-linked glycosylation sites.

Pharmacologic characterization of the recombinant gastrin receptor expressed in COS-7 cells demonstrated agonist binding specificity typical of CCK-B/gastrin

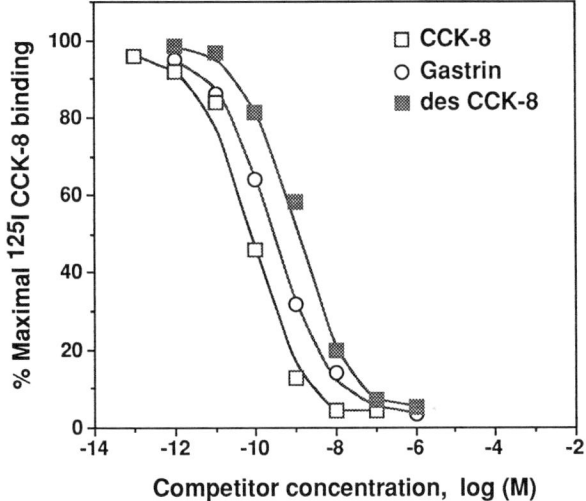

FIGURE 3. Agonist binding to the recombinant canine gastrin receptor expressed in COS-7 cells. The calculated IC$_{50}$ values (means from $n = 3$) for CCK-8, gastrin, and CCK-8-desulfate are 0.09, 0.26, and 1.4 nM, respectively.

receptors. FIGURE 3 shows agonist competition binding experiments using 40 pM ^{125}I CCK-8 as radioligand. The calculated IC$_{50}$s for CCK-8, gastrin, and CCK-8-desulfate were 0.09, 0.26, and 1.4 nM, respectively. The relatively high affinity of the recombinant protein for the latter two agonists confirmed that this receptor was a gastrin/CCK-B subtype rather than an A subtype.

In addition to binding different ligands with the correct specificity, a cloned receptor must signal through appropriate second messenger pathways. COS-7 cells were loaded with the calcium-sensitive dye Fura-2, and fluorescence emission ratios were used to monitor free cytosolic calcium. As shown in FIGURE 4, gastrin (10^{-6} M) triggered a marked increase in free cytosolic calcium, [Ca^{+2}]$_i$, only in cells expressing the recombinant receptor. In these cells, [Ca^{+2}]$_i$ increased from a basal level of 46.5 ± 6.9 nM to a gastrin-stimulated level of 142.4 ± 16.2 nM. This pattern of [Ca^{2+}]$_i$ response suggests activation of phospholipase C, in agreement with previous

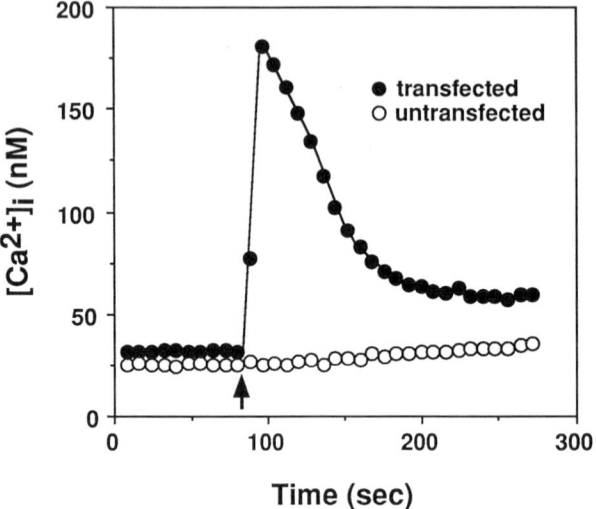

FIGURE 4. Gastrin stimulates calcium increase in COS-7 cells expressing the recombinant gastrin receptor. Free cytosolic calcium in COS-7 cells is shown as a function of time. Calcium levels in untransfected COS cells (*open circles*) that do not express the receptor are compared with transfected COS cells that express high numbers of recombinant receptors (*solid circles*). The *arrow* marks the addition of 1 µM gastrin. Data shown are representative of three experiments.

reports of the second messenger pathways linked to the native parietal cell gastrin receptor.[9,10]

The identity of the cloned receptor was also supported by the tissue distribution of the mRNA. High stringency Northern blot analysis (FIG. 5) of RNA isolated from adult canine tissues was probed using a restriction fragment of GR-1 as the hybridization probe. Receptor mRNA was found in gastric parietal cells, pancreas, and cerebral cortex. All of these tissues are reported to have gastrin/CCK-B type receptors.[11,12] The hybridization signal in brain was particularly intriguing. This was

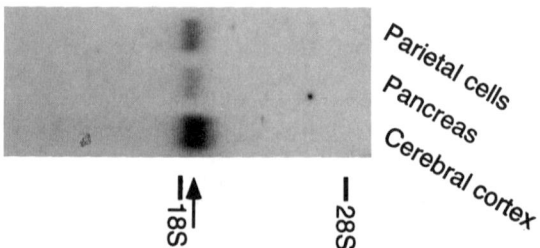

FIGURE 5. Northern blot analysis of gastrin receptor transcripts in mRNA isolated from canine tissues. Poly(A)+ RNA was loaded as follows: parietal cells, 0.3 µg; pancreas, 0.5 µg; and cerebral cortex, 1.0 µg. The transcript corresponding to GR-1 is indicated by an *arrow*. Positions of the 28S and 18S rRNA are indicated.

the first indication at a molecular level that the brain CCK-B receptor was closely related, if not identical, to the gastrin receptor.

To better understand the relation between the brain and the parietal cell receptors, a prototype CCK-B receptor was cloned from human brain. The canine receptor cDNA was used as a hybridization probe to screen a human brain cDNA library. A full-length human clone was identified, purified, subcloned, and sequenced on both strands, revealing an open reading frame encoding a 447 amino acid protein.

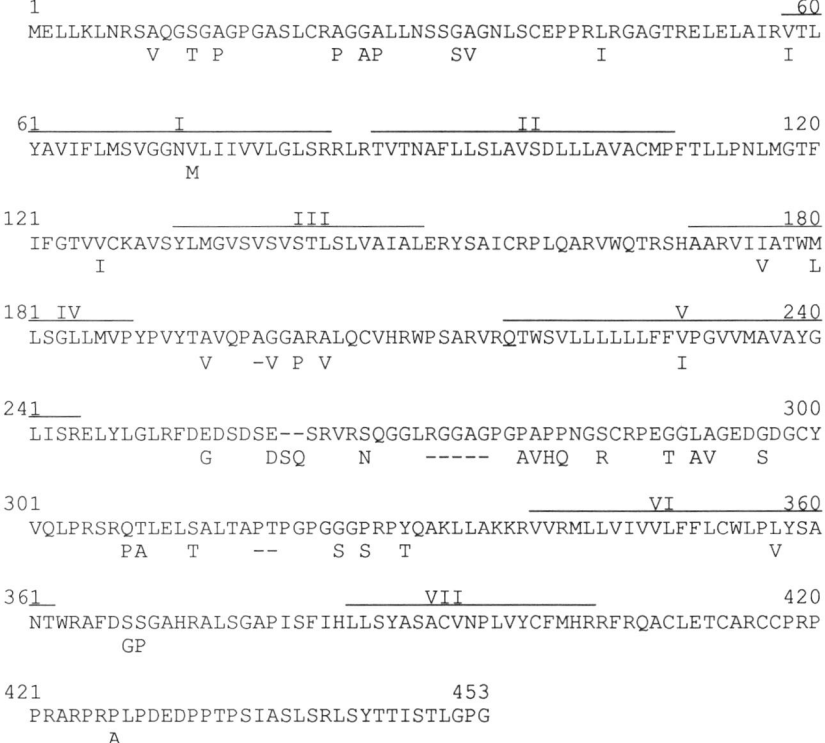

FIGURE 6. The deduced amino acid sequence of the canine and human CCK-B/gastrin receptors. The putative transmembrane domains of the receptor are marked by Roman numerals and bars overlying the sequence. Canine amino acid sequence is indicated in the *top line*; human sequence is shown below only where there is divergence from dog. A *dash* indicates a space, introduced to allow optimal alignment.

The human CCK-B receptor shares 91% amino acid identity with the previously cloned canine gastrin receptor (FIG. 6). All of the structural features discussed above for the dog gastrin receptor are present in the human protein. The high degree of amino acid identity suggested that the "gastrin" and "CCK-B" receptors were most likely the same subtype. This was further supported by the finding that the human receptor resembled the canine in agonist binding, signaling, and tissue distribution.[2]

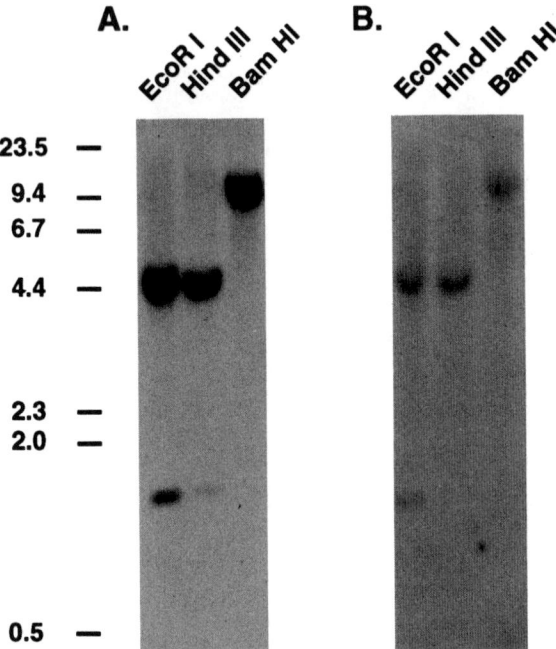

FIGURE 7. Human genomic Southern blot analysis. Ten micrograms of human genomic DNA were digested with either *Eco*RI, *Hind* III, or *Bam*HI, transferred to a nylon membrane, and hybridized with a probe corresponding to (**A**) the full-length human brain CCK-B/gastrin receptor cDNA or (**B**) the full-length canine parietal cell "gastrin" receptor cDNA. Molecular size markers are indicated in kilobases.

To further explore the question of CCK-B/gastrin receptor identity, a human genomic Southern blot was probed with the full-length canine "gastrin" receptor cDNA under conditions that allow cross-hybridization.[2] The canine "gastrin" receptor probe should hybridize to a putative human "gastrin" receptor gene more readily than to the human "CCK-B" receptor gene if separate genes exist. However, the canine gastrin receptor probe recognized only restriction fragments already identified as the human brain CCK-B/gastrin receptor gene (FIG. 7). Therefore, it is most likely that a single gene encodes both the brain "CCK-B" and the stomach "gastrin" receptors and that these two proteins represent the same receptor subtype.

Although the canine and human proteins appear to represent the same receptor, the binding of nonpeptide antagonists L365,260 and L364,718 markedly differed between species. Classically, L365,260 is a CCK-B/gastrin specific antagonist, whereas L364,718 has higher affinity for the CCK-A receptor.[13,14] The human receptor bound L364,718 and L365,260 with IC_{50} values of 145 and 3.8 nM, respectively.[2] L365,260 bound with approximately 40-fold higher affinity than did L364,718, well within the 6–125-fold range described in the literature.[14,15] The canine homolog, however, showed a reversal in the affinity rank order of these antagonists, with higher affinity for L364,718 (IC_{50} = 19 nM) than for L-365,260 (IC_{50} = 130 nM).[6] Since the human and canine receptors are 91% identical, 51 amino acids were candidates to explain this dramatic difference in antagonist binding. This variation in nature presented a unique opportunity to map a critical determinant of antagonist affinity.

As an initial step, receptor chimeras were used to identify the domain conferring high affinity binding of L365,260. Portions of the cDNAs encoding the human and canine receptors were ligated together *in vitro* and expressed in COS-7 cells, and the respective affinities for L365,260 were determined by competition binding experiments. As shown in FIGURE 8, the *Bam*HI chimera revealed that the segment of the human receptor extending from the distal end of the third intracellular loop through the carboxy terminus was sufficient to maintain high affinity for L365,260.

Amino acid sequence alignment of this domain among the human (high affinity for L365,260),[2] rat (high affinity for L365,260),[16] and canine receptors (low affinity for L365,260)[6] revealed five amino acids that were unique to the canine receptor and were therefore candidate residues to explain the interspecies variation in antagonist affinity. These five canine amino acids were sequentially replaced with the corresponding human residues using site-directed mutagenesis. Each construct was expressed in COS-7 cells and tested for L365,260 affinity by ^{125}I CCK-8 competition binding experiments (FIG. 9). Amino acid substitutions in four positions resulted in IC$_{50}$ values comparable to the canine wild-type receptor. However, replacement of ^{355}Leu in the canine receptor with ^{349}Val, the corresponding amino acid in the human receptor, increased the affinity for L365,260 to the human wild-type value. A direct comparison of the canine wild-type and can ^{355}L $\Rightarrow$ V receptor affinities is shown in FIGURE 10, bottom panel. To confirm the importance of the residue in the position corresponding to canine ^{355}Leu, the converse experiment was carried out and is shown in FIGURE 10, top panel. The homologous amino acid in the human receptor, ^{349}Val, was changed to a Leu residue. The affinity of hum ^{349}V $\Rightarrow$ L for L365,260 was reduced to the canine wild-type value. Therefore, a single amino acid substitution between the canine and human receptors confers species-specific binding of L365,260.

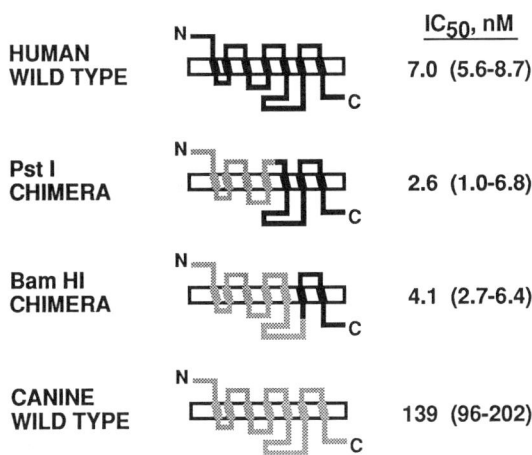

FIGURE 8. Determinants for high affinity binding of L365,260 are found at the carboxy end of the human CCK-B/gastrin receptor. IC$_{50}$ values for L365,260 were calculated from ^{125}I CCK-8 competition studies of recombinant wild-type and chimeric CCK-B/gastrin receptors. The *Pst*I chimera was constructed using the naturally occurring *Pst*I sites which are found in the same relative position in both receptors. Construction of the *Bam*HI chimera required the introduction of a *Bam*HI restriction site (nucleotides 970–975) into the canine cDNA.

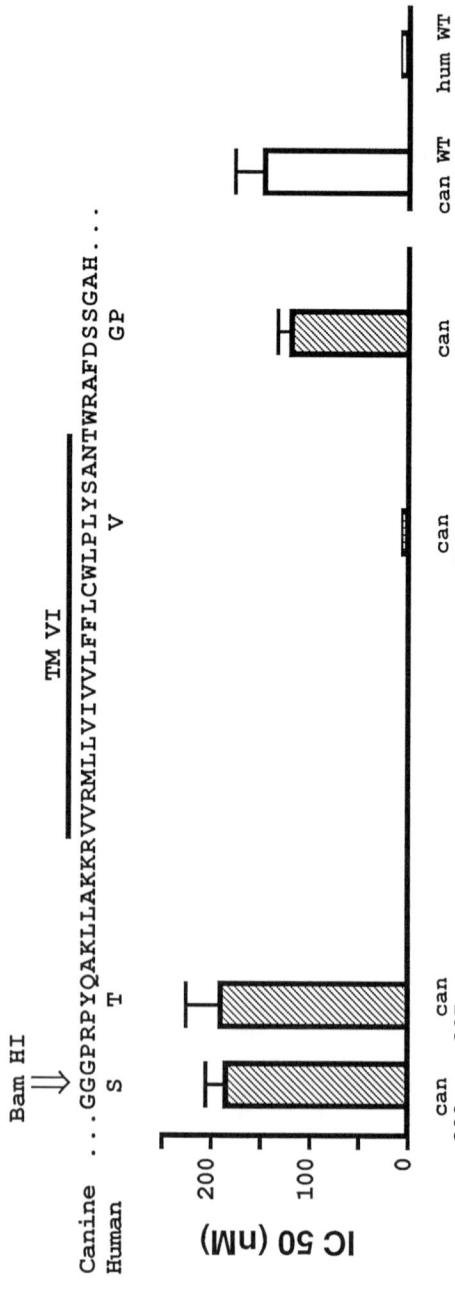

FIGURE 9. Identification of the amino acid residue of the CCK-B/gastrin receptor which determines affinity for L365,260. Amino acids (single letter code) of the canine CCK-B/gastrin receptor are compared with the corresponding human sequence; only human residues that diverge are shown. Using site-specific mutagenesis, the nucleotides encoding the human amino acids were introduced into the homologous location of the canine cDNA. Wild-type and mutant receptors were expressed in COS-7 cells and characterized by ^{125}I CCK-8 competition binding experiments with L365,260 (means ± SEM, $n \geq 2$). Cross-hatched and open columns represent mutant and wild-type receptors, respectively. WT = wild type; can = canine; hum = human; TM = transmembrane domain.

FIGURE 10. ^{125}I CCK-8 competition experiments comparing L365,260 binding to human and canine wild-type and mutant receptors (see text for details). IC$_{50}$ values and 95% confidence intervals for L365,260 (mean of at least four experiments) were: hum WT, 4.5 nM (4.3–4.8), hum ^{349}V ⇒ L, 90 nM (54–151), can WT, 80 nM (65–100), and can ^{355}L ⇒ V, 3.6 nM (3.0–4.3). Control experiments (^{125}I CCK-8 competition with unlabeled CCK-8) confirmed that the radioligand affinity was identical in wild-type and mutant receptors (not shown). Hum = human; can = canine; WT = wild type.

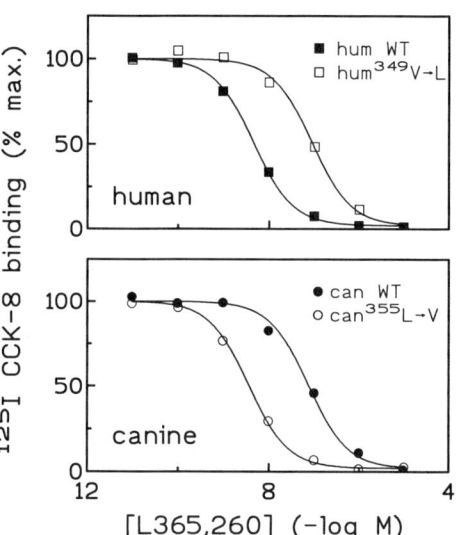

The same transmembrane domain VI amino acid appears to define specificity for L364,718. The bottom panel in FIGURE 11 compares the canine wild-type receptor, which has relatively high affinity for L364,718, with the single can ^{355}L ⇒ V substitution mutant which has lower affinity for L364,718, comparable to the human wild-type receptor. The converse experiment is shown in the top panel. The wild-type human receptor has relatively low affinity for L364,718. The hum ^{349}V ⇒ L substitution results in a receptor with higher affinity for L364,718, comparable to canine wild-type value. It is apparent from these data that the amino acid correspond-

FIGURE 11. ^{125}I CCK-8 competition experiments comparing L364,718 binding to human and canine wild-type and mutant receptors (see text for details). IC$_{50}$ values and 95% confidence intervals for L364,718 (mean of at least four experiments) were: hum WT, 147 nM (123–191), hum ^{349}V ⇒ L, 21 nM (11–40), can WT, 14 nM (12–17), and can ^{355}L ⇒ V, 95 nM (40–223). Hum = human; can = canine; WT = wild type.

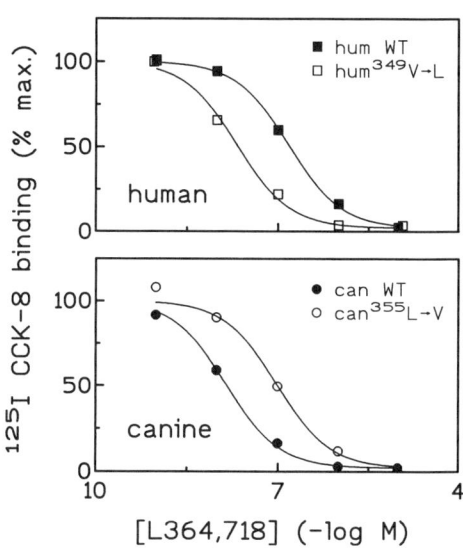

ing to human [349]Val (canine [355]Leu) is a critical determinant of antagonist affinity for both benzodiazepine-based compounds.

When the amino acid sequences of all known CCK/gastrin receptors are compared, the residue corresponding to human [349]Val is uniformly found to be a branched chain aliphatic amino acid (FIG. 12). The human and rat CCK-B/gastrin receptors both have a valine residue in this position and, as predicted from our findings, have comparable affinities for L365,260 as well as for L364,718.[2,16] A Leu markedly alters the affinities for both L365,260 and L364,718, as illustrated by the canine wild-type receptor.[6] In the mastomys receptor[17] and in the rat CCK-A receptor,[18] an Ile corresponds to human [349]Val. Although antagonist affinities for the recombinant mastomys receptor have not yet been reported, it is well established that the rat CCK-A receptor binds L364,718 with >100-fold higher affinity and L365,260 with >100-fold lower affinity than does the human CCK-B/gastrin receptor. To determine if an isoleucine is sufficient to confer CCK-A type antagonist selectivity, an isoleucine was substituted in place of human [349]Val. As shown in FIGURE 13, the isoleucine substitution did not change the affinity for L365,260. However, this substitution selectively increased the affinity for L364,718. The changes

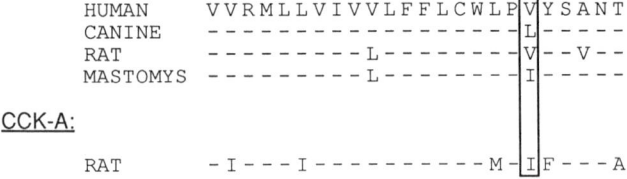

FIGURE 12. Comparison of the amino acid sequences (single letter code) corresponding to transmembrane domain VI of the human, canine, rat, and mastomys CCK-B/gastrin and the rat CCK-A receptors, as deduced from the corresponding cDNAs. *Dashes* indicate identity with the human receptor. The boxed amino acids correspond to human [349]Val.

in IC_{50} values were considerably less pronounced than those expected for a CCK-A receptor, suggesting that other residues contribute to the differences in antagonist affinities between the CCK-B/gastrin and the CCK-A receptors.

These results indicate that the aliphatic side chain of the amino acid in the position corresponding to human valine 349 at least in part determines the affinity for both L364,718 and L365,260. In the human receptor, a leucine for valine substitution alters affinities for both 364,718 and 365,260 to values comparable to those of the canine wild-type receptor. An isoleucine in the same position selectively alters L364,718 affinity. Although the benzodiazepine-derived antagonists appear extremely sensitive to changes in the amino acid corresponding to human valine 349, aliphatic amino acid substitutions in this position (valine, leucine, or isoleucine) do not affect the binding of gastrin or CCK-8 (data not shown). The affinity determinants of agonists and nonpeptide antagonists must therefore, at least in part, be different. On this basis, one might predict that the site corresponding to human valine 349 would not be important in the binding of a new type of agonist-derived peptoid antagonists.[19] To test this hypothesis, the affinity of the peptoid compound PD136,450 was determined for each of the wild-type (canine, human) and mutant

FIGURE 13. Comparison of non-peptide antagonist binding to the wild-type human and the mutant human, $^{349}V \Rightarrow I$, receptors. ^{125}I CCK-8 competition experiments were performed with L365,260 (*bottom panel*) and L364,718 (*top panel*). See text for details. IC_{50} values and 95% confidence intervals for L365,260 and L364,718 (mean of at least four experiments) were, respectively: hum WT, 4.5 nM (4.3–4.8) and 147 nM (123–191); hum $^{349}V \Rightarrow I$, 5.3 nM (4.7–6.0) and 26 nM (18–40). Hum = human; WT = wild type.

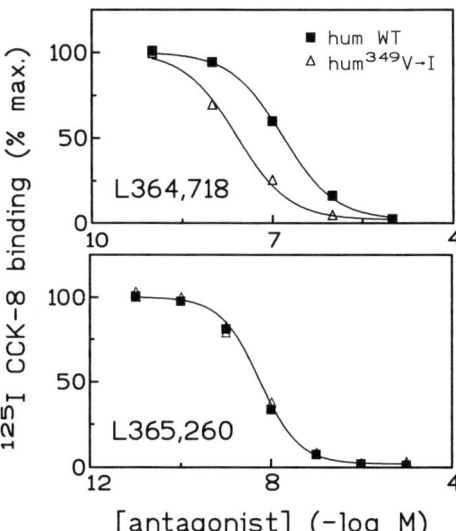

(can $^{355}L \Rightarrow V$, hum $^{349}V \Rightarrow L$) receptors. As shown in FIGURE 14, the affinity of this antagonist remains essentially constant and does not reflect the change in amino acid occupying either position 349 in the human or 355 in the dog receptor.

In summary, our results suggest that the parietal cell "gastrin" receptor and the brain "CCK-B" receptor are the product of a single gene and most likely represent the same receptor subtype. A single conservative amino acid change (human ^{349}Val *versus* canine ^{355}Leu) in the CCK-B/gastrin receptor underlies species differences in affinity for nonpeptide antagonists. The exquisite sensitivity of some receptor

FIGURE 14. ^{125}I CCK-8 competition experiments comparing PD136,450 binding to human and canine wild-type and mutant receptors (see text for details).

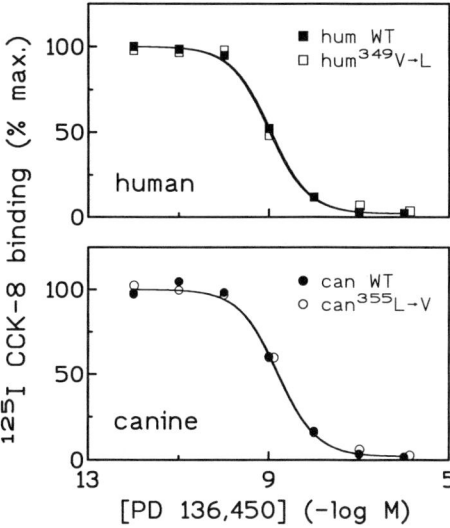

antagonists to even the most conservative of amino acid changes underlines that preclinical antagonist testing in animal models should be limited to species with receptors pharmacologically identical to human receptors.

ACKNOWLEDGMENT

We thank A. Leiter, S. L. Lee, A. Plaut, J. Nishitani, and A. Kane for helpful discussions and support, and L. Rogers and L. Lincicome for technical assistance.

REFERENCES

1. WATSON, S. & A. ABBOTT. 1992. Trends Pharmacol. Sci. Suppl. 11.
2. LEE, Y. M., M. BEINBORN, E. W. MCBRIDE, M. LU, L. F. KOLAKOWSKI, JR. & A. S. KOPIN. 1992. J. Biol. Chem. **268:** 8164–8169.
3. BEINBORN, M., Y. M. LEE, E. W. MCBRIDE, S. M. QUINN & A. S. KOPIN. 1993. Nature **362:** 348–350.
4. SOLL, A. H., D. A. AMIRIAN, L. P. THOMAS, T. J. REEDY & J. D. ELASHOFF. 1984. J. Clin. Invest. **73:** 1434–1447.
5. PEARSON, R. K., S. P. POWERS, E. M. HADAC, H. GAISANO & L. J. MILLER. 1987. Biochem. Biophys. Res. Commun. **147:** 346–353.
6. KOPIN, A. S., Y. M. LEE, E. W. MCBRIDE, L. J. MILLER, M. LU, H. Y. LIN, L. F. KOLAKOWSKI, JR. & M. BEINBORN. 1992. Proc. Natl. Acad. Sci. USA **89:** 3605–3609.
7. KARNIK, S. S., T. P. SAKMAR, H. B. CHEN & H. G. KHORANA. 1988. Proc. Natl. Acad. Sci. USA **85:** 8459–8463.
8. DOHLMAN, H. G., J. THORNER, M. G. CARON & R. J. LEFKOWITZ. 1991. Annu. Rev. Biochem. **60:** 653–688.
9. MUALLEM, S. & G. SACHS. 1984. Biochim. Biophys. Acta **805:** 181–185.
10. CHEW, C. S. & M. R. BROWN. 1986. Biochim. Biophys. Acta **888:** 116–125.
11. JENSEN, R. T., S. C. HUANG, T. V. SCHRENCK, S. A. WANK & J. D. GARDNER. 1990. In Gastrointestinal Endocrinology: Receptors and Post-Receptor Mechanisms. J. C. Thompson, ed.: 95–113. Harcourt Brace Jovanovich. San Diego, CA.
12. MAGOUS, R., J. C. GALLEYRAND & J. P. BALI. 1989. Biochim. Biophys. Acta **1010:** 357–362.
13. CHANG, R. S. & V. J. LOTTI. 1986. Proc. Natl. Acad. Sci. USA **83:** 4923–4926.
14. LOTTI, V. J. & R. S. CHANG. 1989. Eur. J. Pharmacol. **162:** 273–280.
15. HUGHES, J., P. BODEN, B. COSTALL, A. DOMENEY, E. KELLY, D. C. HORWELL, J. C. HUNTER, R. D. PINNOCK & G. N. WOODRUFF. 1990. Proc. Natl. Acad. Sci. USA **87:** 6728–6732.
16. WANK, S. A., J. R. PISEGNA & A. DE WEERTH. 1992. Proc. Natl. Acad. Sci. USA **89:** 8691–8695.
17. NAKATA, H. et al. 1992. Biochem. Biophys. Res. Commun. **187:** 1151–1157.
18. WANK, S. A., R. HARKINS, R. T. JENSEN, H. SHAPIRA, A. DE WEERTH & T. SLATTERY. 1992. Proc. Natl. Acad. Sci. USA **89:** 3125–3129.
19. HORWELL, D. C., J. HUGHES, J. C. HUNTER, M. C. PRITCHARD, R. S. RICHARDSON, E. ROBERTS & G. N. WOODRUFF. 1991. J. Med. Chem. **34:** 404–414.
20. MATHEWS, L. S. & W. W. VALE. 1991. Cell **65:** 973–982.

Biological Evaluation of JMV180 Cholecystokinin Analogs

M. AMBLARD,[a] M. F. LIGNON,[a] N. BERNAD,[a]
A. M. NOEL-ARTIS,[a] L. HAUAD,[a] J. LAUR,[a]
M. RODRIGUEZ,[a] M. C. GALAS,[a] D. FOURMY,[b]
AND J. MARTINEZ[a]

[a]*Chimie et Pharmacologie de Molécules d'Intérêt Biologique*
EP CNRS 51
Faculté de Pharmacie
15 avenue C. Flahault
34060 Montpellier, France

[b]*INSERM U151*
CHU Rangueil
31054 Toulouse, France

The dose-response curve for cholecystokinin (CCK)-stimulated enzyme secretion in isolated pancreatic acini from different species is biphasic. With increasing doses of CCK, amylase secretion increases to a maximum and then decreases at higher concentrations. The CCK analog Boc-Tyr(SO_3H)-Nle-Gly-Trp-Nle-Asp-O-CH_2-CH_2-C_6H_5 (JMV180), lacking the C-terminal amide function, in which the phenylalanine residue was replaced by 2-phenylethyl alcohol[1] and both methionines in position 28 and 31 were substituted by norleucines, exhibited "partial agonist activity" of CCK in rat pancreatic acini. C-terminal JMV180 did not produce a decrease in amylase stimulation at supramaximal concentrations in rat pancreatic acini,[2] but it showed a plateau of maximal stimulation. It has been hypothesized that compound JMV180 interacts with both low- and high-affinity peripheral CCK binding sites. It acts as an agonist at CCK high-affinity binding sites and as an antagonist at low-affinity binding sites.[3] Compound JMV180 has been used extensively to determine the relations between occupation of each class of the CCK binding sites and their linkage to various transduction systems and resulting biological activities and it is still widely used in various studies.[4–7] Interestingly, replacing L-tryptophan by D-tryptophan in compound JMV180 produced Boc-Tyr(SO_3H)-Nle-Gly-D-Trp-Nle-Asp-O-CH_2-CH_2-C_6H_5 (JMV179) which proved to be a full and potent CCK receptor antagonist.[8] When compound JMV180 or the corresponding D-tryptophan analog was used in *in vivo* studies, larger doses than expected from *in vitro* results had to be used to obtain biological activity.[9,10] We also observed that although the corresponding 2-phenylethyl-amide analog of compound JMV180, such as Boc-Tyr(SO_3H)-Nle-Gly-Trp-Nle-Asp-NH-CH_2CH_2-C_6H_5, was less potent *in vitro* than JMV180, it was equally potent in *in vivo* studies. These observations suggested that compounds JMV180 and JMV179 were probably not very stable *in vivo;* we were particularly concerned about the stability of the ester linkage. One of our goals was to synthesize an analog of compound JMV180 that would have enhanced stability, particularly for *in vivo* studies, and maintain high *in vitro* activity. In the first part of this work, we report on the biological activity of analogs of compound JMV180 in which the ester bond was replaced by a "carba" linkage (CH_2-CH_2) (FIG. 1). This modification implied the synthesis of 3-amino 7-phenyl heptanoic acid (β-homo-Aph) with the R configura-

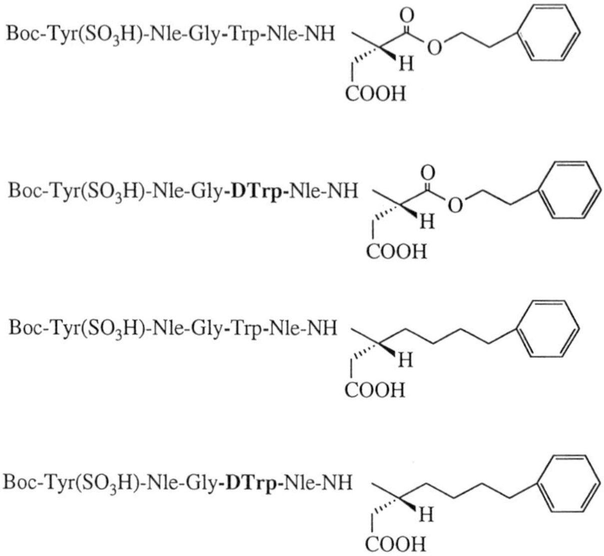

Boc-Tyr(SO₃H)-Nle-Gly-Trp-Nle-NH—CH(COOH)—C(=O)—O—CH₂CH₂—C₆H₅   JMV180

Boc-Tyr(SO₃H)-Nle-Gly-**DTrp**-Nle-NH—CH(COOH)—C(=O)—O—CH₂CH₂—C₆H₅   JMV179

Boc-Tyr(SO₃H)-Nle-Gly-Trp-Nle-NH—CH(COOH)—CH₂CH₂CH₂—C₆H₅   JMV300

Boc-Tyr(SO₃H)-Nle-Gly-**DTrp**-Nle-NH—CH(COOH)—CH₂CH₂CH₂—C₆H₅   JMV301

FIGURE 1. Chemical formula of compounds Boc-Tyr(SO₃H)-Nle-Gly-Trp-Nle-Asp-2-phenylethyl ester (JMV180), Boc-Tyr(SO₃H)-Nle-Gly-DTrp-Nle-Asp-2-phenylethyl ester (JMV179), Boc-Tyr(SO₃H)-Nle-Gly-Trp-Nle-(R)-β-homo-Aph-OH (JMV300), and Boc-Tyr(SO₃H)-Nle-Gly-DTrp-Nle-(R)-β-homo-Aph-OH (JMV301).

tion, in order to mimic the Asp-O-CH_2-CH_2-C_6H_5 moiety with the correct side chain orientation. We undertook the synthesis of compounds Boc-Tyr(SO₃H)-Nle-Gly-Trp-Nle-(R)-β-homo-Aph-OH (JMV300) and of its analog having a D-tryptophan, Boc-Tyr(SO₃H)-Nle-Gly-D-Trp-Nle-(R)-β-homo-Aph-OH (JMV301), and we evaluated their biological activities on rat pancreatic acini. In the second part of this work, we report on the particular pharmacological profile of sulfated and nonsulfated analogs of compounds JMV180 and JMV179 in rat pancreatic acini expressing the CCK-A receptor type and in guinea pig brain membranes and Jurkat T cells expressing the CCK-B receptor type.

RESULTS AND DISCUSSION

Boc-Tyr(SO₃H)-Nle-Gly-Trp-Nle-(R)-β-homo-Aph-OH (JMV300) and Boc-Tyr(SO₃H)-Nle-Gly-D-Trp-Nle-(R)-β-homo-Aph-OH (JMV301) were synthesized as recently described.[11] These compounds were tested for their ability to stimulate *in vitro* amylase secretion from rat pancreatic acini (FIG. 2) and to inhibit the binding of (^{125}I)BH-CCK-8 to isolated rat pancreatic acini (FIG. 3), to guinea pig brain membranes (FIG. 4), and to Jurkat cells (FIG. 5).[12,13] In the same experiments they were compared with compounds JMV180 or JMV179. The CCK analog JMV300 was able to inhibit binding of labeled CCK-8 to rat pancreatic acini with an IC_{50} of about 12 ± 8 nM. Compound JMV301 with a D-tryptophan was almost equally potent, with an IC_{50} of 14 ± 4 nM. These results indicated that in CCK analogs lacking the C-terminal amide function replacement of L-tryptophan by D-tryptophan did not affect the affinity for the CCK receptor in rat pancreatic acini, in contrast to what occurred with CCK-8.[14] On stimulation of amylase secretion from rat pancreatic acini, compound JMV300 acted like JMV180, exhibiting maximal stimulation with no decrease in response at high concentrations ($EC_{50} = 6 \pm 2$ nM). As with previous results showing that replacement of L-tryptophan by D-tryptophan in such analogs resulted in full CCK-receptor antagonists,[8] compound JMV301 was unable to stimulate amylase secretion from rat pancreatic acini (FIG. 1). However, compound JMV301 was able to dose-dependently inhibit CCK-8–stimulated amylase secretion from rat pancreatic acini with an IC_{50} of 0.5 ± 0.2 μM (FIG. 6). This result confirms that in CCK analogs exhibiting a plateau of stimulation of amylase secretion at high concentrations, replacement of L-tryptophan by D-tryptophan led to full CCK receptor antagonists. As expected, compound JMV300 and particularly JMV301 were less potent than CCK-8 in inhibiting binding of labeled CCK-8 to guinea pig brain membranes (IC_{50} of 32 ± 2 and $1,150 \pm 30$ nM, respectively) and to Jurkat T cells ($IC_{50} = 75 \pm 15$ and $1,100 \pm 52$ nM), both expressing CCK-B/gastrin receptors. These results are in accord with the observation that the C-terminal tetrapeptide is crucial for interaction with CCK-B receptors.

As is well known, the sulfate group of CCK is crucial for the interaction of CCK analogs with CCK-A receptors, whereas it is not important for the interaction with CCK-B/gastrin receptors.[15] In fact, the C-terminal tetrapeptide of CCK is the minimal fragment having high affinity for CCK-B receptors.[16,17] After finding that the configuration of the tryptophan residue was not crucial to recognizing CCK-A receptors in CCK analogs lacking the C-terminal amide function, we decided to study

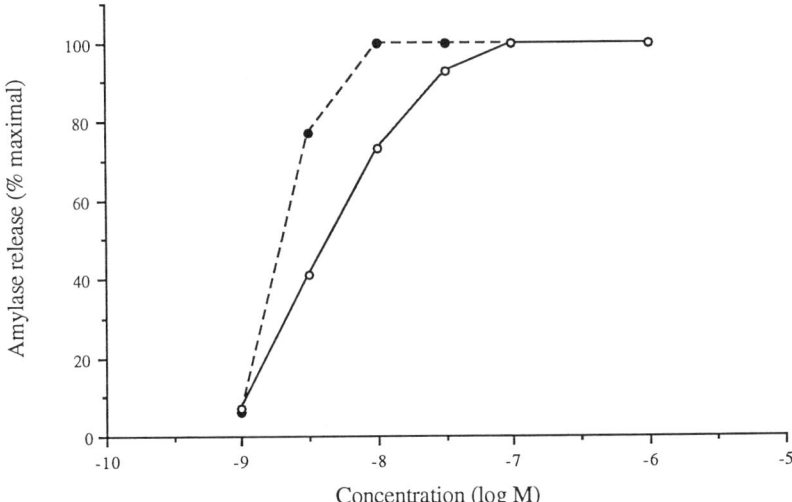

FIGURE 2. Effect of compounds JMV180 (●) and JMV300 (○) on amylase release from rat pancreatic acini. Dispersed pancreatic acini from rat were prepared, and amylase release was measured according to previously described procedures.[8] Amylase release was measured as the difference of amylase activity at the end of incubation that was released into the extracellular medium with and without secretagogue and expressed as the percentage of maximal stimulation. In each experiment, each value was determined in duplicate, and the results given are the means of at least three separate experiments. JMV179 and JMV301 were unable to stimulate amylase secretion even at concentrations as high as 10 μM.

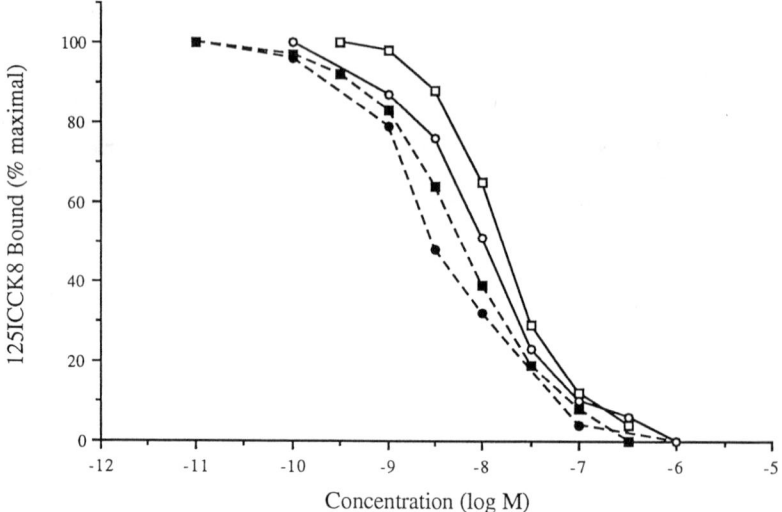

FIGURE 3. Ability of compounds JMV180, JMV179, JMV300, and JMV301 to inhibit binding of labeled CCK8 to rat pancreatic acini. Binding of Bolton-Hunter–labeled CCK8 was performed as described previously.[8] Briefly, acini were incubated for 30 minutes at 37°C with various concentrations of compounds JMV180 (●), JMV179 (■), JMV300 (○), or JMV301 (□) plus 10 pM ^{125}I-BH-CCK8. Values are expressed as the percentage of the value obtained with labeled CCK8 alone. Nonspecific binding was determined in the presence of 1 μM CCK8 and was always less than 15% of the total binding. In each experiment, each value was determined in duplicate, and the results given are the means of at least four separate experiments.

the relations between structure and activity in such CCK analogs and more particularly the influence of the sulfate group. CCK-8, unsulfated CCK-8 (CCK-8NS), and compounds JMV180, JMV180NS, JMV179, and JMV179NS were evaluated for their ability to inhibit the binding of labeled CCK-8 to rat pancreatic acini, to guinea pig brain membranes, and to Jurkat cells. As shown in FIGURE 7, on rat pancreatic acini, compound JMV180 ($IC_{50} \approx 2$ nM), like CCK-8, is largely more potent than its desulfated analog ($IC_{50} \approx 1,000$ nM). Unexpectedly, compound JMV179 ($IC_{50} \approx 8$ nM) had about the same affinity as JMV180, indicating that the stereochemistry of the tryptophan residue is not important for interaction with CCK-A receptors in CCK analogs lacking the C-terminal amide. In comparison, replacement of L-tryptophan by D-tryptophan in CCK-8 resulted in about a 60-fold decrease in affinity.[14] Interestingly, compound JMV179NS ($IC_{50} \approx 25$ nM) is only about three times less potent than its sulfated analog JMV179, indicating that in contrast to CCK-8, sulfation is not a crucial determinant in recognizing the CCK-A receptor in such analogs and does not seem to play the same role as in CCK-8 for interacting with CCK-A receptors. Compounds JMV179 and JMV179NS are CCK-receptor antagonists; it is possible that the sulfate group is not a critical determinant in CCK receptor antagonists for recognizing CCK-A receptors. The potency of compounds JMV180, JMV180NS, JMV179, and JMV179NS in inhibiting the binding of ^{125}I-BH-CCK-8 was evaluated on guinea pig brain membranes (FIG. 8) and Jurkat cells (FIG. 9) expressing the CCK-B/gastrin receptor. Unexpectedly, a great difference in potency was noted between compound JMV180 ($IC_{50} \approx 8$ nM in guinea pig brain membranes and $IC_{50} \approx 2$ nM in Jurkat cells) and its unsulfated form, JMV180NS ($IC_{50} \approx 1,000$ nM in guinea pig brain membranes and $IC_{50} \approx 800$ nM in Jurkat cells). This result indicates that in contrast with CCK-8, in these analogs, the sulfate group is important for recognizing the CCK-B/gastrin receptor. In contrast also to what was observed in rat pancreatic acini, the D-tryptophan analog of compound JMV180 (e.g., JMV179, $IC_{50} \approx 150$ nM in guinea pig brain membranes and $IC_{50} \approx 200$ nM in Jurkat cells) was significantly less potent than that of JMV180 in guinea pig brain membranes and Jurkat cells (about 20 times less potent in guinea pig brain membranes and 100 times less potent in Jurkat cells), pointing out the importance of the side chain orientation of tryptophan in recognizing the CCK-B/gastrin receptor. However, although compound JMV179NS was weakly potent ($IC_{50} \approx 600$ nM in guinea pig brain membranes and $IC_{50} \approx 400$ nM in Jurkat cells), it was about four times less potent in guinea pig brain membranes and two times less potent in Jurkat cells than compound JMV179 and only about two times more potent than JMV180NS.

CONCLUSION

The biological evaluations of a potent analog (JMV300) of compound JMV180 in which the C-terminal ester bond was replaced by a carba bond are described. When

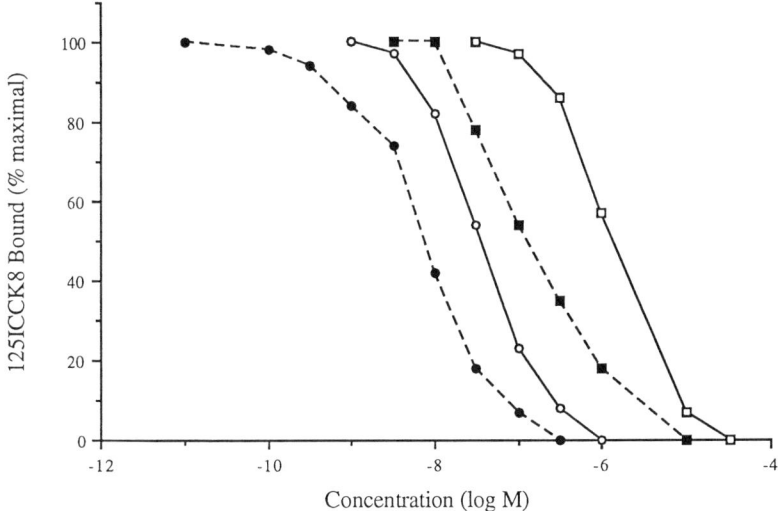

FIGURE 4. Ability of compounds JMV180, JMV179, JMV300, and JMV301 to inhibit binding of labeled CCK8 to guinea pig brain membranes. Binding of Bolton-Hunter–labeled CCK8 was performed as described previously.[8] Briefly, brain membranes (1 mL $\approx$ 0.5 mg protein) were incubated for 60 minutes at 25°C with various concentrations of compounds JMV180 (●), JMV179 (■), JMV300 (○), or JMV301 (□) plus 20 pM ^{125}I-BH-CCK8. Values are expressed as the percentage of the value obtained with labeled CCK8 alone. Nonspecific binding was determined in the presence of 1 μM CCK8 and was always less than 25% of the total binding. In each experiment, each value was determined in duplicate, and the results given are the means of at least four separate experiments.

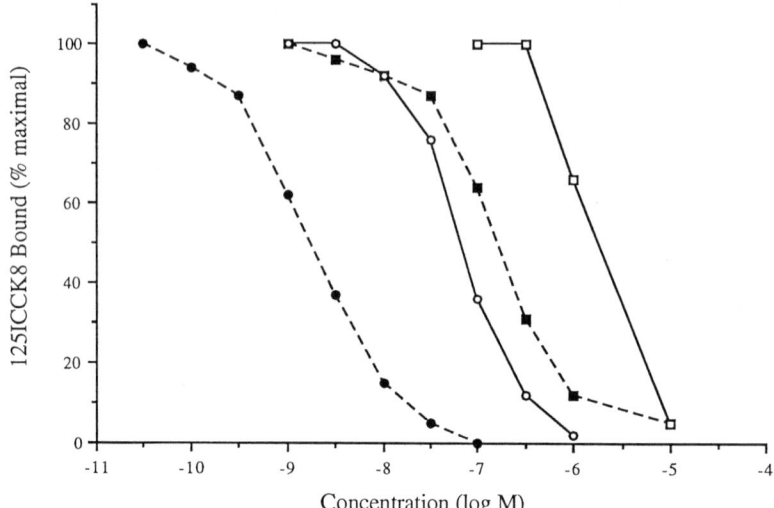

FIGURE 5. Ability of compounds JMV180, JMV179, JMV300, and JMV301 to inhibit binding of labeled CCK8 to Jurkat cells. Binding of Bolton-Hunter–labeled CCK8 was performed as described previously.[12] Briefly, Jurkat cells were incubated for 60 minutes at 37°C with various concentrations of compounds JMV180 (●), JMV179 (■), JMV300 (○), or JMV301 (□) plus 10 pM ^{125}I-BH-CCK8 in a final volume of 0.5 mL containing 4×10^6 cells. Values are expressed as the percentage of the value obtained with labeled CCK8 alone. Nonspecific binding was determined in the presence of 1 μM CCK8 and was always less than 10% of the total binding. In each experiment, each value was determined in duplicate, and the results given are the means of at least three separate experiments.

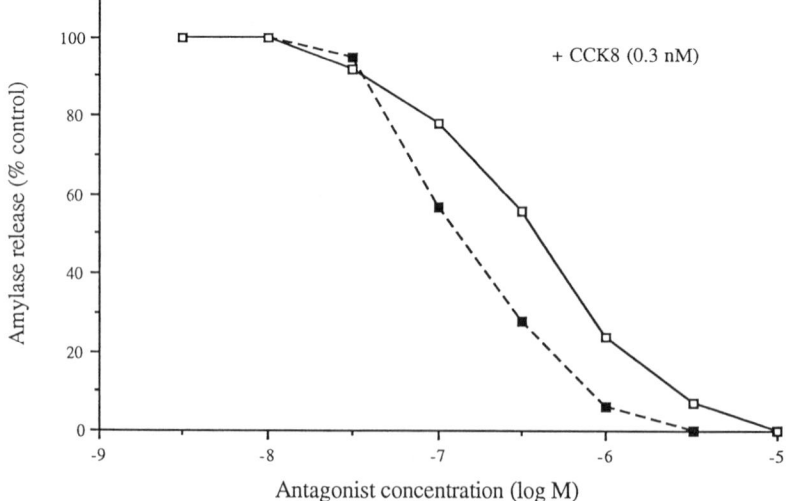

FIGURE 6. Ability of compounds JMV179 (■) and JMV301 (□) to inhibit CCK8-stimulated amylase secretion from rat pancreatic acini. Acini were incubated for 30 minutes at 37°C with various concentrations of compounds JMV179 or JMV301 plus 0.3 nM CCK8. Results are expressed as the percentage of the stimulation of amylase secretion obtained with no added antagonist. In each experiment, each value was determined in duplicate, and the results given are the means of at least three separate experiments.

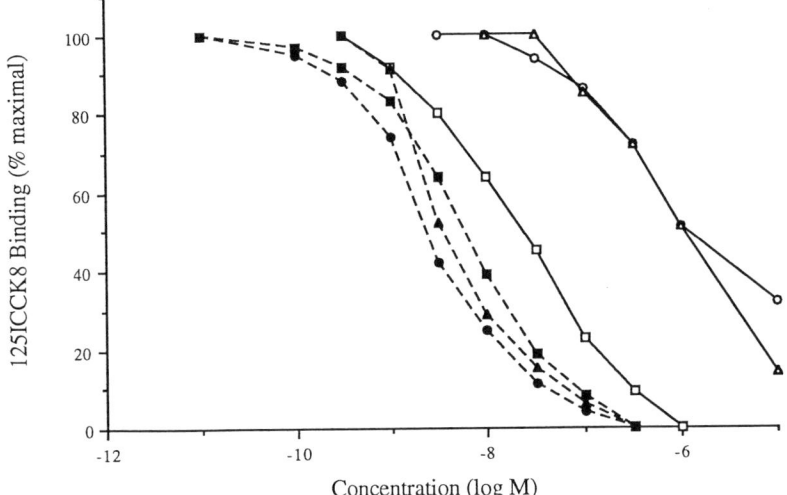

FIGURE 7. Ability of CCK8 (▲), nonsulfated CCK8 (CCK8NS) (△), and compounds JMV180 (●), JMV180NS (○), JMV179 (■), and JMV179NS (□) to inhibit binding of labeled CCK8 to rat pancreatic acini. Binding experiments were performed as described in FIGURE 3. In each experiment, each value was determined in duplicate, and the results given are the means of at least three separate experiments.

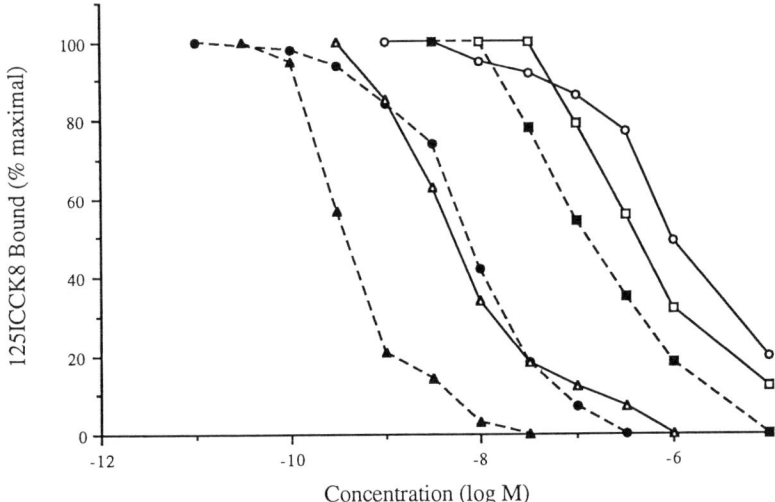

FIGURE 8. Ability of CCK8 (▲), nonsulfated CCK8 (CCK8NS) (△), and compounds JMV180 (●), JMV180NS (○), JMV179 (■), and JMV179NS (□) to inhibit binding of labeled CCK8 to guinea pig brain membranes. Binding experiments were performed as described in FIGURE 4. In each experiment, each value was determined in duplicate, and the results given are the means of at least three separate experiments.

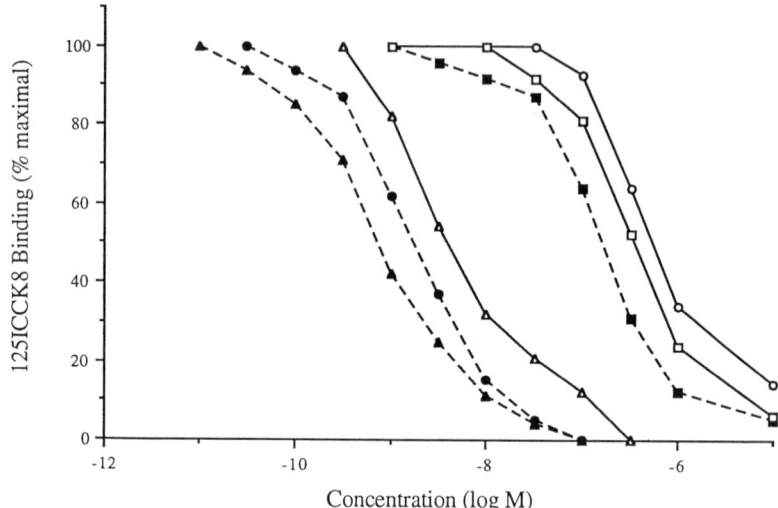

FIGURE 9. Ability of CCK8 (▲), nonsulfated CCK8 (CCK8NS) (△), and compounds JMV180 (●), JMV180NS (○), JMV179 (■), and JMV179NS (□) to inhibit binding of labeled CCK8 to Jurkat cells. Binding experiments were performed as described in FIGURE 5. In each experiment, each value was determined in duplicate, and the results given are the means of at least three separate experiments.

L-tryptophan was replaced by D-tryptophan in such an analog, a full CCK-receptor antagonist (JMV301) was obtained. These analogs might be more stable than compounds JMV180 and JMV179 and suitable for *in vivo* studies. Our studies clearly show that (1) the sulfate ester of tyrosine in compound JMV180, as in CCK-8, is an important determinant for binding to rat pancreatic acini; (2) the sulfate ester of tyrosine in CCK-receptor antagonists is not significant for binding to CCK-A receptors; (3) the sulfate ester of tyrosine in compound JMV180, in contrast with CCK-8, is also an important determinant for binding to CCK-B/gastrin receptors; and (4) the sulfate ester of tyrosine in CCK-receptor antagonists is not significant for binding to CCK-B receptors. These studies confirm the significance of the C-terminal tetrapeptide of CCK in recognizing CCK-B/gastrin receptors, particularly the orientation of the side chain of the tryptophan residue.

REFERENCES

1. FULCRAND, P., M. RODRIGUEZ, M. GALAS, M. C. LIGNON, J. LAUR, A. AUMELAS & J. MARTINEZ. 1988. 2-Phenylethyl ester and 2-phenylethyl amide derivative analogues of the C-terminal hepta- and octapeptide of cholecystokinin. Int. J. Pept. Protein Res. **32:** 384–395.
2. GALAS, M. C., M. F. LIGNON, M. RODRIGUEZ, C. MENDRE, P. FULCRAND, J. LAUR & J. MARTINEZ. 1988. Structure-activity relationship studies on cholecystokinin analogues with partial agonist activity. Am. J. Physiol. **254:** G176–G182.
3. MARTINEZ, J., M. C. GALAS, M. F. LIGNON, M. RODRIGUEZ & P. FULCRAND. 1991. Boc-Tyr(SO₃H)-Nle-Gly-Trp-Nle-Asp-2-Phenylethyl Ester-JMV180: A unique CCK analogue with different actions on high- and low-affinity CCK-receptors. *In* Cholecysto-

kinin Antagonists in Gastroenterology. G. Adler & C. Beglinger, eds.: 80–90. Springer-Verlag.
4. SALUJA, A. K., R. K. DAWRA, M. LERCH & M. L. STEER. 1992. CCK-JMV-180, an analog of cholecystokinin, releases intracellular calcium from an inositol triphosphate-independent pool in rat pancreatic acini. J. Biol. Chem. **1267:** 11202–11207.
5. GARDNER, J. D. 1993. Identification and characterization of three different affinity states of the CCK receptor in pancreatic acini. *In* Cholecystokinin. Ann. N.Y. Acad. Sci., this volume.
6. WILLEMS, P. H. G. M., H. J. M. VAN HOOF, M. G. H. VAN MACKELENBERGH, J. G. J. HOENDEROP, S. E. VAN EMST DE VRIES & J. J. H. H. M. DE PONT. 1993. CCK_8-evoked Ca^{2+} mobilization in pancreatic acinar cells: Evidence for a regulatory role of protein kinase C by phosphorylation-dependent inhibition of signalling through the high affinity CCK receptor. *In* Cholecystokinin. Ann. N.Y. Acad. Sci., this volume.
7. RIVARD, N., G. RYDZEWSKA & J. MORRISSET. 1993. Cholecystokinin-induced pancreatic growth involves the high-affinity CCK receptor and concomitant activation of tyrosine kinase and phospholipase D. *In* Cholecystokinin. Ann. N.Y. Acad. Sci., this volume.
8. LIGNON, M. F., M. C. GALAS, M. RODRIGUEZ, J. LAUR, A. AUMELAS & J. MARTINEZ. 1987. A synthetic peptide derivative that is a cholecystokinin receptor antagonist. J. Biol. Chem. **262:** 7226–7231.
9. NAGAIN, C., M. C. GALAS, M. F. LIGNON, M. RODRIGUEZ, J. MARTINEZ & C. ROZE. 1991. Synthetic CCK8 analogs with antagonist activity on pancreatic receptors: *In vivo* study in the rat, compared to non-peptidic antagonists. Pancreas **32:** 275–281.
10. NAGAIN, C., M. F. LIGNON, M. C. GALAS, M. RODRIGUEZ, J. MARTINEZ & C. ROZE. 1992. Large and prolonged *in vivo* response of pancreatic secretion to phenethylamide and phenethylester derivatives of Boc-(Nle^{28}, Nle^{31})CCK(26-33) in the rat. Peptides **13:** 1127–1132.
11. AMBLARD, M., M. RODRIGUEZ, M. F. LIGNON, M. C. GALAS, N. BERNAD, A. M. NOEL-ARTIS, L. HAUAD, J. LAUR, A. AUMELAS, J. C. CALIFANO & J. MARTINEZ. 1993. Synthesis and biological evaluation of cholecystokinin analogs in which the Asp-Phe-NH_2 moiety has been replaced by a 3-amino-7-phenylheptanoic acid or a 3 amino-6-(phenyloxy)-hexanoic acid. J. Med. Chem. **36:** 3021–3028.
12. LIGNON, M. F., N. BERNAD & J. MARTINEZ. 1991. Pharmacological characterization of type B cholecystokinin binding sites on the human JURKAT T lymphocyte cell line. Mol. Pharmacol. **39:** 615–620.
13. LIGNON, M. F., N. BERNAD & J. MARTINEZ. 1993. Cholecystokinin increases intracellular Ca^{2+} concentration in the human JURKAT T lymphocyte cell line. Eur. J. Pharmacol. **245:** 241–246.
14. ROLLAND, M., M. RODRIGUEZ, M. F. LIGNON, M. C. GALAS, J. LAUR, A. AUMELAS & J. MARTINEZ. 1991. Synthesis and biological activity of 2-phenylethyl ester analogs of the C-terminal heptapeptide of cholecystokinin modified in the Tryptophan 30 region. Int. J. Pept. Protein Res. **38:** 181–192.
15. VILLANUEVA, M. L. S., M. COLLINS, R. T. JENSEN & J. D. GARDNER. 1982. Structural requirements for action of cholecystokinin on enzyme secretion from pancreatic acini. Am. J. Physiol. **242:** G416–G422.
16. KNIGHT, M., C. A. TAMMINGA, L. STEARDO, M. E. BECK, P. BARONE & T. N. CHASE. 1984. Cholecystokinin-octapeptide fragments: Binding to brain cholecystokinin receptors. Eur. J. Pharmacol. **105:** 49–55.
17. INNIS, R. B. & S. H. SNYDER. 1980. Distinct cholecystokinin receptors in brain and pancreas. Proc. Natl. Acad. Sci. USA **77:** 6917–6921.

Distinguishing Multiple CCK Receptor Subtypes

Studies with Guinea Pig Chief Cells and Transfected Human CCK Receptors

ROBERT T. JENSEN,[a] JIA-MING QIAN, JAW-TOWN LIN,
SAMUEL A. MANTEY, JOSEPH R. PISEGNA, AND
STEPHEN A. WANK

Digestive Diseases Branch
National Institute of Diabetes and Digestive and Kidney Diseases
National Institutes of Health
Bethesda, Maryland 20892

Functional, pharmacological, and recent cloning studies have now established that two classes of receptors exist for cholecystokinin (CCK)/gastrin-related peptides (TABLE 1). One class, the CCK_A receptor, has a high affinity only for the naturally occurring CCK/gastrin-related peptides that are sulfated in the seventh position from the COOH-terminus which includes all forms of CCK (CCK-58, CCK-39, CCK-33, and CCK-8), caerulein, and the invertebrate peptide cionin.[1-9] In contrast, the CCK_B receptor has high affinity for both CCK peptides and gastrin with sulfation in either the sixth position (cionin, gastrin-17-II) or the seventh position from the COOH-terminus (CCK peptides, caerulein, and cionin), increasing potency less than 10-fold in most studies (TABLE 1).[2,5,8-15] Both selective agonists and antagonists were described for each of these receptors (TABLE 1).[2,3,16-30]

Functional and binding studies as well as studies of the distribution of mRNA for these receptors show that they are widely distributed in the CNS and peripheral tissues (TABLE 1).[3,31] In an increasing number of tissues such as guinea pig and dog pancreatic acinar cells, guinea pig chief cells, somatostatin-releasing cells of the stomach, gastrointestinal smooth muscle from stomach and gallbladder, in the CNS, and on the pancreatic acinar tumor cell line AR42J, both CCK_A and CCK_B receptors exist on the same cells.[15,31-38] In other tissues such as the gastric mucosa, tissue containing both CCK/gastrin receptor subtypes exists in close proximity.[39,40] Therefore, in assessing changes in biological responses frequently even in single cells, but particularly in assessing *in vivo* responses to CCK, it is becoming increasingly important to differentiate which effect is mediated by which receptor subtype, because CCK interacts with high affinity with both CCK receptor subtypes.[8,10,15] Furthermore, activation of CCK_A and CCK_B receptors may lead to similar responses in some tissues such as somatostatin release from isolated fundi D cells[35] or increases in inositol phosphates and $[Ca^{2+}]_i$ in AR42J cells,[34] whereas in other tissues such as effects on gastric acid secretion,[40] their activation in the gastric mucosa may have opposing effects. It is therefore becoming increasingly important to differentiate the ability of CCK to activate either subtype.

---

[a] Address for correspondence: Dr. Robert T. Jensen, National Institutes of Health, Building 10, Room 9C-103, Bethesda, Maryland 20892.

To differentiate these receptors in *in vivo* studies in humans, it is important to establish which of the various proposed CCK/gastrin receptor agonists and antagonists are selective for CCK_A and CCK_B receptors in humans, which agonists have full efficacy, as well as which proposed antagonists have no agonist activity. Recent studies demonstrate considerable differences for a number of these proposed agonists and antagonists in affinity in different species as well as efficacy.[41-44] For example, L-365,260 has shown a high affinity and selectivity for CCK_B over CCK_A receptors in rat and human, but not in the dog.[1,4,11,12,42] Similarly, a number of peptides function as agonists in one species and antagonists in another.[43,44] It is therefore important to establish which of these various proposed antagonists function as pure antagonists in various species and in humans. In the present study we report the usefulness of some of the selective CCK receptor agonists and antagonists in establishing if both CCK_A and CCK_B receptors are functional in the same cell, the

TABLE 1. Characteristics of Classes of CCK Receptors

Characteristic	CCK_A Receptor	CCK_B Receptor
Structure (human)	428 amino acids (4)	447 amino acids (13, 14)
Natural agonists	CCK-8, cionin, caerulein >>> gastrin ≈ CCK-4	CCK-8, gastrin, cionin > CCK-4
Location	CNS (limited), islets, pancreatic acini, gallbladder, neurons (GI tract), gastric mucosal cells (D-cells, chief), AR42J cells	CNS (widespread), GI smooth muscle, gastric mucosal (parietal, D-cell, chief), pancreatic acini, AR42J cells, SCLC cells
Selective agonists	A-71378 [0.4 nM] (19)	A-72962 [0.2 nM] (19) SNF-8702 [0.2 nM] (29) Gastrin [1 nM] (8, 10) BC-264 [0.2 nM] (18)
Selective antagonists	L-364,718 (devazepide) [1 nM] (22, 25, 28) Tetronothiodin [4 nM] (26) PD-140548 [10 nM] (2, 21, 27) Lorglumide (CR-1409) [150 nM] (15, 20, 24) SR-27897 [1 nM] (17)	CI-988 (PD-134,308) [10 nM] (2, 21, 27) L-365,260 [2 nM] (22, 23, 30) LY262691 [30 nM] (2)
Transduction	IP_3/Ca^{2+} (4, 59, 60, 65)	IP_3/Ca^{2+} (12, 36, 52-54)

NOTE: Numbers in brackets are affinities. Modified from references 2, 16, 41, and 57.

guinea pig chief cell.[36] Also, because of the importance of establishing the potencies and efficacies of the various putative CCK receptor agonists/antagonists for human CCK receptors, we report the results of preliminary studies investigating their abilities to interact with and activate human CCK_A and CCK_B receptors transfected into COS-7 cells.

STUDIES ON DISPERSED GUINEA PIG CHIEF CELLS: BINDING AND INITIAL FUNCTIONAL STUDIES

As just discussed, frequently both subtypes of CCK receptors exist on the same cell[15,31,32,34-38] (TABLE 1). In different tissues, occupation and activation of both subtypes have different effects. Both receptors can cause either similar changes in some cells such as contraction caused by CCK_A and CCK_B receptors on isolated gastrointestinal smooth muscle cells[33] or stimulation of somatostatin release from fundic D cells.[35] In other cells, occupation of either receptor has different functions such as CCK_A and CCK_B receptors on guinea pig pancreatic acini where only occupation of the CCK_A receptor stimulates secretion and activation of phospholipase C.[10] In other cells, such as rat pituitary, activation of CCK_A receptors in anterior pituitary corticotrophs[45] stimulates β-endorphin release, whereas activation of CCK_B receptors inhibits CCK-stimulated β-endorphin release.

The role of CCK_A and CCK_B receptors in mediating pepsinogen release by CCK/gastrin-related peptides is a particularly good example of the difficulty in resolving the role of activation of each receptor in altering cell function. CCK and gastrin have both been shown to stimulate pepsinogen release from isolated gastric chief cells and glands.[37,46–50] CCK-related peptides also have been shown to activate phospholipase C, increase cytosolic calcium, and stimulate the breakdown of phosphoinositides.[36,50–54] However, in numerous cell systems, CCK and gastrin both can interact with CCK_A and CCK_B receptors if sufficiently high concentrations are used.[8,10,15] Previous binding studies on chief cells have given variable results, with some studies suggesting a single class of receptors[38,48] and another study[55] suggesting heterogeneity of CCK/gastrin binding sites. Some functional studies have provided evidence for one subtype[46] and others for two subtypes.[37,56] It is also unclear if both subtypes are present, if they alter cell function by a similar transduction mechanism, or if the intracellular mechanisms have similar relationships.

Detailed binding studies using either ^{125}I-BH-CCK-8 or ^{125}I-gastrin with various selective agonists (FIG. 1) or selective antagonists (FIG. 2) failed to provide evidence for both subtypes of CCK receptors. For agonists, for both ligands the relative potencies were CCK-8 = 3 × gastrin-17-I = 30 × desulfated CCK-8 = 60 × CCK-4 (FIG. 1), which is typical for interaction with a CCK_B receptor (TABLE 1). Similarly,

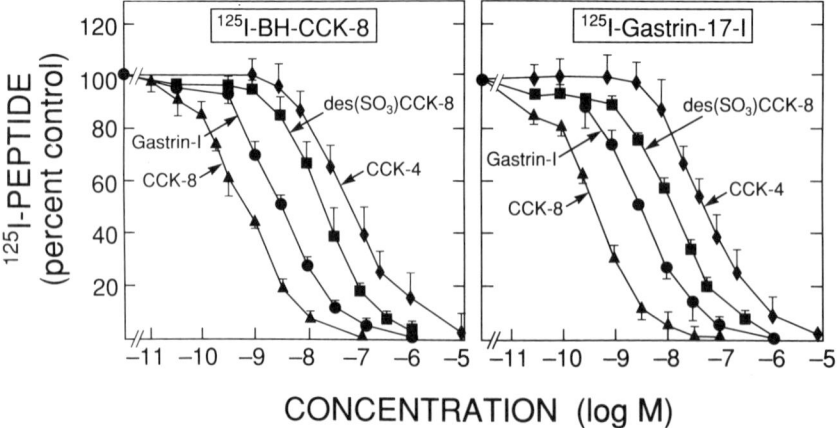

FIGURE 1. Ability of various CCK and gastrin-related peptides to inhibit binding of ^{125}I-BH-CCK-8 or ^{125}I-gastrin-17-I to dispersed chief cells from guinea pig pancreas. Dispersed chief cells were incubated with 50 pM ^{125}I-BH-CCK-8 or ^{125}I-gastrin-17-I for 30 minutes at 37°C. Results are expressed as the percentage of saturable binding in the presence of no unlabeled peptide added. Results are from three experiments, and in each experiment each point was determined in duplicate.

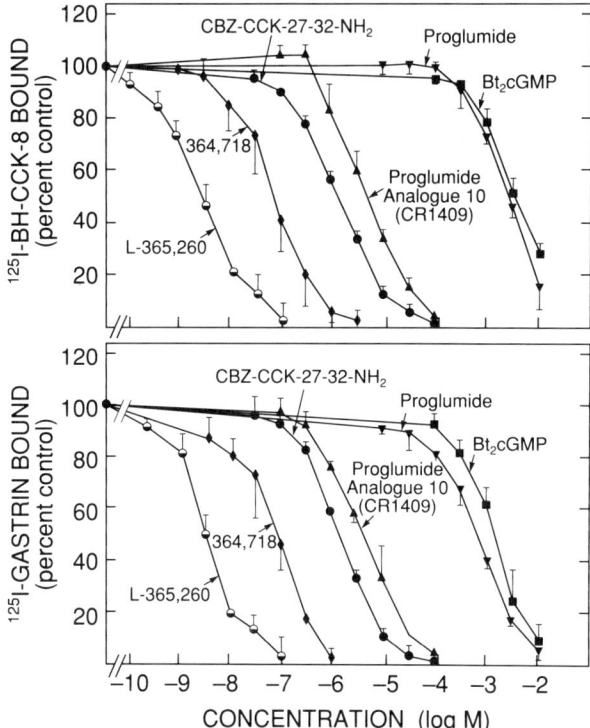

FIGURE 2. Ability of various CCK_A and CCK_B receptor antagonists to inhibit binding of ^{125}I-BH-CCK-8 or ^{125}I-gastrin-17-I to dispersed chief cells from guinea pig pancreas. Dispersed chief cells were incubated with 50 pM ^{125}I-BH-CCK-8 or ^{125}I-gastrin-17-I for 30 minutes at 37°C. Results are expressed as the percentage of saturable binding in the presence of no unlabeled peptide added. Results are from three experiments, and in each experiment each point was determined in duplicate.

with the selective antagonists (FIG. 2), for each ligand potencies were L-365,260 (IC_{50} = 2 nM) = 30 × L-364,718 = 300 × CBZ-CCK-27-32-NH$_2$ = 1,000 × CR-1409 = 1,000,000 × proglumide, Bt$_2$ cGMP. These data are similar to those reported for CCK_B receptors in other cell preparations[3,10,57] (TABLE 1). Therefore, binding studies give no evidence for CCK_A receptors; however, this does not disprove their existence because they might be present in such small numbers that they are not being detected in the binding studies.

By contrast to the binding studies, functional studies measuring pepsinogen release suggest that both CCK_A and CCK_B receptors might be involved in mediating pepsinogen release by CCK/gastrin peptides in guinea pig chief cells.[37] CCK-8 caused detectable pepsinogen release at 0.01 nM, half-maximal release at 0.3 nM, and maximal release at 10 nM (FIG. 3). By contrast, gastrin-17-I was 180-fold less potent, desulfated CCK-8 was 900-fold less potent, and CCK-4 4,000-fold less potent. Furthermore, similar to findings in another study,[37] even maximally effective concentrations of CCK-4 or gastrin-17-I were less efficacious than CCK-8 or desulfated CCK-8. These data suggest that a CCK_A receptor is mediating some of the

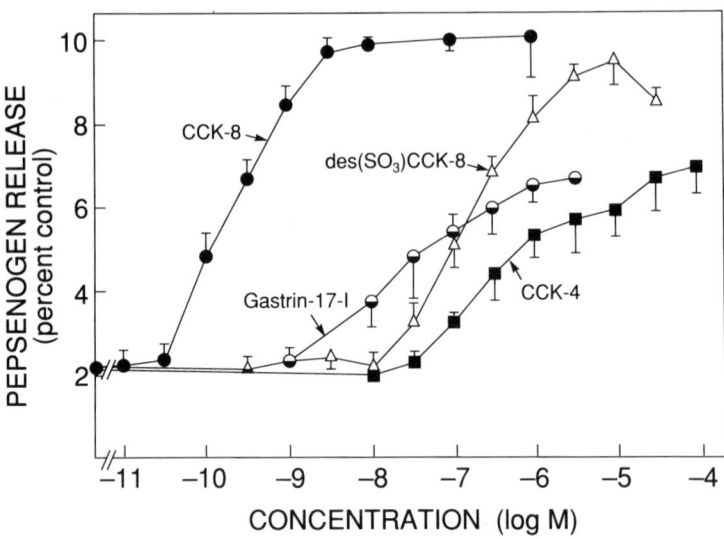

FIGURE 3. Ability of CCK and gastrin-related peptides to stimulate pepsinogen release from dispersed chief cells from guinea pig stomach. Pepsinogen release was measured after a 30-minute incubation at 37°C. Results are expressed as the percentage of cellular pepsinogen release during incubation. Data are modified from references 36 and 37.

pepsinogen secretion seen with these peptides because of the marked effect of the presence of a sulfate moiety in CCK on potency. Similar to pepsinogen release, both CCK-8 and gastrin-17-I stimulated changes in $[Ca^{2+}]_i$ and inositol phosphates (FIG. 4), with gastrin being less efficacious than CCK-8. In other cell systems, CCK_A and CCK_B receptors have both been coupled to activation of phospholipase C, resulting in stimulation of increases in $[Ca^{2+}]_i$ and inositol phosphates.[53,58–60] However, the fact that gastrin-17-I is less efficacious suggests that it is either a partial agonist at the CCK_A receptor or is stimulating changes in cellular function interacting with a CCK_B receptor. To explore this possibility further, increasing concentrations of gastrin-17-I were combined with a maximally effective concentration of CCK-8 (FIG. 5). If gastrin-17-I was a partial agonist at the CCK_A receptor, it should inhibit the action of CCK-8 at this receptor with high concentrations, as shown in the figure by the dotted line which shows the predicted curve. The maximal effect of CCK-8 was not altered by increasing concentrations of gastrin-17-I, suggesting that CCK-8 and gastrin-17-I are stimulating pepsinogen release through distinct receptors, activation of which results in different efficacies (FIG. 5).

In summary, the binding studies provided evidence for only a CCK_B receptor subtype despite the use of highly selective CCK_A and CCK_B antagonists and selective agonists such as gastrin-17-I. In contrast, the functional studies suggested the presence of a functional CCK_A receptor and perhaps a CCK_B receptor, but the data were inconclusive. To resolve this more clearly, studies were done using the highly selective CCK_A receptor agonist A-71378[19] and the CCK_A specific antagonist L-364,718 (TABLE 1).

STUDIES ON DISPERSED CHIEF CELLS: USING SELECTIVE CCK$_A$ RECEPTOR AGONIST AND ANTAGONISTS

A-71378 was equally as potent as CCK-8 in stimulating increases in [^{3}H]IP, [Ca^{2+}]$_i$, or pepsinogen release; however, A-71378 was 15–20% less efficacious than CCK-8[36] (FIGS. 6 and 7; TABLE 2). Furthermore, with higher concentrations of gastrin-17-I, the dose-response curves for changes in [^{3}H]IP were clearly biphasic (FIG. 6). The data suggested that both CCK-8 and gastrin-17-I might be interacting with two different classes of receptors to stimulate changes in cellular function with activation of CCK$_A$ receptors, resulting in a significantly more efficacious response than that with activation of CCK$_B$ receptors.

To explore this possibility further, the effect of a selective CCK$_A$ (A-71378) or CCK$_B$ (gastrin-17-I) agonist on cell function in the presence of the CCK$_A$ receptor antagonist L-364,718 was determined[36] (FIGS. 7 and 8; TABLE 2). This concentration

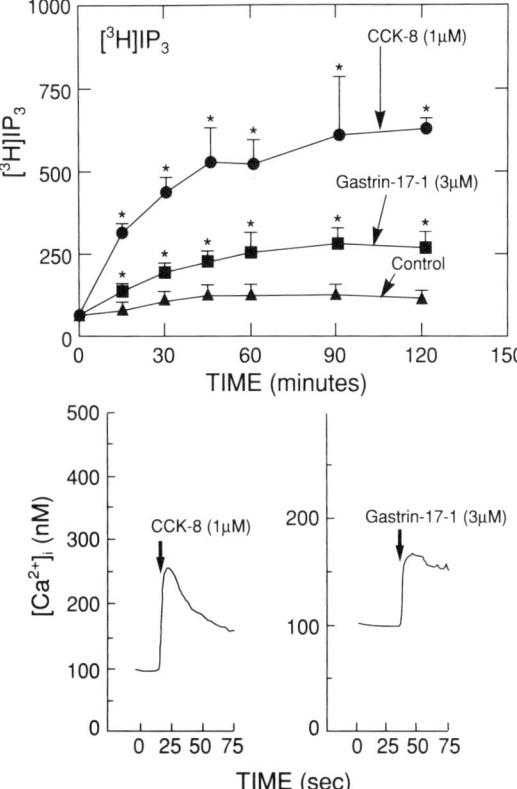

FIGURE 4. Ability of CCK and gastrin to increase [^{3}H]IP$_3$ (*top panel*) and alter cytosolic calcium [Ca^{2+}]$_i$ levels (*bottom panel*) in dispersed chief cells from guinea pig stomach. *Top panel* shows the time course of changes in [^{3}H]IP$_3$ after loading dispersed chief cells with myo-[2-^{3}H]-inositol. Data are modified from ref. 36. The *bottom panel* shows the change in [Ca^{2+}]$_i$ after loading chief cells with 1 μM fura-2/AM for 30 minutes at 37°C.

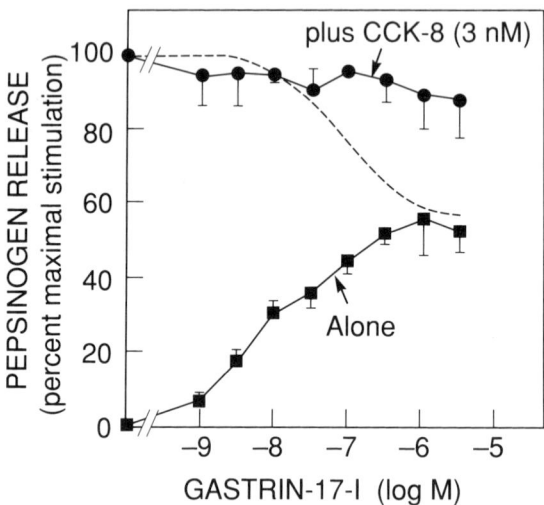

FIGURE 5. Lack of effect of gastrin-17-I on CCK-8-stimulated pepsinogen release from dispersed gastric chief cells. Pepsinogen secretion is expressed as the percentage of stimulation caused by 3 nM CCK-8 alone. *Dashed line* refers to hypothetical values assuming gastrin-17-I interacts with the same receptors as CCK-8 calculated using the $R = [(R_1C/K_1) + (R_2B/K_2)]/[C/K_1 + (B/K_2) + 1]$, where R is the calculated response, R_1 is the maximal stimulation by CCK-8 alone, R_2 is the maximal stimulation by gastrin-17-I alone, C is the concentration of CCK-8, B is the concentration of gastrin-17-I, K_1 is the concentration of CCK-8 that causes half-maximal stimulation of pepsinogen release, and K_2 is the concentration of gastrin-17-I that causes half-maximal stimulation of pepsinogen release. Data are modified from reference 37.

of L-364,718 was used because in previous studies it caused 90% inhibition of binding to CCK_A receptors with no effect on interaction with CCK_B receptors.[10,15] L-364,718 (0.1 μM) completely inhibited the ability of A-71378 up to concentrations of 10 nM for increases in [^{3}H]IP or 1 nM A-71378 for pepsinogen release (FIG. 7), A-71378 concentrations that caused maximal stimulation when L-364,718 was not present (FIG. 7). In contrast, CCK-8 continued to cause 10–20% maximal stimulation over

TABLE 2. Ability of Various CCK/Gastrin-Related Peptides to Stimulate Pepsinogen Release, Increase [Ca^{2+}]$_i$, and Stimulate Accumulation of [^{3}H]IP$_3$ in Dispersed Chief Cells from Guinea Pig Stomach

Agent	EC_{50} (nM)		
	Pepsinogen Release	Increase in [Ca^{2+}]$_i$	Increase in [^{3}H]IP$_3$
A-71378	0.2 ± 0.1	1.4 ± 0.5	2.0 ± 0.1
CCK-8	0.3 ± 0.1	1.8 ± 0.3	1.7 ± 0.3
des(SO$_3$)CCK-8	280 ± 65	1,300 ± 120	420 ± 70
Gastrin-17-I	55 ± 20	3,600 ± 70	>5,000
Gastrin-17-I + L-364,718 (0.1 μM)	12 ± 5	15 ± 9	40 ± 23

NOTE: Data are mean ± 1 SEM from at least four separate experiments. Data are modified from reference 36.

this concentration range (FIG. 7), demonstrating that this proportion of its stimulation was due to occupation of CCK_B receptors by CCK-8. Similarly, with gastrin-17-I stimulated increases in [^{3}H]IP or pepsinogen release (FIG. 8), all stimulation caused by gastrin-17-I concentrations < 1 μM was unaffected by 0.1 μM L-364,718, whereas further stimulation by gastrin-17-I concentrations > 1 μM was inhibited to the extent seen with a 1 μM gastrin-17-I concentration (FIG. 8). These data demonstrate that gastrin-17-I causes stimulation through the CCK_B receptor at low concentrations and through the CCK_A receptor at high concentrations. Approximately 15% of the maximal stimulation of pepsinogen release by CCK-8 at low concentrations is due to occupation of CCK_B receptors and the remaining 85% to occupation of CCK_A receptors. These results are in close agreement with results of another recent study[56] using primarily guinea pig gastric glands and a series of selective CCK_A and CCK_B

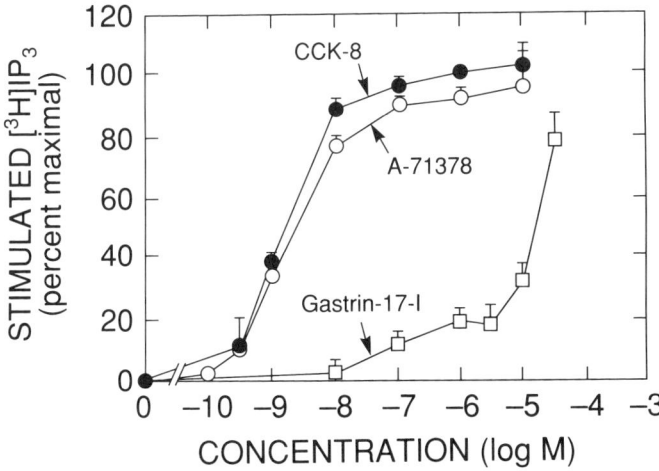

FIGURE 6. Ability of CCK-8, the selective CCK_A receptor agonist A-71378, and the selective CCK_B receptor agonist gastrin-17-I to stimulate [^{3}H]inositol phosphate accumulation in dispersed gastric chief cells. Accumulation of [^{3}H]IP$_3$ is expressed as percentage of stimulation caused by a maximally effective concentration of CCK-8 (i.e., 1 μM). Data are modified from reference 36.

receptor agonists and the CCK_A selective antagonist L-364,718 and the CCK_B selective antagonist CI-988. Similar to the present study, a close correlation was found between the ability of various agonists to stimulate pepsinogen release and cause PI hydrolysis.[56] In this gastric gland preparation, 30–40% of the gastrin-stimulated increase in pepsinogen release was not inhibited by L-364,718, but was inhibited by the CCK_B antagonist CI-988.[56] This study[56] concluded that 60–70% of the stimulation caused by CCK-8 was due to occupation of CCK_A receptors and 30–40% to occupation of CCK_B receptors.

In addition to clearly establishing the ability of occupation of CCK_A and CCK_B receptors on guinea pig chief cells to cause pepsinogen release, because of the selectivity of the CCK_A and CCK_B receptor agonists and antagonists, it was possible to compare the stoichiometric relationships between increases in [Ca^{2+}]$_i$, [^{3}H]IP, and

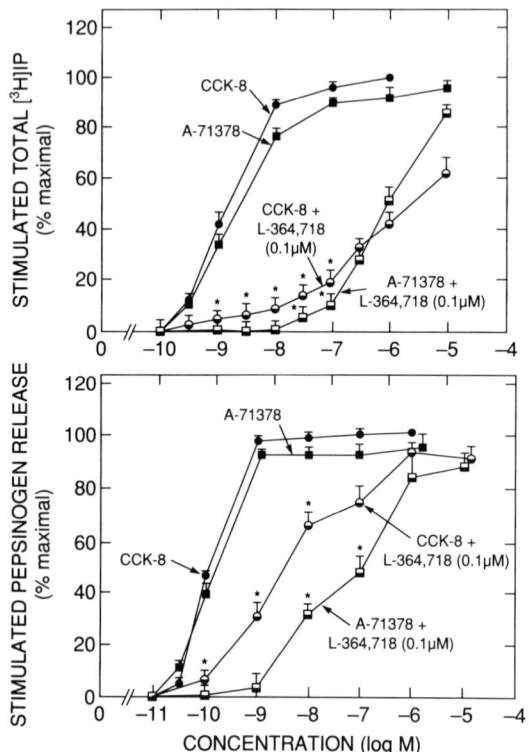

FIGURE 7. Effect of L-364,718 on CCK-8 or A-71378 stimulated increases in [^{3}H]IP (*top*) or pepsinogen release (*bottom*). Chief cells were incubated with the indicated concentration of CCK-8 or A-71378 with 0.1 μM L-364,718 present or absent. Accumulation of [^{3}H]IP is expressed as the percentage of stimulation caused by a maximally effective concentration of CCK-8 (i.e., 1 μM). Significant increase over incubation containing no additives. Data are modified from reference 36.

pepsinogen release with each receptor.[36] Because the ability of A-71378 to increase [^{3}H]IP or [Ca^{2+}]$_i$ up to a concentration of 10 nM could be completely inhibited by L-364,718, this represented only stimulation by occupation of the CCK_A receptor (FIG. 7). In contrast, because the CCK_A-specific antagonist L-364,718 did not inhibit stimulation of the initial component of the biphasic dose-response curve with gastrin-17-I for any changes in cellular function, this represented activation entirely of the CCK_B receptor (FIG. 8). CCK_A receptor activation resulted in superimposible dose-response curves for changes in [Ca^{2+}]$_i$ and [^{3}H]IP$_3$ (FIG. 9, bottom) with half-maximal effects at 1–2 nM, whereas the dose-response curve for pepsinogen release was to the left with a half-maximal effect at 0.2 nM (FIG. 9, bottom). Therefore, maximal stimulation of pepsinogen release was seen with a 30% maximal increase in the intracellular mediators. For gastrin-17-I, the dose-response curves for changes in [^{3}H]IP$_3$, [Ca^{2+}]$_i$, and pepsinogen release were almost superimposible; therefore, maximal changes in pepsinogen release by CCK_B receptor activation occurred with maximal stimulation of intracellular mediators (FIG. 9, top). These data demonstrate that amplification of the calcium/IP_3 signal differs markedly for activation of CCK_A and CCK_B receptors in the same cell.[36] The results with the CCK_B receptor on chief cells are similar to those reported for changes in inositol phosphates and acid secretion in rabbit parietal cells which possess only CCK_B receptors[61-63] and for the ability of muscarinic cholinergic agents to stimulate glycoprotein release and changes in $[Ca^{2+}]_i$ and inositol phosphates in isolated gastric mucous cells.[64] The results with activation of the CCK_A receptor on chief cells are both similar and different from those for activation of CCK_A receptors on pancreatic acini.[3,65] Similar to chief cells with activation of CCK_A receptors in pancreatic acini, both the dose-response curve for changes in $[Ca^{2+}]_i$ and [^{3}H]IP are to the right of the enzyme release curve; however, the [^{3}H]IP curve is further to the right than are the changes in $[Ca^{2+}]_i$, demonstrating that intracellular amplification

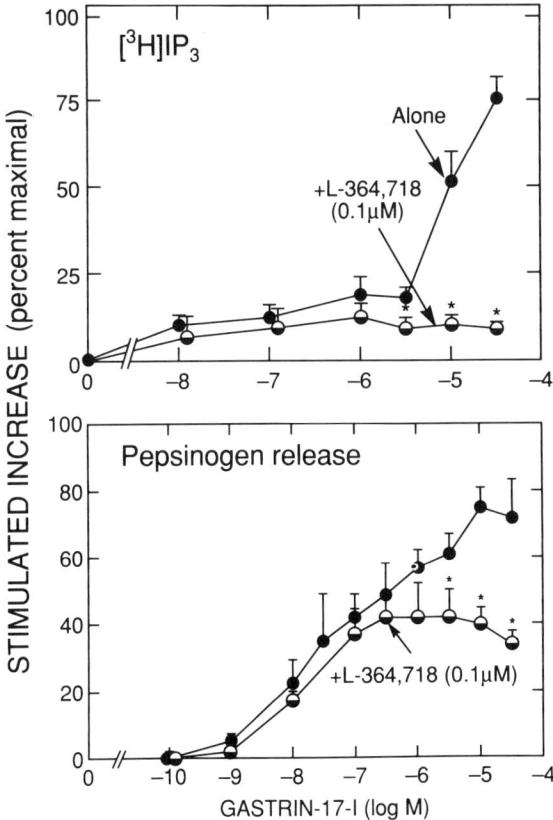

FIGURE 8. Effect of L-364,718 on the ability of various concentrations of gastrin-17-I to stimulation and accumulation of [^{3}H]IP_3 (*top panel*) or pepsinogen release (*bottom panel*) in dispersed chief cells. Chief cells were incubated with the indicated concentration of gastrin-17-I with or without 0.1 μM L-364,718. Accumulation of [^{3}H]IP_3 and pepsinogen release are expressed as percentage of stimulation caused by a maximally effective concentration of CCK-8 (i.e., 1 μM). *Significantly different ($p < 0.05$) from incubation containing no L-364,718. Data are modified from reference 36.

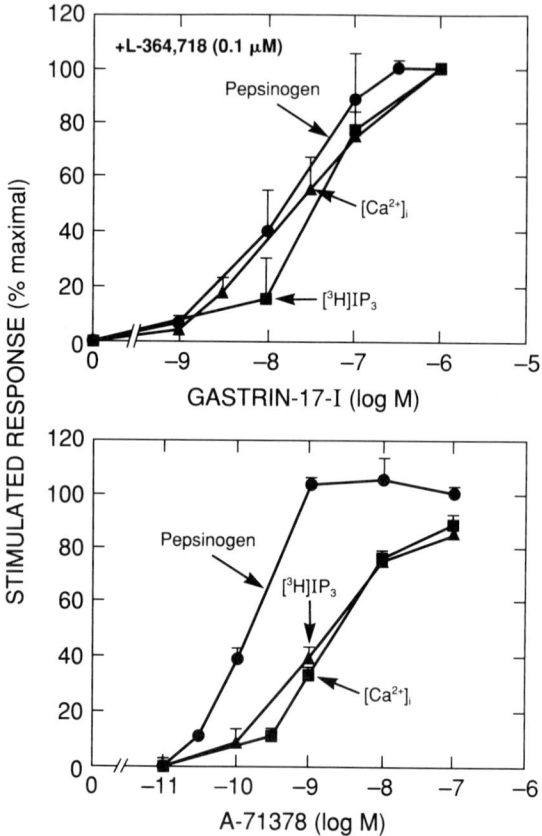

FIGURE 9. Comparison of the ability to stimulate pepsinogen release changes in $[Ca^{2+}]_i$ and accumulation of $[^3H]IP_3$ by gastrin-17-I or CCK-8. Stimulation was determined after incubation of chief cells with the indicated concentration of gastrin-17-I or A-71378 with 0.1 μM L-364,718. Data with gastrin-17-I are expressed as percentage of maximal stimulation caused by 1 μM gastrin-17-I, and data with A-71378 are expressed as the percentage of maximal stimulation caused by A-71378. Data are modified from reference 36.

with activation of this receptor differs in different cell types or could possibly represent species differences.

In conclusion, by the use of highly selective agonists and antagonists for CCK_A and CCK_B receptors, this study demonstrates that it is possible, even when both receptors are present on the same cell, altering similar intracellular mediators and both causing a similar change in cellular function (i.e., pepsinogen release), to determine the consequences of activation of either receptor. Similar results should be obtainable *in vivo* when both receptor subtypes may also be involved in causing the changes studied, if the agonists and antagonists are sufficiently stable *in vivo* and can penetrate the areas of interest. However, in human studies as in other species, it will be important to establish which CCK receptor antagonists/agonists are selective and have either no agonist activity for an antagonist or full agonist activity for an agonist.

This may be particularly true for CCK_A/CCK_B receptors, because recent studies demonstrate that some synthetic analogs such as CCK-JMV-180 can have almost no agonist activity and function as an antagonist in the guinea pig pancreas, as a partial agonist in rat, and a full agonist in mouse.[43,65,66] Similarly, the antagonist L-365,260 has high selectivity for CCK_B receptors in some species (rat, guinea pig, and man), but not in the dog.[11–14,42] Therefore, to address this issue, we have begun to assess the ability of reported CCK_A and CCK_B receptor selective agonists and antagonists to interact with and activate human CCK_A and CCK_B receptors transfected into COS-7 cells.

STUDIES ON TRANSFECTED HUMAN CCK_A AND CCK_B RECEPTORS

Preliminary data from binding studies to human CCK_A and CCK_B receptors transfected in COS-7 cells are presented in FIGURES 10 and 11 and for changes in [^{3}H]IP with human CCK_B receptors in FIGURE 12. To first establish the ability of naturally occurring agonists to interact with human CCK_A and human CCK_B receptors, their ability to inhibit binding of ^{125}I-BH-CCK-8 to each receptor transiently transfected into COS-7 cells was determined and compared with results with the highly selective CCK_A agonist A-71378 (FIG. 10; TABLE 3). ^{125}I-BH-CCK-8 was used as the ligand because it has high affinity for both CCK_A and CCK_B receptors

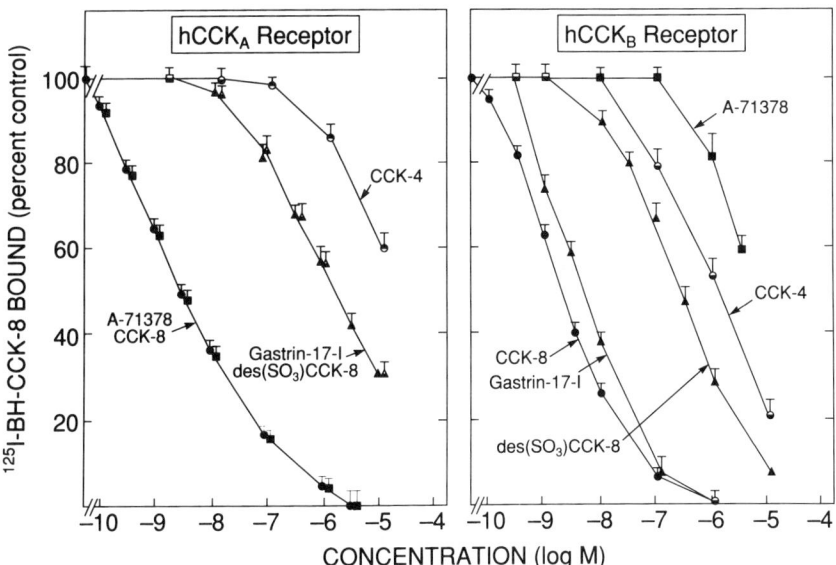

FIGURE 10. Ability of CCK-8, gastrin-17-I, and related peptides to inhibit binding of ^{125}I-BH-CCK-8 to COS-7 cells transfected with human CCK_A or human CCK_B receptors. COS-7 cells were transiently transfected with a full-length human CCK_A[4] or CCK_B receptor clone[13] using DEAE/Dextran as described previously.[4,13] Binding was determined using 50 pM ^{125}I-BH-CCK-8 and was for 30 minutes at 37°C. Results are expressed as the percentage of the saturable binding seen with no unlabeled peptide present. Data are mean ± 1 SEM of four separate experiments.

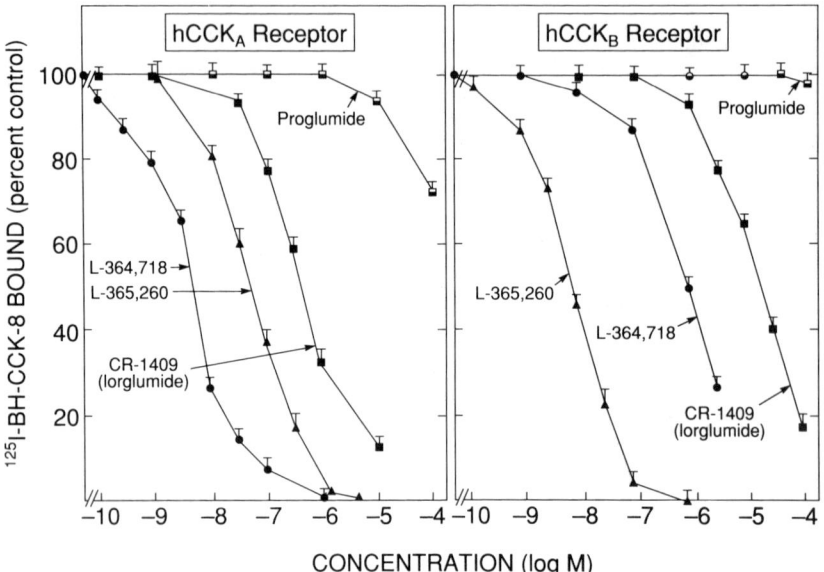

FIGURE 11. Ability of various CCK_A and CCK_B receptor antagonists to inhibit binding of ^{125}I-BH-CCK-8 to COS-7 cells transfected with human CCK_A or human CCK_B receptors. COS-7 cells were transiently transfected with a full-length human CCK_A[4] or CCK_B receptor clone[13] using DEAE/Dextran as described previously.[4,13] Binding was determined using 50 pM ^{125}I-BH-CCK-8 and was for 30 minutes at 37°C. Results are expressed as the percentage of the saturable binding seen with no unlabeled peptide present. Data are mean ± 1 SEM of four separate experiments.

(TABLES 1 and 3), and similar results are obtained with CCK_B receptors in animal studies (FIGS. 1 and 2) whether ^{125}I-gastrin-17-I or ^{125}I-BH-CCK-8 is used. CCK-8, similar to that previously reported with CCK_A and CCK_B receptors in guinea pig (TABLE 3), had a high affinity for both human CCK_A and CCK_B receptors (IC_{50} − 2 nM). In contrast, the selective CCK_A agonist A-71378 had an equally high affinity for CCK-8 for human CCK_A receptors, but a 1,600-fold lower affinity for human CCK_B receptors. These data, similar to studies in guinea pig (TABLE 3), demonstrate that this CCK analog has marked selectivity for human CCK_A receptors and thus should be a useful selective CCK_A agonist in human studies. In contrast, gastrin-17-I had high affinity for human CCK_B receptors (TABLE 3; IC_{50} − 6 nM) and had a 260-fold higher affinity for human CCK_B than CCK_A receptors. These data, similar to previous studies in guinea pig (TABLE 3) and other species,[6] demonstrate that gastrin-17-I is a relatively specific natural ligand for CCK_B receptors. For human CCK_A receptors the relative order of potency was CCK-8 ≫ des(SO_3)CCK-8 = gastrin-17-I ≫ CCK-4 with absolute potencies of 1:608:7,138. This relative order is, in general, close to that reported previously in guinea pig pancreas (TABLE 3). For human CCK_B receptors the relative order was CCK-8 > gastrin-17-I > des(SO_3)CCK-8 > CCK-4 with absolute potencies of 1:3:51:582. This relative order of potencies for these agonists is, in general, very close to that previously reported for CCK_B receptors in guinea pig pancreas and in other species.[8,10]

For the reported CCK_B receptor antagonists, preliminary studies suggest that the affinities will be similar to those reported on guinea pig pancreatic acinar cells (TABLE 3). L-364,718 had a high affinity for human CCK_A receptors (IC_{50} − 5 nM) and had a 200-fold lower affinity for human CCK_B receptors (FIG. 11). For human CCK_B receptors, L-365,260 had a similar affinity to that found on guinea pig pancreatic acini (IC_{50} − 10 nM) and was 90-fold more potent than L-364,718 (TABLE 3). These data demonstrate that similar to recent reports, the human CCK_B receptor resembles that reported in rat, guinea pig, and mouse in having a higher affinity for L-365,260 than L-364,718 and differs from the canine CCK_B receptor which has a higher affinity for L-364,718 than L-365,260.[4,11–14,42] The comparative affinity data of L-364,718 and L-365,260 for human CCK receptors in TABLE 3 suggest that L-364,718 will be a highly selective CCK_A receptor antagonist and useful for human studies. However, L-365,260 has only a fivefold greater affinity for human CCK_B than CCK_A receptors and in another study[4,13] only a twofold greater affinity; therefore, its selectivity for the human CCK_B receptor is sufficiently low that it will likely not be useful for *in vivo* human studies.

To determine if the proposed antagonists actually function as CCK receptor antagonists in human CCK receptors, studies on the ability of the various antagonists to inhibit stimulated increases in [^{3}H]IP were started. Preliminary data from studies with human CCK_B receptors are shown in FIGURE 12. Neither L-364,718 nor L-365,260 had activity at concentrations up to 1 μM. However, each inhibited gastrin-17-I stimulated increases in [^{3}H]IP (FIG. 12). L-365,260 was 50-fold more

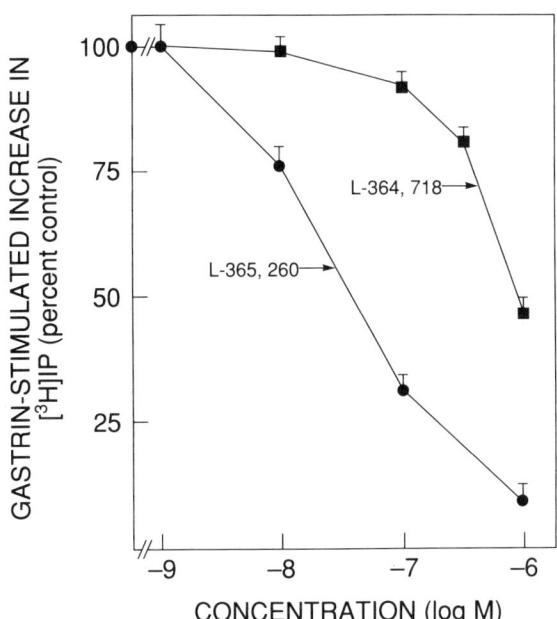

FIGURE 12. Ability of various CCK receptor antagonists to inhibit gastrin-17-I-stimulated increases in [^{3}H]IP in COS-7 cells transfected with a full-length human CCK_A[4] or CCK_B[13] receptor clone using DEAE/Dextran. [^{3}H]IP was measured as described previously.[4,65] [^{3}H]IP is expressed as the percentage of stimulation caused by 10 nM gastrin-17-I alone. Data are means ± 1 SEM from four separate experiments.

TABLE 3. Comparison of the Affinities of Various CCK Receptor Agonists and Antagonists for Human CCK_A and CCK_B Receptors Transfected into COS-7 Cells and for CCK_A and CCK_B Receptors in Guinea Pig Pancreas

	IC_{50} (nM)			
	CCK_A Receptor		CCK_B Receptor	
	Human	Guinea Pig Pancreatic Acini	Human	Guinea Pig Pancreatic Acini
Antagonists				
L-364,718	5 ± 2	4 ± 1	890 ± 150	500 ± 100
CR-1409 (lorglumide)	520 ± 120	200 ± 10	12,800 ± 1,200	30,200 ± 12,900
Proglumide	660,000 ± 120,000	3,000,000 ± 1,500,000	4,130,000 ± 1,350,000	ND
L-365,260	55 ± 15	570 ± 50	10 ± 1	7 ± 1
Agonists				
A-71378	2.6 ± 1.2	0.4 ± 0.1	4,260 ± 456	300 ± 45
CCK-8	2.8 ± 1.2	0.7 ± 0.1	5.7 ± 0.6	1.5 ± 1.0
Gastrin-17-I	1,580 ± 490	1,000 ± 100	1,280 ± 217	508 ± 155
CCK-4	18,600 ± 2,000	29,000 ± 3,100	112 ± 46	28 ± 6
des(SO_3)CCK-8	1,580 ± 559	352 ± 36	2.2 ± 0.2	0.4 ± 0.01

NOTE: COS-7 cells were transiently transfected with human CCK_A or CCK_B receptors. Data for human receptors are from FIGURES 10 and 11. Data for guinea pig receptors are from references 8, 10, 15, and 19.

potent than L-364,718 in inhibiting 10 nM gastrin-17-I-stimulated [^{3}H]IP, and these data are in close agreement with the results of the binding studies (TABLE 3).

These preliminary data suggest that, using this transfected cell system, it will be possible to obtain good pharmacological data about the relative affinities of the different CCK receptor agonists and antagonists for human CCK_A and CCK_B receptors. Furthermore, it will be possible to determine if they have full or partial agonist activity or behave as pure antagonists. Therefore, it should be possible to identify which compounds should be useful to distinguish CCK_A and CCK_B receptors in humans even when present on the same cell.

REFERENCES

1. WANK, S. A., R. HARKINS, R. T. JENSEN, H. SHAPIRA, D. E. DEWEERTH & T. S. SLATTERY. 1992. Purification, molecular cloning and functional expression of the CCK receptor from rat pancreas. Proc. Natl. Acad. Sci. USA **89:** 3125–3129.
2. RECEPTOR NOMENCLATURE SUPPLEMENT. TRENDS. PHARMACOL. SCI., JAN. 1991.
3. JENSEN, R. T., S. A. WANK, W. H. ROWLEY, S. SATO & J. D. GARDNER. 1989. Interactions of cholecystokinin with pancreatic acinar cells: A well-studied model of a peripheral action of CCK. Trends Pharmacol. Sci. **10:** 418–423.
4. DeWeerth, A., J. R. Pisegna & S. A. Wank. 1993. Gallbladder and pancreas possess identical CCKA receptor subtypes: Receptor cloning and expression. Am. J. Physiol., in press.
5. SCHJOLDAGER, B., J. PARK, A. H. JOHNSEN, T. YAMADA & J. F. REHFELD. 1991. Cionin, a protochordean hybrid of cholecystokinin and gastrin: Biological activity in mammalian systems. Am. J. Physiol. **260:** G977–G982.
6. SANKARAN, H., I. D. GOLDFINE, C. W. DEVENEY, K. Y. WONG & J. A. WILLIAMS. 1980. Binding of cholecystokinin to high affinity receptors on isolated rat pancreatic acini. J. Biol. Chem. **255:** 1849–1853.
7. JENSEN, R. T., G. F. LEMP & J. D. GARDNER. 1980. Interaction of cholecystokinin with specific membrane receptors on pancreatic acinar cells. Proc. Natl. Acad. Sci. USA **77:** 2079–2083.
8. HUANG, S. C., D.-H. YU, S. A. WANK, S. A. MANTEY, J. D. GARDNER & R. T. JENSEN. 1989. Importance of sulfation of gastrin or cholecystokinin (CCK) in determining affinity for gastrin and CCK receptors. Peptides **10:** 785–789.
9. JORPES, J. E. & V. MUTT, Eds. 1973. Handbook of Experimental Pharmacology. Secretin, Cholecystokinin, Pancreozymin.: 1–376. Springer-Verlag. Berlin, Heidelberg.
10. YU, D.-H., M. NOGUCHI, Z.-C. ZHOU, M. L. VILLANUEVA, J. D. GARDNER & R. T. JENSEN. 1987. Characterization of gastrin receptors on guinea pig pancreatic acini. Am. J. Physiol. (Gastrointest. Liver Physiol. 16) **253:** G793–G801.
11. WANK, S. A., J. R. PISEGNA & A. DEWEERTH. 1992. Brain and gastrointestinal cholecystokinin receptor family: Structure and functional expression. Proc. Natl. Acad. Sci. USA **89:** 8691–8695.
12. KOPIN, A. S., Y. M. LEE, E. W. MCBRIDE, L. J. MILLER, M. LU, H. Y. LIN, L. F. KOLAKOWSKI, JR. & M. BEINBORN. 1992. Expression cloning and characterization of the canine parietal cell gastrin receptor. Proc. Natl. Acad. Sci. USA **89:** 3605–3609.
13. PISEGNA, J. R., A. DEWEERTH, K. HUPPI & S. A. WANK. 1992. Molecular cloning of the human brain and gastric cholecystokinin receptor; structure, functional expression and chromosomal localization. Biochem. Biophys. Res. Comm. **189:** 296–303.
14. LEE, Y. M., M. BEINBORN, E. W. MCBRIDE, M. LU, L. F. KOLAKOWSKI, JR. & A. S. KOPIN. 1993. The human brain cholecystokinin-B/gastrin receptor. Cloning and characterization. J. Biol. Chem. **268:** 8164–8169.
15. YU, D.-H., S.-C. HUANG, S. A. WANK, S. A. MANTEY, J. D. GARDNER & R. T. JENSEN. 1990. Pancreatic receptors for cholecystokinin: Evidence for interaction with 3 receptor classes. Am. J. Physiol. **258** (GLP 21): G86–G95.
16. JENSEN, R. T. & J. D. GARDNER. 1991. Cholecystokinin receptor antagonists *in vivo*. *In*

Cholecystokinin Antagonists in Gastroenterology: Basic and Clinical Studies. G. Adler & C. Beglinger, eds.: 93–111. Springer-Verlag GmbH and Co. Heidelberg, Germany.
17. GULLY, D., D. FREHEL, C. MARCY, A. SPINAZZE, L. LESPY, G. NELIAT, J. P. MAFFRAND & G. LE FUR. 1993. Peripheral biological activity of SR 27897: A new potent non-peptide antagonist of CCKA receptors. Eur. J. Pharmacol. **232:** 13–19.
18. ROQUES, B. P., B. CHARPENTIER, I. MARSEIGN, et al. 1989. Development of CCK-related compounds as probes for biochemical and pharamcological characteristics of CCK binding site heterogeneity. In The Neuropeptide Cholecystokinin. J. Hughes, G. Dockery & G. Woodruff, eds.: 133–142. Ellis Horwood Limited. Chichester, UK.
19. LIN, C. W., M. W. HOLLADAY, D. G. WITTE, T. R. MILLER, C. A. W. WOLFRAM, B. R. BIANCHI, M. J. BENNETT & A. M. NADZAN. 1990. A71378: A CCK agonist with high potency and selectivity for CCK-A receptors. Am. J. Physiol. **258:** G648–G651.
20. MAKOVEC, F., R. CHRISTE, M. BANI, M. A. PACINI, I. SETNIKAR & L. A. ROVATI. 1985. New glutaramic acid derivatives with potent competitive and specific cholecystokinin-antagonistic activity. Arzneimittelforschung **35:** 1048–1051.
21. HUGHES, J., P. BODEN, B. COSTALL, A. DOMENEY, E. KELLY, D. C. HORWELL, J. C. HUNTER, R. D. PIMNOCK & G. N. WOODRUFF. 1990. Development of a class of selective cholecystokinin type B receptor antagonists having potent anxiolytic activity. Proc. Natl. Acad. Sci. USA **87:** 6728–6732.
22. HUANG, S. C., L. ZHANG, S. A. WANK, P. N. MATON, J. D. GARDNER & R. T. JENSEN. 1989. Comparison of benzodiazepine analogues L-365,260 and L-364,718 as gastrin and pancreatic CCK receptor antagonists. Am. J. Physiol. **257** (GLP 20): G169–G174.
23. BOCK, M. G., R. M. DIGARDO, B. E. EVANS, K. E. RITTLE, W. E. WHITTER, D. F. VEBER, P. S. ANDERSON & R. M. FREIDINGER. 1989. Benzodiazepine gastrin and cholecystokinin receptor ligands: L-365 260. J. Med. Chem. **32:** 13–16.
24. NIEDERAU, C., M. NIEDERAU, J. A. WILLIAMS & J. H. GRENDELL. 1986. New proglumide-analogue CCK receptor antagonists: Very potent and selective for peripheral tissues. Am. J. Physiol. **251:** G856–G860.
25. LOUIE, D. S., J.-P. LIANG & C. OWYANG. 1988. Characterization of a new antagonist, L-364,718 in vitro and in vivo studies. Am. J. Physiol. **255:** G261–G266.
26. OHTSUKA, T., H. KOTAKI, N. NAKAYAMA, Y. ITEZONO, N. SHIMMA, T. KUDOH, T. KUWAHARA, M. ARISAWA, K. YOKOSE & H. SETO. 1993. Tetronothiodin, a novel cholecystokinin type-B receptor antagonist produced by *Streptomyces* sp. NR0489. II. Isolation, characterization and biological activities. J. Antibiot. (Tokyo) **46:** 11–17.
27. HOWELL, D. C. 1991. Development of CCK-B antagonists. Neuropeptides **19**(suppl): 57–64.
28. CHANG, R. S. L. & V. J. LOTTI. 1986. Biochemical and pharmacological characterization of an extremely potent and selective nonpeptide cholecystokonin antagonist. Proc. Natl. Acad. Sci. USA **83:** 4923–4926.
29. KNAPP, R. J., L. K. VAUGHN, S. N. FANG, C. L. BOGERT, M. S. YAMAMURA, V. J. HRUBY & H. I. YAMAMURA. 1990. A new, highly selective CCK-B receptor radioligand ([^{3}H][N-methyl-Nle^{28,31}]CCK$_{26-33}$): Evidence for CCK-B receptor heterogeneity. J. Pharmacol. Exp. Ther. **255:** 1278–1286.
30. LOTTI, V. J. & R. S. L. CHANG. 1989. A new potent and selective non-peptide gastrin antagonist and brain cholecystokinin receptor (CCK-B) ligand: L-365 260. Eur. J. Pharmacol. **162:** 273–280.
31. HONDA, T., E. WADA, J. F. BATTEY & S. A. WANK. 1993. Differential gene expression of CCKA and CCKB receptors in the rat brain. Mol. Cell. Neurosci. **4:** 143–154.
32. FOURMY, D., A. ZAHIDI, R. FABRE, M. GUIDET, L. PRADAYROL & A. RIBET. 1987. Receptors for cholecystokinin and gastrin peptides display specific binding properties and are structurally different in guinea-pig and dog pancreas. Eur. J. Biochem. **165:** 683–692.
33. GRIDER, J. R. & G. M. MAKHLOUF. 1990. Distinct receptors for cholecystokinin and gastrin on muscle cells of stomach and gallbladder. Ann. N. Y. Acad. Sci. **259:** G184–G190.
34. LAMBERT, M., N. D. BUI & J. CHRISTOPHE. 1991. Functional and molecular characteriza-

tion of CCK receptors in the rat pancreatic acinar cell line AR 4-2J. Regul. Pept. **32:** 151–167.
35. DELVALLE, J., T. CHIBA, J. PARK & T. YAMADA. 1993. Distinct receptors for cholecystokinin and gastrin on canine fundic D-cells. Am. J. Physiol **264:** G811–G815.
36. QIAN, J.-M., W. H. ROWLEY & R. T. JENSEN. 1993. Gastrin and CCK activate phospholipase C and stimulate pepsinogen release by interacting with two distinct receptors. Am. J. Physiol. (Gastrointest. Liver Physiol. #27) **264:** G718–G727.
37. CHERNER, J. A., V. E. I. SUTLIFF, D. A. GRYBOWSKI, R. T. JENSEN & J. D. GARDNER. 1988. Functionally distinct receptors for cholecystokinin and gastrin on dispersed chief cells from guinea pig stomach. Am. J. Physiol. (Gastrointest. Liver Physiol. 17) **254:** G151–G155.
38. SUTLIFF, V. E. I., J. A. CHERNER, R. T. JENSEN & J. D. GARDNER. 1990. Binding of ^{125}I-CCK and ^{125}I-gastrin to dispersed chief cells from guinea pig stomach. Biochem. Biophys. Acta **1052:** 9–16.
39. LLOYD, D. C., H. E. RAYBOULD & J. H. WALSH. 1992. Cholecystokinin inhibits gastric acid secretion through type "A" cholecystokinin receptors and somatostatin in rats. Am. J. Physiol **263** (3 Pt 1): G287–G292.
40. WALSH, J. H. 1992. Gastrin physiology. Regul. Pept. Lett. **IV:** 21–26.
41. ADLER, G. & C. BEGLINGER, Eds. 1991. Cholecystokinin antagonists in gastroenterology.: 1–233. Springer-Verlag. Berlin, Heidelberg.
42. BEINBORN, M., Y. M. LEE, E. W. MCBRIDE, S. M. QUINN & A. S. KOPIN. 1993. A single amino acid of the cholecystokinin-B/gastrin receptor determines specificity for nonpeptide antagonists. Nature **362:** 348–350.
43. MATOZAKI, T., B. GOKE, Y. TSUNODA, M. RODRIGUEZ, J. MARTINEZ & J. A. WILLIAMS. 1990. Two functionally distinct cholecystokinin receptors show different modes of action on Ca^{2+} mobilization and phospholipid hydrolysis in isolated rat pancreatic acini. J. Biol. Chem. **265:** 6247–6254.
44. VINAYEK, R., R. T. JENSEN & J. D. GARDNER. 1987. The role of the sulfate ester in influencing the biologic activity of cholecystokinin-related peptides. Am. J. Physiol. (Gastrointest. Liver Physiol. 15) **252:** G178–G181.
45. MILLINGTON, W. R., G. P. MUELLER & G. J. LAVIGNE. 1992. Cholecystokinin type A and type B receptor antagonists produce opposing effects on cholecystokinin-stimulated beta-endorphin secretion from the rat pituitary. J. Pharmacol. Exp. Ther. **261:** 454–461.
46. HERSEY, S. J., D. MAY & D. SCHYBERG. 1983. Stimulation of pepsinogen release from isolated gastric glands by cholecystokinin-like peptides. Am. J. Physiol. **244:** G192–G197.
47. KASBEKAR, D. K., R. T. JENSEN & J. D. GARDNER. 1983. Pepsinogen secretion from dispersed glands from rabbit stomach. Am. J. Physiol. (Gastrointest. Liver Physiol. 7) **244:** G392–G396.
48. NOGUCHI, M., H. ADACHI, S. SATO, T. HONDA, S. OHNISHI, E. AOKI & K. TORIZUKA. 1987. Cholecystokinin-stimulated pepsinogen secretion and cholecystokinin receptors on gastric chief cells in guinea pigs. Endocrinol. Jpn. **34:** 727–736.
49. RAUFMAN, J.-P., V. E. SUTLIFF, D. K. KASBEKAR, R. T. JENSEN & J. D. GARDNER. 1984. Pepsinogen secretion from dispersed chief cells from guinea pig stomach. Am. J. Physiol. (Gastrointest. Liver Physiol. 10) **247:** G95–G104.
50. SAKAMOTO, C., T. MATOZAKI, H. NISHISAKI, Y. KONDA, M. NAGAO & O. NAKANO. 1990. Effects of CCK-receptor antagonists on CCK-stimulated pepsinogen secretion and calcium increase in isolated guinea pig gastric chief cells. Dig. Dis. Sci. **35:** 873–878.
51. CHEW, C. S. & M. R. BROWN. 1986. Release of intracellular Ca^{2+} and elevation of inositol trisphosphate by secretagogues in parietal and chief cells isolated from rabbit gastric mucosa. Biochim. Biophys. Acta **888:** 116–125.
52. TSUNODA, Y., H. TAKEDA, T. OTAKI, M. ASAKA, I. NAKAGAKI & S. SASAKI. 1988. A role for Ca^{2+} in mediating hormone-induced biphasic pepsinogen secretion from the chief cell determined by luminescent and fluorescent probes and X-ray microprobe. Biochim. Biophys. Acta **941:** 83–101.
53. TSUNODA, Y., J. A. WILLIAMS & J. DELVALLE. 1991. Secretagogue-induced Ca^{2+} oscillations in isolated canine gastric chief cells. Biochim. Biophys. Acta **1091:** 251–254.

54. CHANG, R. S., V. J. LOTTI & T. B. CHEN. 1985. Cholecystokinin receptor mediated hydrolysis of inositol phospholipids in guinea pig gastric glands. Life Sci. **36:** 965–971.
55. MATOZAKI, T., C. SAKAMOTO, M. NAGAO, H. NISHISAKI, Y. KONDA, O. NAKANO, K. MATSUDA, K. WADA, T. SUZUKI & M. KASUGA. 1991. Characterization of cholecystokinin receptors on guinea pig gastric chief cell membranes. Biochem. Biophys. Res. Commun. **174:** 1055–1063.
56. LIN, C. W., B. R. BIANCHI, T. R. MILLER, D. G. WITTE & C. A. WOLFRAM. 1992. Both CCK-A and CCK-B/gastrin receptors mediate pepsinogen release in guinea pig gastric glands. Am. J. Physiol. **262:** G1113–G1120.
57. JENSEN, R. T., S. C. HUANG, T. VON SCHRENCK, S. A. WANK & J. D. GARDNER. 1990. Cholecystokinin receptor antagonists: Ability to distinguish various cholecystokinin receptor classes. *In* Gastrointestinal Endocrinology: Receptors and Postreceptor Mechanisms. J. C. Thompson, C. M. Townsend, Jr., G. A. Greeley, Jr., *et al.*: 95–114. Academic Press, Inc. New York, NY.
58. STALEY, J., R. T. JENSEN & T. W. MOODY. 1990. CCK antagonists interact with CCK-B receptors on human small cell lung cancer cells. Peptides **11:** 1033–1036.
59. JENSEN, R. T. 1993. Receptors on pancreatic acinar cells. *In* Physiology of the Gastrointestinal Tract. 3rd ed. L. R. Johnson, E. D. Jacobsen, J. Christensen, D. H. Alpers & J. H. Walsh. Raven Press Publishing Co. New York, NY, in press.
60. WILLIAMS, J. A. & D. I. YULE. 1993. Stimulus-secretion coupling in pancreatic acinar cells. *In* The Pancreas. Biology, Pathobiology and Disease. 2nd ed. V. L. W. Go, E. P. DiMagno, J. D. Gardner, E. Lebenthal, H. A. Reber & G. A. Scheele.: 167–189. Raven Press. New York.
61. MAGOUS, R., J. C. GALLEYRAND & J. P. BALI. 1989. Common or distinct receptors for gastrin and cholecystokinin in gastric mucosa? Biochim. Biophys. Acta **1010:** 357–362.
62. ROCHE, S., J. P. BALI, J. C. GALLEYRAND & R. MAGOUS. 1991. Characterization of a gastrin-type receptor on rabbit gastric parietal cells using L365,260 and L364,718. Am. J. Physiol. **260:** G182–G188.
63. ROCHE, S. & R. MAGOUS. 1989. Gastrin and CCK-8 induce inositol 1,4,5-trisphosphate formation in rabbit gastric parietal cells. Biochim. Biophys. Acta **1014:** 313–318.
64. SEIDLER, U. & A. PFEIFFER. 1991. Inositol phosphate formation and [Ca2+]i in secretagogue-stimulated rabbit gastric mucous cells. Am. J. Physiol. **260:** G133–G141.
65. ROWLEY, W. H., S. SATO, S.-C. HUANG, D. M. COLLADO-ESCOBAR, M. A. BEAVEN, L.-H. WANG, J. MARTINEZ, J. D. GARDNER & R. T. JENSEN. 1990. Cholecystokinin-induced formation of inositol phosphates in pancreatic acini. Am. J. Physiol. (Gastrointest. Liver Physiol. 22) **259:** G655–G665.
66. SATO, S., H. A. STARK, J. MARTINEZ, M. A. BEAVEN, R. T. JENSEN & J. D. GARDNER. 1989. Receptor occupation, calcium mobilization and amylase release in pancreatic acini: effect of CCK-JMV-180. Am. J. Physiol. (Gastrointest. Liver Physiol. 20) **257:** G202–G209.

Novel CCK Analogs for Studying CCK-B Receptor

CHIZUKO YANAIHARA,[a,e] ATSUKAZU KUWAHARA,[b]
MUTSUAKI SUZUKI,[c] MINORU HOSHINO,[c] MIN LI,[d]
LI QIN ZHENG,[d] KAZUHISA KASHIMOTO,[d] YASUO
TAKEDA,[d] KAZUAKI IGUCHI,[d] TOHORU MOCHIZUKI,[d]
AND NOBORU YANAIHARA[d]

[a]*Laboratory of Pharmaceutical Sciences*
Osaka University School of Medicine
Suita-shi, Osaka, Japan

[b]*National Institute for Physiological Sciences*
Okazaki-shi, Aichi, Japan

[c]*Laboratory of Environmental Metabolism*
Graduate School of Nutritional and Environmental Sciences and
[d]*Laboratory of Bioorganic Chemistry*
School of Pharmaceutical Sciences
University of Shizuoka
Shizuoka-shi, Shizuoka, Japan

Cholecystokinin (CCK) is a typical brain-gut peptide that localizes not only in the endocrine system but also in the central and peripheral nervous systems and that exhibits various biological activities in different mammalian tissues and organs. Although tissue forms of CCK-related peptides have been identified and sequenced, it has still not been established which forms are released into blood as proper hormone and/or transmitter. CCK-8 possesses the full biological properties of CCK, and structure-activity studies of CCK, which have been carried out in several laboratories worldwide, have been devoted mainly to CCK-8 or CCK-7.

In an earlier study,[1] we demonstrated dissociation of pancreatic exocrine-stimulating (PZ) activity from gallbladder-contracting (CCK) activity in N$^\alpha$-succinylated [D-Trp^3]-CCK-7 (Suc-[D-Trp^3]-CCK-7) in anesthetized dogs. Several other synthetic analogs of CCK-7 and CCK-8, in which the Gly residue was substituted, as well as the [D-Trp^3] analog were also shown to possess full or almost full PZ activities in anesthetized rats as compared with CCK-8, whereas they were considerably less potent in CCK activity in anesthetized guinea pigs. These observations suggested the possible existence of multi-subtypes of CCK receptor in the gut. We then proposed the usefulness of synthetic analogs of CCK-7 and CCK-8 as tools for distinguishing between receptors associated with CCK and PZ activities. Subsequently, we succeeded in differentiating CCK binding properties of rat pancreatic and brain receptors with the use of various synthetic CCK COOH-terminal-related peptides and analogs.[2] Our results, together with recent progress in research on CCK receptors in other laboratories, encouraged us to extend our study on characterization of CCK receptors in various tissues specifically with the use of synthetic CCK

---

[e]Present address: 2-2 Yamadaoka, Suita-shi, Osaka-fu 565, Japan.

analogs. We thus continued our efforts to develop synthetic analogs of CCK-7 and CCK-8 which are considered appropriate for the study.

CCK-8–RELATED PEPTIDES AND RAT BRAIN AND PANCREATIC RECEPTORS

We had clearly demonstrated differences in binding affinities of rat brain and pancreatic acini plasma membrane preparations for various synthetic peptides and analogs related to CCK-8 and CCK-7.[2] Typical inhibition curves of some of our synthetic peptides against ^{3}H-propionyl CCK-8 binding to the brain and pancreas membrane preparations are shown in FIGURE 1. The relative potencies of the peptides examined to inhibit ^{3}H-propionyl CCK-8 binding paralleled those in the cerebral cortex, striatum, hypothalamus, and hippocampus membrane preparations.[2] TABLE 1 indicates IC$_{50}$ values of the inhibitory activities of synthetic peptides

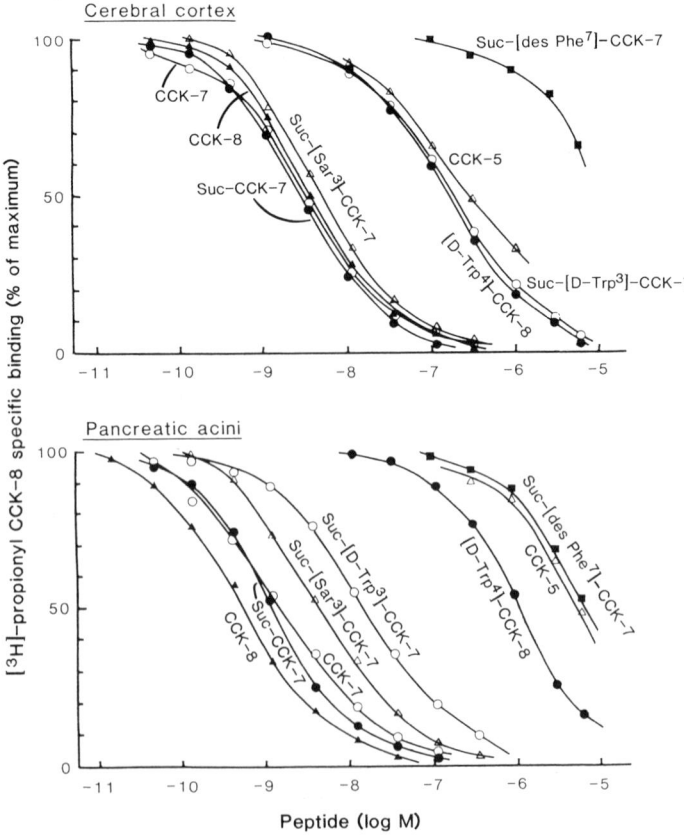

FIGURE 1. Displacement curves of CCK-8–related peptides against ^{3}H-propionyl CCK-8 binding to rat cerebral cortex and pancreatic acini plasma membrane preparations.[2]

TABLE 1. IC_{50} Values[a] for Inhibitory Activities of Synthetic CCK-8–Related Peptides on ³H-Propionyl CCK-8 Specific Binding to Rat Brain and Pancreatic Plasma Membrane Preparations

Peptide	IC_{50} Value (nM)	
	Cerebral Cortex	Pancreas
CCK-8	4.3 ± 0.3	0.63 ± 0.05
CCK-7	3.5 ± 0.5	1.7 ± 0.1
CCK-5	215 ± 38	$>10^3$
CCK-4	138 ± 10	$>10^3$
Suc-CCK-7	3.5 ± 0.3	1.5 ± 0.1
Suc-[des Phe⁷]-CCK-7	$>10^3$	$>10^3$
NS-CCK-8	39.4 ± 3.7	577 ± 50
Suc-[Phe(NHSO$_3^-$)¹]-CCK-7	8.2 ± 1.2	656 ± 57
Suc-[Sar³]-CCK-7	6.1 ± 1.2	4.9 ± 0.1
Suc-[D-Trp³]-CCK-7	152 ± 13	18.4 ± 1.0
Suc-[D-Ala³]-CCK-7	47.7 ± 7.9	69.6 ± 9.9
[D-Trp⁴]-CCK-8	176 ± 47	992 ± 17
[D-Ala⁴]-CCK-8	64.7 ± 8.4	$>10^3$

[a]Values are mean ± SEM for IC_{50} values calculated by Hill analysis in independent experiments.

in rat cerebral cortex and pancreatic acini plasma membrane preparations. The binding potencies of CCK-8–related analogs in the pancreatic acini preparation are relatively parallel to the *in vivo* PZ activities of the corresponding peptides.[1]

Suc-CCK-7 was as potent as CCK-8 in both brain and pancreas assay systems. The NH$_2$-terminal Asp of CCK-8 is not essentially involved in CCK-8 binding to either receptor. Steigerwalt and Williams[3] reported that CCK-4 is the minimum fully active agonist for CCK-B receptor. The relative binding potencies of CCK-5 and CCK-4 against CCK-8 in our systems were two to three orders of magnitude greater in the brain than in the pancreas. In the brain system, IC_{50} values of the two shortened peptides were 30–50 times as high as that of CCK-8. It is already known that the potencies of tetragastrin (CCK-4) are about one tenth those of gastrin-17 in various gastrin actions. Suc-[des Phe⁷]-CCK-7, lacking the COOH-terminal Phe moiety of CCK, showed little activity in both brain and pancreatic receptors, indicating, as already known,[4] the crucial role of the Phe residue for CCK-8 binding to both receptors.

With the use of nonsulfated CCK-8 (NS-CCK-8), the critical role of O-sulfated Tyr of CCK-8 was confirmed in recognition of the pancreatic binding site, but not the cerebral cortex binding site. We had thus synthesized Suc-CCK-7 analogs in which O-sulfated Tyr was substituted. In fact, Suc-[Phe(NHSO$_3^-$)¹]-CCK-7 showed significantly high selectivity for the brain cortical receptor. The peptide retains substantially full binding activity for the brain receptor as compared with CCK-8, whereas the potency of its binding to the pancreatic receptor is four orders of magnitude less than that of CCK-8. More recently, McCort-Tranchepain *et al.*[5] reported that replacement of Tyr O-sulfate by *p*-carboxylmethyl-Phe in CCK-8 retained considerably high affinity for CCK-B receptor.

Dibutyryl (db) cGMP is known to be a potent CCK-A receptor antagonist, and Miller *et al.*[6] described that the db-cGMP might interact directly with CCK, thereby blocking the region of the peptide, probably COOH-terminal portion, that binds to the receptor. We observed a distinct discrepancy in the inhibiting activities of db-cGMP and some other nucleotides against ³H-propionyl CCK-8 binding to the

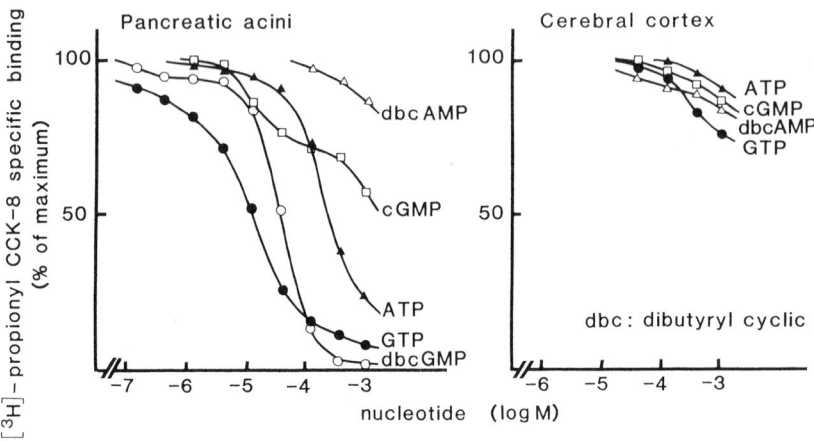

FIGURE 2. Inhibition curves of nucleotides against ^{3}H-propionyl CCK-8 binding to rat cerebral cortex and pancreatic acini plasma membrane preparations. Experiments were carried out according to procedures described in reference 2.

pancreatic acini and cerebral cortex plasma membrane preparations (FIG. 2). The nucleotides inhibited dose-dependently the binding of ^{3}H-propionyl CCK-8 to the pancreatic receptor but not to the brain receptor. On the basis of this observation together with our results showing binding selectivity of CCK-5, CCK-4, nonsulfated CCK-8, and Suc-[Phe(NHSO$_3^-$)^1]-CCK-7 to the brain receptor, it is assumed that a major part of the CCK-8 molecule that participates in interaction of the molecule with the brain cortical receptor is confined rather to its COOH-terminal half portion, whereas that for the pancreatic receptor is localized in the NH$_2$-terminal half portion of the molecule. Therefore, in combination with the explanation by Miller et al.,[6] the nucleotides may interact with the NH$_2$-terminal region of CCK-8 molecule so that the peptide can no longer bind to the pancreatic receptor.

The hypothesis that the NH$_2$-terminal part of CCK-8 participates in the direct interaction of the molecule with the pancreatic receptor is further supported by our observation with synthetic analogs of CCK-8 and CCK-7 in which Gly residue was substituted. That is, synthetic analogs in which Gly in CCK-8 or CCK-7 was substituted by D-Trp, D-Ala, or Sar showed more widely varied activities to displace ^{3}H-propionyl CCK-8 in the pancreatic acini preparation than in the cerebral cortex preparation (FIG. 1) (TABLE 1). The pancreatic receptor distinguishes more sensitively the changes in the amino acid side chain in Gly position or/and in conformation which is determined by the substituent for Gly, whereas the brain cortical receptor is less sensitive to such changes. The relative potency of Suc-[D-Trp^3]-CCK-7 against CCK-8 in inhibition of labeled CCK-8 binding to the brain cortical receptor was almost comparable to that in the pancreatic receptor. This supports a discrepancy in CCK-8 binding properties of the brain and gallbladder receptors, because Suc-[D-Trp^3]-CCK-7 has little CCK activity, though in vivo.

Substitution of Gly with D-Trp or D-Ala affects the inhibitory activity of labeled CCK-8 binding to the pancreatic receptor to a greater extent in the CCK-8 molecule than in Suc-CCK-7. Among the Gly-substituted analogs examined, [D-Ala^4]-CCK-8 possesses the highest selectivity for the cerebral cortex receptor. Here we showed the significance of Gly, in addition to Tyr O-sulfate, as a key target for designing synthetic CCK-8 analogs that possess high selectivity for the brain (CCK-B) receptor and are useful in identifying possible subtypes of the receptor.

ACYLATED CCK-8 AND CCK-7 ANALOGS

Synthetic analogs related to CCK-8 that were recently prepared in several laboratories are mostly in an NH_2-terminal acetyl- or *t*-butyloxycarbonyl (Boc)-blocked form which are expected to be enzyme-resistant (TABLE 2). Stability of biologically active peptides towards proteolytic enzymes is especially required for their *in vivo* use. When we found that Suc-CCK-8 and Suc-CCK-7 are as active as CCK-8 in binding to the brain receptor,[2] we designed synthetic CCK-8 and CCK-7 in which NH_2-termini are protected with various acyl or carboxyacyl groups, such as glutaryl (Glt), pyroglutamyl (pGlu), phtharyl (Pht), and benzyloxycarbonyl groups.

Infusion of Glt-CCK-8 or pGlu-CCK-8 into rat suprachiasmatic nucleus resulted in significant suppression of total daily food intake, while CCK-8 showed little effect.[7] Glt-CCK-8 was significantly more potent than pGlu-CCK-8 in the suppressive activity on food intake.

Close intraarterial injection of CCK-8 into the gastroepiploic artery supplying the antral region of the stomach induced, in nanomolar concentration, dose-dependent stimulation on antral smooth muscle contraction in anesthetized dogs.[8] The injection technique had the advantage of examining local peptide actions *in vivo* rather than systemic effects. Atropine abolished the gastric contraction by CCK-8, whereas hexamethonium failed to block the contraction, suggesting that the peptide acts on the intramural cholinergic innervation of the smooth muscle cells and not directly on the muscle. Fox *et al.*[9] suggested that the pentagastrin receptor is present on

TABLE 2. Synthetic CCK-8–Related Peptides Recently Reported

Synthetic CCK-8–Related Peptides		Ref.
A. CCK Analogs Active to Both CCK-A and CCK-B Receptors		
Boc-[Nle^{28,31}]-CCK(27–33)	(BDNL)	14
Ac-[Nle^{28,31}, Sar^{29}]-CCK(26–33)		14
[L-Phe(*p*-CH$_2$SO$_3$H)^{27}]-CCK(26–33)		15
[D-Phe(*p*-CH$_2$SO$_3$H)^{27}]-CCK(26–33)		15
Ac-[2-Nal^{30}]-CCK(27–33)		16
Ac-[X-Ala^{33}]-CCK(27–33)		17
X = cyclophenyl, cyclohexyl, cyclooctyl, 1-naphthyl		
B. CCK Analogs for CCK-B Receptor		
[N-MeNle^{28,31}]-CCK(26–33)	(SNF8702)	18
Boc-[Nle^{28}, N-MeNle^{31}]-CCK(27–33)		19
Boc-[gNle^{28}, mGly^{29}, Nle^{31}]-CCK(27–33)	(BC264)	19
Boc-[gNle^{28}, mGly^{29}, N-MeNle^{31}]-CCK(27–33)		19

Ac-Tyr(SO$_3^-$)-Lys-Gly-Trp-Lys-Asp-Phe-NH$_2$
              | |
              CO—(CH$_2$)—CO
	(JMV310)	20

Boc-γ-D-Glu-Tyr(SO$_3^-$)-Nle-D-Lys-Trp-Nle-Asp-Phe-NH$_2$		21
C. CCK Analogs with Antagonistic Activity		
Boc-Tyr(SO$_3^-$)-Nle-Gly-D-Trp-Nle-Asp-O-CH$_2$-CH$_2$-C$_6$H$_5$		22
Boc-Try(SO$_3^-$)-Nle-Gly-D-Trp-Nle-Asp-NH-CH$_2$-CH$_2$-*p*-F-C$_6$H$_5$		22
Boc-[Phg^{31}, 1-Nal-N(CH$_3$)$_2$^{33}]-CCK(30–33)		23

TABLE 3. ED_{50} Values[a] for Stimulating Effects of Intraarterially Injected CCK-8 Analogs on Gastric Motility in Anesthetized Dogs[8]

Peptide	ED_{50}(ng/ml)
CCK-8	2.97 ± 0.63
Glt-CCK-8	4.86 ± 0.62
pGlu-CCK-8	4.43 ± 0.55
Suc-[MePhe^7]-CCK-7	11.87 ± 1.15[b]

[a]Values are mean ± SEM ($n = 8$).
[b]$p < 0.05$ (vs CCK-8).

cholinergic nerves of the canine gastric corpus. We therefore examined the effects of synthetic CCK-8 analogs in this system. Glt-CCK-8 and pGlu-CCK-8 were less active, but not significantly so, than CCK-8 in the local stimulating effect on gastric motility in anesthetized dogs (TABLE 3). This indicates that NH_2-terminal blocking of the CCK-8 molecule does not necessarily cause enhancement of the actions of CCK-8 in *in vivo* experiments.

It remains to be established if the discrepancy in the relative potencies among CCK-8 and its acylated analogs, Glt-CCK-8 and pGlu-CCK-8, in the aforementioned two assay systems is attributable, at least in part, to differences in ligand recognition mechanisms between CCK receptors in the suprachiasmatic nucleus and those in the stomach muscle cell associated with the suppressive effect on food intake and the local stimulating effect on gastric smooth muscle contraction, respectively; however, the animal species used were different.

CCK-8 ANALOGS AND GASTRODUODENAL MOTILITY

Our synthetic CCK-8 analogs were also examined for their stimulatory effect on gastroduodenal motility in anesthetized dogs.[10] Peptides were infused through the femoral vein, and the gastric and duodenal mechanical activities were simultaneously recorded. Doyle *et al.*[11] observed that CCK-8–related peptides traverse the liver without significant degradation. The response reached a maximum level in about 5 minutes in the gastric region and immediately in the duodenal region after the initiation of peptide infusion, but the possibility of central effects of CCK-8 cannot be thoroughly excluded in this system. The results are summarized in TABLES 4 and 5. NH_2-terminal modification of CCK-8 did not affect the stimulatory activity of CCK-8 on either gastric or duodenal motility. Nonsulfated CCK-8 showed little effect in this

TABLE 4. ED_{50} Values[a] for Stimulating Effects of Intravenously Infused CCK-8 Analogs on Gastroduodenal Motility in Anesthetized Dogs[10]

Peptide	ED_{50} (ng/kg/h)	
	Stomach	Duodenum
CCK-8	439 ± 58.5	209 ± 81.5
Glt-CCK-8	448 ± 60.5	202 ± 73.5
pGlu-CCK-8	475 ± 60.5	186 ± 50.0
Suc-[MePhe^7]-CCK-7	653 ± 52.0[b]	248 ± 50.5

[a]Values are mean ±SEM ($n = 6$).
[b]$p < 0.05$ (vs CCK-8).

system. Displacement of Phe in Suc-CCK-7 with N-methylated Phe (Suc-[MePhe[7]]-CCK-7) significantly decreased the stimulating effect on gastric motility as seen in intraarterial injection as mentioned in the preceding section, but its activity on duodenal motility was not changed (TABLE 4) (FIG. 3). This analog, Suc-[MePhe[7]]-CCK-7, also retained essentially full potency in pancreatic exocrine activity in rats (volume: 91 ± 23% [mean ± SEM] vs CCK-8) and in gallbladder contraction activity in guinea pigs (83% [62 ~ 105%], mean [95% confidence limit], vs CCK-8). On the other hand, removal of COOH-terminal Phe from Suc-CCK-7, namely, Suc-[des Phe[7]]-CCK-7, disrupted the stimulating activity on gastroduodenal motility (FIG. 3), as seen in most biological assay systems for CCK-8.

Suc-[D-Trp[3]]-CCK-7 was already mentioned as an interesting analog that selectively stimulates pancreatic exocrine secretion in anesthetized dogs.[1] Moreover, the binding activities of this peptide to rat pancreatic and brain cortical receptors were approximately one thirtieth and one fortieth of those of CCK-8, respectively (TABLE 1). This [D-Trp[3]] analog was substantially inactive to gastroduodenal motility in the system used (FIG. 3). It is noteworthy that Suc-[Sar[3]]-CCK-7 showed little activity on gastroduodenal motility (TABLE 5) even though it was almost as potent as CCK-8 in rat cerebral cortex receptor binding assay (TABLE 1).

TABLE 5. Effects of Intravenously Injected CCK-8–Related Peptides on Gastroduodenal Motility in Anesthetized Dogs[10]

Peptide (800 ng/kg/h)	Motility	
	Stomach	Duodenum
CCK-8	+	+
Glt-CCK-8	+	+
pGlu-CCK-8	+	+
NS-CCK-8	±	±
Suc-[MePhe[7]]-CCK-7	+	+
Suc-[des Phe[7]]-CCK-7	−	−
Suc-[D-Trp[3]]-CCK-7	−	−
Suc-[Sar[3]]-CCK-7	−	−

These observations suggest possible differences between CCK receptors linked to stimulation of gastric and duodenal smooth muscle contractions, respectively, and also between the gastric and/or duodenal receptors and the cerebral cortex receptor.

CCK-8 ANALOGS AND GUINEA PIG ILEUM CONTRACTION

A recent study by Forno et al.[12] provides evidence that two CCK receptors, CCK-A and CCK-B/gastrin, mediate contraction of guinea pig isolated ileal longitudinal muscle. We used some of our synthetic CCK-8 analogs to characterize neuronal CCK receptors in guinea pig ileum preparation. In the experiment, L-shaped muscle strips were used to simultaneously record circular and longitudinal muscle contractions.[13] These preparations contain all elements of the gastrointestinal tract (enteric nervous system, muscle layers, and mucosa). CCK-8 showed distinct contractile activities on both circular and longitudinal muscles (FIG. 4). In these preparations, atropine completely blocked CCK-8–induced longitudinal, but not circular, muscle

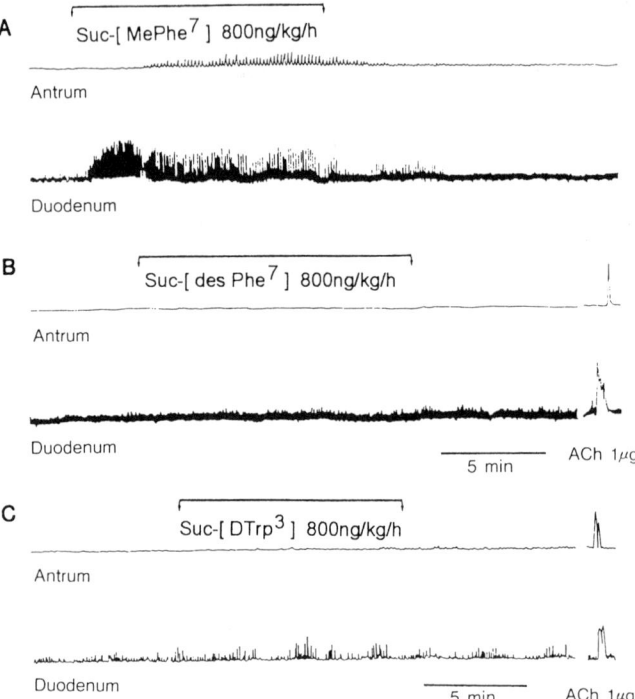

FIGURE 3. Effects of intravenously infused Suc-[MePhe⁷]-CCK-7 (**A**), Suc-[des Phe⁷]-CCK-7 (**B**), and Suc-[D-Trp³]-CCK-7 (**C**) on gastroduodenal contracting activity in dogs. A cannula was placed at the gastroepiploic artery supplying the antral region of the stomach and at the cranial pancreaticoduodenal artery supplying the proximal duodenum, respectively. All experiments were carried out during the quiescent period of the interdigestive state under anesthetic conditions.[10]

contraction, indicating distinct differences in the innervation of the two muscle layers; the longitudinal muscle layer of guinea pig ileum is innervated mainly by the cholinergic nervous system, and the circular muscle predominantly by the noncholinergic system.

As in TABLE 6, contracting activities of the CCK-8–related peptides listed are parallel in the circular and longitudinal muscles. Deletion of COOH-terminal Phe of

TABLE 6. Stimulating Effects of CCK-8 Analogs on the Circular and Longitudinal Muscle Preparation of Guinea Pig Ileum

	Muscle Preparation	
Peptide (10^{-6} M)	Circular	Longitudinal
[Sar¹]-CCK-8	+	+
[des Phe⁸]-CCK-8	−	−
[D-Ala⁴]-CCK-8	+	+
Suc-[Thr², Leu⁵, MePhe⁷]-CCK-7	+	+

CCK-8 again caused complete loss of both contracting activities on the two muscle layers. Neither NH$_2$-terminal modification of CCK-8 ([β-Asp^1]-, [Sar^1]-, and [D-Asp^1]-CCK-8) nor substitution of Gly in CCK-8 by D-Ala ([D-Ala^4]-CCK-8) did not affect the contracting activity of CCK-8 on either muscle layer; both [β-Asp^1]-CCK-8 and [D-Ala^4]-CCK-8 were as active as CCK-8 in the two muscle assay systems (FIG. 4).

Suc-[Thr^2, Leu^5, MePhe^7]-CCK-7, a compound that possessed relatively high potencies in pancreatic exocrine stimulation in rats (volume: $31 \pm 16\%$, mean $\pm$ SEM, vs CCK-8) and in gallbladder contraction activity in guinea pigs (53% [26 ~ 75], mean [95% confidence limit], vs CCK-8), was also appreciably active in these systems (TABLE 6).

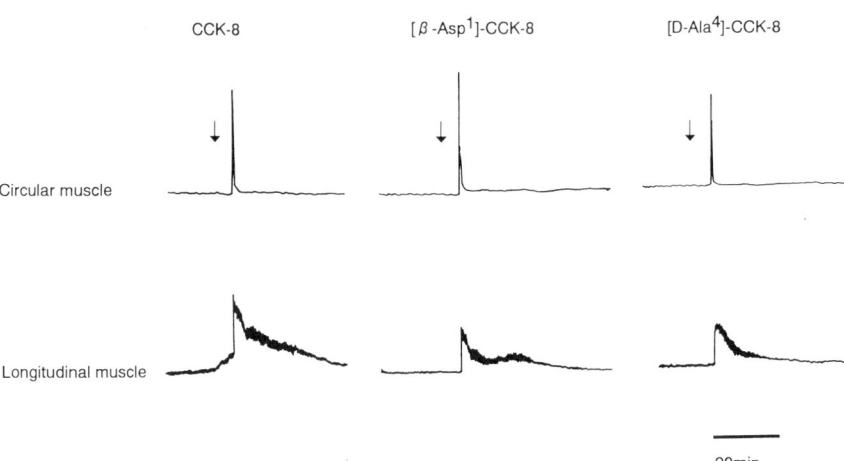

FIGURE 4. Effects of CCK-8 analogs on contracting activity of isolated guinea pig ileal muscle preparations. Experiments were carried out essentially according to the procedures described in reference 13. Muscle preparations were equilibrated in warm oxygenated Krebs solution for at least 40 minutes before initiation of the experiment. Each peptide (10^{-6} M) was added at the time indicated by an *arrow*.

Although [D-Ala^4]-CCK-8 was almost fully active in ileal muscle systems, the binding affinity of this analog for rat cerebral cortex receptor was about one fifteenth that of CCK-8 (TABLE 1). Again, with the use of CCK-8 analogs, we presented data suggesting a possible difference between CCK receptors in the cerebral cortex and ileal muscles. However, no difference between CCK binding sites in the circular and longitudinal muscle layers of guinea pig ileum was detected in this experiment; innervation of the two layers, however, is completely different.

CONCLUSION

We have synthesized over 50 kinds of CCK-8–related peptides. Some of them proved useful for direct or indirect characterization of CCK receptors in brain and gut. In fact, with the use of synthetic analogs, we succeeded in providing data that support the existence of subtypes of neuronal CCK receptors (CCK-B) in the gut. These data will be clues for further detailed study of CCK-B/gastrin receptor.

From pharmacological and pharmaceutical points of view, several recently developed elegant nonpeptide CCK receptor antagonists are most promising in CCK research. Molecular biology is disclosing amino acid sequences of CCK receptor molecules. However, for differential analysis of CCK receptors, especially in ligand-binding states, various CCK analogs are indispensable, and development of peptide analogs that can differentiate each subtype receptor, if any, in the CCK-B family is an important target for synthesis of CCK-8 analogs.

REFERENCES

1. YANAIHARA, C., N. SUGIURA, K. KASHIMOTO, M. KONDO, M. KAWAMURA, S. NARUSE, A. YASUI & N. YANAIHARA. 1985. Dissociation of pancreozymin (PZ) activity from cholecystokinin (CCK) activity by N^{α}-carboxyacyl CCK7 and CCK8 analogues with a substituted glycine. Biomed. Res. **6:** 111–115.
2. TAKEDA, Y., M. HOSHINO, N. YANAIHARA, C. YANAIHARA, J. ISOBE, N. SUGIURA, K. KASHIMOTO, Y. TAKANO & H. KAMIYA. 1989. Comparison of CCK-8 receptors in the pancreas and brain of rats using CCK-8 analogues. Japan. J. Pharmacol. **49:** 471–481.
3. STEIGERWALT, R. W. & J. A. WILLIAMS. 1981. Characterization of cholecystokinin receptors on rat pancreatic membranes. Endocrinology **109:** 1746–1753.
4. GALAS, M.-C., M.-F. LIGNON, M. RODRIGUEZ, C. MENDRE, P. FULCRAND, J. LAUR & J. MARTINEZ. 1988. Structure-activity relationship studies on cholecystokinin: Analogues with partial agonist activity. Am. J. Physiol. **254:** G176–G182.
5. MCCORT-TRANCHEPAIN, I., D. FICHEUX, C. DURIEUX & B. P. ROGUES. 1992. Replacement of Tyr-SO$_3$H by a p-carboxymethyl-phenylalanine in a CCK8-derivative preserves its high affinity for CCK-B receptor. Int. J. Peptide Protein Res. **39:** 48–57.
6. MILLER, L. J., W. M. REILLY, S. A. ROSENZWEIG, J. D. JAMIESON & V. L. W. GO. 1983. A soluble interaction between dibutyryl cyclic guanosine 3':5'-monophosphate and cholecystokinin: A possible mechanism for the inhibition of cholecystokinin activity. Gastroenterology **84:** 1505–1511.
7. MORI, T., K. NAGAI, H. NAKAGAWA & N. YANAIHARA. 1986. Intracranial infusion of CCK-8 derivatives suppresses food intake in rats. Am. J. Physiol. **251:** R718–R723.
8. KUWAHARA, A., K. OZAWA & N. YANAIHARA. 1986. Effects of cholecystokinin-octapeptide on gastric motility of anesthetized dogs. Am. J. Physiol. **251:** G678–G681.
9. FOX, J. E. T., E. E. DANIEL, J. JURY, A. E. FOX & S. M. COLLINS. 1983. Sites and mechanisms of action of neuropeptides on canine gastric motility differ *in vivo* and *in vitro*. Life Sci. **33:** 817–825.
10. KUWAHARA, A., N. SUGIURA & N. YANAIHARA. 1989. Structure-function relationship of cholecystokinin to canine gastroduodenal motility. Biomed. Res. **10:** 123–130.
11. DOYLE, J. W., M. M. WOLFE & J. E. MCGUIGAN. 1984. Hepatic clearance of gastrin and cholecystokinin peptides. Gastroenterology **87:** 60–68.
12. FORNO, G. D., C. PIETRA, M. URCIUOLI, F. T. M. V. AMSTERDAM, G. TOSON, G. GAVIARAGHI & D. TRIST. 1992. Evidence for two cholecystokinin receptors mediating the contraction of the guinea pig isolated ileum longitudinal muscle myenteric plexus. J. Pharmacol. Exp. Ther. **261:** 1056–1063.
13. KUWAHARA, A., T. OZAKI & N. YANAIHARA. 1989. Galanin suppresses the neurally-evoked circular muscle contractions in the guinea-pig ileum. Eur. J. Pharmacol. **164:** 175–178.
14. RON, D., C. GILON, M. HANANI, A. VROMEN, Z. SELINGER & M. CHOREV. 1992. N-methylated analogs of Ac[Nle^{28,31}]CCK(26-33): Synthesis, activity, and receptor selectivity. J. Med. Chem. **35:** 2806–2811.
15. GONZALEZ-MUNIZ, R., F. CORNILLE, F. BERGERON, D. FICHEUX, J. POTHIER, C. DURIEUX & B. P. ROGUES. 1991. Solid phase synthesis of a fully active analogue of cholecystokinin using the acid-stable Boc-Phe (p-CH$_2$) SO$_3$H as a substitute for Boc-Tyr(SO$_3$H) in CCK8. Int. J. Peptide Protein Res. **37:** 331–340.

16. DANHO, W., J. W. TILLEY, S.-J. SHIUEY, I. KULESHA, J. SWISTOK, R. MAKOFSKE, J. MICHALEWSKY, R. WAGNER, J. TRISCARI, D. NELSON, F. Y. CHIRUZZO & S. WEATHERFORD. 1992. Structure activity studies of tryptophan^{30} modified analogs of Ac-CCK-7. Int. J. Peptide Protein Res. **39:** 337–347.
17. TILLEY, J. W., W. DANHO, S.-J. SHIUEY, I. KULESHA, R. MAKOFSKE, G. L. OLSON, E. CHIANG, V. K. RUSIECKI, R. WAGNER, J. MICHALEWSKY, J. TRISCARI, D. NELSON, F. Y. CHIRUZZO & S. WEATHERFORD. 1992. Structure activity of C-terminal modified analogs of Ac-CCK-7. Int. J. Peptide Protein Res. **39:** 322–336.
18. HRUBY, V. J., S. FANG, R. KNAPP, W. KAZMIERSKI, G. K. LUI & H. I. YAMAMURA. 1990. Cholecystokinin analogues with high affinity and selectivity for brain membrane receptors. Int. J. Peptide Protein Res. **35:** 566–573.
19. CHARPENTIER, B., C. DURIEUX, D. PELAPRAT, A. DOR, M. REIBAUD, J.-C. BLANCHARD & B. P. ROQUES. 1988. Enzyme-resistant CCK analogs with high affinities for central receptors. Peptides **9:** 835–841.
20. RODRIGUEZ, M., M. AMBLARD, M.-C. GALAS, M.-F. LIGNON, A. AUMELAS & J. MARTINEZ. 1990. Synthesis of cyclic analogues of cholecystokinin highly selective for central receptors. Int. J. Peptide Protein Res. **35:** 441–451.
21. CHARPENTIER, B., A. DOR, P. ROY, P. ENGLAND, H. PHARM, C. DURIEUX & B. P. ROQUES. 1989. Synthesis and binding affinities of cyclic and related linear analogues of CCK8 selective for central receptors. J. Med. Chem. **32:** 1184–1190.
22. FULCRAND, P., M. RODRIGUEZ, M.-C. GALAS, M.-F. LIGNON, J. LAUR, A. AUMELAS & J. MARTINEZ. 1988. 2-Phenylethyl ester and 2-phenylethyl amide derivative analogues of the C-terminal hepta- and octapeptide of cholecystokinin. Int. J. Peptide Protein Res. **32:** 384–395.
23. CORRINGER, P. J., J. H. WENG, B. DUCOS, C. DURIEUX, P. BOUDEAU, A. BÖHME & B. P. ROQUES. 1993. CCK-B agonist or antagonist activities of structurally hindered and peptidase-resistant Boc-CCK4 derivatives. J. Med. Chem. **36:** 166–172.

The Ureidoacetamides, a Novel Family of Non-peptide CCK-B/Gastrin Antagonists

G. A. BÖHME, P. BERTRAND, C. GUYON,[a] M. CAPET,[a]
C. PENDLEY,[b] J. M. STUTZMANN, A. DOBLE,
M. C. DUBROEUCQ,[a] G. MARTIN,[b]
AND J. C. BLANCHARD

Rhône-Poulenc Rorer S.A.
Departments of Biology and [a]Chemistry
Centre de Recherches de Vitry-Alfortville
94403 Vitry-Sur-Seine, France

[b]Department of General Pharmacology
Collegeville Research Center
Collegeville, Pennsylvania 19426

The predominant form of cholecystokinin (CCK) in the central nervous system (CNS) is the sulfated octapeptide CCK-8 which shares a common COOH-terminal sequence with gastrin. Although the digestive functions of CCK are well established, its function in the brain remains largely unknown. It has been suggested that CCK is involved in a variety of pathophysiological processes in the CNS such as schizophrenia,[1] panic attacks,[2] nociception,[3] and memory formation.[4,5] The actions of CCK-8 in the CNS are mediated by specific receptors termed CCK-A and CCK-B receptors, the former being identical to the gastrointestinal receptors mediating most of the digestive actions of CCK and the latter corresponding to peripheral gastrin receptors. cDNAs encoding both receptor types were recently cloned.[6,7] Understanding the respective roles of CCK receptors in the physiology of this peptide requires the availability of potent, selective, and easy to handle antagonists. Here we describe the properties of several representative members of the ureidoacetamides, a new family of selective and soluble non-peptide CCK-B antagonists.[8]

Affinity of the ureidoacetamides for CCK-A and CCK-B/gastrin receptors was measured on guinea pig pancreas, cortex, and gastric gland membrane preparations as a displacement of [^{3}H]-propionylated CCK$_8$ or [^{125}I]-(leu$_{15}$)-Gastrin$_{17}$. As shown in TABLE 1, the ureidoacetamides are endowed with nanomolar affinity for CCK-B receptors and exhibit greater than hundredfold lower affinity for CCK-A receptors. Nanomolar affinity was also observed for gastrin receptors in guinea pig stomach, and there was a close correlation between affinities for CCK-B and gastrin receptors among several representative ureidoacetamides and chemically unrelated standards, providing another example of the pharmacological similarity between these receptors. RP 69758 and RP 72540 had no affinity (IC$_{50}$ greater than 10^{-6} M) for a variety of other neurotransmitter or hormone receptors including α_1-adrenoceptors, histamine H$_1$, dopamine D$_2$, muscarinic, benzodiazepine, opiate, serotonin 5-HT$_2$, tachykinin NK$_1$, neurotensin, VIP, neuropeptide Y, vasopressin V$_1$, and PAF receptors. Furthermore, RP 69758 and RP 72540 did not interact with dihydropyridine or verapamil binding to voltage-dependent calcium channels, [^{3}H]batrachotoxin binding to voltage-dependent sodium channels, or [^{3}H]3-PPP binding to sigma binding sites. The brain penetration of the ureidoacetamides was predicted using *ex vivo* binding techniques on mouse brain membranes following intraperitoneal or oral administration of the compounds (see Dubroeucq *et al.*, this volume).

The antagonist activity of the ureidoacetamides was assessed electrophysiologically against CCK_8-evoked excitation of hippocampal neurons in rat brain slices. Nontachyphylactic CCK-sensitive neurons were recorded in the CA1 cell body area and selected by repeated bath applications of a test concentration of CCK_8. The potency of the antagonists was evaluated by measuring the extent to which the

TABLE 1. Structure-Activity Relationships in the Ureidoacetamides Family of CCK-B Antagonists

Compound	NR$_1$R$_2$	Ar, HetAr	X	In Vitro Binding^a (guinea pig)			Electrophysiology^b (rat)
				CCK-A	CCK-B	Gastrin	
RP 69758			CH$_2$CO$_2$H	730	9.2	3.7	250
RP 71267			CO$_2$H	354	3.6	2.4	21
RP 71483			CH=NOH	97	0.76	1.2	720
RP 72540			CH(Me)CO$_2$H	1342	2.4	1.2	45
RP 73870A			CH(Me)SO$_3$K	837	0.45	0.89	3
L-365,260				510	11	4.9	2700
CI-988				797	5.7	2	980

^{a}K$_i$ in nM except gastrin, IC$_{50}$.
^{b}IC$_{50}$ in nM.

control excitatory integrated response is reduced in the presence of the antagonist. The ureidoacetamides showed no CCK_8-like excitatory intrinsic activity on CCK-sensitive neurons and concentration dependently blocked responses to co-applied CCK_8 in a reversible manner. The IC$_{50}$ values of these compounds and standards are shown in TABLE 1. This confirms the involvement of CCK-B receptors in the excitatory effects of CCK_8 in the hippocampus, as was suggested by the excitatory potency rank order seen among selective CCK-B agonists.[9]

These results establish the ureidoacetamides as a novel family of chemically original CCK-B antagonists, of which RP 69758 and RP 72540 are representative members.

REFERENCES

1. CRAWLEY, J. N. 1991. Trends. Pharmacol. Sci. **12:** 232.
2. BRADWEJN, J., D. KOSZYCKI, A. CÖUETOUC DU TERTRE, M. BOURIN, R. PALMOUR & F. ERWIN. 1992. J. Psychopharmacol. **6:** 345.
3. BABER, N. S., C. T. DOURISH & D. R. HILL. 1989. Pain **39:** 307.
4. LEMAIRE, M., O. PIOT, B. P. ROQUES, G. A. BÖHME & J. C. BLANCHARD. 1992. NeuroReport **3:** 929.
5. ITOH, S. & H. LAL. 1990. Drug. Dev. Res. **21:** 257.
6. LEE, Y.-M., M. BEINBORN, E. W. MCBRIDE, M. LU, L. F. KOLAKOWSKI, JR. & A. S. KOPIN. 1993. J. Biol. Chem. **268:** 8164.
7. WANK, S. A., J. R. PISEGNA & A. DE WEERTH. 1992. Proc. Natl. Acad. Sci. USA **89:** 8691.
8. RHÔNE-POULENC RORER, patent applications WO91/13874 and WO91/13907.
9. BÖHME, G. A., C. DURIEUX, J. M. STUTZMANN, B. CHARPENTIER, B. P. ROQUES & J. C. BLANCHARD. 1989. Peptides **10:** 407.

CCK Elicits and Modulates Vagal Afferent Activity Arising from Gastric and Duodenal Sites

GARY J. SCHWARTZ[a] AND TIMOTHY H. MORAN

Department of Psychiatry & Behavioral Sciences
Johns Hopkins University School of Medicine
Baltimore, Maryland 21205

The brain-gut peptide cholecystokinin (CCK) is a potent suppressant of food intake in a variety of species,[1-3] and a role for endogenously released CCK in the control of food intake is supported by a range of recent studies.[4-6] The vagus nerve, the primary neural link between gastrointestinal structures handling the nutrient products of ingestion and the central nervous system structures that mediate the control of food intake, appears to play a significant role in mediating CCK's effects on food intake. Specifically, a role for afferent gastrointestinal vagal fibers supplying gastrointestinal targets has emerged from a variety of lesion studies. These studies have used selective neural transections or the neurotoxin capsaicin to damage a subpopulation of vagal afferents. Such manipulations have been demonstrated to significantly attenuate CCK's feeding inhibitory actions.[7,8]

Neurophysiological studies of the activity of afferent vagal fibers arising from the gastrointestinal tract have begun to identify and characterize responses to local exogenous administration of CCK, providing potential mechanisms for vagally mediated CCK-induced suppression of food intake. In this discussion, we summarize some results from our recent *in vivo* studies of the vagus nerve in the rat. These results will be placed in a context relating CCK-induced vagal afferent activity to CCK-induced suppression of food intake.

GASTRIC VAGAL AFFERENT RESPONSES TO CCK

Davison and Clarke[9] were the first to demonstrate vagal afferent responses to exogenous application of CCK in fibers innervating the gastrointestinal tract. They showed that intravenous administration of CCK elicited an increase in spike rate in single vagal fibers with gastric mechanoreceptive fields. Raybould and Davison[10] expanded on this initial finding to suggest that these responses to CCK were occurring in capasaicin-sensitive vagal afferents. We have used these findings as the basis for providing a more complete characterization of the response properties of these CCK-sensitive fibers.

We have characterized rat gastric vagal afferent fibers sensitive to both CCK and gastric loads.[11] They are spontaneously active and respond with an increase in spike rate above baseline levels during inflation of a gastric balloon or in response to a gastric saline infusion (FIG. 1). These elevated firing rates do not dissipate once the

---

[a] Address for correspondence: Gary J. Schwartz, Department of Psychiatry & Behavioral Sciences, Johns Hopkins University School of Medicine, 720 Rutland Ave., Ross Bldg., Rm 618, Baltimore, MD 21205-2196.

final load volume has been achieved; thus, these fibers do not rapidly adapt to the load stimulus. Rather, the activity in these fibers appears to be nonadapting, in that it persists as long as the load is maintained in the stomach. On deflation of the balloon or withdrawal of the load, firing abruptly ceases completely for a few seconds, below spontaneous baseline levels. All of the gastric fibers we have identified have small (<3 mm), circular receptive fields located in forestomach and antral regions determined by gentle probing of the serosal surface. In addition, these fibers all have conduction velocities <2 m/s, consistent with their categorization as small unmyelinated C fibers, typical of visceral afferents. These fibers are dynamically responsive to a range of loads in a dose-dependent fashion; the larger the load volume, the greater the firing rate, up to 7 ml.

We examined the responses of these fibers to exogenous administration of CCK by positioning catheters in the descending aorta where the celiac artery branches off to supply the vascular bed of the stomach and small intestine.[11] Close celiac arterial

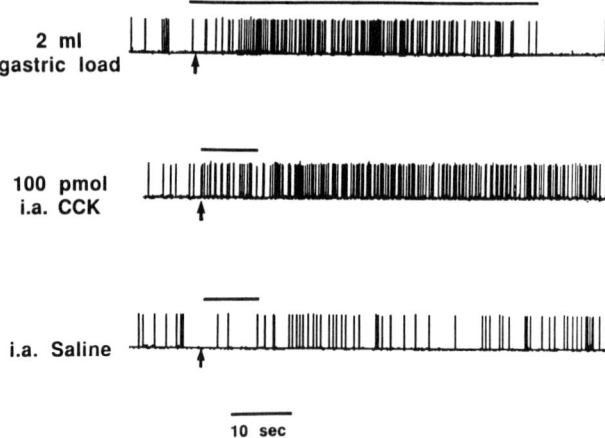

FIGURE 1. Representative example of neural activity recorded from a single gastric vagal afferent fiber in response to a 2-ml gastric load and 100-pmol intraarterial (i.a.) administration of CCK. *Bars above traces* indicate duration of stimulus application.

administration of CCK yields a significant increase in spike rate in these mechanoresponsive gastric vagal afferent fibers (FIG. 1). The increase in response rate to 100 pmol CCK lasts from 5–12 minutes. Furthermore, the 30-second firing rates generated by this dose are statistically identical to those elicited by 2-ml gastric saline loads.[11] These fibers respond to CCK in a dose-dependent fashion, with increasing doses eliciting greater spike rates, and firing rates in response to CCK vary across the same dynamic range as that seen in response to varying gastric loads. Thus, consistent with the findings of Davison and Clarke,[9] we have identified single vagal afferent fibers with gastric mechanoresponsive fields that share responsivity to both distending gastric loads and close arterial administration of CCK.

Not only are these fibers directly responsive to CCK and gastric loads, but also CCK alters the response to these loads. A single pretreatment with CCK significantly enhances the subsequent response to gastric saline loads, *after* the response to CCK administration has completely dissipated[11] (FIG. 2). Although we have not investi-

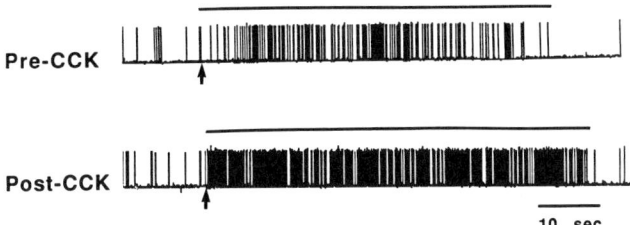

FIGURE 2. Representative example of neural activity recorded from a single gastric vagal afferent fiber in response to a 2-ml gastric saline load before (Pre-CCK) and after (Post-CCK) intraarterial administration of 100 pmol CCK. *Bars above traces* indicate duration of stimulus application.

gated the duration of this sensitization, our finding suggests that CCK acts to alter signal transduction mechanisms involved in visceral mechanoreception. Furthermore, simultaneous administration of CCK and gastric saline loads yields greater spike rates than does either gastric load or CCK alone.[12] Load volumes that are subthreshold for the production of an increase in spike rate will generate significant increases if paired with subthreshold doses of CCK. Load volumes that alone will generate significant increases in spike rate will produce even greater spike rates if paired with CCK. Thus, CCK and gastric loads act *synergistically* to excite this population of vagal afferent fibers. In fact, the dose-response curve relating vagal afferent activity to gastric load volume can be left-shifted by simultaneous application of a fixed dose of CCK (FIG. 3), demonstrating that CCK increases the potency

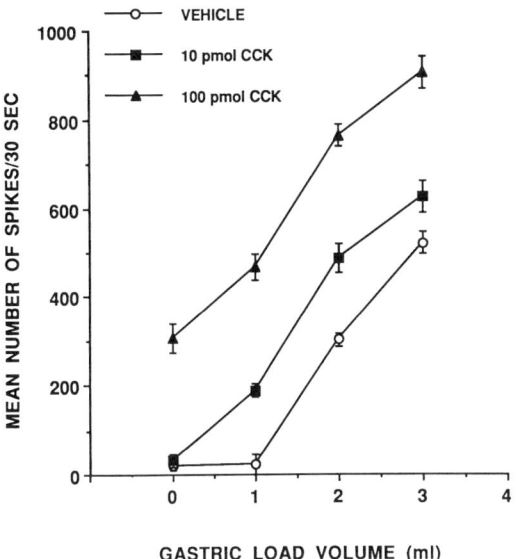

FIGURE 3. Dose-response curve relating the activity of gastric vagal afferent fibers to varying gastric saline load volumes alone (*open symbols*) and in the presence of CCK (*filled symbols*).

of gastric load stimuli. The greater the dose of CCK, the more left-shifted the dose-response curve for loads becomes.

These results of CCK-induced sensitization to gastric loads and the synergistic interaction of CCK and gastric load stimuli demonstrate that the activity of these vagal afferent fibers reflects an integration of signals arising from distinct sources. This integration could occur in a variety of ways that rely on the fact that CCK binding sites are found both in the circular muscle layer of the pylorus[13] and in vagal afferent fibers.[14] One possibility is that CCK could affect vagal activity by producing changes in the gastric musculature similar to those produced by an intragastric load. Alternatively, gastric distention may produce a local release of endogenous CCK around a vagal afferent terminal, and our exogenous CCK administration might merely mimic this local release. Finally, responses to CCK and gastric load may be independently transduced but have similar effects on vagal afferent activity. We have begun to investigate these possibilities.

The vagal afferent response to CCK may be secondary to some local contractile action that deflects its mechanosensitive ending. CCK contracts the pyloric sphincter *in vitro* and *in vivo*,[15] and this contraction is transmitted in the form of further contractions in gastric and duodenal muscle.[16] If the gastric vagal afferent response to CCK is secondary to pyloric and subsequent gastric muscle contraction, then surgical elimination of the gastroduodenal region including the pylorus (pylorectomy) should eliminate the ability of CCK to stimulate gastric vagal afferent fibers.[17] In fact, pylorectomy failed to alter the vagal afferent response to gastric loads or 100 pmol close arterial CCK. Thus, an intact pylorus is not necessary for the gastric vagal afferent response to CCK.

An adjunct of the foregoing hypothesis is that CCK may stimulate gastric vagal afferents indirectly through vagal cholinergic efferent activation of gastric muscle, which would deflect mechanoreceptive vagal afferent endings. If the vagal afferent response to CCK is secondary to cholinergic vagally mediated contraction of gastric muscle, then cholinergic blockade should eliminate the CCK response. Cholinergic blockade produced by 15 mg/rat intraarterially of atropine sulfate failed to attenuate the vagal afferent response to close celiac artery infusions of CCK, demonstrating that cholinergic vagal efferent activation is not necessary for the CCK response.

We have also begun to investigate the potential role of vagal CCK binding sites in the transduction of the vagal afferent responses to CCK and intragastric loads. CCK binding sites have been identified and undergo axonal transport in afferent subdiaphragmatic vagal branches. These binding sites may become functional CCK receptors incorporated in the membranes of gastric vagal afferent fiber terminations, where they could mediate the responses to local CCK.[14] Thus, CCK may have a direct effect on vagal afferent endings by interacting with membrane-bound CCK receptors linked to transduction mechanisms involved in the production of action potentials. We have addressed this "vagal receptor" possibility in a number of ways. Local intraarterial administration of increasing doses of the CCK_A receptor antagonist devazepide progressively attenuates and, at higher doses, completely eliminates the vagal afferent response to CCK. The effects of devazepide may be reversed by application of higher doses of CCK, resulting in a rightward shift in the dose-response curve for devazepide.[17] Thus, devazepide acts to reduce the potency of CCK and appears to act as a competitive antagonist. The parallel shift in the CCK dose response curve is consistent with competitive interaction at a single type of CCK receptor.[17]

In contrast to the ability of devazepide to block the vagal afferent response to CCK, the selective CCK_B antagonist L-365,260 failed to block the CCK response at doses up to three orders of magnitude higher than those of the A antagonists that completely blocked the CCK response.[17] Thus, these gastric vagal afferent responses appear to be mediated through an interaction with CCK_A receptors.

Neither devazepide nor L-365,260 had any effect on the vagal afferent response to 2 ml gastric loads, demonstrating some independence between the transduction mechanisms underlying the gastric afferent responses to loads and CCK.[17] Consequently, it appears that a local release of CCK is not an intermediate step in the production of vagal afferent response by intragastric loads.

In summary, we have outlined the response profile of a population of gastric vagal afferent fibers in the rat. These unmyelinated fibers have small receptive fields, respond with comparable increases in firing rate to gastric loads and CCK, and these responses do not depend on CCK's actions at the pyloric sphincter. CCK mimics and amplifies the response to gastric loads in these fibers, and selective type A receptor blockade competitively attenuates CCK responses.

The fact that vagal afferent responses to gastric loads remain while CCK responses are blocked following administration of the CCK_A receptor antagonist suggests that independent mechanisms are mediating the transduction of CCK and gastric load responses. The possibility of a structural basis for this independent transduction is supported by recent anatomical studies of Berthoud and Powley.[18] They identified single gastric vagal afferent fibers that terminate in the rat fundus in two morphologically distinct endings. One type of ending is a long lattice-like arborization that runs in parallel with longitudinal or circular muscles, seemingly ideally suited to detect changes in gastric wall muscle tension during distention. The second type of ending lies in calyx-like arborizations surrounding myenteric neurons. These two types of endings may provide an anatomical separation of functional transduction sites, one mediating distention signals and the other mediating neuropeptide activation, that would account for our ability to dissociate neurophysiological responses to loads from responses to CCK in the same vagal afferent fiber.

DUODENAL VAGAL AFFERENT RESPONSES TO CCK

Recently we expanded our search for gastrointestinal vagal targets for the actions of CCK to include the small intestine. Previous neurophysiological studies in the ferret identified small intestinal vagal afferent fibers driven by mucosal stimulation that also respond to CCK.[19] Mucosal fibers were not usually spontaneously active, they were rapidly adapting in response to mucosal probing, and the duration of the response to intravenous CCK administration was brief. In contrast, we identified a population of fibers with response profiles to loads and CCK that are very similar to those found in the gastric vagal afferents just described.[20] These fibers *are* spontaneously active and respond with a significant increase in firing rate above baseline levels when a duodenal balloon or saline load is applied (FIG. 4). The load-induced increased firing rate persists as long as the load is maintained in the duodenal lumen, and withdrawal of the load results in a brief cessation of spike activity, similar to the "off" response seen in gastric vagal afferents. Receptive fields of these units can be localized by probing the serosal duodenal surface, and these fibers have small circular receptive fields (<3 mm) along the proximal duodenum. These duodenal receptive fields did not extend to the stomach, because inflation of the gastric balloon failed to increase duodenal fiber firing rates.

Close celiac artery infusions of CCK elicited a significant increase in firing rate in these duodenal vagal afferents, lasting 5–7 minutes following a 100 pmol CCK infusion (FIG. 4). Atropine treatment failed to alter the duodenal afferent response to CCK or loads. Pretreatment with 100 pmol CCK enhanced the subsequent response to duodenal loads in these fibers, *after* the response to CCK itself had dissipated, as shown for gastric vagal afferents above. Thus, CCK also sensitized this duodenal population of vagal afferents to distending loads. Furthermore, simultaneous administration of CCK and duodenal loads resulted in greater firing rates in these fibers than did those produced by either stimulus alone, demonstrating that

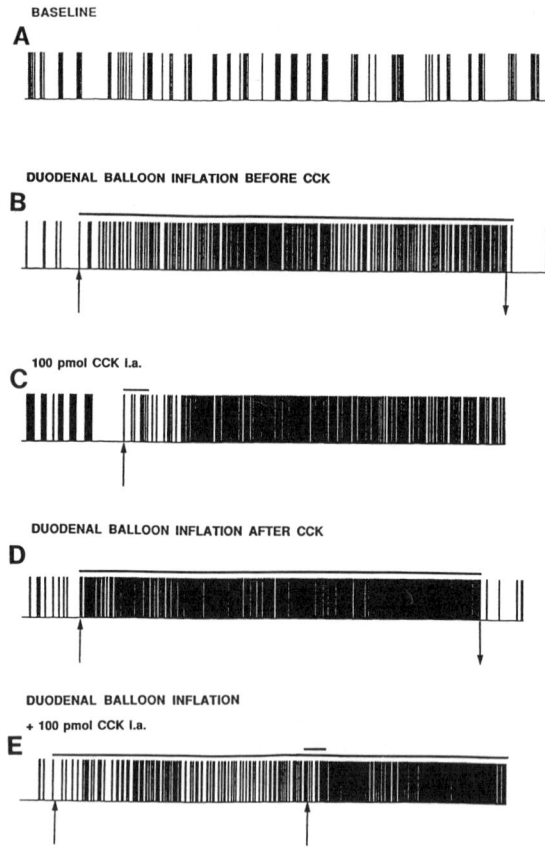

FIGURE 4. Representative examples of neural activity recorded from a single duodenal vagal afferent fiber in response to no stimulation (**A**), duodenal balloon inflation (**B**), 100 pmol CCK (**C**), or a combination of the two (**E**). In E, duodenal balloon inflation occurred at the *leftmost arrow* and CCK was administered at the *arrow* to the right. In (**D**), the duodenal balloon was inflated 10 minutes after 100 pmol CCK infusion. *Bars above traces* indicate duration of stimulus application.

CCK and load stimuli act synergistically to stimulate duodenal load-sensitive rat vagal afferents (FIG. 4). Although we do not yet know the pharmacological specificity of these duodenal vagal afferent responses, it seems likely that they, like the gastric responses just discussed, are mediated by CCK_A receptors.

Together, these data demonstrate load-sensitive vagal afferents supplying the rat duodenum respond to CCK. These fibers, which terminate at sites where CCK is likely to be released following a meal, have the ability to integrate signals arising from both the volume and composition of duodenal loads.

SUMMARY

We have begun to identify and characterize the locations and response profiles of vagal afferent fibers sensitive to CCK in the rat upper gastrointestinal tract. We found gastric and duodenal vagal afferent fibers that respond to CCK and to intraluminal loads. CCK both sensitizes and amplifies the response to loads in these fibers but may do so through separate transduction mechanisms. Thus, meal-related signals arising from the presence of gastroduodenal loads and the release of endogenous CCK can be integrated at the level of the peripheral afferent vagus nerve. These findings are consistent with behavioral results, demonstrating that combinations of gastric loads and exogenous CCK are more effective in suppressing food intake than is either stimulus presented alone.[21]

Our findings that both gastric and duodenal vagal afferent fibers are sensitive to CCK suggest that meal-related CCK may act at a range of peripheral neural sites linking the upper gastrointestinal tract to the central nervous system substrates underlying the control of food intake. The mode of activation of gastric vagal afferent by endogenously released CCK may be an endocrine action of intestinally derived CCK. Alternatively, the novel finding of duodenal load-sensitive vagal afferents close to a site of CCK release provides a potential for local paracrine actions of endogenous CCK in the mediation of satiety.

REFERENCES

1. GIBBS, J., R. C. YOUNG & G. P. SMITH. 1973. Cholecystokinin decreases food intake in rats. J. Comp. Physiol. Psychol. **84:** 488–495.
2. MORAN, T. H. & P. R. MCHUGH. 1982. Cholecystokinin suppresses food intake by inhibiting gastric emptying. Am. J. Physiol. **242:** R491–R497.
3. KISSILEFF, H. R., F. X. PI-SUNYER, J. THORNTON & G. P. SMITH. 1981. Am. J. Clin. Nutr. **34:** R154–R160.
4. DOURISH, C. T., W. RYCROFT & S. D. IVERSEN. 1989. Postponement of satiety by blockade of brain cholecystokinin (CCK-B) receptors. Science **245:** 1509–1511.
5. REIDELBERGER, R. D. & M. F. O'ROURKE. 1989. Potent cholecystokinin antagonist L-364,718 stimulates food intake in rats. Am. J. Physiol. **257:** R1512–R1518.
6. MORAN, T. H., P. J. AMEGLIO, G. J. SCHWARTZ & P. R. MCHUGH. 1992. Blockade of type A, not type B, cholecystokinin (CCK) receptors attenuates the satiety actions of both exogenous and endogenous CCK. Am. J. Physiol. **262:** R46–R50.
7. SMITH, G. P., C. JEROME & R. NORGREN. 1985. Afferent axons in abdominal vagus mediate satiety effects of cholecystokinin in rats. Am. J. Physiol. **249:** R638–R641.
8. SOUTH, E. H. & R. C. RITTER. 1988. Capsaicin application to central or peripheral vagal fibers attenuates CCK satiety. Peptides **9:** 601–612.
9. DAVISON, J. S. & G. D. CLARKE. 1988. Mechanical properties and sensitivity to CCK of vagal slowly adapting mechanoreceptors. Am. J. Physiol. **255:** G55–G61.
10. RAYBOULD, H. E. & J. S. DAVISON. 1989. Perivagal application of capsaicin abolishes response of vagal gastric mechanoreceptors to cholecystokinin. Neurosci. Abstr. **15:** 973.
11. SCHWARTZ, G. J., P. R. MCHUGH & T. H. MORAN. 1991. Integration of vagal afferent responses to gastric loads and cholecystokinin. Am. J. Physiol. **261:** R64–R69.

12. SCHWARTZ, G. J., P. R. MCHUGH & T. H. MORAN. 1993. Gastric loads and cholecystokinin synergistically stimulate rat gastric vagal afferents. Am. J. Physiol. **265:** R872–R876.
13. SMITH, G. T., T. H. MORAN, J. T. COYLE, M. J. KUHAR, T. L. O'DONOHUE & P. R. MCHUGH. 1984. Anatomical localization of cholecystokinin receptors in the pyloric sphincter. Am. J. Physiol. **246:** R127–R130.
14. MORAN, T. H., R. NORGREN, R. J. CROSBY & P. R. MCHUGH. 1990. Central and peripheral transport of vagal cholecystokinin binding sites occurs in afferent fibers. Brain Res. **526:** 95–102.
15. MURPHY, R. B., G. P. SMITH & J. GIBBS. 1987. Pharmacological examination of cholecystokinin (CCK-8) induced contractile activity in the rat isolated pylorus. Peptides **8:** 127–134.
16. SCHEURER, U., L. VARGA, E. DRACK, H. R. BURKI & F. HALTER. 1983. Measurement of cholecystokinin octapeptide-induced motility of rat antrum, pylorus and duodenum in vitro. Am. J. Physiol. **244:** G261–G265.
17. SCHWARTZ, G. J., P. R. MCHUGH & T. H. MORAN. 1992. Characterization of gastric vagal afferent mechanoreceptor responses to close arterial infusions of CCK in the rat. Neurosci Abstr. **18:** 1068.
18. BERTHOUD, H. R. & T. L. POWLEY. 1992. Vagal afferent innervation of the rat fundic stomach: Morphological characterization of the gastric tension receptor. J. Comp. Neurol. **319:** 261–276.
19. BLACKSHAW, L. A. & D. GRUNDY. 1990. Effects of cholecystokinin (CCK-8) on two classes of gastroduodenal vagal afferent fibers. J. Auton. Nerv. Sys. **31:** 191–202.
20. SCHWARTZ, G. J., G. TOUGAS & T. H. MORAN. 1993. Integration of responses to duodenal loads and CCK in rat single vagal afferent fibers. Neurosci. Abstr. **19:** 816.
21. SCHWARTZ, G. J., L. A. NETTERVILLE, P. R. MCHUGH & T. H. MORAN. 1991. Gastric loads potentiate and magnify the inhibition of food intake produced by a cholecystokinin analog. Am. J. Physiol. **261:** R1141–R1146.

Ionic Mechanisms Underlying Cholecystokinin Action in Rat Brain

P. BODEN AND G. N. WOODRUFF

Parke-Davis Neuroscience Research Centre
Addenbrookes Hospital
Hills Road
Cambridge, CB2 2QB, England

Cholecystokinin (CCK) is widely distributed in rat brain, but its physiological role until recently has been poorly understood. The development of potent and selective CCK antagonists[1] has led to clues as to the function of the peptide in the central nervous system. Particular interest has focused on the anxiolytic-like action of CCK antagonists. Using these antagonists in combination with autoradiographic studies, it was shown that most CCK receptors in brain are of the CCK_B type, but CCK_A receptors occur in discrete brain regions.[2-5]

Electrophysiological recordings from neurons contained within brain slice preparations have revealed that CCK can influence the activity of cells in a wide variety of brain nuclei. Initial studies focusing on the hippocampus showed that the peptide could depolarize both CA1 and dentate gyrus neurons.[6-8] The advent of a hypothalamic slice preparation brought the finding that CCK increased the firing rate of spontaneously active hypothalamic neurons.[9-11] More recently, CCK effects were recorded from 5-HT neurons of rat dorsal raphe,[12] neurons of rat supraoptic hypothalamus,[13] rat *nucleus tractus solitarius*,[14] and type 2 and 3 neurons of rat lateral amygdala.[15] The importance of the neuropeptide in brain function is exemplified by the most recent findings that functional CCK receptors exist in regions involved in processing of nociceptive information such as the periaqueductal gray and at either end of the *retroflexus fasciculus* of Meynert in the medial habenula and interpeduncular nucleus (Boden, unpublished data). One feature common to these reports is that the predominant action of the neuropeptide is excitatory with depolarization of the neuronal membrane leading to an increase in firing rate, but there is little information on the ionic mechanism involved or, in some instances, on the exact nature of the CCK receptor that underlies the response. The following sections discuss the principal findings in the aforementioned studies with respect to CCK receptor definition using agonist and antagonist pharmacology and mode of action.

AGONIST PHARMACOLOGY

The vast majority of CCK responses reported in the current literature have used CCK-8s as the agonist despite its nonspecific profile for CCK receptors. One feature of CCK_B receptors is their relatively high affinity for nonsulfated CCK-8 and also the smaller fragments pentagastrin (BOC-β alanine-CCK-4) and CCK-4 when compared with the more stringent requirements of the CCK_A receptor. Early studies therefore relied heavily on the use of these ligands to define the CCK receptor involved. The pioneering efforts of Dodd and Kelly[6] showed that CCK-8s and CCK-4 (but not nonsulfated CCK-8) were potent agonists when applied to CA1 hippocampal neurons. With the same preparation, pentagastrin was also found to be a potent agonist, and the demonstration of cross-desensitization between CCK-8s and pentagastrin suggested that both agonists shared a common receptor in the CA1 region of the hippocampus.[8]

Studies from Sugita et al.[15] showed that both pentagastrin and CCK-8s evoked identical responses from type 2 and 3 neurons in the rat lateral amygdala, while Boden and Hill[11] showed equivalent data from intracellular recordings of CCK responses from rat ventromedial hypothalamic neurons.

ANTAGONIST PHARMACOLOGY

Selective Antagonist Studies

The development of selective antagonists for both the CCK_A and CCK_B receptor has led to the characterization of CCK receptor types in several brain regions and perhaps more significantly it has shown that in most of these nuclei, both types of CCK receptor coexist (TABLE 1). Interestingly, it is the CCK_A receptor density that varies from region to region, while the CCK_B receptor density remains constant. For example, in the rat ventromedial hypothalamus (VMH), the vast majority of responses are a result of CCK_B receptor activation, but neurons that possess only CCK_A receptors or a mixture of the two can be found.[16] In the solitary tract nucleus of the rat[14] and the periaqueductal gray (Boden, unpublished observations), there appears to be a roughly equal density of both receptor types.

To date we know of only three brain regions that possess functional CCK_A receptors and are devoid of CCK_B receptor influence. Extracellular recordings made from a subpopulation (15%) of neurons in the medial habenula revealed that these were excited by CCK-8s but not by pentagastrin. Further proof for involvement of a CCK_A receptor in this response came from antagonist studies that showed no effect of the CCK_B antagonist CI-988 at concentrations up to 1 μM, but a block of the CCK-8s response by devazepide with an equilibrium constant (Ke) of 130 pM. The rat interpeduncular nucleus possesses neurons that are hyperpolarized by dopamine, an effect that is potentiated by CCK-8s. This modulation can be blocked by prior administration of the CCK_A receptor antagonist devazepide, but not by CI-988. In the rat dorsal raphe we showed that CCK-8s (but not pentagastrin) can depolarize some 5-HT sensitive neurons. In this instance, the CCK-8s effect could be blocked by devazepide with a Ke value of 130 pM. Two CCK_B antagonists were either inactive (CI-988 to 1 μM) or weakly active (L365,260, Ke of 724 nM) at blocking the CCK-8s response, in agreement with the presence of CCK_A receptors in this nucleus.[12]

The rat VMH is the most well-characterized brain region in terms of both CCK agonist and antagonist specificity. CCK-8s and pentagastrin are both full agonists in this preparation, and early studies showed that agonist responses were only reduced by micromolar concentrations of the highly selective CCK_A antagonist devazepide, providing further evidence for a functional CCK_B receptor in the rat VMH.[11] Novel CCK_B antagonists, notable for their structural dissimilarities, are now available. Nonpeptide CCK_B antagonists have been derived from three different approaches. The gastrin antagonist L365,260 was produced after modification of the selective CCK_A receptor antagonist devazepide.[17,18] L365,260 displays between 50-[19] and a 100-fold[20] greater affinity for the CCK_B receptor over the CCK_A receptor. Research at Lilly has produced a series of CCK_B antagonists following screening and structure-activity work based on early lead compounds, culminating in the synthesis of LY262691. This compound shows improved selectivity for the CCK_B receptor when compared with L365,260 (400-fold cf. 100-fold), but its affinity for the CCK_B receptor

TABLE 1. Summary of Pharmacology and Electrophysiology of CCK Responses in Rat Brain *in Vitro*

Brain Region	Receptor Type	Agonist	Antagonist (Ke)	Mode of Action	References
Ventromedial hypothalamus (VMH)	B	8s = 5 = 4	CI-988 (6 nM)	Block of K^+ current	Boden & Hill,[11] Boden[33]
Dorsal raphe	A	8s	Devazepide (130 pM)	Block of K^+ current	Boden et al.[12]
Supraoptic nucleus	B	8s = 4	L365260[a]	Increase in nonselective cation conductance	Jarvis et al.[13]
Lateral amygdala	B	8s = 5	Not known	Increase in resistance	Sugita et al.[15]
CA1 hippocampus	B	8s = 4	Not known	Increase in resistance	Boden and Hill[8]
CA1 hippocampus	B	8s = 4	Not known	Decrease in resistance	Dodd and Kelly[6]
CA1 (cultured) hippocampus	Not known	Not specified	Not known	Block of K^+ current	Buckett and Saint[34]
Dentate gyrus hippocampus	Not known	Not specified	Not known	Increase in resistance	Brooks and Kelly[7]
Nucleus tractus solitarius	B	8s = 4	L365260[a]	Not known	Branchereau et al.[14]
Nucleus tractus solitarius	A	8s	Devazepide[a]	Not known	Branchereau et al.[14]
Ventromedial hypothalamus (VMH)	A	8s	Devazepide (225 pM)	Not known	Pinnock et al.[41]
Interpeduncular nucleus	A	8s	Devazepide[a]	Not known	Boden, unpublished data
Medial habenula	A	8s	Devazepide (130 pM)	Not known	Boden, unpublished data
Periaqueductal gray	A	8s	Devazepide (190 pM)[b]	Not known	Boden, unpublished data
Periaqueductal gray	B	8s = 5	CI-988[a]	Not known	Boden, unpublished data

[a] No Ke obtained in these series of experiments.
[b] Ke value obtained in the presence of 300 nM CI-988 to eliminate CCK_B receptor.

per se is lower.[21] Horwell[22] used a peptoid approach to modify the smallest active fragment of CCK, CCK-4, to produce CI-988. This compound has the highest CCK_B binding affinity compared with the aforementioned compounds and is the most selective CCK_B receptor antagonist to date.[23] It is also an effective anxiolytic in a number of animal models[19,23] and enhances morphine-induced analgesia in rats.[24] We compared these three antagonists using *in vitro* electrophysiological methods to obtain Ke values for their block of pentagastrin-induced excitation of VMH neurons and our studies reveal a Ke value for CI-988 of 6.5 nM compared to 39 nM for L365,260 and 150 nM for LY262691 in this model (Boden and Woodruff, in preparation).

Benzodiazepine-CCK Interactions

Inhibition of both central and peripheral CCK responses by benzodiazepines has been reported. In the periphery, the benzodiazepines diazepam and chlordiazepoxide both inhibited CCK-induced contractions of guinea pig gallbladder[25] where the CCK response is traditionally associated with CCK_A receptor activation. In mice, flurazepam and the benzodiazepine antagonist Ro15-1788 have also both been shown to block the antinociceptive actions of intracisternal CCK.[26] Iontophoretic application of the water-soluble benzodiazepine flurazepam produced a selective block of CCK-induced increases in firing rate of CA1 and CA3 hippocampal neurons *in vivo*,[27] an effect that was reversed by application of Ro15-1788. Furthermore, long-term treatment of rats with flurazepam (15 mg/day ip) reduced the neuronal responsiveness to CCK of rat CA3 hippocampal neurons.[28] In behavioral studies, cessation of chronic diazepam administration produced an increase in CCK-8 binding in cortex and hippocampus,[29] and recent *in situ* hybridization studies showed that CCK mRNA levels in nonpyramidal cells (where CCK and GABA coexist) increased after a single injection of diazepam (2 mg/kg.) or withdrawal from chronic diazepam treatment.[30] We have addressed the possible interactions between benzodiazepine moieties and CCK at the receptor level using *in vitro* electrophysiological studies with pentagastrin as the selective CCK_B agonist and CI-988 as the CCK_B antagonist. Extracellular recordings and analyses were made from rat ventromedial hypothalamic neurons and the effects of the benzodiazepines were compared with those of the CCK_B antagonist on the same neurons.

We were unable to find any effect of either flurazepam or Ro15-1788 at concentrations up to and including 10 μM. With higher concentrations (100 μM) of flurazepam a competitive block of the pentagastrin response was found yielding a Ke of approximately 12 μM. The flurazepam effect was selective for pentagastrin and reversible on washing in drug-free saline solution, after which time the preparation could be treated with CI-988 to produce the predicted block of pentagastrin. However, no change in the ability of flurazepam to attenuate pentagastrin-induced excitations was seen when the preparation was pretreated with the benzodiazepine antagonist Ro15-1788 (100 μM). From these series of experiments we conclude that the only interaction between flurazepam and CCK_B receptors occurs at high concentrations when the benzodiazepine interacts competitively with CCK_B agonists at the CCK_B receptor. The low probability that such high concentrations of benzodiazepines would occur at CCK_B receptors to block the CCK_B response when anxiolytic doses of benzodiazepines are given would preclude us from suggesting a common pathway between CCK_B antagonist and benzodiazepine agonist-induced anxiolysis.

We have begun to explore a possible interaction between benzodiazepines and

CCK_A receptors using the rat dorsal raphe preparation. Our preliminary results show that flurazepam is more effective at blocking CCK responses from CCK_A receptor activation, but the block appears noncompetitive. These data suggest that any central benzodiazepine-CCK receptor interaction would occur at CCK_A sites before CCK_B receptors are affected. Further studies are underway to determine the exact nature of the inhibition produced by benzodiazepines at CCK_A sites in the rat dorsal raphe.

MODE OF ACTION OF CCK

Much of the early work on the ionic mechanisms underlying CCK-induced excitation of brain neurons *in vitro* came from studies of hippocampal neurons. Unfortunately, CCK responses in this preparation do show pronounced desensitization, eliminating the use of long-term application of the peptide, and possible conclusions regarding the currents involved are contradictory. Dodd and Kelly[6] showed that CCK-8s depolarized CA1 neurons by an apparent decrease in input resistance with a net equilibrium potential closer to zero than the cell resting membrane potential and suggestive of involvement of one or more ionic species. Other workers have noted that CCK-like peptides produced an increase in input resistance of CA1 neurons[8,31] and suggested that blockage of a potassium current could be responsible. The proposal that CCK depolarizes hippocampal neurons by reducing outward current is supported by Brooks and Kelly[7] who showed a decrease in input resistance of dentate gyrus neurons following CCK application. However, further research using selective antagonists to identify the CCK receptor involved in the generation of the depolarization clearly will be required before a firm conclusion can be reached on the ionic nature of the CCK response recorded from hippocampal neurons.

Selective antagonists have been used to identify a CCK_B receptor whose activation leads to depolarization of rat supraoptic neurons. Jarvis *et al.*[13] reported that this CCK effect was mediated through activation of a nonselective cation conductance akin to that described by Petersen[32] in rat pancreatic acinar cells (TABLE 2).

Much of our work on the mechanism of action of CCK has centered around the CCK_B receptor in the rat VMH and the CCK_A receptor in the rat dorsal raphe. In the former, we showed that CCK excitations persisted in tetrodotoxin-containing solutions and were not dependent on external calcium. Under voltage-clamp conditions the effect of CCK was seen as a net inward current resulting from a reduction in a voltage-dependent outward current.[33] Voltage-current relationships showed this current to become activated as the neuron was depolarized from resting membrane potential and that CCK inhibited the activation of the current. However, CCK also reduced instantaneous inward current, implying that at least two mutually reinforcing effects on separate currents produced the pronounced excitation seen with the peptide under normal physiological conditions. The results resembled those seen with muscarinic agonists and other peptides in a variety of preparations.[34] One surprising feature was the uncovering of a third effect of CCK under conditions in which the voltage-dependent outward current was blocked using either carbachol or phorbol ester-12,13-dibutyrate (PdBu) which is known to activate protein kinase C.[35] Treatment of CCK-sensitive VMH neurons with either of these agents produced effects akin to those seen when the peptide itself was applied, but application of CCK during the response to PdBu (or carbachol) now produced an outward current. Under current-clamp conditions without tetrodotoxin, this was seen as membrane

TABLE 2. Summary of Mechanism of Action Studies for CCK Responses *in Vitro*[a]

Block of Potassium Current	Increase in Cation Current	Activation of Calcium-Dependent Potassium Current	Decrease in Calcium Current
Rat ventromedial hypothalamus (B receptor)	Rat supraoptic nucleus (B receptor)	Guinea pig acinar cell	Rat spinal cord[b]
Rat CA1 (B receptor)	Rat nodose ganglia "fast" response		
Rat CA1/culture (B receptor)	Rat acinar cell		
Rat lateral amygdala (B receptor)			
Rat dentate gyrus			
Rat dorsal raphe (A receptor)			
Rat nodose ganglia "slow" response			

[a] Pharmacological characterization of CCK receptor type, where known, is given in brackets.
[b] Willetts et al.[42]

hyperpolarization leading to a reduction in the PdBu-induced increase in firing of the cell. Thus, it appears that, under normal conditions, CCK acts by inhibition of two separate outward currents to increase neuronal excitability. Under conditions of increased neuronal excitation when this CCK-sensitive current is blocked, the peptide then activates an outward current. A model of such a scheme is shown in FIGURE 1.

Modulation of this nature by activation of two opposing currents by one peptide (e.g., bradykinin) has been reported previously.[36] The excitatory effects of CCK are also seen when pentagastrin is used as the agonist, but we have not yet determined the CCK receptor involved in the third effect nor have we used selective antagonists to block the individual CCK effects. We are currently undertaking single channel recording from VMH neurons *in situ* in an attempt to determine the channel type(s) involved and the possible role of second messengers in the CCK response.

In tha rat dorsal raphe, CCK excites a subpopulation of 5-HT neurons[12] that differ from those responsive to the neuropeptide bombesin[16] through activation of a CCK_A receptor. We have undertaken experiments designed to see if the transduction mechanism linked to this CCK receptor type is similar to that found in the periphery. Unfortunately in peripheral assays for CCK, the receptor type and ionic mechanism both appear to be species dependent. For example, in the rat and mouse acinar cell preparation, the depolarizing effects of secretagogues can be seen with a rank order corresponding to the presence of a mixture of CCK_B/gastrin and CCK_A receptors,[37] and CCK depolarizes pancreatic acinar cells by increasing calcium to activate a calcium-dependent nonselective monovalent cation channel. In the guinea pig, pig (and probably human) CCK evokes amylase secretion, with a profile corresponding to action at a CCK_A receptor only[38] by increasing intracellular calcium to activate a calcium- and voltage-dependent potassium channel.[32,39]

Our voltage-clamp experiments in brain slice preparations have revealed that activation of the CCK_A receptor reduces a potassium current to excite raphe neurons (Boden and Woodruff, in preparation). The potassium current involved is not dependent on extracellular calcium, because the inward current produced by CCK was not affected by removal of calcium ions or by the calcium-dependent channel blockers charybdotoxin (100 nM) and apamin (100 nM). The response was unaffected by blockers of I_A (dendrotoxin 100–300 nM) or inward rectifier currents (rubidium, 5 mM; caesium, 2 mM) but was blocked by barium (1–2 mM).

TABLE 2 summarizes the findings of mechanistic studies of CCK responses *in vitro*. Although the table is incomplete with respect to identification of receptor types involved in a particular response, one feature that does emerge from the studies so far undertaken is that invariably the ionic mechanism linked to the CCK receptor is either a potassium current or a nonselective cation current, irrespective of a central or peripheral location of the receptor. In some instances CCK acts on both in the same preparation, such as rat nodose ganglia cells where CCK produces a fast depolarization by increasing a cation conductance followed by a slow response as a result of potassium current block.[40]

In conclusion, our own investigations of the ionic mechanisms involved following activation of central CCK receptors point overwhelmingly to a discrete population of potassium currents. Data from dorsal raphe neurons show that a difference exists between the linkage of peripheral and central CCK_A receptors and their ionic counterpart, while the CCK_B receptor studies reveal that neuromodulators such as CCK can be linked to several different transduction mechanisms on the same neuron, enabling fine tuning of neuronal output to take place.

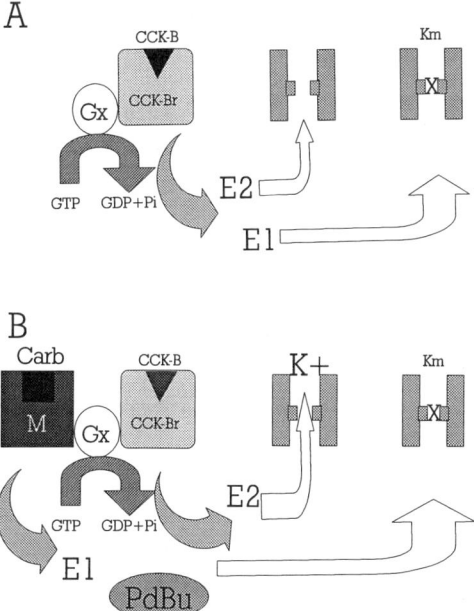

FIGURE 1. (**A**) CCK binds to its G-protein (pertussis toxin-insensitive Gx)-linked receptor (CCK-Br) to excite ventromedial hypothalamus neurones by blocking a voltage-dependent potassium current (Km). The nature of the effector involved (E1) is unknown, but block of the same current can be mimicked by protein kinase C activator PdBu or by carbachol (**B**). In this situation CCK acts through a second effector (E2) to open a different potassium current.

REFERENCES

1. WOODRUFF, G. N. & J. HUGHES. 1991. Ann. Rev. Pharmacol. & Toxicol. **31:** 473–491.
2. HILL, D. R., N. J. CAMPBELL, T. M. SHAW & G. N. WOODRUFF. 1987. J. Neurosci. **7:** 2967–2976.
3. HILL, D. R., T. M. SHAW & G. N. WOODRUFF. 1987. Neurosci. Letts. **79:** 286–289.
4. HILL, D. R. & G. N. WOODRUFF. 1990. Brain Res. **526:** 276–283.
5. HILL, D. R., T. M. SHAW, W. GRAHAM & G. N. WOODRUFF. 1990. J. Neurosci. **10:** 1070–1081.
6. DODD, J. & J. S. KELLY. 1981. Brain Res. **205:** 337–350.
7. BROOKS, P. A. & J. S. KELLY. 1985. Ann. N. Y. Acad. Sci. **448:** 361–374.
8. BODEN, P. R. & R. G. HILL. 1988. Neuropeptides **12:** 95–103.
9. KOW, L. M. & D. W. PFAFF. 1986. Peptides **7:** 473–479.
10. BODEN, P. R. & R. G. HILL. 1987. Brit. J. Pharmacol. **92:** 585P.
11. BODEN, P. R. & R. G. HILL. 1988. Brit. J. Pharmacol. **94:** 246–252.
12. BODEN, P. R., R. D. PINNOCK & G. N. WOODRUFF. 1991. Brit. J. Pharmacol. **102:** 635–638.
13. JARVIS, C. A., C. W. BOURQUE & L. P. RENAUD. 1992. J. Physiol. **458:** 621–632.
14. BRANCHEREAU, P., G. A. BOHME, J. CHAMPAGNAT, M-P. MORIN-SAUVIN, C. DURIEUX, J. C. BLANCHARD, B. P. ROQUES & M. DENAVIT-SAUBIE. 1992. J. Pharm. Exp. Ther. **260:** 1433–1440.
15. SUGITA, S., E. TANAKA & R. A. NORTH. 1993. J. Physiol. **460:** 705–718.
16. PINNOCK, R. D., R. S. RICHARDSON, P. R. BODEN & G. N. WOODRUFF. 1992. Mol. Neuropharmacol. **1:** 211–218.
17. EVANS, B. E., M. G. BOCK, R. M. DIPARDO, K. E. RITTLE, W. L. WHITTER, V. D. VEBER, P. S. ANDERSON & R. M. FREIDINGER. 1986. Proc. Natl. Acad. Sci. USA **83:** 4918–4922.
18. EVANS, B. E., K. E. RITTLE, M. G. BOCK, R. M. DIPARDO, R. M. FREIDINGER, W. L. WHITTER, G. F. LUNDELL, D. F. VEBER, P. S. ANDERSON, R. S. L. CHANG, V. L. LOTTI, P. J. KLING, K. A. KUNKEL, J. P. SPRONGER & J. HIRSCHFELD. 1988. J. Med. Chem. **31:** 2235–2246.
19. HUGHES, J., P. BODEN, B. COSTALL, A. DOMENEY, E. KELLY, D. C. HORWELL, J. C. HUNTER, R. D. PINNOCK & G. N. WOODRUFF. 1990. Proc. Natl. Acad. Sci. USA **87:** 6728–6732.
20. LOTTI, V. J. & R. S. L. CHANG. 1989. Eur. J. Pharmacol. **162:** 273–280.
21. BOCK, M. G. 1991. Drugs of the Future. **16:** 631–640.
22. HORWELL, D. C. 1991. Neuropeptides **19** (suppl.): 57–64.
23. WOODRUFF, G. N., D. R. HILL, P. R. BODEN, R. D. PINNOCK, L. SINGH & J. HUGHES. 1991. Neuropeptides **19** (suppl.): 56.
24. WEISENFELD-HALLIN, Z., X.-J. XU, J. HUGHES, D. C. HORWELL & T. HOKFELT. 1990. Proc. Natl. Acad. Sci. USA **87:** 7105–7109.
25. KUBOTA, K., K. SUGAYA, N. SUNAGANE, I. MATSUDA & T. URUNO. 1985. Eur. J. Pharmacol. **110:** 225–231.
26. KUBOTA, K., K. SUGAYA, M. MATSUDA, Y. MATSUOKA & Y. TERAWAKI. 1985. Jap. J. Pharmacol. **37:** 101–105.
27. BRADWEJN, J. & C. DE MONTIGNY. 1984. Nature **312:** 363–364.
28. BOUTHILLIER, A. & C. DE MONTIGNY. 1988. Eur. J. Pharmacol. 135–138.
29. HARRO, J., A. LANG & E. VASAR. 1990. Eur. J. Pharmacol. **180:** 77–83.
30. RATTAY *et al.* 1993.
31. BUCKETT, K. J. & D. A. SAINT. 1989. Neurosci. Letts. **107:** 162–166.
32. PETERSEN, O. H. 1987. *In* Gastrin and Cholecystokinin, Chemistry, Physiology and Pharmacology. J.-P. Bali & J. Martinez, eds.: 93–97. Elsevier Scientific Pub. Co. New York.
33. BODEN, P. 1991. Mol. Neuropharmacol. **1:** 155–161.
34. BROWN, D. A. 1988. Trends in Neurosci. **11:** 294–299.
35. NISHIZUKA, Y. 1984. Nature **308:** 693–698.
36. HIGASHIDA, H. & D. A. BROWN. 1986. Nature **323:** 333–335.
37. IWATSUKI, N., K. KATO & A. NISHIYAMA. 1977. Brit. J. Pharmacol. **60:** 147–154.

38. JENSEN, R. T., T. VON SCHRENCK, D.-H. YU, S. A. WANK & J. D. GARDNER. 1989. In The Neuropeptide Cholecystokinin (CCK). Anatomy and Biochemistry, Receptors, Pharmacology and Physiology. J. Hughes, G. Dockray & G. Woodruff, eds.: 150–162. N. Ellis Horwood.
39. PETERSEN, O. H. & I. FINDLAY. 1987. Physiol. Rev. **67:** 1054–1116.
40. DUN, N. J., S. Y. WU & C.-W. LIN. 1991. Brain Res. **556:** 161–164.
41. PINNOCK, R. D. & G. N. WOODRUFF. 1991. J. Physiol. **440:** 55–66.
42. WILLETTS, J., L. URBAN, K. MURASE & M. RANDIC. 1985. Ann. N. Y. Acad. Sci. **448:** 385–402.
43. CHANG, R. S. L. & V. J. LOTTI. 1986. Proc. Natl. Acad. Sci. USA **83:** 4923–4926.

Cholecystokinin Modulates Dopamine-Mediated Behaviors

Differential Actions in Medial Posterior *versus* Anterior Nucleus Accumbens

JACQUELINE N. CRAWLEY

Section on Behavioral Neuropharmacology
Experimental Therapeutics Branch
National Institute of Mental Health
Building 10, Room 4N214
Bethesda, Maryland 20892

Cholecystokinin (CCK) coexists with dopamine (DA) in the mammalian midbrain (FIG. 1).[1-6] Immunoreactivity and/or messenger RNA for CCK and for tyrosine hydroxylase, the rate-limiting enzyme in the synthesis of dopamine, is visible within the same neuronal cell bodies in the ventral tegmentum and substantia nigra of rat, cat, and monkey.[1-7] At least 40% of dopaminergic neurons in the A10 ventral tegmental area of the rat contain CCK.[7] One major terminal field of the CCK-DA coexistence lies within the medial posterior region of the nucleus accumbens. CCK immunoreactivity is visible in the anterior accumbens and caudate nucleus; however, the majority of these CCK-containing fibers arise from neurons located elsewhere, for example, nearby cortical areas such as the claustrum.[1,2,3,7]

Two subtypes of CCK receptors have been identified by pharmacological properties and cDNA sequences.[8-10] The CCK-A receptor binds the sulfated CCK octapeptide with at least 1,000-fold greater affinity than the unsulfated octapeptide or the COOH-terminal tetrapeptide, is localized in peripheral organs including pancreas and gallbladder, and is seen in a small number of brain sites.[8-10] The CCK-B receptor binds the sulfated CCK octapeptide, the unsulfated CCK octapeptide, and the COOH-terminal tetrapeptide, with almost equimolar affinity, is localized throughout the central nervous system, and appears to be the same cDNA sequence as the gastrin receptor, which is localized in the stomach.[8-10]

In the nucleus accumbens, high concentrations of CCK-B receptors are seen, and low levels of CCK-A receptors have been reported.[9,11-13]

Anatomical findings suggest that afferents and efferents of the nucleus accumbens differentiate the medial posterior region, termed the shell, from the anterior regions of the nucleus accumbens and most of the caudate nucleus, termed the core.[14,15] The shell distinction corresponds to the terminal field of the CCK-DA coexistence.[1-3] This unique location of CCK in the medial posterior nucleus accumbens, in terminals from ventral tegmental dopaminergic neurons, raises the possibility that CCK interacts with DA at the shell region in a manner different from CCK actions in brain regions which do not demonstrate CCK-DA coexistence.

Behavioral studies designed to investigate the functional interactions between CCK and DA reveal opposite effects of CCK on DA-mediated behaviors in the medial posterior *versus* the anterior nucleus accumbens of the rat. CCK, microinjected bilaterally at doses from 20 pg to 200 ng, potentiated DA-induced hyperlocomotion in a Digiscan automated open field, when CCK was administered in combination with DA into the rat medial posterior nucleus accumbens.[16–18] In the anterior nucleus accumbens, CCK had no effect or inhibited DA-induced hyperlocomotion.[17,18] Similarly, CCK potentiated amphetamine-induced hyperlocomotion when microinjected into the medial posterior nucleus accumbens, whereas CCK inhibited amphetamine-induced hyperlocomotion when microinjected into the anterior nucleus accumbens.[19] Intracranial self-stimulation, a reward-related behavior, was potentiated by CCK microinjected into the medial posterior nucleus accumbens and was inhibited by CCK microinjected into the rat anterior nucleus accumbens.[20,21]

The CCK receptor subtypes mediating the dichotomous effects of CCK in the medial posterior *versus* anterior nucleus accumbens were investigated, using several of the CCK-A and CCK-B receptor subtype selective analogs and antagonists which are described in detail elsewhere in this volume. In the Digiscan open field exploratory locomotion paradigm, sulfated CCK octapeptide was active, whereas unsulfated CCK octapeptide, CCK tetrapeptide, and the CCK-B agonist BC264 were

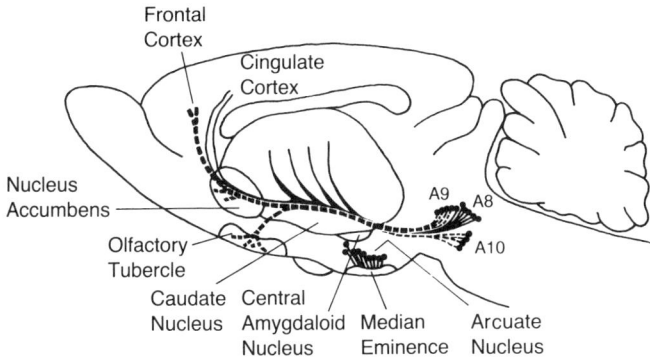

FIGURE 1. Schematic representation of dopamine pathways in the rat brain (saggital view). Cholecystokinin (CCK) coexists with dopamine in the A10 ventral tegmental neurons projecting to the nucleus accumbens and olfactory tubercles.[1–6] A10 neurons containing neurotensin coexisting with dopamine project to the frontal cortex.[4] A9 substantia nigra neurons contain CCK mRNA coexisting with tyrosine hydroxylase mRNA;[5,6] however, lesion studies indicate that most CCK in the caudate nucleus arises from local cortical projections rather than from the A9 dopamine neurons.[1–3,7]

inactive at the medial posterior nucleus accumbens microinjection site.[22,23] The CCK-A antagonist L-364,718 (MK 329 or devazepide, 10 ng administered 5 minutes before vehicle, DA, or CCK + DA) significantly blocked the facilitatory effect of CCK microinjected into the medial posterior nucleus accumbens, whereas CCK-B antagonists L-365,260 (10 ng) and CI-988 (20 ng or 2 μg) did not.[18] In the anterior nucleus accumbens, sulfated CCK octapeptide significantly attenuated DA-induced hyperlocomotion.[18] The CCK-B antagonists L-365,260 and CI-988 significantly blocked the inhibitory effect of CCK microinjected into the anterior nucleus accumbens, whereas the CCK-A antagonist L-364,718 did not.[18] These results, summarized in FIGURE 2, suggest that CCK potentiates DA-mediated behaviors in the medial posterior nucleus accumbens of the rat by a CCK-A receptor subtype mechanism, whereas CCK inhibits DA-mediated behaviors in the anterior nucleus accumbens of the rat by a CCK-B receptor subtype mechanism.

These behavioral findings are consistent with data from *in vitro* release experiments. In tissue slices from rat posterior nucleus accumbens, CCK potentiated potassium-stimulated DA release, an effect blocked by L-364,718, indicating a CCK-A receptor subtype.[24,25] In tissue slices from rat anterior nucleus accumbens, CCK attenuated potassium-stimulated DA release, an effect blocked by L-365,260, indicating a CCK-B receptor subtype.[25] In addition, in tissue homogenates from the rat posterior nucleus accumbens region, CCK potentiated DA-stimulated adenylate cyclase activity, whereas in the anterior accumbens region, CCK inhibited DA-stimulated adenylate cyclase activity.[26]

Taken together, these behavioral and biochemical data support an interpretation that CCK has opposite actions, mediated by different receptor subtypes, in the two subdivisions of the rat nucleus accumbens. Topographical analysis indicates that the facilitatory actions of CCK on DA-induced hyperlocomotion occur within the anatomical region containing terminals from ventral tegmental neurons in which

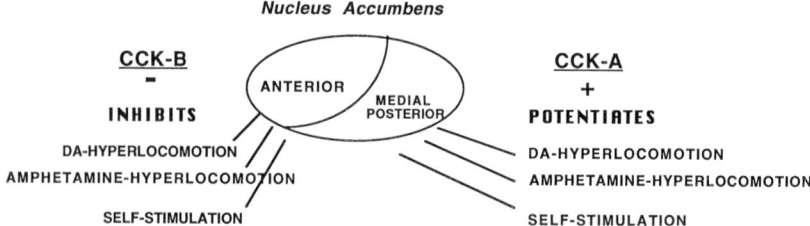

FIGURE 2. Summary of the actions of cholecystokinin (CCK) in modulating dopamine (DA) on behavioral paradigms in rats. In the medial posterior nucleus accumbens, a terminal field of the A10 CCK-DA coexistence,[1-7] CCK potentiates dopamine-induced exploratory locomotion,[16-18] CCK potentiates amphetamine-induced locomotion,[19] and CCK potentiates self-stimulation, particularly in the A10 dopamine cells.[20,21] In the anterior nucleus accumbens, where CCK is present but arises from cells other than the A10 CCK-DA coexistence,[1-7] CCK has no effect or inhibits dopamine-induced exploratory locomotion,[17,18] CCK inhibits amphetamine-induced locomotion,[19] and CCK has no effect or inhibits self-stimulation.[20,21] The facilitatory effect of CCK on DA-induced hyperlocomotion in the medial posterior nucleus accumbens demonstrates a CCK-A receptor subtype pharmacology,[18] whereas the inhibitory effect of CCK on DA-induced hyperlocomotion in the anterior nucleus accumbens demonstrates a CCK-B receptor subtype pharmacology.[18]

CCK and DA coexist.[17] It is interesting to speculate that a special mechanism of CCK-DA interaction exists in the mesolimbic neurons that contain the CCK-DA coexistence, perhaps at the level of second messengers, presynaptic localization of receptors, or anatomical outputs.

Midbrain dopaminergic neurons have been implicated in human neuropsychiatric disorders. The nigrostriatal pathway, projecting from the substantia nigra to the striatum, has been linked to the motor dysfunctions in Parkinson's disease, whereas the mesocorticolimbic pathway, projecting from the ventral tegmentum to the nucleus accumbens, olfactory tubercles, and prefrontal cortex, has been linked to approach behaviors, appetitive behaviors, rewarded behaviors, anxiety, drug abuse, stress syndromes, and schizophrenia.[27] Clinical studies are investigating the levels of CCK-like immunoreactivity, CCK mRNA, and CCK-A and CCK-B receptors in dopaminergic pathways in postmortem samples from victims of drug abuse and schizophrenia. An intriguing report recently demonstrated high levels of CCK mRNA in midbrain dopamine neurons of schizophrenics as compared to low or undetectable levels of CCK mRNA in midbrain dopamine neurons of normal controls.[28] Although it is possible that the chronic neuroleptic treatment of the schizophrenic group was responsible for the high CCK expression, subchronic neuroleptic treatment did not increase CCK mRNA levels in midbrain dopamine neurons of rats.[29] If further investigations demonstrate unusual levels of CCK or CCK receptors in specific subregions of dopaminergic pathways, specific to a clinical disease state, then CCK-based non-peptide agonists or antagonists, administered alone or in combination with dopaminergic drugs, may provide novel therapeutic tools for the treatment of neuropsychiatric disorders.

REFERENCES

1. HÖKFELT, T., J. F. REHFELD, L. SKIRBOLL, B. IVEMARK, M. GOLDSTEIN & K. MARKEY. 1980. Evidence for coexistence of dopamine and CCK in mesolimbic neurons. Nature **285:** 476–478.
2. HÖKFELT, T., L. SKIRBOLL, J. F. REHFELD, M. GOLDSTEIN, K. MARKEY & O. DANN. 1980. A subpopulation of mesencephalic dopamine neurons projecting to limbic areas containing cholecystokinin-like peptides: Evidence from immunohistochemistry combined with retrograde tracing. Neuroscience **5:** 2093–2124.
3. STUDLER, J.-M., H. SIMON, F. CESSELIN, J. C. LEGRAND, J. GLOWINSKI & J.-P. TASSIN. 1981. Biochemical investigation on the localization of the cholecystokinin octapeptide in dopaminergic neurons originating from the ventral tegmental area of the rat. Neuropeptides **2:** 131–139.
4. SEROOGY, K. B., A. MEHTA & J. FALLON. 1987. Neurotensin and cholecystokinin coexistence within neurons of the ventral mesencephalon: Projections to forebrain. Exp. Brain Res. **68:** 277–289.
5. SEROOGY, K., M. SCHALLING, S. BRENE, A. DAGERLIND, S. Y. CHAI, T. HÖKFELT, H. PERSSON, M. BROWNSTEIN, R. HUAN, J. DIXON, D. FILER, D. SCHLESSINGER & M. GOLDSTEIN. 1989. Cholecystokinin and tyrosine hydroxylase messenger RNAs in neurons of rat mesencephalon: Peptide/monoamine coexistence studies using *in situ* hybridization combined with immunocytochemistry. Exp. Brain Res. **74:** 149–162.
6. SAVASTA, M., E. RUBERTE, J. M. PALACIOS & G. MENGOD. 1989. The colocalization of cholecystokinin and tyrosine hydroxylase mRNAs in mesencephalic dopaminergic neurons in the rat brain examined by in situ hybridization. Neuroscience **29:** 363–369.
7. HÖKFELT, T., L. SKIRBOLL, B. EVERITT, B. MEISTER, M. BROWNSTEIN, T. JACOBS, A. FADEN, S. KUGA, M. GOLDSTEIN, R. MARKSTEIN, G. DOCKRAY & J. REHFELD. 1985. Distribution of cholecystokinin-like immunoreactivity in the nervous system: Coexistence with classical neurotransmitters and other neuropeptides. Ann. N. Y. Acad. Sci. **448:** 255–274.
8. MORAN, T. H., P. ROBINSON, M. S. GOLDRICH & P. R. MCHUGH. 1986. Two brain cholecystokinin receptors: Implications for behavioral actions. Brain Res. **362:** 175–179.
9. HILL, D. R., N. J. CAMPBELL, T. M. SHAW & G. N. WOODRUFF. 1987. Autoradiographic localization and biochemical characterization of peripheral type CCK receptors in rat CNS using highly selective ligands. J. Neurosci. **7:** 2967–2976.
10. WANK, S. A., J. R. PISEGNA & A. DE WEERTH. 1992. Brain and gastrointestinal cholecystokinin receptor family: Structure and functional expression. Proc. Natl. Acad. Sci. USA **89:** 8691–8695.
11. GAUDREAU, P., R. QUIRION, S. ST-PIERRE & C. B. PERT. 1983. Tritium-sensitive film autoradiography of [^{3}H]cholecystokinin-5/pentagastrin receptors in rat brain. Eur. J. Pharmacol. **87:** 173–174.
12. PELEPRAT, D., Y. BROER, J. M. STUDLER, M. PECHANSKI, J. P. TASSIN, J. GLOWINSKI, W. ROSTENE & B. P. ROQUES. 1987. Autoradiography of CCK receptors in the rat brain using [^{3}]BOC[Nle28-31]-CCK-27-33 and [^{125}I]Bolton Hunter CCK-8. Functional significance of subregional distributions. Neurochem. Int. **10:** 495–508.

13. BARRETT, R. W., M. E. STEFFEY & C. A. W. WOLFRAM. 1989. Type-A cholecystokinin binding sites in cow brain: Characterization using (−)[^{3}H]L364718 membrane binding assays. Mol. Pharmacol. **36:** 285–290.
14. HEIMER, L., D. S. ZAHM, L. CHURCHILL, P. W. KALIVAS & C. WOHLTMANN. 1991. Specificity in the projection pattern of accumbal core and shell. Neuroscience **41:** 89–126.
15. DEUTCH, A. Y. & D. S. CAMERON. 1992. Pharmacological characterization of dopamine systems in the nucleus accumbens core and shell. Neuroscience **46:** 49–56.
16. CRAWLEY, J. N., J. A. STIVERS, L. K. BLUMSTEIN & S. M. PAUL. 1984. Cholecystokinin potentiates dopamine-mediated behaviors: Evidence for modulation specific to a site of coexistence. J. Neurosci. **5:** 1972–1983.
17. CRAWLEY, J. N., D. W. HOMMER & L. R. SKIRBOLL. 1985. Topographical analysis of nucleus accumbens sites at which cholecystokinin potentiates dopamine-induced hyperlocomotion in the rat. Brain Res. **335:** 337–341.
18. CRAWLEY, J. N. 1992. Subtype-selective cholecystokinin receptor antagonists block cholecystokinin modulation of dopamine-mediated behaviors in the rat mesolimbic pathway. J. Neurosci. **12:** 3380–3391.
19. VACCARINO, F. J. & J. RANKIN. 1989. Nucleus accumbens cholecystokinin (CCK) can either attenuate or potentiate amphetamine-induced locomotor activity: Evidence for rostral-caudal differences in accumbens CCK function. Behav. Neurosci. **103:** 831–836.
20. VACCARINO, F. J. & A. L. VACCARINO. 1989. Antagonism of cholecystokinin function in the rostral and caudal nucleus accumbens: Differential effects on brain stimulation reward. Neurosci. Lett. **97:** 151–156.
21. DE WITTE, P., C. HEIDBREDER, B. ROQUES & J.-J. VANDERHAEGHEN. 1987. Opposite effects of cholecystokinin octapeptide (CCK-8) and tetrapeptide (CCK-4) after injection into the caudal part of the nucleus accumbens or into its rostral part and the cerebral ventricles. Neurochem. Int. **4:** 473–479.
22. CRAWLEY, J. N., J. A. STIVERS, D. W. HOMMER, L. R. SKIRBOLL & S. M. PAUL. 1986. Antagonists of central and peripheral behavioral actions of cholecystokinin. J. Pharmacol. Exp. Therap. **236:** 320–330.
23. DAUGE, V., G. A. BOHME, J. N. CRAWLEY, C. DURIEUX, J. M. STUTZMANN, J. FEGER, J. C. BLANCHARD & B. P. ROQUES. 1990. Investigations of behavioral and electrophysiological responses induced by selective stimulation of CCKB receptors by using a new highly potent CCK analog: BC 264. Synapse **6:** 73–80.
24. VICKROY, T. W. & B. R. BIANCHI. 1989. Pharmacological and mechanistic studies of cholecystokinin-facilitated [^{3}H]-dopamine efflux from rat nucleus accumbens. Neuropeptides **13:** 43–50.
25. MARSHALL, F. H., S. BARNES, J. HUGHES, G. N. WOODRUFF & J. C. HUNTER. 1991. Cholecystokinin modulates the release of dopamine from the anterior and posterior nucleus accumbens by two different mechanisms. J. Neurochem. **56:** 917–922.
26. STUDLER, J. M., M. REIBAUD, D. HERVE, G. BLANC, J. GLOWINSKI & J. P. TASSIN. 1986. Opposite effects of sulfated cholecystokinin on DA-sensitive adenylate cyclase in two areas of the rat nucleus accumbens. Eur. J. Pharmacol. **126:** 125–128.
27. KALIVAS, P. W. & C. B. NEMEROFF, Eds. 1988. The Mesocorticolimbic Dopamine System. Vol. 537. Ann. N. Y. Acad. Sci. New York.
28. SCHALLING, M., K. FRIBERG, K. SEROOGY, P. RIEDERER, E. BIRD, S. N. SCHIFFMANN, P. MAILLEUX, J.-J. VANDERHAEGHEN, S. KUGA, M. GOLDSTEIN, K. KITAHAMA, P. H. LUPPI, M. JOUVET & T. HÖKFELT. 1990. Analysis of expression of cholecystokinin in dopamine cells in the ventral mesencephalon of several species and in humans with schizophrenia. Proc. Natl. Acad. Sci. USA **87:** 8427–8431.
29. COTTINGHAM, S. L., D. PICKAR, T. K. SHIMOTAKE, P. MONTPIED, S. M. PAUL & J. N. CRAWLEY. 1990. Tyrosine hydroxylase and cholecystokinin mRNA levels in the substantia nigra, ventral tegmental area, and locus coeruleus are unaffected by acute and chronic haloperidol administration. Cell Mol. Neurobiol. **10:** 41–50.

Integration of Postprandial Function in the Proximal Gastrointestinal Tract

Role of CCK and Sensory Pathways[a]

HELEN E. RAYBOULD[b] AND K. C. KENT LLOYD

CURE/UCLA Digestive Diseases Research Center
VA West Los Angeles
Department of Medicine and Brain Research Institute
UCLA School of Medicine
Los Angeles, California 90073

The rate of delivery of nutrients into the proximal small intestine is regulated, along with pancreatic secretion and gallbladder contraction, to maximize the efficiency of digestion and absorption in the small intestine. That nutrients in the intestine exert negative feedback control over gastric function has been recognized for many years, and although the mechanisms are not well defined, there is evidence for both neural and hormonal pathways. This chapter reviews the evidence for a role of cholecystokinin (CCK) and neural pathways in this regulation. Specifically, we examine the hypothesis that nutrients in the intestine release CCK that then acts on neural pathways to produce reflex changes in gastric function.

EVIDENCE FOR NEURAL PATHWAYS IN THE REGULATION OF GASTRIC MOTOR FUNCTION

Aspiroz and Malagelada[1] demonstrated in the conscious dog that vagal blockade reversed the ability of intestinal nutrients to inhibit motility of the proximal stomach. However, this study does not indicate whether afferent or efferent nerves are involved. It is possible that the efferent pathway plays a permissive role in the regulation of gastric motility, and its blockade could alter the sensitivity to other influences, such as hormones. More recently, direct involvement of visceral afferent pathways has been demonstrated using the sensory neurotoxin capsaicin. Chemical ablation of vagal and spinal sensory pathways either by topical application to the vagus nerves or celiac/mesenteric ganglia or by systemic capsaicin treatment significantly attenuates inhibition of gastric emptying in response to different nutrients in rats.[2–4]

Selective chemical ablation using capsaicin of the vagal and spinal afferent pathway reveals that different nutrients act to inhibit gastric emptying through distinct afferent pathways. Inhibition of gastric emptying induced by intestinal perfusion with fat was inhibited by selective ablation of the vagal, but not the spinal, capsaicin-sensitive pathway[2] (FIG. 1). In contrast, inhibition of gastric emptying

---

[a] This work was supported by NIH Grant DDK 41004 to H. E. R. and by NIH Grant to the CURE/UCLA Digestive Diseases Core Center (DK 41301). K. C. K. L. is a recipient of an NIH Fellowship Award.

[b] Address for correspondence: Helen E. Raybould, PhD, Bldg 115, Room 115, VA Wadsworth Medical Center, Wilshire and Sawtelle Blvds, Los Angeles, CA 90073.

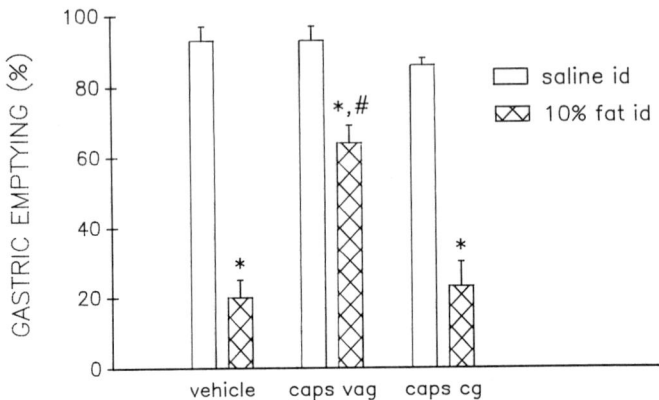

FIGURE 1. Effect of perineural application of capsaicin of either the vagus nerves (caps vag) or the celiac/superior mesenteric ganglia (caps cg) on inhibition of gastric emptying induced by intraduodenal infusion with fat. Gastric emptying of a non-nutrient liquid was measured in awake rats with chronic gastric and duodenal cannulas during intraduodenal infusion with saline or lipid (10% Intralipid). *$p < 0.01$ saline vs lipid; #$p < 0.05$ vehicle vs capsaicin. Functional ablation of vagal capsaicin-sensitive afferents attenuated fat-induced inhibition of gastric emptying by around 60%.

induced by intestinal carbohydrate (300 mM maltose) was inhibited by selective ablation of either the vagal or spinal capsaicin-sensitive pathway[3] (FIG. 2).

These experiments clearly show a role for sensory nervous pathways in transmitting essential signals from the intestine regulating gastric emptying. However, several

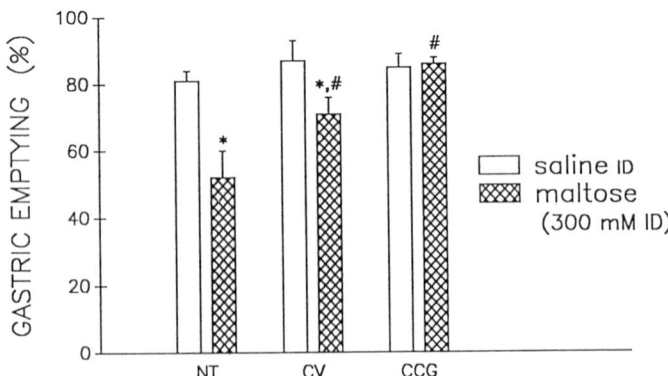

FIGURE 2. Inhibition of gastric emptying by intestinal perfusion with maltose (300 mM) in awake rats. NT = no treatment; CV = capsaicin on vagus; CCG = capsaicin on celiac/superior mesenteric ganglia. Gastric emptying of a non-nutrient liquid was measured in awake rats with chronic gastric and duodenal cannulas during intraduodenal infusion with saline or maltose (300 mM, 10%). *$p < 0.01$ saline vs maltose; #$p < 0.05$ vehicle vs capsaicin. Functional ablation of vagal capsaicin-sensitive afferents attenuated maltose-induced inhibition of gastric emptying by around 60%, whereas functional ablation of spinal afferents completely abolished the response to maltose. (Reprinted from ref. 3 with permission.)

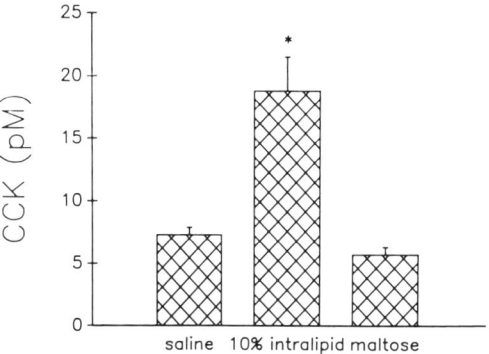

FIGURE 3. Administration of the CCK A receptor antagonist L364718 (MK329) reverses around 70% of the lipid-induced inhibition of gastric emptying. Gastric emptying was measured in awake rats following intraperitoneal injection of either vehicle or antagonist 30 minutes before gastric emptying was measured. $^*p < 0.05$ saline vs lipid; $p < 0.01$ vehicle vs L364718.

hormones, including CCK, are released by nutrients in the intestine, and when administered exogenously, they mimic some of the effects of intestinal nutrients. It is well established that exogenous administration of CCK inhibits gastric emptying, and it now seems clear that CCK mediates its effect in a neurally dependent fashion. Inhibition of gastric emptying induced by CCK is attenuated by systemic capsaicin treatment[4] and by functional ablation of the vagal afferent pathway.[5] The proposed mechanism is that CCK decreases tone in the proximal stomach, which tends to delay the emptying of gastric contents. This effect of CCK to inhibit proximal gastric motility is also abolished by vagotomy and is hexamethonium-sensitive, suggesting it activates a vagal reflex pathway.[6,7]

EVIDENCE FOR A ROLE FOR CCK

The availability of potent CCK receptor antagonists over the last 5 years has provided evidence for a role for CCK in the regulation of postprandial gastric

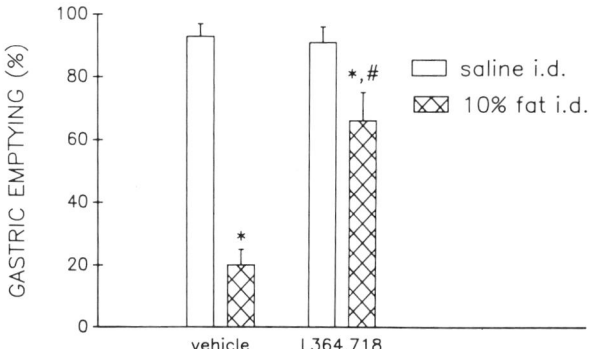

FIGURE 4. Intraduodenal perfusion of 10% lipid increased plasma levels of CCK in the portal blood in rats, whereas maltose (300 mM, 10%) had no effect. The duodenum of awake rats was perfused with saline, lipid, or maltose (300 mM) for 10 minutes and then blood was taken from the portal vein under pentobarbitone anesthesia. CCK in plasma was measured by Drs. Turkelson and Solomon (VA Kansas City, Kansas).

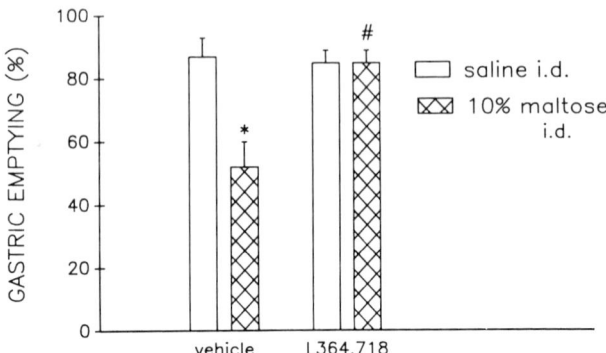

FIGURE 5. Effect of administration of L364718 on inhibition of gastric emptying induced by maltose (10%, 300 mM). Gastric emptying was measured in awake rats after intraperitoneal injection of either vehicle or antagonist 30 minutes before gastric emptying was measured. $^*p < 0.05$ saline vs maltose; $p < 0.01$ vehicle vs L364718.

function.[8–10] In experimental animals, administration of the selective CCK A receptor antagonist devazepide (MK-329) accelerated the emptying of a liquid mixed nutrient meal[11] and reversed the delay in gastric emptying induced by hydrolyzed protein, but not acid or hyperosmolar saline solution.[12] In addition, inhibition of

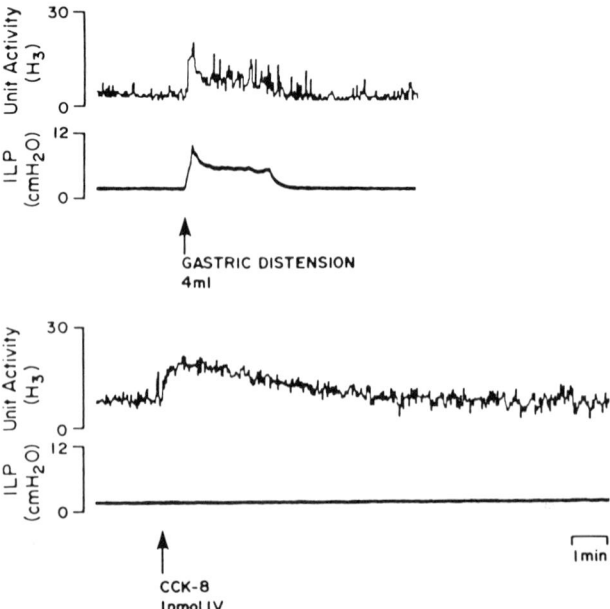

FIGURE 6. Cholecystokinin (CCK) stimulates gastric mechanoreceptor discharge in the anesthetized rat. Integrated record of firing from a single unit from the cervical vagus shows stimulation of afferent fiber discharge by gastric distention and CCK.

gastric emptying in response to a protease inhibitor that is thought to release endogenous CCK by inhibiting negative feedback control by lumenal proteases was also inhibited by MK329.[12] Inhibition of gastric emptying induced by intralipid in rats was attenuated by administration of MK329[2] (FIG. 3). However, this drug had no effect on inhibition of gastric emptying induced by fat in dogs.[13,14] In man, the use of CCK antagonists has produced evidence both for and against a role for CCK in the regulation of gastric emptying. Administration of loxiglumide accelerated the emptying of liquid meal in man,[15] but it had no effect on emptying of a standard meal.[16] Administration of MK329 inhibited gallbladder contraction in response to a stan-

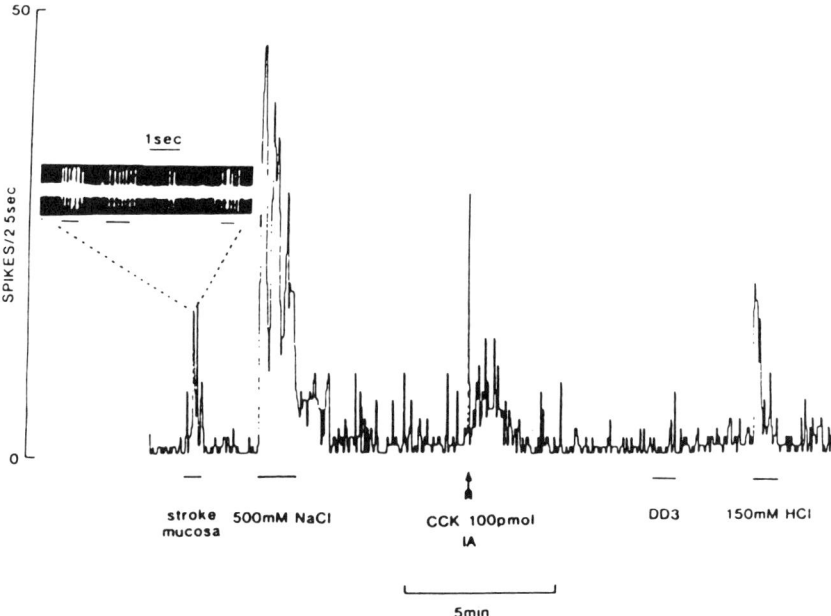

FIGURE 7. Integrated record of firing of duodenal mucosal afferent. Stimulation of discharge in this afferent fiber in response to duodenal stimulation and CCK. This unit exhibits the characteristics of a mucosal receptor, because it is activated by mucosal stroking, hyperosmotic saline solution, and intraduodenal infusion of acid, but it is unaffected by duodenal distention with 3 ml of saline solution (DD3). This unit also responds vigorously to local injection of CCK. (From reference 23 with permission.)

dard, mixed nutrient meal, but it had no effect on the emptying of either the liquid or the solid phase of the meal.[17]

The effect of the CCK antagonist is not always limited to nutrients that result in an increase in circulating concentrations of CCK. Nutrients such as maltose and other carbohydrates do not increase plasma levels of CCK in the peripheral or portal plasma (FIG. 4), but their effects on gastric emptying are mediated via a CCK-dependent pathway[3] (FIG. 5). It is our hypothesis that CCK may be released by fat or carbohydrate and achieve locally high concentrations that stimulate CCK receptors on sensory nerve endings situated in the duodenal mucosa. Thus, measurable

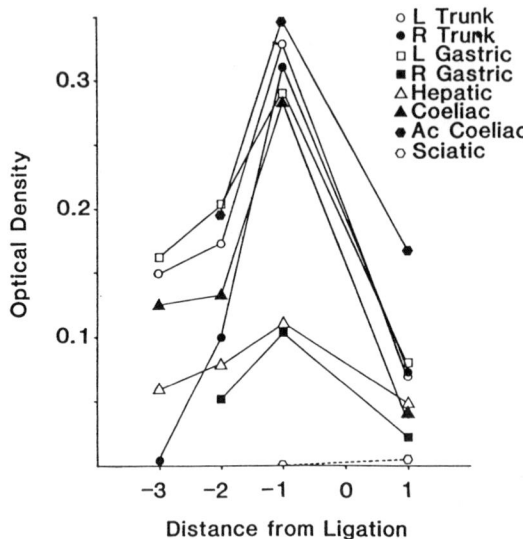

FIGURE 8. Relative density of CCK binding sites accumulated proximal to a ligature on the left and right vagal trunks, on different branches of the subdiaphragmatic vagus, and on the sciatic nerve. Receptors for CCK visualized by autoradiography accumulate proximal to the ligature, indicating that they are transported from the cell bodies towards the periphery. Binding sites occur in greatest density on the accessory celiac and celiac branches of the subdiaphragmatic vagus. (Reprinted from reference 27 with permission.)

circulating levels of CCK are not indicative of the importance of a physiological effect of peripheral CCK in gastric emptying. Alternatively, fat releases CCK, which achieves high enough plasma concentrations to act via the circulation to stimulate vagal sensory endings in the stomach to produce a vagovagal reflex decrease in gastric motility and hence delay gastric emptying.

In inhibition of feeding experiments, a similar finding has been described. The potency of nutrients to inhibit feeding is not related to their ability to increase circulating levels of CCK. Thus, casein, which increases circulating levels of CCK, has a weak effect on real or sham feeding, whereas maltose potently inhibits feeding. In addition, the response to these different nutrients, fat, protein, and carbohydrate is blocked by peripheral, but not central, administration of MK329. This is discussed in more detail by Ritter (this volume).

If we are suggesting that endogenous CCK acts by a neural pathway, we must examine evidence from electrophysiological recording of visceral afferents and from studies of the receptor distribution for CCK on visceral afferents that might support our hypothesis.

INTESTINAL SENSORY INNERVATION

Studies have confirmed the existence of gastrointestinal mechanoreceptors and chemoreceptors in the gut wall.[18] Muscle endings with vagal afferent fibers detect tension within the muscle generated either by passive distention or actively by contraction. Afferent fibers, both vagal and spinal, with mucosal terminal fields form a heterogeneous group. Specific amino acid receptors, glucoreceptors, liporeceptors, and acid receptors have been described in several species. However, several groups find that these mucosal receptors are polymodal, responding to a number of lumenal stimulants and also to light brushing of the mucosa.

It is not known how changes in lumenal contents alter afferent fiber discharge.

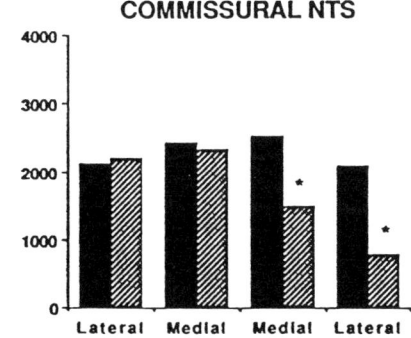

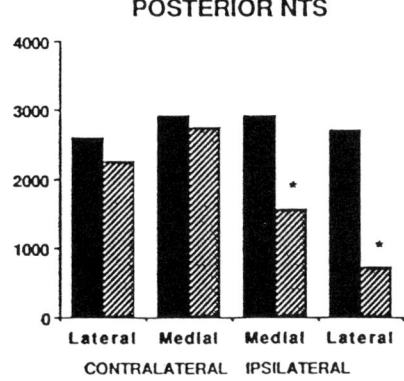

FIGURE 9. Effect of efferent and afferent vagal rootlet transection on density of CCK binding sites in the nucleus of the solitary tract. Afferent transection significantly reduced the density of binding sites only in the ipsilateral NTS at all levels examined, suggesting that the receptors are on vagal afferent fibers. (From reference 28 with permission.)

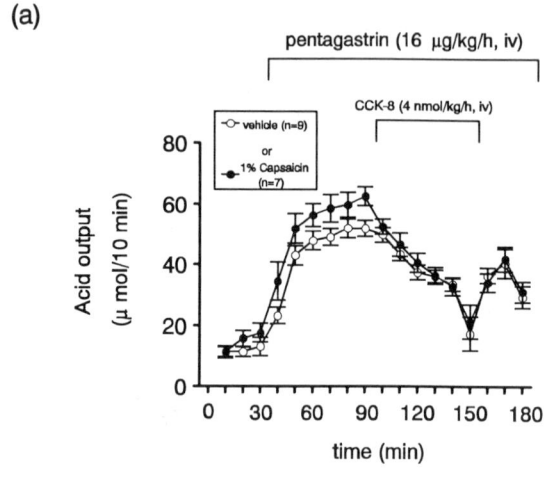

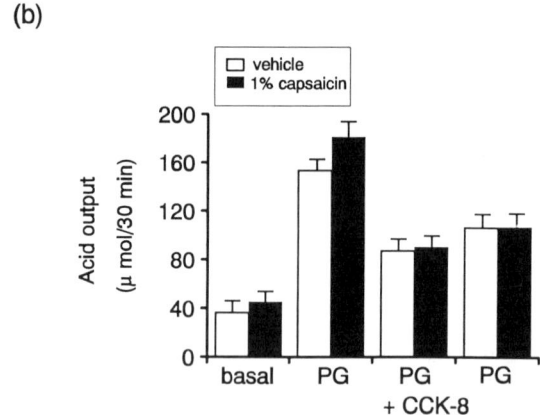

FIGURE 10. Effect of perivagal capsaicin treatment on the inhibition of gastric acid secretion induced by exogenous CCK. Intravenous infusion of CCK inhibits pentagastrin-stimulated gastric acid secretion in urethane-anesthetized rats. This response was unaltered by functional ablation of the vagal sensory pathway using capsaicin. (From reference 35 with permission.)

The available evidence from morphological studies suggests that afferent terminals lie in the lamina propria, below epithelial cells.[19] Therefore, it is not clear how changes in lumenal content are signaled to afferent terminals that are not directly exposed to these lumenal contents.

PRIMARY AFFERENT RESPONSES TO CCK

It is now well established that gastric mechanoreceptor discharge is stimulated by circulating CCK in rats.[20–22] In experiments recording from single vagal afferent fibers, over 90% of afferent fibers responding to gastric distention also respond to CCK given close-arterial to the stomach (FIG. 6). However, in the ferret, it seems that antral and duodenal mucosal receptors, not muscle mechanoreceptors, are responsive to CCK.[23] These units are also responsive to intestinal perfusion with acid and with solutions of high osmolarity (FIG. 7).

The afferent response to CCK is capsaicin sensitive in rats.[20] In recordings from vagal afferent fibers in rats in which the vagus has been pretreated with capsaicin, units responding to distention can still be found, but no units respond to CCK. These observations support functional data showing that inhibition of gastric motility and emptying in response to CCK is abolished by perivagal capsaicin.[5]

TRANSDUCTION PROCESS IN AFFERENT ENDINGS

If the afferents terminate in the lamina propria or epithelium, what is the "sensory transduction" mechanism by which lumenal contents alter afferent discharge? It is possible that the transduction mechanism for mucosal receptors lies in some kind of mechanical distortion of the receptive field. However, for stimuli-

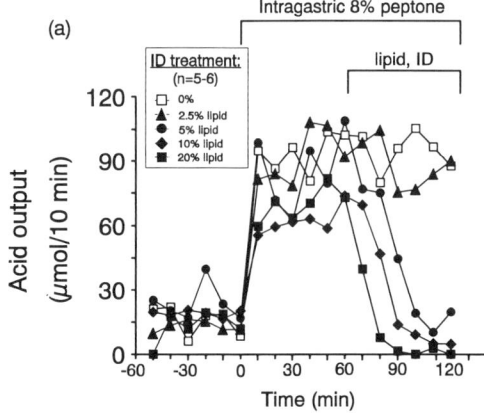

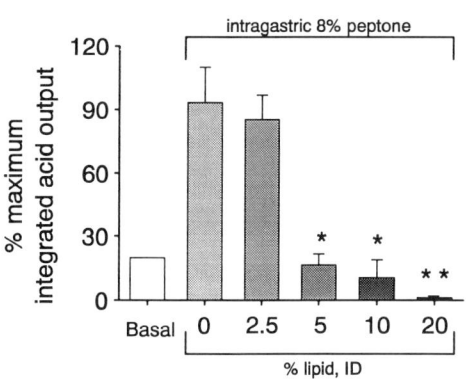

FIGURE 11. Effect of intraduodenal lipid infusion on gastric acid secretion in awake rats. Gastric acid secretion stimulated by intragastric peptone was measured continuously by extragastric titration in awake rats fitted with chronic gastric and duodenal cannulas. Gastric acid secretion was dose-dependently inhibited by intraduodenal perfusion with lipid. (From reference 36 with permission.)

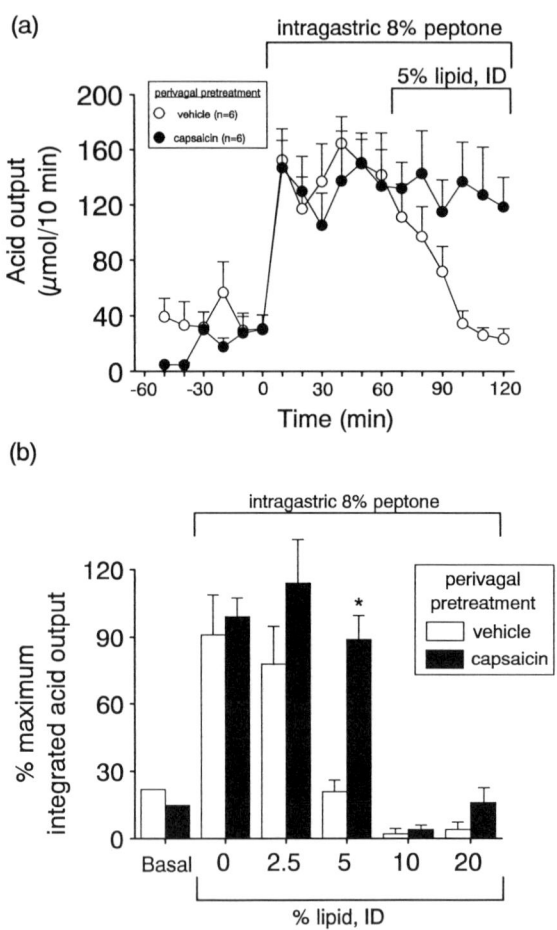

FIGURE 12. Effect of functional ablation of the vagal afferent pathway on lipid-induced inhibition of gastric acid secretion in the conscious rat. Inhibition of gastric acid secretion induced by intraduodenal perfusion with 5% lipid is completely abolished by perivagal application of capsaicin. (From reference 36 with permission.)

specific receptors, an alternate hypothesis has to be put forward. Mucosal receptors may be activated secondarily to paracrine release of a peptide or amine.[24,25] It is in this way that CCK is proposed to play a role. Mucosal epithelial cells have apical finger-like projections into the gut lumen that would be ideally placed to taste the lumenal contents, then release a neuroactive agent that then diffuses to stimulate afferent fiber discharge. This arrangement is similar to that found in tastebuds.[25]

RECEPTORS FOR CCK ON VAGAL AND SPINAL AFFERENTS

That CCK binding sites could be detected on vagal nerves was shown by autoradiography by Zarbin et al.[26] in 1981. Moran et al.[27] showed that these putative

CCK receptors exhibit selectivity for sulfated *versus* nonsulfated CCK-8, indicating that they are type A receptors, that they are transported on vagal fibers both centrally and peripherally,[28] and that they occur on all subdiaphragmatic vagal branches (FIG. 8). These receptors have been shown to be on afferents; unilateral afferent but not efferent vagal rootlet transection[28] or nodosectomy[29] decreases CCK bindings sites in the ipsilateral nucleus of the solitary tract (FIG. 9); and infraganglionic but not supraganglionic section abolished peripheral transport of receptors, demonstrating that they are on afferent fibers.[29] Recent studies with nonpeptide antagonists for CCK (MK329 and L365260) provide evidence for both type A and B CCK receptors on the vagus nerve.[30] The density of these receptors is reduced by 50% after neonatal capsaicin treatment.[31]

In addition to CCK binding sites on abdominal vagal afferents, binding sites for CCK are also present on dorsal root ganglia cells.[32,33] At this point it is not clear if they are on a subpopulation of cell bodies that innervates the viscera.

FUNCTIONAL IMPORTANCE OF CCK AND NEURAL PATHWAYS IN FEEDBACK REGULATION

We have discussed evidence that CCK, released by nutrients in the intestine, may act either locally or via the circulation to stimulate afferent fiber discharge to regulate the emptying of gastric contents. In addition, evidence also indicates that CCK may play a similar role in the regulation of food intake (Ritter, this volume). Moreover, there is evidence that CCK acting on neural pathways plays a role in the regulation of gastric acid and pancreatic secretion in the postprandial period.

Experimental evidence suggests that CCK may be one of the principal enterogastrones that mediates fat-induced inhibition of gastric acid secretion. However, the

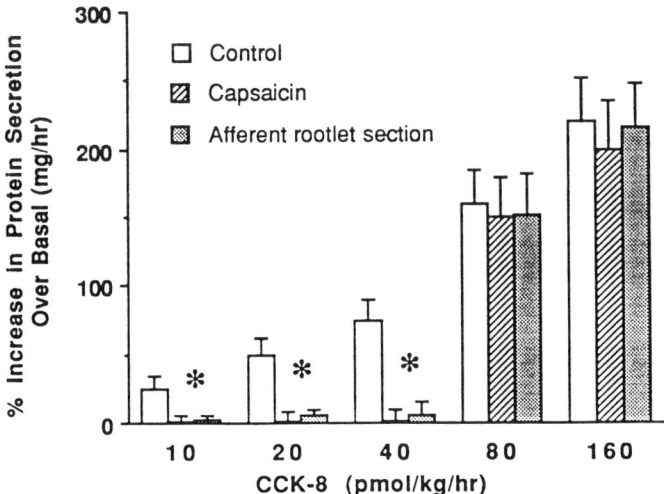

FIGURE 13. Perivagal application of capsaicin or vagal afferent rootlet transection completely abolished the increase in pancreatic protein secretion in response to exogenous CCK. Pancreatic protein secretion was measured in anesthetized rats treated either with capsaicin infused into the gastroduodenum or after vagal afferent root transection. (From reference 37 with permission.)

mechanism by which CCK acts is not completely determined. CCK-induced inhibition of meal-stimulated gastric acid secretion is blocked by administration of MK329 in dogs[13] and, in some cases, in man.[34] In the rat, administration of MK329 blocks CCK-induced inhibition of agonist-induced gastric acid secretion.[35] This inhibition seems to involve release of somatostatin, because administration of a monoclonal antibody against somatostatin inhibits the CCK-induced inhibition of gastric acid secretion.[35] However, perivagal capsaicin pretreatment had no effect on CCK-induced inhibition of gastric acid secretion, suggesting that exogenous, circulating CCK does not act by way of a vagal afferent pathway to inhibit gastric acid secretion[35] (FIG. 10).

How does endogenous CCK act to inhibit gastric acid secretion? In conscious dogs and rats, inhibition of meal-stimulated gastric acid secretion by intestinal perfusion with intralipid was abolished by the administration of MK329,[13,36] suggesting a physiological role for CCK in mediating intestinal feedback inhibition of gastric

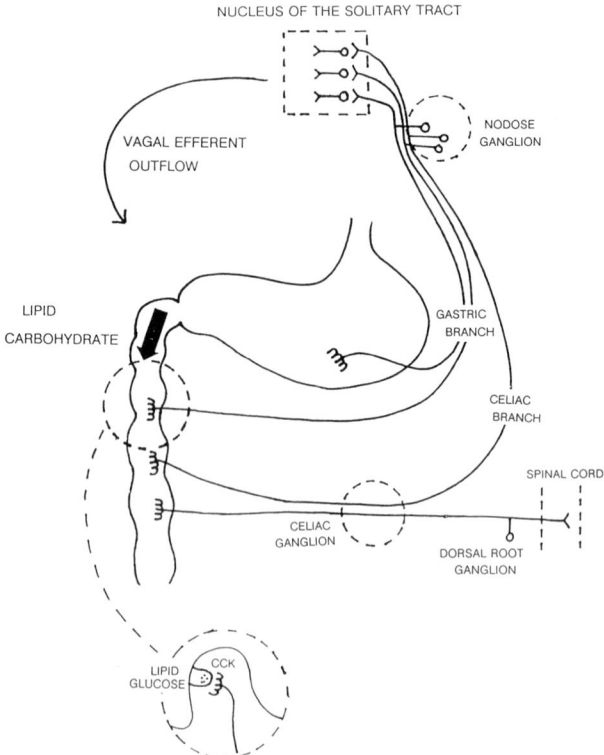

FIGURE 14. Proposed pathway by which nutrients in the intestine may inhibit gastric emptying. Because maltose delays gastric emptying via CCK-dependent pathways and yet does not increase circulating CCK, we propose that maltose releases CCK locally, which then stimulates vagal and spinal afferents to produce changes in function. Lipid may act in this way, but it may also act by releasing CCK into the circulation, stimulating gastric mechanoreceptors. These effects are mediated by afferents passing to the central nervous system in both the vagus nerve and the splanchnic nerves, some of which pass through the celiac/superior mesenteric ganglion.

acid secretion. In addition, in rats the lipid-induced inhibition of gastric acid secretion was markedly attenuated by functional ablation of the vagal, but not spinal, visceral afferent pathway[36] (FIGS. 11 and 12). Thus, endogenous release of CCK by fat in the intestine acts to inhibit gastric acid secretion by way of a capsaicin-sensitive pathway, similar to the pathway to inhibit gastric emptying. This result supports the hypothesis that CCK acts in the intestine to stimulate vagal afferent fiber discharge.

Intestinal nutrients also increase pancreatic secretion as part of the intestinal feedback regulation of proximal gut function. CCK released by intestinal nutrients is thought to act directly on acinar cells to stimulate pancreatic enzyme secretion. However, recent evidence from Owyang's group[37] suggests that CCK, at physiologically relevant doses, can act via a vagal afferent pathway, originating in the intestine, to increase pancreatic secretion. In anesthetized rats, stimulation of pancreatic secretion in response to small doses of exogenous CCK, similar to those seen after a meal, was abolished by hexamethonium or bilateral cervical vagotomy, suggesting that a reflex pathway is involved. Pancreatic protein secretion in response to small doses of CCK was also abolished by gastroduodenal infusion of capsaicin or vagal afferent rootlet transection (FIG. 13), suggesting that the response comes from the intestinal mucosa. In addition, endogenous CCK released by intestinal infusion with soybean trypsin inhibitor stimulates pancreatic protein secretion; this response was also abolished by intraluminal capsaicin.

SUMMARY

Cholecystokinin (CCK) stimulates vagal afferent fiber discharge, both gastric and intestinal, which seems to result in reflex decrease in gastric motility, gastric acid secretion, and stimulation of pancreatic protein secretion. Endogenous release of CCK by fat or soybean trypsin inhibitor also alters function by way of a capsaicin-sensitive pathway. We suggest that CCK is released locally from the intestine and acts locally or systemically to stimulate vagal afferent fiber discharge to alter proximal gastrointestinal function (FIG. 14). In this way, in addition to its effect on food intake, CCK and the neural pathway integrate function in the proximal gastrointestinal tract, regulating the entry of food into the duodenum to ensure effective digestion and absorption.

REFERENCES

1. ASPIROZ, F. & J. M. MALAGELADA. 1986. Am. J. Physiol. **251:** G727–G735.
2. HOLZER, H. H., C. M. TURKELSON, T. E. SOLOMON & H. E. RAYBOULD. 1991. Gastroenterology **100:** A451.
3. RAYBOULD, H. E. & H. H. HOLZER. 1992. Neurosci. Letts. **141:** 236–238.
4. FORSTER, E. R., T. GREEN, M. ELIOT, A. BREMNER & G. J. DOCKRAY. 1991. Am. J. Physiol. **258:** G552–G556.
5. RAYBOULD, H. E. & Y. TACHE. 1988. Am. J. Physiol. **255:** G242–G246.
6. RAYBOULD, H. E., M. E. ROBERTS & G. J. DOCKRAY. 1987. Am. J. Physiol. **253:** G165–G170.
7. BLACKSHAW, L. A. & D. GRUNDY. 1991. J. Auton. Nerv. Syst. **36:** 129–138.
8. EVANS, B. E., M. G. BOCK, K. E. RITTLE, R. M. DIPARDO, W. L. WHITTER, D. F. VEBER, P. S. ANDERSON & R. M. FREIDEINGER. 1986. Proc. Natl. Acad. Sci. USA **83:** 4918–4922.
9. CHANG, R. S. L. & V. J. LOTTI. 1986. Proc. Natl. Acad. Sci. USA **83:** 4923–4926.
10. LOTTI, V. J., R. G. PENDLETON, R. J. GOULD, H. M. HANSON, R. S. L. CHANG & B. V. CLINESCHMIDT. 1987. J. Pharmacol. Exp. Ther. **241:** 103–109.

11. SHILABEER, G. & J. S. DAVISON. 1987. Am. J. Physiol. **252:** G353–G360.
12. GREEN, T., R. DIMALINE, S. PEIKIN & G. J. DOCKRAY. 1988. Am. J. Physiol. **255:** G685–G689.
13. LLOYD, K. C. K., V. MAXWELL, T. O. G. KOVACS, J. MILLER & J. H. WALSH. 1992. Gastroenterology **102:** 131–138.
14. PENDLETON, R. G., R. J. BENDENSKY, L. SCHAFFER, T. E. NOLAN, R. J. GOULD & B. V. CLINESCHMIDT. 1987. J. Pharmacol. Exp. Ther. **241:** 110–116.
15. MEYER, B. M., C. BEGLINGER, J. B. M. J. JANSEN, L. C. ROVATI, B. A. WERTH, P. HILDEBRAND, D. ZACH & G. A. STADLER. 1989. Lancet **8653:** 12–15.
16. CORAZZIARI, E., R. RICCI, D. BILIOTTI, I. BONTEMPO, A. DE'MEDICI, N. PALLOTTA & A. TORSOLI. 1990. Dig. Dis. Sci. **35:** 50–54.
17. LIDDLE, R. A., B. J. GERTZ, S. KANAYAMA, L. BECCARIA, L. D. COKER, T. A. TURNBULL & E. T. MORITA. J. Clin. Invest. **84:** 1220–1225.
18. GRUNDY, D. & T. SCRATCHERD. 1989. *In* Handbook of Physiology. Section 6. Volume 1. Motility and circulation. S. G. Schultz, J. D. Wood & B. B. Rauner, eds.: 593–620. American Physiology Society. Bethesda.
19. SATO, M. & H. KOYANO. 1987. Brain Res. **400:** 101–109.
20. RAYBOULD, H. E. & J. S. DAVISON. 1989. Soc. Neurosci. Abstr. **15:** 973.
21. DAVISON, J. S. & G. D. CLARKE. 1988. Am. J. Physiol. **255:** G55–G61.
22. SCHWARTZ, G. J., P. R. MCHUGH & T. H. MORAN. 1991. Am. J. Physiol. **261:** R64–R69.
23. BLACKSHAW, L. A. & D. GRUNDY. 1990. J. Auton. Nerv. System **31:** 191–202.
24. GRUNDY, D. 1988. J. Auton. Nerv. System **22:** 175–180.
25. FUJITA, T. 1991. Physiol. Behav. **49:** 883–885.
26. ZARBIN, M. A., J. K. WALMSLEY, R. B. INNIS & M. J. KUHAR. Life Sci. **29:** 697–705.
27. MORAN, T. H., G. P. SMITH, A. M. HOSTETLER & P. R. MCHUGH. 1987. Brain Res. **415:** 149–152.
28. MORAN, T. H., R. NORGREN, R. J. CROSBY & P. R. MCHUGH. 1990. Brain Res. **526:** 95–102.
29. LADENHEIM, E. E., R. C. SPETH & R. C. RITTER. 1988. Brain Res. **474:** 125–129.
30. MERCER, J. G. & C. B. LAWRENCE. 1992. Neurosci. Letts. **137:** 229–231.
31. MERCER, J. G., D. A. H. FARNINGHAM & C. B. LAWRENCE. 1992. Brain Res. **569:** 311–316.
32. MANTYH, P. W., M. D. CATTON, C. J. ALLEN, M. E. LABENSKI, J. E. MAGGIO & S. R. VIGNA. 1992. Neuroscience **46:** 739–754.
33. GHILARDI, J. R., C. J. ALLEN, S. R. VIGNA, D. C. MCVEY & P. W. MANTYH. 1992. J. Neurosci. **12:** 4854–4866.
34. KONTUREK, S. J., N. KWIECIEN, W. OBTULOWICZ, B. KOPP, J. OLESKY & L. ROVATI. 1990. Digestion **45:** 1–8.
35. LLOYD, K. C. K., H. E. RAYBOULD & J. H. WALSH. 1992. Am. J. Physiol. **262:** G287–G292.
36. LLOYD, K. C. K., H. H. HOLZER, T. T. ZITTEL & H. E. RAYBOULD. 1993. Am. J. Physiol. **264:** G659–G663.
37. LI, Y. & C. OWYANG. 1993. J. Clin. Invest., **92:** 418–424.

CCK in Cerebral Cortex and at the Spinal Level[a]

T. HÖKFELT,[b] P. MORINO,[b] V. VERGE,[b] M.-N. CASTEL,[b]
C. BROBERGER,[b] X. ZHANG,[b]
M. HERRERA-MARSCHITZ,[c] J. J. MEANA,[c]
U. UNGERSTEDT,[c] X.-J. XU,[d] J.-X. HAO,[d] M. J. C. PUKE,[d]
ZS. WIESENFELD-HALLIN,[d] Å. SEIGER,[e] J. HUGHES,[f]
A. VARRO,[g] AND G. DOCKRAY[g]

Departments of [b]Neuroscience and [c]Pharmacology
Karolinska Institutet
Stockholm, Sweden

[d]*Department of Clinical Physiology*
Section of Clinical Neurophysiology
Karolinska Institutet
Stockholm, Sweden

[e]*Department of Geriatric Medicine*
Huddinge University Hospital
Karolinska Institutet
Stockholm, Sweden

[f]*Parke-Davis Neuroscience Research Centre*
Cambridge, UK

[g]*Department of Physiology*
University of Liverpool
Liverpool, UK

Cholecystokinin (CCK), the gut hormone,[1] is present in the rat central nervous system,[2] mainly in the form of the sulfated COOH-terminal octapeptide CCK-8S,[3] and it has a wide distribution as revealed with radioimmunoassay,[4] immunohistochemistry,[5,6] and *in situ* hybridization.[7,8] Moreover, CCK has been shown to coexist with classic transmitters such as dopamine in the ventral mesencephalon[9] and GABA in cortical interneurons.[10] In our laboratory we have mainly analyzed CCK-like immunoreactivity (LI) with immunohistochemistry and CCK mRNA with *in situ* hybridization, and more recently CCK with *in vivo* microdialysis, and have focused our attention on several systems in cortex, basal ganglia, and spinal cord including sensory neurons. Progress in this work has been reported at several meetings on CCK.[11–14] Here we briefly summarize our recent findings on cortical systems and on neurons at the spinal cord level. We will not deal with CCK-dopamine coexistence now, but refer to a recent review article.[14]

---

[a]This work was supported by the Swedish MRC, the National Institute of Mental Health, the Bank of Sweden Terecentenary Foundation, the Wenner Gren Center Foundation, the King Gustav V and Queen Victoria Foundation, and the Miami Project Foundation.

CCK IN CORTEX

Cortical areas have very high concentrations of CCK-LI.[4] Despite this, even detailed immunohistochemical studies have only revealed small numbers of CCK-positive neurons in rat cortex, constituting less than 1% of the neuronal population in this brain region.[15-17] These CCK-positive cells are nonpyramidal neurons with the highest numbers in layers II and III. It therefore came as both a surprise and a partial explanation when *in situ* hybridization studies revealed extensive populations of cortical cells, including pyramidal neurons, containing CCK mRNA.[7,8,18-21] This raises the question whether in these neurons there is a translation into CCK peptides recognized by the commonly used antisera or whether CCK peptide levels in the individual cells are too low to be detected with immunohistochemistry. A partial explanation was obtained when it was shown that intraventricular colchicine reduces CCK mRNA levels in cortical areas.[22] Colchicine is assumed to act on microtubles, in this way preventing centrifugal transport of the peptide. It is routinely used to elevate peptide levels in cell bodies in rat brain in order to make them detectable with immunohistochemistry.

Recently we used a novel antibody directed against a COOH-terminal fragment of rat pro-CCK to further investigate this question.[23] With this antiserum two populations of cortical CCK-immunoreactive neurons could be observed even in normal animals, that is, those without colchicine treatment. A small population of neurons was strongly fluorescent and of nonpyramidal type. Double staining experiments using monoclonal antibodies against CCK-8 revealed that these strongly pro-CCK–positive cells also contain CCK-8-LI. The other population represented a large number of cells, the majority being pyramidal neurons. Here the immunoreactive product was mostly confined to the Golgi apparatus and thus appeared as a faint globular or fibrous immunoreactivity surrounding the nucleus. These cells were found in layers II, III, V, and VI, thus showing a distinct overlap with the CCK mRNA-positive cell bodies. Although double labeling experiments have so far not been carried out, it is highly likely that the CCK mRNA-positive cells at least express a CCK precursor peptide.[23] This pro-CCK-LI was also found in all other regions previously shown to contain CCK-positive cell bodies and also to a certain extent in fibers.[23] For example, the bed nucleus of the stria terminalis and certain areas of the posterior, medial nucleus accumbens exhibited a weakly fluorescent fiber plexus, overlapping with strongly CCK-immunoreactive fibers seen with the common CCK-8 antisera. Whether the antibodies recognize a free peptide fragment or react with an amino acid sequence within the precursor is not yet known.

CORTICOSTRIATAL CCK SYSTEMS

It is well known that cortical neurons project to the striatum in the rat with both ipsilateral and crossed projections.[24] The presence of numerous CCK neurons in cortex including pyramidal cells therefore raises the question of a corticostriatal CCK pathway. Combined lesions and radioimmunoassay of CCK-LI have provided evidence for such a pathway and subsequently also that some of these fibers are crossed.[25,26] Burgunder and Young[27] injected tracer into the striatum and observed retrogradely labeled, CCK mRNA-positive neurons bilaterally in cortical areas, providing further evidence for a crossed corticostriatal CCK pathway. Many CCK neurons in cortex may also represent association fibers projecting to the contralateral cortex, because CCK-positive fibers have been described in corpus callosum[6] and because of a marked accumulation of CCK-LI in corpus callosum after colchicine injection[13] or after mechanical transection.[28] Furthermore, in combined lesion and immunohistochemical experiments, complete disappearance of CCK immunoreactive patches in the medial aspects of the caudate nucleus was observed after cortical kainic acid injections combined with callosotomy.[28] This effect was only seen on the ipsilateral side. Taken together, these findings strongly suggest that a corticostriatal CCK pathway exists that is partly crossed.

The corticostriatal pathway has also been analyzed in studies on CCK release using *in vivo* microdialysis combined with cortical lesions[29,30] (see also ref. 31). Low basal, extracellular CCK levels could be measured with the microdialysis probe, and a 30-fold increase in CCK levels was noted after potassium depolarization. The CCK release was calcium-dependent (see also ref. 31). After unilateral decortication (multiple kainic acid injections), no differences were found between basal levels detected on intact and lesioned side or between the two sides after potassium stimulation. However, when unilateral decortication was combined with callosotomy, CCK was significantly decreased to about 30% (basal) or 40% (KCl stimulation) of control levels. This decrease was only seen on the ipsilateral side. The authenticity of the monitored CCK was established by HPLC of the recovered peptide showing coelution with CCK-8, with no or only minute amounts of immunoreactivity at the positions of CCK-4 and CCK-5.[30] These results further support the occurrence of a corticostriatal CCK pathway which contains releasable CCK-8 in terminal ramifications in the striatum.

The presence of a corticostriatal glutamatergic pathway in rats has been demonstrated in many studies.[32–37] A further interesting question concerns therefore the relation between the corticostriatal CCK pathway and those corticostriatal neurons containing glutamate. More precisely, is it possible that CCK and glutamate coexist in a corticostriatal pathway? This question was in part addressed in the *in vivo* microdialysis experiments, because in parallel also glutamate and aspartate release was monitored.[29,30] In fact, after unilateral decortication plus callosotomy a less strong decrease in the glutamate level was observed as for CCK, that is, by 35% under basal conditions and by 45% after K^+ depolarization. With regard to aspartate, a bilateral decrease was observed in our first study,[29] but no significant changes were seen in the subsequent one.[30] Further histochemical evidence is needed however to establish the coexistence of CCK and glutamate in corticostriatal neurons.

CCK IN SENSORY AND SPINAL NEURONS

In the early 1980s several studies reported that primary sensory neurons contain CCK-LI (see ref. 13). However, subsequent analysis raised the possibility that COOH-terminally directed CCK antisera may cross-react with calcitonin gene-related peptide (CGRP),[38] presumably due to the identity of two amino acids in the COOH-terminal part of the two peptides. (For a discussion see ref. 13.) In agreement, several *in situ* hybridization studies have reported the lack of CCK mRNA-positive neurons in dorsal root ganglia or at most in single cells.[39–41] This situation may be unique for rat, because genuine CCK-LI has been described in guinea pig[42] and high levels of CCK mRNA have been reported in sensory ganglia in monkey.[43] The latter findings are in good agreement with physiological studies on the eye, demonstrating the potent effects of CCK on the iris in monkey, presumably related to sensory neurons.[44–46] Recently we analyzed lumbar 4 and 5 dorsal root ganglia in the rat after peripheral axotomy. Three weeks after nerve section, up to 30% of the remaining neurons expressed low but significant levels of CCK mRNA.[43] Thus, it is possible that after nerve lesion CCK also in the rat may have a role as mediator released from central branches of sensory neurons in the dorsal horn. High numbers of CCK and CCK mRNA-positive neurons can however be detected in the dorsal horn in the rat under normal circumstances,[11,39,47] suggesting that the effects of CCK at the spinal level under normal conditions mainly are related to these interneurons (see ref. 13).

There is multiple evidence of an involvement of CCK in pain mechanisms. Early studies suggested an antinociceptive effect of centrally administered CCK peptides,[48,49] but more recent studies show that CCK may be an endogenous inhibitor of opioid-induced analgesia. (For review see ref. 50.) This new view is based on the use of smaller doses of CCK as well as CCK antagonists. Thus, exogenously administered CCK reduces the analgesic effect of both morphine and endogenous opioids.[51–58] Furthermore, intrathecal CCK counteracts the depressive effect of morphine on a nociceptive flexor reflex,[59] and the morphine-induced inhibition of C-fiber–evoked discharges of dorsal horn nociceptive neurons is attenuated by CCK.[60] Finally, CCK receptor antagonists potentiate morphine's analgesic effects and prevent tolerance to morphine.[55,61–69] Similar mechanisms may operate in man, because a CCK antagonist enhances analgesia induced by morphine.[54,70]

In two recent studies we explored the possible relation between CCK and chronic pain. Thus, the effect of morphine and a CCK_B antagonist on the self-mutilating behavior (autotomy) of rats was analyzed after axotomy.[71] Autotomy is possibly a sign of neurogenic pain and/or dysesthesia.[72–74] Only small effects were observed, when morphine or the CCK_B antagonist CI-988[75] was individually administered intrathecally.[71] However, when the two compounds were given together, a marked reduction was observed in both the number of rats exhibiting autotomy and the severity of the behavior.[74] We have speculated that the aforementioned increase in CCK mRNA levels after axotomy may result in increased CCK levels and increased CCK release, perhaps counteracting the analgesic action of morphine. The parallel administration of the CCK_B antagonist may then abolish the effect of such endogenously released CCK and allow morphine to reduce the autotomy behavior. These findings may be clinically relevant, as it is known that chronic neurogenic pain is usually difficult to treat[76,77] and is insensitive to opioid analgesics.[78,79]

Involvement of CCK in chronic pain was also observed in a recently developed model based on photochemically induced spinal cord ischemia.[80–82] Two phases were reported, one of tonic allodynia lasting less than a week, followed by a chronic pain-related syndrome. This syndrome was only seen in some rats with severe ischemia and extensive spinal cord lesions. Thus, severe mechanical allodynia was observed in skin areas at the rostral border of the sensory loss. Whereas a number of drugs with analgesic effects failed to affect this allodynia, the recently developed CCK_B receptor antagonist CI-988[75] effectively relieved the allodynia-like symptoms seen in these rats.[83] This effect was reversed by the opioid receptor antagonist naloxone.[83] By contrast, neither the CCK_A antagonist CAM1481 nor diazepam was effective, suggesting that the anxiolytic property of CI-988 is not important for the antiallodynia effect.[81] The mechanisms underlying the apparent analgesic effect of CI-988 in this type of chronic pain model are not known. It is possible that the ischemic lesion initiates an abnormal sensory processing involving up-regulation of CCK systems counteracting the analgesic effect of endogenous opioids and that the CCK_B antagonist blocks these systems. In any case, these results also suggest that CCK_B antagonists should be taken into consideration in the treatment of chronic pain.

REFERENCES

1. MUTT, V. & G. E. JORPES. 1968. Eur. J. Biochem. **6:** 156–162.
2. VANDERHAEGHEN, J. J., P. SIGNEAU & W. GEPTS. 1975. Nature **257:** 604–605.
3. DOCKRAY, G. J. 1980. Brain Res. **188:** 155–165.
4. BEINFELD, M. C., D. K. MEYER, R. L. ESKAY, R. T. JENSEN & M. J. BROWNSTEIN. 1981. Brain Res. **212:** 51–57.
5. INNIS, R. B., F. M. A. CORREA, G. R. UHL, B. SCHNEIDER & S. H. SNYDER. 1979. Proc. Natl. Acad. Sci. USA **76:** 521–525.
6. VANDERHAEGHEN, J. J., F. LOTSTRA, J. DE MEY & C. GILLES. 1980. Proc. Natl. Acad. Sci. USA **77:** 1190–1194.
7. INGRAM, S. M., R. G. KRAUSE, I. F. BALDINO, JR., L. C. SKEEN & M. E. LEWIS. 1989. J. Comp. Neurol. **287:** 260–272.
8. SCHIFFMAN, S. N. & J.-J. VANDERHAEGHEN. 1991. J. Comp. Neurol. **304:** 219–233.
9. HÖKFELT, T., L. SKIRBOLL, J. F. REHFELD, M. GOLDSTEIN, K. MARKEY & O. DANN. 1980. Neuroscience **5:** 2093–2124.
10. JONES, E. G. & S. H. C. HENDRY. 1986. TINS **9:** 71–76.
11. HÖKFELT, T., L. SKIRBOLL, B. J. EVERITT, B. MEISTER, M. BROWNSTEIN, T. JACOBS, A. FADEN, S. KUGA, M. GOLDSTEIN, R. MARKSTEIN, G. DOCKRAY & J. REHFELD. 1985. *In* Neuronal Cholecystokinin. J.-J. Vanderhaeghen & J. N. Crawley, eds. Ann. N.Y. Acad. Sci. **448:** 255–274.
12. HÖKFELT, T., M. SCHALLING, K. SEROOGY, M. HERRERA-MARSCHITZ, R. CORTÉS, S. BRENÉ, Å. DAGERLIND, G. JU, M. ERIKSDOTTER-NILSSON, L. OLSON, B. MEISTER, H. PERSSON, A. ERICSSON, J. REHFELD, C. UNSON, P. GOLDSMITH, A. SPIEGEL & M. GOLDSTEIN. 1989. *In* The Neuropeptide Cholecystokinin (CCK). Anatomy and Biochemistry, Receptors, Pharmacology and Physiology. J. Hughes, G. Dockray & G. Woodruff, eds.: 11–23. John Wiley & Sons. New York.
13. HÖKFELT, T., R. CORTÉS, M. SCHALLING, S. CECCATELLI, M. PELTO-HUIKKO, H. PERSSON & M. J. VILLAR. 1991. Neuropeptides **19:** 31–43.
14. HÖKFELT, T., M. SCHALLING, K. SEROOGY, P. FREY, J. WALSH & M. GOLDSTEIN. 1992. *In* Multiple Cholecystokinin Receptors in the CNS. C. Dourish, S. Cooper, S. Iversen & L. Iversen, eds.: 331–353. Oxford University Press. Oxford.
15. MCDONALD, J. K., J. G. PARNAVELAS, A. KARAMANLIDIS, N. BRECHA & G. ROSENQUIST. 1982. J. Neurocytol. **11:** 881–895.
16. PETERS, A., M. MILLER & L. M. KIMERE. 1983. Neuroscience **8:** 431–448.
17. HENDRY, S. H. C., E. G. JONES & M. C. BEINFELD. 1983. Proc. Natl. Acad. Sci. USA **80:** 2400–2404.
18. BURGUNDER, J. M. & W. S. YOUNG, III. 1988. Mol. Brain Res. **4:** 179–189.
19. SAVASTA, M., J. M. PALACIOS & G. MENGOD. 1988. Neurosci. Lett. **93:** 132–138.
20. VOIGT, M. M. & G. R. UHL. 1988. Mol. Brain Res. **4:** 247–253.
21. LANAUD, P., T. POPOVICI, E. NORMAND, C. LEMOINE, B. BLOCH & B. P. ROQUES. 1989. Neurosci. Lett. **104:** 38–42.
22. CORTÉS, R., S. CECCATELLI, M. SCHALLING & T. HÖKFELT. 1990. Synapse **6:** 369–391.
23. MORINO, P., M. HERRERA-MARSCHITZ, M. N. CASTEL, U. UNGERSTEDT, A. VARRO, G. DOCKRAY & T. HÖKFELT. 1994. Eur. J. Neurosci., in press.
24. MCGEORGE, A. J. & R. L. M. FAULL. 1989. Neuroscience **29:** 503–538.
25. MEYER, D. K., M. C. BEINFELD, W. H. OERTEL & M. J. BROWNSTEIN. 1982. Science **215:** 187–188.
26. MEYER, D. K. & Z. PROTOPAPAS. 1985. Ann. N.Y. Acad. Sci. **448:** 133–143.
27. BURGUNDER, J.-M. & W. S. YOUNG, III. 1990. J. Comp. Neurol. **300:** 26–46.
28. MORINO, P., M. HERRERA-MARSCHITZ, J. J. MEANA, U. UNGERSTEDT & T. HÖKFELT. 1992. Neurosci. Lett. **148:** 133–136.
29. HERRERA-MARSCHITZ, M., J. J. MEANA, T. HÖKFELT, Z.-B. YOU, P. MORINO, E. BRODIN & U. UNGERSTEDT. 1992. NeuroReport **3:** 905–908.
30. YOU, Z.-B., M. HERRERA-MARSCHITZ, E. BRODIN, J. J. MEANA, P. MORINO, T. HÖKFELT, R. SILVEIRA, M. GOINY & U. UNGERSTEDT. 1994. J. Neurochem., in press.

31. MAIDMENT, N. T., B. J. SIDDALL, V. D. RUDOLPH, E. ERDELYI & C. J. EVAN. 1991. Neuroscience **45:** 81–93.
32. FONNUM, F., J. STORM-MATHISEN & I. DIVAC. 1981. Neuroscience **6:** 863–873.
33. MCGEER, P. L., E. G. MCGEER, V. SCHERER & K. SINGH. 1977. Brain Res. **128:** 369–373.
34. REUBI, J. C. & M. CUÉNOD. 1980. Brain Res. **176:** 185–188.
35. ROWLANDS, G. J. & P. J. ROBERTS. 1980. Exp. Brain Res. **39:** 239–240.
36. FAGG, G. E. & A. C. FOSTER. 1983. Neuroscience **9:** 701–719.
37. STREIT, P. 1984. *In* Cerebral Cortex, Vol. 2. Functional Properties of Cortical Cells. E. G. Jones & A. Peters, eds.: 119–143. Plenum. New York.
38. JU, G., T. HÖKFELT, J. A. FISCHER, P. FREY, J. F. REHFELD & G. J. DOCKRAY. 1986. Neurosci. Lett. **68:** 305–310.
39. CORTÉS, R., U. ARVIDSSON, M. SCHALLING, S. CECCATELLI & T. HÖKFELT. 1990. J. Chem. Neuroanat. **3:** 467–485.
40. SEROOGY, K. B., N. K. MOHAPATRA, P. K. LUND, M. RÉTHELYI, D. S. MACGEHEE & E. R. PERL. 1990. Molec. Brain Res. **7:** 171–176.
41. SCHIFFMAN, S. N., E. TEUGELS, P. HALLEUX, R. MENU & J.-J. VANDERHAEGHEN. 1991. Neurosci. Lett. **123:** 123–126.
42. LINDH, B., T. HÖKFELT & L.-G. ELFVIN. 1988. Neuroscience **26:** 1037–1071.
43. VERGE, V. M. K., Z. WIESENFELD-HALLIN & T. HÖKFELT. 1993. Eur. J. Neurosci. **5:** 240–250.
44. ALMEGÅRD, B. & S. E. ANDERSSON. 1990. Exp. Eye Res. **51:** 685–689.
45. BILL, A., S. E. ANDERSSON & B. ALMEGÅRD. 1990. Acta Physiol. Scand. **138:** 479–485.
46. ALMEGÅRD, B., J. STJERNSCHANTZ & A. BILL. 1992. Eur. J. Pharmacol. **211:** 183–187.
47. FUJI, K., E. SENBA, S. FUJI, I. NOMURA, J.-Y. WU, U. UEDA & M. TOHYAMA. 1985. Neuroscience **14:** 881–894.
48. ZETLER, G. 1980. Neuropharmacology **19:** 415–422.
49. JURNA, I. & G. ZETLER. 1981. Eur. J. Pharmacol. **73:** 323–331.
50. BARBER, N. S., C. T. DOURISH & D. R. HILL. 1989. Pain **39:** 307–328.
51. ITOH, S., G. KATSUURA & Y. MAEDA. 1982. Eur. J. Pharmacol. **80:** 421–425.
52. FARIS, P. L., B. R. KOMISARUK, L. R. WATKINS & D. J. MAYER. 1983. Science **219:** 310–312.
53. TANG, J., J. CHOU, M. IADAROLA, H.-Y. T. YANG & E. COSTA. 1984. Neuropharmacology **23:** 715–718.
54. PRICE, D. D., A. VONDERGRUEN, J. MILLER, A. RAFII & C. PRICE. 1985. Anesth. Analg. **64:** 52–60.
55. O'NEILL, M. F., C. T. DOURISH & S. D. IVERSEN. 1989. Neuropharmacology **28:** 243–248.
56. SUH, H. H. & L. F. TSENG. 1990. Eur. J. Pharmacol. **179:** 329–338.
57. SUH, H. H., K. A. COLLINS & T. TSENG. 1992. Neuropeptides **21:** 131–137.
58. TSENG, L. F. & K. A. COLLINS. 1992. J. Pharmacol. Exp. Ther. **260:** 1086–1092.
59. WIESENFELD-HALLIN, Z. & R. DURANTI. 1987. Peptides **8:** 153–158.
60. KELLSTEIN, D. E., D. D. PRICE & D. J. MAYER. 1991. Brain Res. **540:** 302–306.
61. WATKINS, L. R., I. B. KINSCHECK, E. F. S. KAUFMAN, J. MILLER, H. FRENK & D. J. MAYER. 1985. Brain Res. **327:** 181–190.
62. WATKINS, L. R., I. B. KINSCHECK & D. J. MAYER. 1985. Brain Res. **327:** 169–180.
63. PANERAI, A. E., L. C. ROVATI, E. COCCO, P. SACERDOTE & P. MANTEGAZZA. 1987. Brain Res. **40:** 52–60.
64. DOURISH, C. T., M. L. CLARK & S. D. IVERSEN. 1988. Soc. Neurosci. Abstr. **14.** 290.
65. DOURISH, C. T., D. HAWLEY & S. D. IVERSEN. 1988. Eur. J. Pharmacol. **147:** 469–472.
66. DOURISH, C. T., M. F. O'NEILL, J. COUGHLAN, S. J. KITCHENER, D. HAWLEY & S. D. IVERSEN. 1990. Eur. J. Pharmacol. **176:** 35–44.
67. KELLSTEIN, D. E. & D. J. MAYER. 1990. Brain Res. **516:** 263–270.
68. WIESENFELD-HALLIN, Z., X.-J. XU, J. HUGHES, D. C. HORWELL & T. HÖKFELT. 1990. Proc. Natl. Acad. Sci. USA **87:** 7105–7109.
69. XU, X. J., Z. WIESENFELD-HALLIN, J. HUGHES, D. C. HORWELL & T. HÖKFELT. 1992. Br. J. Pharmacol. **105:** 591–596.
70. LAVIGNE, G., K. M. HARGREAVES, E. S. SCHMIDT & R. A. DIONNE. 1989. Clin. Pharmacol. Ther. **45:** 666–673.

71. XU, X.-J., M. J. C. PUKE, V. M. K. VERGE, Z. WIESENFELD-HALLIN, J. HUGHES & T. HÖKFELT. 1993. Neurosci. Lett. **152:** 129–132.
72. WALL, P. D., M. DEVOR, R. INBAL, J. W. SCADDING, D. SCHONFIELD, Z. SELTZER & M. M. TOMKIEWIOCZ. 1979. Pain **7:** 103–113.
73. WIESENFELD-HALLIN, Z. & U. LINDBLOM. 1980. Pain **8:** 285–298.
74. CODERRE, T. J., R. W. GRIMES & R. MELZACK. 1986. Pain **26:** 61–84.
75. HUGHES, J., P. BODEN, B. COSTALL, A. DOMENEY, E. KELLY, D. C. HORWELL, J. C. HUNTER, R. D. PINNOCK & G. N. WOODRUFF. 1990. Proc. Natl. Acad. Sci. USA **87:** 6728–6732.
76. SUNDERLAND, S. 1978. Nerves and Nerve Injuries. Churchill-Livingstone. London.
77. TASKER, R. R. 1990. *In* The Management of Pain. Bonica J. J., ed.: 264–283. Lea & Febiger. Philadelphia.
78. ARNÉR, S. & B. A. MEYERSON. 1988. Pain **33:** 11–23.
79. PORTENOY, R. K., K. M. FOLEY & C. E. INTURRISI. 1991. Pain **43:** 273–286.
80. HAO, J.-X., X.-J. XU, H. ALDSKOGIUS, Å. SEIGER & Z. WIESENFELD-HALLIN. 1991. Pain **45:** 175–185.
81. HAO, J.-X., X.-J. XU, H. ALDSKOGIUS, Å. SEIGER & Z. WIESENFELD-HALLIN. 1992. Exp. Neurol. **118:** 187–194.
82. XU, X.-J., J.-X. HAO, H. ALDSKOGIUS, Å. SEIGER & Z. WIESENFELD-HALLIN. 1992. Pain **48:** 279–290.
83. XU, X.-J., J.-X. HAO, Å. SEIGER, J. HUGHES, T. HÖKFELT & Z. WIESENFELD-HALLIN. 1993. Pain, in press.

Gastric Distention Induces c-Fos Immunoreactivity in the Rat Brain Stem

KATHLEEN A. FRASER AND JOSEPH S. DAVISON

Department of Medical Physiology
University of Calgary
3330 Hospital Dr. N.W.
Calgary, Alberta, Canada, T2N 4N1

Recently, it was demonstrated that c-fos activation can be used as a metabolic marker for tracing polysynaptic pathways in brain and spinal cord. The c-fos oncoprotein can be detected in neurons by immunohistochemistry 20–90 minutes after depolarization. Using this technique, we showed that exogenously administered CCK-8 (100 µg/kg intraperitoneally) activates neurons in the area postrema, the dorsal motor nucleus of the vagus, and the nucleus of the tractus solitarius in the rat brain stem.[1] Furthermore, ingestion of a normal meal, which elevates cholecystokinin (CCK) levels endogenously, induces c-fos immunoreactivity in the nucleus of the tractus solitarius, dorsal motor nucleus of the vagus, and area postrema.[2] However, meal-induced c-fos expression was not blocked by the CCK-A antagonist L-364,718, which will block exogenous CCK-induced fos expression. These findings indicate that feeding induces c-fos expression by a pathway that is largely independent of CCK release. Consequently, the role of alternative gastrointestinal cues activated during the course of feeding was assessed by a sham feeding procedure in which gastric contents emptied through a gastric fistula. Sham feeding produced significantly less c-fos expression in the more caudal aspects of the dorsal vagal complex than did feeding rats with the fistula closed.[3] Furthermore, c-fos immunoreactivity at more rostral levels of the dorsal vagal complex appeared to be comparable to that of fistula closed and fed rats.

The purpose of the present study was to determine if gastric distention is a signal contributing to the pattern of c-fos expression seen after ingestion of a meal. Modified pediatric Foley catheters served as gastric balloons and were chronically implanted in male Sprague-Dawley rats (250–350 g). The non-balloon end of the Foley catheter was drawn beneath the skin and exposed at the back of the neck. Two weeks later, after rats recovered from surgery, the catheters were connected to an infusion pump, and the balloon portion of the catheter was inflated with saline solution and subsequently deflated over a 70-minute period, to reflect physiological distention ($n = 4$). Controls rats were implanted with gastric balloons but were not inflated or deflated ($n = 4$) on the test day. To determine and then mimic the manner in which the stomach normally distends and empties following ingestion of a meal, another group of rats were provided access to the same liquid diet over a 10-minute period. Rats were sacrificed at various intervals (5, 10, 20, and 70 minutes) after the start of the meal, stomachs were removed, and the volume of gastric contents measured. We then used these data to inflate and deflate the balloon catheters according to the following infusion parameters. From 0–5 minutes, 7 ml of saline solution was infused into the catheter at a rate of 1.4 ml/min. An additional 2 ml was infused at a rate of 0.4 ml/min over the next 5 minutes. From 10–20 minutes 0.5 ml of saline solution was withdrawn from the balloon (0.05 ml/min). The last 50 minutes of infusion involved the withdrawal of 1.5 ml of saline solution at a rate of 0.03 ml/min.

Gastric distention produced by inflation of the gastric balloon evoked c-fos expression primarily in the medial nucleus of the tractus solitarius, a region where gastric vagal afferents terminate (FIG. 1b). Furthermore, distention induced either

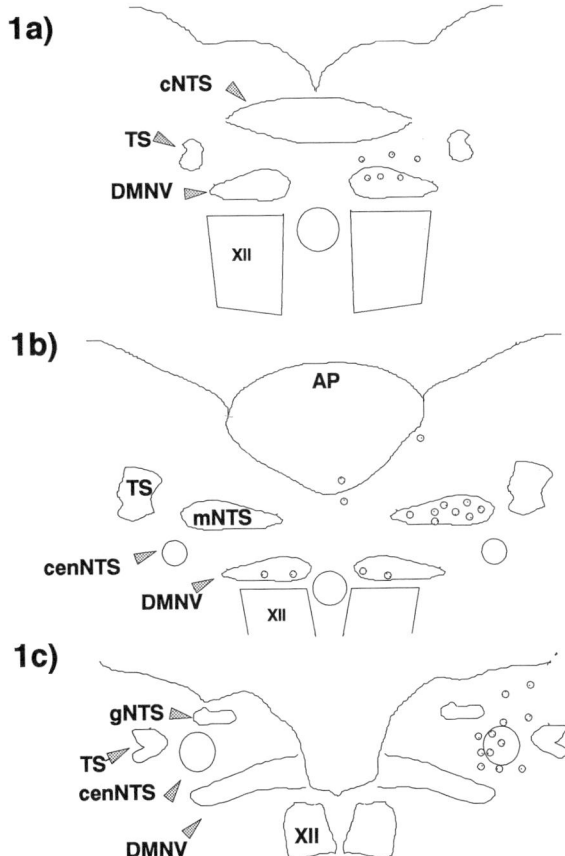

FIGURE 1. Cartoon representations of distention-induced c-fos immunoreactivity at interaural levels: −5.15 mm (a), −4.68 mm (b), and −4.55 mm (c). AP = area postrema; eenNTS = nucleus centralis; cNTS = commissural nucleus of the tractus solitarius; gNTS = nucleus gelatirosis; DMNV = dorsal motor nucleus of the vagus; NTS = nucleus of the tractus solitarius; TS = tractus solitarius. (From Paxinos and Watson.[4])

minimal or no c-fos immunoreactivity in the area postrema. Moderate levels of c-fos expression were evident at the more caudal levels of the dorsal motor nucleus of the vagus (FIG. 1a), whereas more rostral levels stained minimally following distention (FIG. 1c).

Controls failed to stain positively for c-fos immunoreactivity in the area postrema and nucleus of the tractus solitarius. However, two nondistended controls showed minimal c-fos expression in the dorsal motor nucleus of the vagus. These results indicate that the signals arising from the ingestion of a meal activate specific subregions of the nucleus of the tractus solitarius in the rat, which may include the neural pathways involved in signaling satiety.

REFERENCES

1. FRASER, K. A. & J. S. DAVISON. 1992. Exp. Physiol. **77:** 225–228.
2. FRASER, K. A. & J. S. DAVISON. 1993. Am. J. Physiol. **265:** R235–R239.
3. FRASER, K. A., E. RAIZADA & J. S. DAVISON. 1992. Physiol. Canada **23:** 74.
4. PAXINOS G. & C. WATSON. 1986. The Rat Brain in Stereotaxic Coordinates. Academic Press Limited. London.

Feedback Inhibition of Cholecystokinin Secretion by Bile Acids and Pancreatic Proteases

GARY M. GREEN

Department of Physiology
University of Texas Health Science Center at San Antonio
San Antonio, Texas 78284

Gastrointestinal secretions stimulated by the intestinal peptide cholecystokinin (CCK) include pancreatic exocrine secretion and bile, the latter due to contraction of the gallbladder by CCK. The question of whether these secretions act back in a negative feedback fashion to suppress CCK release, and possible mechanisms involved, are the subjects of this review.

INHIBITION OF CCK RELEASE BY BILE AND BILE ACIDS

Three kinds of studies strongly support the concept that bile acids physiologically suppress CCK release: (1) studies in which nutrient-stimulated pancreatic or biliary secretion is inhibited by exogenous bile or bile acids; (2) studies in which CCK release or pancreatic/biliary secretion that is stimulated by luminal nutrients is further augmented by the bile acid binding resin cholestyramine; and (3) studies in which administration of CCK receptor antagonists causes exaggerated CCK release in the presence of luminal nutrients.

Thomas and Crider[1] were the first to report that bile in the intestine had a predominantly inhibitory effect on nutrient-stimulated pancreatic secretion in dogs. Their study was prompted by earlier reports that bile had a stimulatory effect on pancreatic secretion. Studies in dogs provided with chronic gastric and duodenal fistulas permitted sampling of pure pancreatic secretion. Initially, they sought to determine if the introduction of bile alone into the duodenum could stimulate pancreatic secretion, as had previously been reported. They noted that only 7 of 62 injections of bile into the duodenum caused an increase in the rate of pancreatic secretion (only fluid output was measured). They also noted the appearance "at unpredictable times of spontaneous secretion from the pancreas," presaging the discovery of cyclic interdigestive pancreatic secretion. Satisfied that bile had no important stimulatory role in pancreatic secretion, they undertook a systematic study to determine if bile had inhibitory actions on the pancreatic response to other stimuli. They noted that peptone, soap, or hydrochloric acid caused less secretion when given in the presence of bile in the intestine than when given alone, commenting that "Peptone or soap often failed to cause any secretion when bile was present and almost invariably failed if only moderate amounts of the stimulus . . . were used," and they concluded that "In contrast with the doubtful character of the evidence suggesting an excitatory effect of bile on pancreatic secretion, the evidence for an inhibitory effect on the response to various stimuli is clear and consistent."[1]

For three decades after the 1943 report by Thomas and Crider, studies on the effects of bile or bile acids on pancreatic secretion were roughly evenly divided between those showing an inhibitory effect and those showing a stimulatory effect. Convincing confirmation of the views expressed by Thomas and Crider occurred in two publications by Malagelada and coworkers,[2,3] in which they demonstrated in healthy human subjects that bile acids at physiological concentrations could inhibit or abolish gallbladder contraction or pancreatic enzyme secretion stimulated by luminal fatty acids or amino acids. FIGURE 1, taken from their 1973 paper, illustrates the effect of intraduodenal infusion of 10 mM sodium taurocholate on gallbladder contraction (indicated by bilirubin output) and pancreatic enzyme secretion (trypsin output) stimulated by intraduodenal perfusion of an essential amino acid (EAA) solution. Intraduodenal taurocholate strongly inhibited EAA-stimulated pancreatic and biliary secretion. Withdrawal of the taurocholate infusion rapidly elicited gallbladder contraction and pancreatic secretion again. Similar results occurred

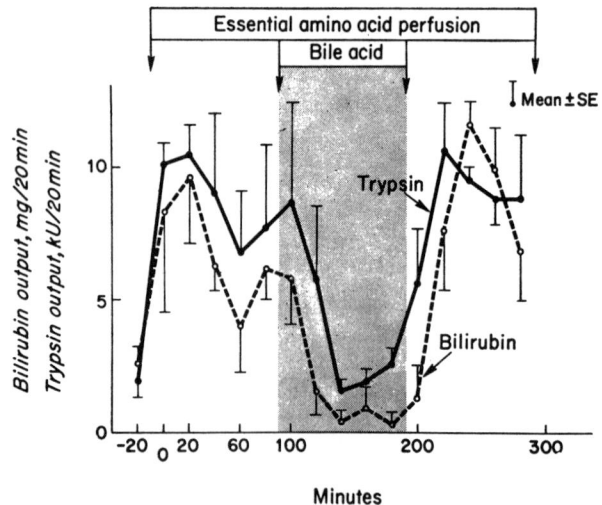

FIGURE 1. Trypsin and bilirubin outputs during continuous intraduodenal perfusion of essential amino acids before, during, and after the addition of sodium taurocholate in human subjects. Sodium taurocholate (10 mM) and essential amino acids (78 mM) were infused intraduodenally at 10 ml/min. (From Malagelada et al.[2])

when monooleate (10 mM) was infused in place of EAA. Taurocholate alone had no effect on basal pancreatic enzyme output. The inhibitory effect of taurocholate was local, because release of CCK activity by EAA in the duodenum was not affected when taurocholate was perfused in the jejunum, nor did intraduodenal perfusion of taurocholate influence exogenous CCK stimulation of pancreatic enzyme output or gallbladder contraction. These results indicated that intraluminal bile acid did not produce a systemic inhibitory action on the target organs.

Malagelada et al.[2] interpreted their results as indicating that the inhibitory effect of bile acid in their study was due to inhibition of CCK release. They concluded that the results reflected events occurring during digestion of a normal meal, because bile acid concentrations in the proximal small bowel after a test meal in man approach or exceed 9 mM after gallbladder contraction.

Studies that used the bile acid binding resin cholestyramine to deplete the bile acid pool provide further evidence that bile acids physiologically inhibit CCK release. Brand and Morgan[4] demonstrated in rats that feeding cholestyramine increased pancreatic size and DNA content similar to that caused by feeding trypsin inhibitors (raw soy flour). Chronic bile diversion had a similar effect. Cholestyramine added to raw soy flour stimulated further pancreatic growth (above that caused by raw soy flour alone), indicating that the effect of cholestyramine was at least in part independent of the protective effect of bile acids on trypsin activity in the intestine. Koop et al.[5] showed that CCK mediated the effect of cholestyramine on the rat pancreas.

Gomez and coworkers[6] used cholestyramine to demonstrate the suppressive effect of endogenous bile acids on CCK release in dogs and humans. Fasted conscious dogs with pancreatic fistulas were infused intraduodenally with an amino acid solution, and pancreatic protein output and plasma CCK response were determined in the presence and absence of cholestyramine (infused intraduodenally). Cholestyramine alone had no effect on pancreatic secretion or CCK release but dose dependently augmented amino acid-stimulated pancreatic protein output and plasma CCK levels. Maximal augmentation ($\sim$twofold in protein secretion, $\sim$threefold in integrated plasma CCK) occurred with a dose of cholestyramine that bound the entire bile salt pool. In separate experiments, bile diversion had the same effect as did cholestyramine, that is, marked enhancement of amino acid-stimulated CCK release and pancreatic protein secretion. Replacement of the bile acid pool by intraduodenal infusion of taurocholate completely reversed the effects of cholestyramine and bile diversion. In the same report, the investigators showed in humans that cholestyramine markedly augmented CCK release stimulated by oral triglyceride or amino acid test meals. Nustede et al.[7] recently confirmed the effect of cholestyramine in augmenting nutrient-stimulated (20% lipid emulsion) pancreatic protein secretion and CCK release in dogs, and additionally showed that neurotensin release was similarly augmented under these conditions.

By demonstrating that amino acid-stimulated pancreatic secretion in the absence of bile acids in the intestine (i.e., by bile diversion or cholestyramine treatment) was equivalent to that produced by maximally effective doses of intravenous CCK-8, Gomez et al.[5] helped explain the well-established observation[8] that the pancreatic enzyme response to meals or to intraduodenal perfusion with amino acids is submaximal when compared to the response to exogenous CCK. In brief, the pancreatic response to intraluminal stimulants is submaximal because bile acids secreted in response to these stimulants limit the amount of CCK released, preventing a maximal pancreatic response.

The third type of study strongly supporting a physiological role for bile acids in feedback inhibition of CCK release is that in which CCK receptor antagonists were used to examine the role of CCK in gastrointestinal functions. In every study in humans in which CCK receptor antagonists were administered with a meal or with luminal nutrients, CCK release was exaggerated, sometimes as much as fourfold.[9-12] This observation has frequently been interpreted as evidence of feedback inhibition of CCK release by bile acids or pancreatic proteases, because CCK antagonists block the stimulation of these secretions by CCK. However, CCK receptor antagonists inhibit gallbladder contraction to a greater extent than pancreatic enzyme secretion in humans, indicating that the exaggeration of CCK release by CCK receptor antagonists is primarily due to reduced bile acids in the intestine. These relationships are illustrated in FIGURES 2 and 3, taken from Cantor et al.[12] In this study, six normal subjects consumed a mixed meal 2 hours after treatment with MK-329 or placebo. Plasma CCK concentrations (FIG. 2) in response to the mixed meal were increased to

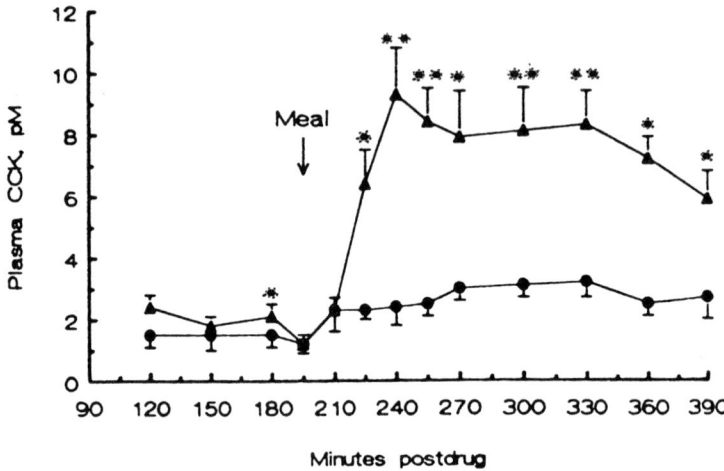

FIGURE 2. Plasma CCK concentrations after a mixed meal in six normal subjects during treatment with MK-329 (*triangles*) and placebo (*circles*). Experimental conditions are described in the legend for Figure 3. $*p < 0.05$; $**p < 0.01$; MK-329 vs placebo. (From Cantor et al.[12])

a far greater degree during treatment with MK-329. Measurements of bile acids and trypsin (FIG. 3) in these experiments showed a reduction in postprandial bile acid output of 77%, whereas trypsin output was reduced by only 15% (nonsignificant). These data support the hypothesis that the augmentation of plasma CCK concentration by MK-329 treatment was due to removal of the inhibitory effect of bile acids on CCK release, and not to removal of an inhibitory effect of trypsin on CCK release, inasmuch as intraluminal trypsin was not significantly decreased. The results also confirmed that meal-stimulated gallbladder contraction is much more dependent on CCK than is pancreatic enzyme secretion. Interestingly, their study showed that MK-329 significantly decreased duodenal pH, suggesting that pancreatic bicarbonate secretion during a meal may be more dependent on CCK (e.g., through potentiation of secretin) than is pancreatic enzyme secretion.

MECHANISM OF INHIBITION OF CCK RELEASE BY BILE ACIDS

The studies just described support the view that bile acids inhibit nutrient-stimulated CCK release. The mechanism by which bile acids inhibit amino acid-stimulated CCK release is not known, but inhibition of fatty acid-stimulated CCK release by bile acids has a straightforward explanation. In their 1976 paper, Malagelada and coworkers[3] examined the effects of increasing intraluminal bile acid concentrations on gallbladder contraction and pancreatic enzyme secretion stimulated by intraduodenal infusion of fatty acids in healthy human subjects. Additionally, fatty acid intraluminal concentrations and absorption rates were determined. Illustrated in FIGURE 4 are the effects of increasing the concentration of taurocholate in the duodenal perfusate (1, 10, and 20 mM) on duodenal bile acid concentrations and on gallbladder contraction (indicated by bilirubin output) stimulated by intraduodenal infusion of 10 mM oleic acid. These figures were constructed from data presented in tabular form in their paper. Increasing the concentration of taurocholate in the duodenal perfusate caused proportional increases in duodenal bile acid concentrations (FIG. 4A). Bilirubin output (FIG. 4B) in response to oleic acid infusion was maximal when the concentration of taurocholate in the perfusate

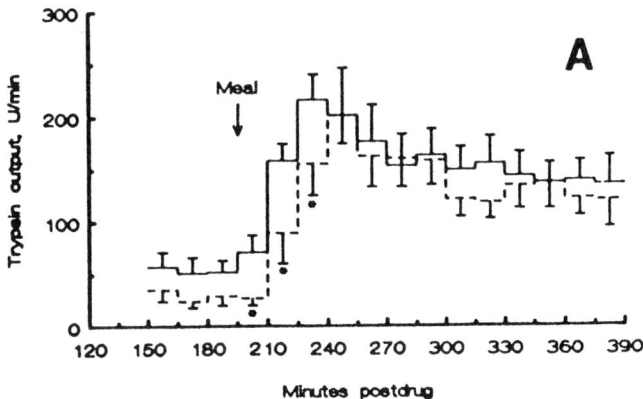

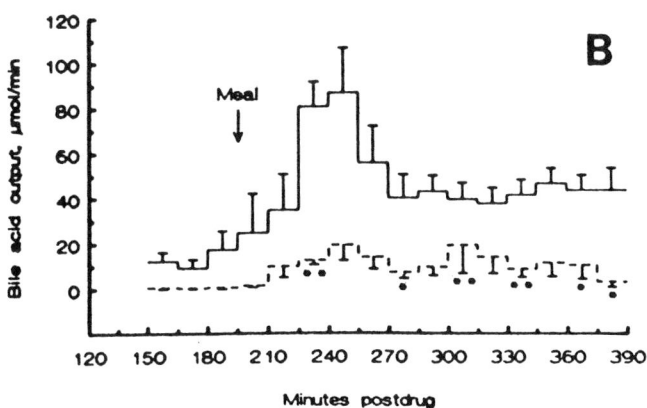

FIGURE 3. Trypsin secretion (**A**) and bile acid output (**B**) after a mixed meal in six normal subjects during treatment with MK-329 (*dashed line*) and placebo (*solid line*). On separate days, fasting subjects ingested either 10 mg MK-329 or placebo. Starting 120 minutes after administration of the drug, duodenal contents were continuously aspirated in 15-minute periods through a multilumen tube using ^{57}Co-B$_{12}$ as recovery marker. After an equilibrium period of 30 minutes, basal aspirates were obtained over the next 45 minutes; 195 minutes after drug administration, a standard meal was ingested. *$p < 0.05$; **$p < 0.01$; MK-329 *vs* placebo. (From Cantor *et al.*[12])

was lowest. Increasing the concentration of taurocholate in the perfusate from 1–10 mM (producing duodenal bile acid concentrations of ~10 mM) virtually abolished gallbladder contraction, as indicated by reduction of bilirubin output to values equivalent to those produced by perfusion with saline solution in place of oleic acid. Surprisingly, increasing the concentration of taurocholate in the perfusate from 10–20 mM *reduced* the suppression of gallbladder emptying, resulting in a biphasic pattern of inhibition with respect to the dose of taurocholate infused.

To explain the biphasic response of the gallbladder to increasing bile acid concentrations during oleic acid infusion, Malagelada *et al.*[3] investigated the relation between intraluminal fatty acid absorption rates and the load of bile acid infused into the duodenum. FIGURE 5 shows the concentrations of fatty acids sampled at the

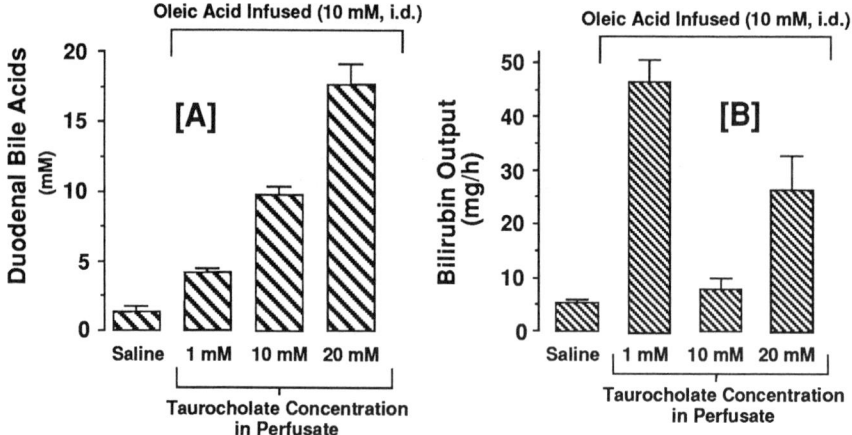

FIGURE 4. Effect of intraduodenal infusion of sodium taurocholate on gallbladder contraction (bilirubin output) in human subjects infused intraduodenally (i.d.) with oleic acid. All solutions were made isotonic with sodium chloride, adjusted to pH 6.3, warmed to 37°C, and infused i.d. at 10 ml/min just proximal to the papilla of Vater. Sodium taurocholate was infused i.d. at 1-, 10-, or 20-mM concentrations. Oleic acid was infused at 10 mM. In **A**, duodenal bile acid concentrations sampled at the ligament of Treitz under basal conditions (saline) or during i.d. infusion of 1, 10, and 20 mM taurocholate with oleic acid infusion are shown. In **B**, peak bilirubin output sampled at the ligament of Treitz during basal conditions (saline) or during taurocholate infusion with oleic acid infusion is shown. (Adapted from Malagelada *et al.*[3])

ligament of Treitz during infusion of 10 mM oleic acid with 1, 10, and 20 mM taurocholate. Intraduodenal concentrations of fatty acids were lowest when 10 mM oleic acid was infused with 10 mM taurocholate, that is, a 1:1 molar ratio, corresponding to the highest fatty acid absorption rates. Changing this ratio by either decreasing or increasing bile acid concentration slowed fatty acid absorption. Thus, the investigators concluded that the "inhibition" of release of CCK activity by effective concentrations of bile acids simply reflected the ability of those concentrations to accelerate the disappearance, by absorption, of the CCK stimulus, that is, fatty acids.

The schematic diagram shown in FIGURE 6 illustrates the relations between intraluminal bile acid concentrations, fatty acid absorption, and CCK release during digestion of a meal, based on the results of studies of Malagelada *et al.*[3] In this

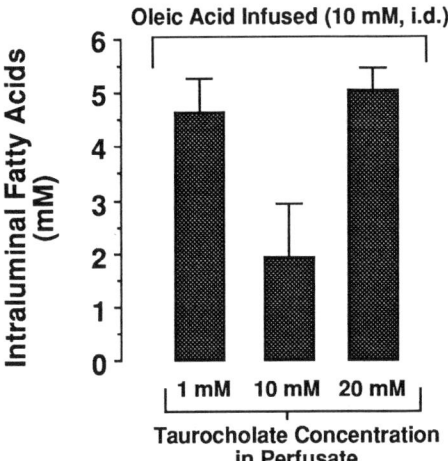

FIGURE 5. Effect of concentration of sodium taurocholate in duodenal perfusate on intraluminal fatty acid concentration in human subjects infused intraduodenally (i.d.) with oleic acid. Fatty acid concentrations determined at the ligament of Treitz. Experimental conditions described in the legend for Figure 4. (Adapted from Malagelada et al.[3])

scheme, fatty acids generated by limited lipolysis in the stomach and/or basal pancreatic secretions initially encounter low bile acid concentrations in the duodenum, indicated in the figure by a high fatty acid to bile acid ratio. Because such ratios hinder fatty acid absorption (presumably due to inadequate micelle formation), luminal fatty acid concentration is high enough to stimulate CCK release, which in turn contracts the gallbladder, bringing about a ratio of fatty acid to bile acid favorable for rapid absorption of fatty acids. Resultant reduction of luminal fatty acid concentration reduces the stimulus for CCK release, permitting gallbladder

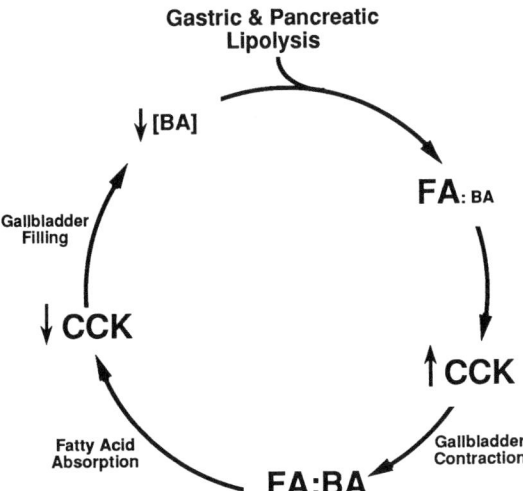

FIGURE 6. Schematic diagram illustrating the relation between the ratio of fatty acids to bile acids (FA:BA) in the intestine on CCK release, fatty acid absorption, and gallbladder contraction. See text for explanation.

refilling and reduction of luminal bile acid concentrations, and the cycle repeats. Gastric emptying would fit into this scheme at the point of increased CCK release (emptying inhibited) and decreased CCK release (emptying increased).

Malagelada et al.[3] speculated that the physiological significance of the inhibition of fatty absorption by excess bile acids may be to disperse fatty acids over a larger segment of intestine.

The mechanism just described does not explain the ability of bile acids to inhibit amino acid-stimulated CCK release, because DiMagno et al.[13] demonstrated that bile acids did not accelerate amino acid absorption in man. Therefore, bile acid suppression of amino acid-stimulated CCK release may occur through a different mechanism, perhaps one related to somatostatin release by bile acids, as suggested by Gomez et al.[6] However, the possibility should not be discounted that bile acids may directly interact with amino acids in such a way as to reduce their ability to stimulate CCK release, and therefore it might be profitable to investigate the relation between CCK release and changes in bile acid:amino acid ratios, analogous to the studies with fatty acid:bile acid ratios reported by Malagelada et al.[3]

FEEDBACK INHIBITION OF CCK RELEASE BY PANCREATIC PROTEASES

Feedback inhibition of CCK release by pancreatic proteases is well established in the rat.[14] In contrast, considerable controversy exists concerning whether such a mechanism operates in man and whether it is physiologically or pathologically significant. Slaff et al.[15] and Owyang et al.[16,17] clearly demonstrated in humans that exogenous trypsin strongly suppressed CCK release and/or pancreatic enzyme secretion stimulated by amino acids or fatty acids. However, other studies in human subjects frequently fail to support the existence of protease-specific feedback regulation of CCK release,[18–21] even though the experimental design, or the pathological condition being studied, regularly validates protease feedback inhibition of CCK release when applied to a rat model.

If we assume that feedback inhibition of CCK release by pancreatic proteases may be an important mechanism in humans, why should it be difficult to demonstrate it, particularly by use of protease inhibitors, which were the compounds that originally unmasked this regulatory mechanism in animals? Three considerations may help explain such difficulty: (1) the presence of inhibitor-resistant trypsins in human pancreatic juice; (2) the necessity to substantially eliminate intraluminal activities of all three pancreatic endopeptidases; and (3) the necessity of providing a positive intraluminal stimulus for CCK release, such as amino acids or fatty acids, to reveal protease inhibitor stimulation of CCK release in humans. These will be considered in turn.

Thorsen et al.[22] described a minor variant of trypsin in human pancreatic juice that retained activity despite a great molar excess of trypsin inhibitor activity from soybean trypsin inhibitor. This variant was distinct from another inhibitor-resistant form of human trypsin described by Rinderknecht et al.[23] Persistence of trypsin inhibitor-resistant trypsin activity may prevent a feedback response to trypsin inhibitors in humans. The reason might be that residual trypsin activity, even though a minor fraction of the total potential trypsin activity, could be sufficient to prevent the release of CCK. However, a more likely reason that residual trypsin activity could prevent a feedback response to trypsin inhibitors may be the ability of the remaining uninhibited trypsin to activate the other pancreatic endopeptidases. This brings up the second point already mentioned, the apparent necessity to substantially eliminate activity from all three endopeptidases, trypsin, chymotrypsin, and elastase. This requirement was not recognized because, in the rat, infusion of "pure" trypsin inhibitors, such as aprotinin or ovomucoid, which have little or no chymotrypsin or elastase inhibitory activity, were highly effective stimulants of pancreatic enzyme secretion. In fact, "pure" trypsin inhibitors administered in large molar excess (over potential trypsin activity) also markedly reduce chymotrypsin activity, and probably elastase activity as well, in the proximal intestine, by preventing their activation from zymogens. This was demonstrated in rats fed ovomucoid trypsin inhibitor[24] and recently in the mouse fed aprotinin.[25]

It should be reasonable to expect that reduction of all three proteases is necessary to evoke a feedback response to protease inhibitors, because all three endopeptidases inhibit CCK release or pancreatic enzyme secretion in the rat. This may explain why the only study in which a trypsin inhibitor clearly augmented nutrient-stimulated pancreatic secretion in man used the unique Bowman-Birk soybean inhibitor, which *directly* inhibits human trypsin, chymotrypsin, and elastase (i.e., by binding with each protease in an inhibitor:enzyme complex). Liener et al.[26] determined the effect of intraduodenally administered Bowman-Birk soybean inhibitor on amino acid-stimulated pancreatic enzyme secretion in healthy human subjects. Pancreatic secretion was collected by endoscopic retrograde cannulation of the pancreatic duct. During the experiment, Bowman-Birk soybean inhibitor or heat-inactivated Bowman-Birk inhibitor was mixed with pancreatic juice collected from the pancreatic duct, and this mixture was returned to the duodenum. The amount of Bowman-Birk soybean inhibitor added to the pancreatic juice was sufficient to inactivate >95% of trypsin and chymotrypsin activities and >50% of elastase activity in human pancreatic juice. Active soybean inhibitor increased amino acid-stimulated pancreatic secretion of four enzymes from two- to threefold compared to heat-inactivated Bowman-Birk inhibitor or saline solution in place of soybean inhibitor. Unfortunately, because plasma CCK was not measured in this study it cannot be concluded that the stimulatory effect of the protease inhibitor was mediated by CCK release.

Other investigators have examined the effect of synthetic protease inhibitors (camostat) on CCK release in humans. Adler et al.[19] reported that camostat did not augment plasma CCK or pancreatic enzyme secretion stimulated by a Lundh meal. This lack of augmentation occurred despite nearly complete inhibition of intraluminal trypsin and chymotrypsin activities (elastase was not measured). In the absence of meal-stimulated or nutrient-stimulated conditions, Adler et al.[19] and Layer et al.[21] found that camostat caused modest but statistically significant increases in pancreatic enzyme secretion that were unaccompanied by increases in plasma endogenous CCK concentrations, suggesting a CCK-independent protease feedback regulation of pancreatic enzyme secretion. However, the latter experiments in which camostat increased human pancreatic secretion but did not increase CCK release are not directly comparable to the study of Liener et al.[26] because they were performed in the absence of a background nutrient stimulant of endogenous CCK release. This brings up the third consideration listed, the necessity for a background positive luminal stimulus to demonstrate protease inhibitor-stimulation of CCK release.

The suggestion that a background stimulus from luminal nutrients is necessary to manifest protease inhibitor-stimulation of CCK release is based on the assumption that protease inhibitors do not directly stimulate CCK release. They only *augment* the stimulation caused by luminal nutrients, by preventing stimulated pancreatic secretions from suppressing the response. This is analogous to the stimulation of CCK release by cholestyramine, in that cholestyramine is ineffective under basal conditions, but it augments CCK release stimulated by luminal nutrients by preventing the feedback suppression of CCK release from bile acids. This may help explain the observation that trypsin inhibitors do not stimulate CCK release or pancreatic enzyme secretion in the absence of luminal nutrients in humans.[16,20] However, this is apparently not the case in the rat, in which trypsin inhibitors consistently stimulate CCK release and/or pancreatic secretion when administered alone, that is, in fasted rats in the absence of luminal exogenous nutrients.[27,28]

To explain why the presence of luminal nutrients may be necessary for protease inhibitor-stimulation of CCK release in humans but not in the rat, it may help to examine the hypotheses proposed for the mechanism of protease inhibition of CCK release. It has been hypothesized that CCK-releasing peptides, either in pancreatic juice[29] or secreted by the small intestine,[30,31] mediate the stimulation of CCK release caused by trypsin inhibitors. FIGURE 7 is a cartoon illustrating the hypothesis[30,31] that an intraluminally secreted, intestinal CCK-releasing peptide mediates protease-specific feedback regulation of CCK release. In the left panel, the cartoon depicts how this mechanism may operate in the rat, and in the right panel, in humans. In the

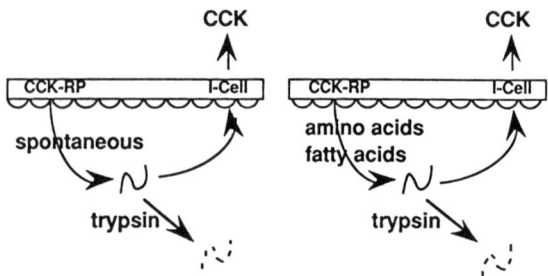

FIGURE 7. Illustration of the hypothesis of regulation of CCK release by an intestinal CCK-releasing peptide (CCK-RP) in rat (*left*) and humans (*right*). In both rat and humans, it is hypothesized that CCK is stimulated by the CCK-RP released into the lumen. In the presence of trypsin, the peptide is degraded, preventing CCK release. In the absence of trypsin activity (and that of other proteases), the CCK-RP survives in the lumen and acts on intestinal "I" cells to release CCK. In the *left panel*, release of the CCK-RP is hypothesized to be tonic, not requiring luminal nutrients. In the *right panel*, luminal nutrients are required to stimulate release of CCK-RP. These two views account for the observations that protease inhibitors stimulate CCK release in fasted rats in the absence of luminal nutrients, but in humans luminal nutrients are required.

left panel, the hypothetical CCK-releasing peptide is secreted tonically by the small intestine, apparently without the need for an exogenous stimulus, and the peptide acts on intestinal "I" cells to release CCK, unless free trypsin is present, in which case the peptide is degraded and CCK release stops. We postulated that "spontaneous" release of the CCK-releasing peptide accounts for the observation that CCK release in the rat occurs maximally simply by removing active proteases from the proximal small intestine, without the necessity of a positive stimulus such as luminal nutrients. The scheme on the right suggests how this mechanism may operate in man. The only difference is that luminal digestive products, such as amino acids or fatty acids, are postulated to be necessary to stimulate secretion of the putative CCK-releasing peptide. This accounts for the observation that inhibition of CCK release by trypsin in healthy humans is manifested by the reversal of *nutrient-stimulated* CCK release.[16] Thus, introduction of trypsin inhibitors into the intestine in man in the absence of luminal nutrients is not expected to cause CCK release. This may explain the negative results of some human studies in which the experimental design did not account for these considerations.

INTERACTION OF BILE ACIDS AND PANCREATIC PROTEASES IN INHIBITION OF CCK RELEASE

Evidence suggests that pancreatic proteases and bile acids may interact in the inhibition of CCK release. Green and Nasset[32] demonstrated that bile acids had a protective effect on pancreatic proteases in the small intestine, and they proposed that bile inhibited pancreatic secretion and CCK release by augmenting feedback inhibition from intraluminal proteases. Nakamura et al.[33] demonstrated that the effect of diversion of pancreatic juice and bile together on CCK release was much greater that the summed effects of diverting bile and pancreatic juice separately, indicating interaction of bile and pancreatic juice in inhibiting CCK release. More recently, Miyasaka et al.[34] demonstrated that bile had a protease-independent (direct) and protease-dependent inhibitory effect on pancreatic secretion and CCK release. In humans and dogs, the inhibitory effects of bile and bile acids appear to be independent of pancreatic proteases, but the possibility of interaction of proteases and bile acids on inhibition of CCK release needs further study in these species.

SUMMARY

Feedback inhibition of CCK release by bile acids and pancreatic proteases is well established in the rat. The question of whether these mechanisms are important in humans has not been completely resolved, but current evidence strongly suggests that feedback regulation of CCK release by bile acids is present in humans and is physiologically significant, whereas the existence and importance of feedback regulation of CCK release by pancreatic proteases in humans are still highly controversial.

REFERENCES

1. THOMAS, J. E. & J. O. CRIDER. 1943. The effect of bile in the intestine on the secretion of pancreatic juice. Am. J. Physiol. **138:** 548–552.
2. MALAGELADA, J.-R., V. L. W. GO, E. P. DIMAGNO & W. H. J. SUMMERSKILL. 1973. Interactions between intraluminal bile acids and digestive products on pancreatic and gallbladder function. J. Clin. Invest. **52:** 2160–2165.
3. MALAGELADA, J.-R., V. L. W. GO, E. P. DIMAGNO & W. H. J. SUMMERSKILL. 1976. Regulation of pancreatic and gallbladder functions by intraluminal fatty acids and bile acids in man. J. Clin. Invest. **58:** 493–499.
4. BRAND, S. J. & R. G. H. MORGAN. 1982. Stimulation of pancreatic secretion and growth in the rat after feeding cholestyramine. Gastroenterology **83:** 851–859.
5. KOOP, I., M. LINDENTHAL, M. SCHADE, M. TRAUTMANN, G. ADLER & R. ARNOLD. 1991. Role of cholecystokinin in cholestyramine-induced changes of the exocrine pancreas. Pancreas **6:** 564–570.
6. GOMEZ, G., J. R. UPP, JR., F. LLUIS, R. W. ALEXANDER, G. J. POSTON, G. H. GREELEY, JR. & J. C. THOMPSON. 1988. Regulation of the release of cholecystokinin by bile salts in dogs and humans. Gastroenterology **94:** 1036–1046.
7. NUSTEDE, R., W. E. SCHMIDT, H. KOHLER, U. R. FOLSCH & A. SCHAFMAYER. 1993. The influence of bile acids on the regulation of exocrine pancreatic secretion and on the plasma concentrations of neurotensin and CCK in dogs. Int. J. Pancreatol. **13:** 23–30.

8. SINGER, M. V. 1986. Neurohormonal control of pancreatic enzyme secretion in animals. *In* The Exocrine Pancreas: Biology, Pathology, and Diseases. V. L. W. Go, E. P. DiMagno & W. H. J. Summerskill, eds.: 315–331. Raven Press. New York, NY.
9. LIDDLE, R. A., B. J. GERTZ, S. KANAYAMA, L. BECCARIA, L. D. COKER, T. A. TURNBULL & E. T. MORITA. 1989. Effects of a novel cholecystokinin (CCK) receptor antagonist, MK-329, on gallbladder contraction and gastric emptying in humans. J. Clin. Invest. **84:** 1220–1225.
10. ADLER, G., C. BEGLINGER, U. BRAUN, M. REINSHAGEN, I. KOOP, A. SCHAFMAYER, L. ROYATI & R. ARNOLD. 1991. Interaction of the cholinergic system and cholecystokinin in the regulation of endogenous and exogenous stimulation of pancreatic secretion in humans. Gastroenterology **100:** 537–543.
11. FRIED, M., U. ERLACHER, W. SCHWIZER, C. LOCHNER, J. KOERFER, C. BEGLINGER, J. B. JANSEN, C. B. LAMERS, F. HARDER, A. BISCHOF-DELALOYE, G. A. STALDER & L. ROVATI. 1991. Role of cholecystokinin in the regulation of gastric emptying and pancreatic enzyme secretion in humans. Gastroenterology **101:** 503–511.
12. CANTOR, P., P. E. MORTENSEN, J. MYHRE, I. GJORUP, H. WORNING, E. STAHL & T. T. SURVILL. 1992. The effect of the cholecystokinin receptor antagonist MK-329 on meal-stimulated pancreaticobiliary output in humans. Gastroenterology **102:** 1742–1751.
13. DIMAGNO, E. P., J.-R. MALAGELADA & V. L. W. GO. 1977. Effects of bile acids, lecithin, and monoolein on amino acid absorption from the human duodenum. Proc. Soc. Exp. Biol. Med. **154:** 325–330.
14. SOLOMON, T. E. 1987. Control of exocrine pancreatic secretion. *In* Physiology of the Gastrointestinal Tract. L. R. Johnson, ed. Vol. **2:** 1173–1207. Raven Press. New York, NY.
15. SLAFF, J., D. JACOBSON, C. R. TILLMAN, C. CURINGTON & P. TOSKES. 1984. Protease-specific suppression of pancreatic exocrine secretion. Gastroenterology **87:** 44–52.
16. OWYANG, C., D. S. LOUIE & D. TATUM. 1986. Feedback regulation of pancreatic enzyme secretion. Suppression of cholecystokinin release by trypsin. J. Clin. Invest **77:** 2042–2047.
17. OWYANG, C., D. MAY & D. LOUIE. 1986. Trypsin suppression of pancreatic enzyme secretion: Differential effect on cholecystokinin release and the enteropancreatic reflex. Gastroenterology **91:** 637–643.
18. DLUGOSZ, J., U. R. FOLSCH & W. CREUTZFELDT. 1983. Inhibition of intraduodenal trypsin does not stimulate exocrine pancreatic secretion in man. Digestion **26:** 197–204.
19. ADLER, G., A. MULLENHOFF, I. KOOP, T. BOZJURT, B. GOKE, C. BEGLINGER & R. ARNOLD. 1988. Stimulation of pancreatic secretion in man by a protease inhibitor (camostate). Eur. J. Clin. Invest. **18:** 98–104.
20. HOTZ, J., S. B. HO, V. L. W. GO & E. P. DIMAGNO. 1983. Short-term inhibition of duodenal tryptic activity does not affect human pancreatic, biliary, or gastric function. J. Lab. Clin. Med. **101:** 488–495.
21. LAYER, P., J. B. M. J. JANSEN, L. CHERIAN, C. B. H. W. LAMERS & H. GOEBELL. 1990. Feedback regulation of human pancreatic secretion. Gastroenterology **98:** 1311–1319.
22. THORSEN, L. I., H. HOLM, J. E. RESELAND, S. BJØRNSEN, L. E. HANSSEN & F. BROSSTAD. 1991. Characterization of a human trypsin resistant to Kunitz soybean trypsin inhibitor. Scand. J. Gastroenterol. **26:** 589–598.
23. RINDERKNECHT, H., I. G. RENNER, S. B. ABRAMSON & C. CARMACK. 1984. Mesotrypsin; a new inhibitor-resistant protease from a zymogen in human pancreatic tissue and fluid. Gastroenterology **86:** 681–692.
24. LYMAN, R. L., B. A. OLDS & G. M. GREEN. 1974. Chymotrypsinogen in the intestine of rats fed soybean trypsin inhibitor and its inability to suppress pancreatic enzyme secretions. J. Nutr. **104:** 105–110.
25. HANSON, D. G., M. J. ROY, S. D. MILLER, E. G. SEIDMAN, M. J. THOMAS, I. R. SANDERSON, J. N. UDALL, I. ELY & G. M. GREEN. 1993. Endopeptidase inhibition and intestinal antigen processing in mice. Reg. Immunol. **5:** 85–93.
26. LIENER, I. E., R. L. GOODALE, A. DESHMUKH, T. L. SATTERBERG, G. WARD, C. M. DIPIETRO, P. E. BANKEY & J. W. BORNER. 1988. Effect of a trypsin inhibitor from

soybeans (Bowman-Birk) on the secretory activity of the human pancreas. Gastroenterology **94:** 419–427.
27. LIDDLE, R. A., I. D. GOLDFINE & J. A. WILLIAMS. 1984. Bioassay of plasma cholecystokinin in rats: Effects of food, trypsin inhibitor, and alcohol. Gastroenterology **87:** 542–549.
28. LEVAN, V. H. & G. M. GREEN. 1986. Effect of atropine on rat pancreatic secretory response to trypsin inhibitors and protein. Am. J. Physiol. **251:** G64–G69.
29. FUSHIKI, T. & K. IWAI. 1989. Two hypotheses on the feedback regulation of pancreatic enzyme secretion. FASEB J. **3:** 121–126.
30. LU, L., D. LOUIE & C. OWYANG. 1989. A cholecystokinin releasing peptide mediates feedback regulation of pancreatic secretion. Am. J. Physiol. **256:** G430–G435.
31. MIYASAKA, K., D. GUAN, R. A. LIDDLE & G. M. GREEN. 1989. Feedback regulation by trypsin: Evidence for intraluminal CCK-releasing peptide. Am. J. Physiol. **257:** G175–G181.
32. GREEN, G. M. & E. S. NASSET. 1980. Importance of bile in regulation of intraluminal proteolytic enzyme activities in the rat. Gastroenterology **79:** 695–702.
33. NAKAMURA, R., K. MIYASAKA, A. FUNAKOSHI & K. KITANI. 1989. Interactions between bile and pancreatic juice diversions on cholecystokinin release and pancreas in conscious rats. Proc. Soc. Exp. Biol. Med. **192:** 182–186.
34. MIYASAKA, K., N. SAZAKI, A. FUNAKOSHI, M. MATSUMOTO & K. KITANI. 1993. Two mechanisms of inhibition by bile on luminal feedback regulation of rat pancreas. Gastroenterology **104:** 1780–1785.

Effects of CCK on Pancreatic Function and Morphology[a]

CLAUS NIEDERAU,[b] REINHARD LÜTHEN,
AND TOBIAS HEINTGES

Department of Medicine
GI-Unit
Heinrich-Heine-University of Düsseldorf
Düsseldorf, Germany

Cholecystokinin (CCK) is a peptide thought to act as both a hormone and a neurotransmitter in the brain, in the enteric nervous system, and at various gastrointestinal organs. Humoral CCK is released from endocrine mucosal cells of the upper small intestine into the circulation in response to a meal.[1] Administration of exogenous CCK or CCK analogs increases gallbladder emptying and pancreatic secretion.[2-5] Exogenous CCK also increases glucose-induced insulin secretion in vitro and in vivo in the experimental animal.[6-9] Recently, it was shown that CCK, given at "physiological" doses that mimic the postprandial increase in plasma concentration of this peptide, does not increase glucose-stimulated insulin secretion in humans but only increases amino acid-stimulated insulin secretion.[10]

It is also well established that exogenous CCK and CCK analogs, such as caerulein, stimulate pancreatic growth in the experimental animal.[11,12] It is also well known that feeding of trypsin inhibitors markedly stimulates pancreatic growth.[13,14] Recently, it was shown that this effect can also be seen in humans.[15] Similarly, it was shown that pancreaticobiliary diversion stimulates pancreatic growth.[16,17] Both feeding of trypsin inhibitors and pancreaticobiliary diversion may stimulate pancreatic growth by the same mechanism of decreasing intraduodenal activity of proteases. Inhibition of intraduodenal proteolytic enzymes by potent protease inhibitors, such as camostate,[18] or their diversion from the duodenum[17] is thought to cause an increase in plasma CCK concentration which is suggested to mediate pancreatic growth under these conditions.[16-18] It has been speculated, however, that other hormones like enteroglucagon may contribute to pancreatic growth after pancreaticobiliary diversion.[19] Mechanisms involved in the feedback mechanisms will not be further analyzed in this review, because a separate report will deal with this specific topic.

Several studies have suggested that CCK increases the growth of pancreatic, gastric, and colonic tumor cells.[20] In some studies CCK also stimulated pancreatic carcinogenesis[21] and induced preneoplastic nodules.[22] As yet, CCK antagonists failed to alter survival in patients with gastric and pancreatic carcinoma (ref. 23 and unpublished observations). This review will not analyze the role of CCK in pancreatic carcinogenesis, but it will focus on its role in regulation and maintenance of pancreatic growth under physiological conditions. In most previous studies pharma-

---

[a] Dr. Niederau was supported by grants from the Deutsche Forschungsgemeinschaft (Ni 224/3-2) and by the Pinguin-Stiftung.
[b] Address for correspondence: Claus Niederau, MD, Medizinische Klinik und Poliklinik, Abteilung für Gastroenterologie, Universität Düsseldorf, Moorenstr. 5, 40255 Düsseldorf, Germany.

cological doses of CCK or CCK-like analogs that exceeded the physiological postprandial rise in plasma CCK had been administered. Indeed, only in recent years has this postprandial rise in plasma CCK been defined more exactly.[24-27] Recent studies, therefore, tried to administer CCK at doses that mimic the increase in plasma concentrations of CCK seen after a meal.[10,25,27,28] However, these studies were still associated with potential pitfalls. There continues to be some controversy about the comparability and quality of radioimmunoassays and bioassays for CCK, and there is a controversy about which molecular forms of CCK are physiologically most important. In addition, an intravenous infusion or injection of a CCK preparation, even considering the dose that best mimics the postprandial increase in plasma CCK, might not reflect the true concentrations of the hormone at its place of action and the kinetics of its release *in vivo*.

The development of new specific CCK-receptor antagonists offers a new approach to evaluate the physiological role of CCK as both a hormone and a neurotransmitter in various gastrointestinal functions, avoiding the pitfalls associated with previous studies. In 1981 proglumide and benzotript were shown to act as specific and competitive CCK-receptor antagonists *in vitro*.[29] However, these compounds had low potencies or were toxic when given in an effective dose *in vivo*.[30] Subsequently, molecules with a proglumide-like structure that were up to 1,000–5,000 times more potent than proglumide in inhibiting the action and binding of CCK *in vitro* and *in vivo* were synthesized.[31,32] More recently, several nonpeptide substances that originate from the substance asperlicin[33] were shown to act as specific CCK antagonists.[34] The most potent nonpeptide substance MK-329 (formerly termed L-364,718) is 25,000–1,000,000 times more potent than proglumide in inhibiting CCK's action and binding *in vitro* and *in vivo*.[32,34] Thus, from the potencies of inhibiting the actions of CCK, both the amino acid derivatives of proglumide and the nonpeptide antagonists are well suitedto *in vivo* studies.

This review analyzes in particular recent studies that employed specific CCK-receptor antagonists to evaluate the physiological role of endogenous CCK in the regulation of pancreatic function and growth.

PHYSIOLOGICAL FUNCTION OF CCK IN REGULATING EXOCRINE PANCREATIC FUNCTION

The CCK-antagonist loxiglumide abolishes the actions of endogenous CCK at the gallbladder and pancreas. When given at doses between 2 and 10 mg/kg · h, loxiglumide even abolishes the actions of pharmacological doses of CCK which increased the plasma concentrations of CCK and CCK analogs to levels markedly exceeding those seen after a meal.[31,32,35-37] Several further lines of evidence suggest that such doses of loxiglumide (about 5 mg/kg · h) completely inhibit the action of postprandially released CCK; loxiglumide at 5–10 mg/kg · h not only abolished gallbladder emptying after intraduodenal infusion of a test meal,[38] after oral food, or after intravenous infusion of caerulein at "physiological" and even suprphysiological doses,[2] but also significantly increased gallbladder volumes compared to prior fasting values (FIG. 1). Results of the imaging studies were corroborated by the secretory studies in which loxiglumide markedly inhibited meal-stimulated secretion of bilirubin[38] (FIG. 2). Despite the effective blockade of the peripheral CCK receptor, loxiglumide caused only a minor decrease in duodenal volume after intraduodenal infusion of a test meal[38] (FIG. 3). This small effect is likely to be caused by inhibition of biliary secretion, because loxiglumide almost abolished bilirubin output.[38] The CCK antagonist significantly reduced the postprandially stimulated

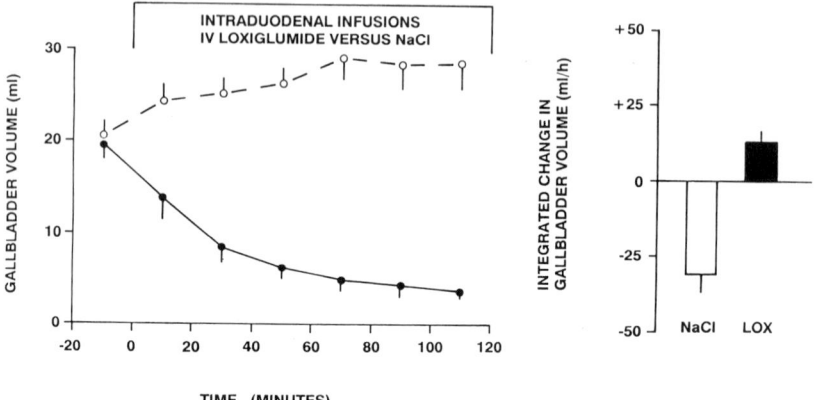

FIGURE 1. Gallbladder volume. Intravenous infusion of 5 mg/kg^{-1} · h^{-1} loxiglumide significantly increased gallbladder volume compared with infusion of NaCl in the control experiment at all individual time intervals from 20–120 minutes after beginning intraduodenal infusion ($p < 0.05$ by ANOVA). Basal values represented measurements performed 30 minutes before intraduodenal infusion was begun. Mean integrated gallbladder volumes after intraduodenal infusion of the test meal were decreased by loxiglumide by more than 90% when compared with the NaCl control (*left*) ($p < 0.001$). Data are given as mean ± SEM for individual time intervals after intraduodenal infusion of nutrients (*left*) and for the integrated change in gallbladder volume (*right*). Data of experiments with intravenous infusion of loxiglumide are shown by the *open circles* and *broken line*, and data of experiments with intravenous infusion of NaCl are shown by the *closed circles* and *solid line*. Mean integrated data for experiments with loxiglumide infusion are shown by *open bars;* mean integrated data for experiments with NaCl infusion are shown by an *open bar;* mean integrated data for experiments with loxiglumide infusion are shown by the *black bars*. Modified from ref. 38.

secretion of pancreatic digestive enzyme, with the integrated enzyme response being decreased by 50–70%[38] (FIG. 4). The inability of the CCK antagonists to completely inhibit postprandial exocrine pancreatic secretion of enzymes suggests that other hormones and neural mechanisms are also involved in the regulation of meal-stimulated pancreatic protein secretion. Therefore, CCK is only one of several factors that mediate stimulation of pancreatic enzyme secretion after a meal. CCK is probably not at all involved in the regulation of pancreatic secretion of fluid (and bicarbonate). Conclusions drawn from the current results are further supported by other recent studies that also showed that blockade of the CCK receptor failed to abolish pancreatic exocrine secretion.[39,40] In contrast to the limited effects on pancreatic secretion, CCK blockade by loxiglumide abolished gallbladder emptying after intraduodenal infusion of a test meal or after oral food and even increased gallbladder volumes compared to prior fasting volumes.[2,38,39] Recently, similar results were obtained with the CCK antagonist MK-329 (formerly termed L-364,718).[41] Thus, in contrast to the regulation of pancreatic secretion, which is only partly mediated by CCK, gallbladder function is mainly regulated by CCK in terms of both its emptying after intestinal absorption of nutrients and the maintenance of its fasting volume.

Recent data suggest that CCK stimulates pancreatic secretion not only through its specific receptors at the acinar cells but also through interaction with the cholinergic system. Both atropine and loxiglumide reduced the enzyme secretory response to meal stimulation. Inhibition of secretion by atropine was more pronounced than was inhibition by loxiglumide.[42] Both antagonists also reduced the enzyme response to exogenous CCK. Inhibition following atropine was more pronounced at low ("physiological") than at high ("pharmacological") CCK doses.[42] A similar phenomenon was observed by Malagelada et al.[43] and by Wormsley[44] in patients after vagotomy; the secretory response to small doses of CCK was reduced, whereas the response to large doses was not changed. These recent results[42] and several previous observations[43-46] strongly suggest that the cholinergic system at least partly mediates the enzyme response to exogenous stimulation by CCK.

In contrast to these findings, Valenzuela et al.[47] failed to show an effect of atropine on stimulation of pancreatic secretion in humans by graded doses of CCK-8 and concomitant infusion of a maximal dose of secretion. As the inhibitory effect of atropine diminishes with increasing doses of secretagogue,[42,46] it is possible that the maximal dose of secretin had masked the inhibitory actions of atropine. Also, nonspecific effects of the large dose of atropine could be responsible for the negative effect.

There may be some species differences concerning the interaction between the cholinergic system and CCK. In dogs, atropine did not affect the pancreatic response to exogenous CCK, and neither extrinsic nor intrinsic pancreatic nerves altered the stimulatory effect of exogenous CCK on pancreatic enzyme secretion.[48,49] In human studies atropine and vagotomy, however, markedly reduced the enzyme response to exogenous pancreatic secretagogues and reduced pancreatic sensitivity to CCK.[43-46] A recent study, however, showed that complete extrinsic denervation of the pancreas

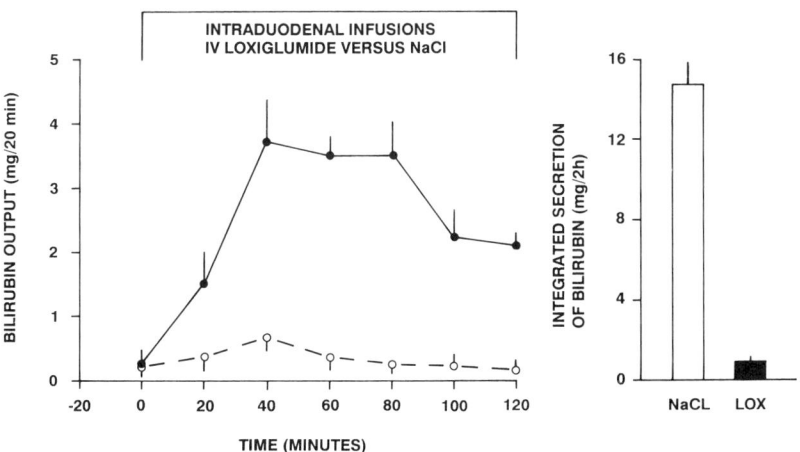

FIGURE 2. Bilirubin output. Intravenous infusion of 5 mg/kg · h loxiglumide significantly decreased output of bilirubin compared with infusion of NaCl in the control experiment at all individual time intervals from 20–120 minutes after beginning intraduodenal infusion ($p < 0.05$ by analysis of variance). Loxiglumide inhibited mean integrated secretion of bilirubin by more than 90% when compared with the NaCl control ($p < 0.001$). Data are given as mean ± SEM for individual time points (*left part*) and for integrated data (*right part*). Data of experiments with intravenous infusion of loxiglumide are shown by *open circles* and *broken line,* and data of experiments with intravenous infusion of NaCl are shown by *closed circles* and *solid line.* Mean integrated data for experiments with loxiglumide infusion are shown by *open bars;* mean integrated data for experiments with NaCl infusion are shown by *black bars.*

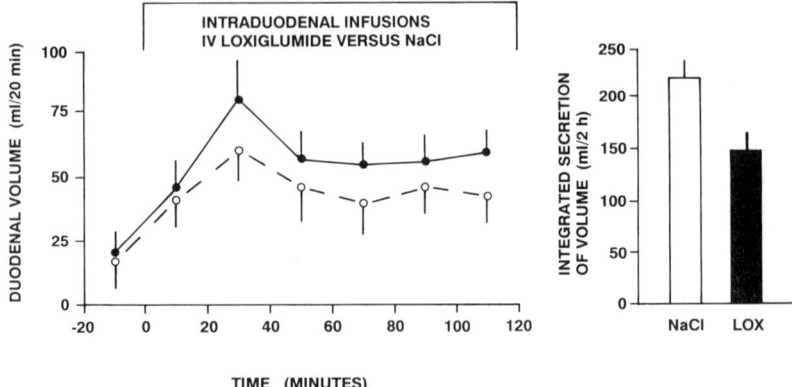

FIGURE 3. Duodenal volume. Intravenous infusion of 5 mg/kg · h loxiglumide did not significantly decrease duodenal volume compared with infusion of NaCl in the control experiment at any time interval after intraduodenal infusion ($p > 0.05$ by analysis of variance). Mean integrated output of volume after intraduodenal infusion of test meal, however, was significantly inhibited by loxiglumide by about 25–30% when compared with NaCl control ($p < 0.05$). Data are given as mean ± SEM both for individual time points (*left part*) and for integrated data (*right part*). Data of experiments with intravenous infusion of loxiglumide are shown by *open circles* and *broken line,* and data of experiments with intravenous infusion of NaCl are shown by *closed circles* and *solid line.* Mean integrated data for experiments with loxiglumide infusion are shown by the *open bar;* mean integrated data for experiments with NaCl infusion are shown by the *black bar.* Modified from ref. 38.

abolished meal-induced pancreatic protein secretion in the dog, whereas the postprandial release of CCK into the plasma was unchanged by the denervation procedure.[50]

In summary, CCK may affect pancreatic acinar cells through several distinct pathways. Two of them mediate stimulation of pancreatic secretion. First, CCK stimulates acinar cell function directly through CCK receptors at the acinar cell membrane. This pathway is blocked by a CCK antagonist, but not by atropine. Second, the effect of CCK on pancreatic enzyme output is modulated by interactions with cholinergic neurons. The second concept could be compatible with recent results and could explain the mechanism of how loxiglumide inhibits secretion that is also blocked by atropine. CCK may act on the exocrine pancreas directly as hormone and indirectly as a modulator of cholinergic neurons.[51] Studies on gallbladder muscle have shown that CCK receptors exist on smooth muscles and at postganglionic cholinergic neurons.[52,53]

PHYSIOLOGICAL FUNCTION OF CCK IN REGULATING ENDOCRINE PANCREATIC FUNCTION

Insulin release after ingestion of nutrients is thought to be faciliated by the release of gut factors, termed insulinotropic factors or incretins.[6,54,55] Since the first report of the insulinotropic effect of extracts of intestinal mucosa,[56] many investigators have shown that CCK is one of the gastrointestinal hormones capable of stimulating insulin secretion.[6–9] By contrast to these observations, some workers have suggested that the insulinotropic effect previously attributed to CCK may be due to contaminating gastric inhibitory polypeptide (GIP), present in crude preparations of CCK, and not to CCK itself.[57,58] Later, however, pure preparations of natural porcine CCK,[59] synthetic COOH-terminal octapeptide of CCK (CCK-OP),[58,60,61] and synthetic caerulein, which contains a COOH-terminal pentapeptide identical to CCK, [59,60,62,63] have also been shown to stimulate insulin and glucagon secretion *in vivo* and *in vitro*. Nevertheless, it has been difficult to determine if the insulinotropic action of these exogenously administered peptides is physiological. Recently, it was shown that CCK, given at physiological doses that mimic the postprandial increase in plasma concentration of this peptide, does not increase glucose-stimulated insulin secretion in humans but only increases amino acid-stimulated insulin secretion.[10] In the rat the CCK antagonist MK-329 reduced the meal-stimulated insulin secretion, suggesting that CCK might play a physiological incretin role in this animal.[64] It was also shown that both the new proglumide derivatives as well as the nonpeptide antagonists MK-329 and asperlicin inhibit CCK-stimulated insulin release at least as potently or even more potently than exocrine secretion from isolated pancreatic islets and acini,[65] and from the isolated perfused rat pancreas,[66,67] respectively. The latter studies strongly suggest that these CCK antagonists will affect the CCK receptor at the endocrine pancreatic tissue at least as effectively as that at the exocrine tissue.

Recent studies do not support the concept that CCK acts as an important incretin factor in humans. Loxiglumide at a dose that completely inhibits the actions of

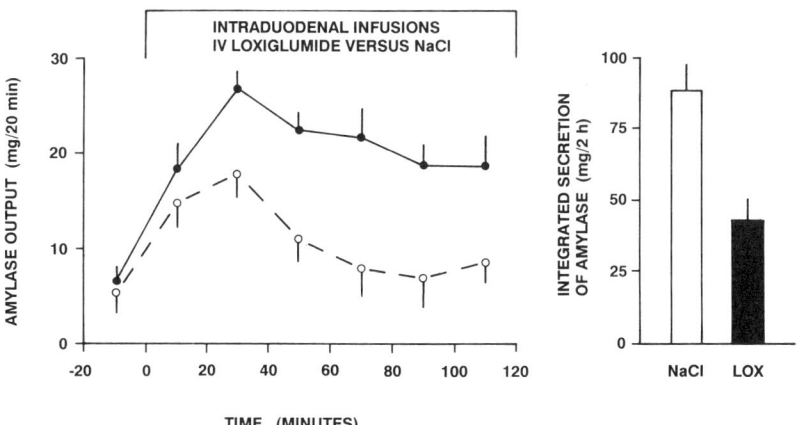

FIGURE 4. Amylase output. Intravenous infusion of 5 mg/kg · h loxiglumide significantly decreased pancreatic output of amylase compared with infusion of NaCl in the control experiment at all individual time intervals from 40–120 minutes after beginning intraduodenal infusion ($p < 0.05$ by analysis of variance). Mean integrated secretion of amylase after intraduodenal infusion of the test meal was inhibited by loxiglumide by more than 50% when compared with the NaCl control ($p < 0.01$). Data shown are given as mean ± SEM both for the individual time points (*left part*) and for the integrated data (*right part*). Data of experiments with intravenous infusion of loxiglumide are shown by *open circles* and *broken line,* and data of experiments with intravenous infusion of NaCl are shown by *closed circles* and *solid line.* Mean integrated data for experiments with loxiglumide infusion are shown by the *open bar;* mean integrated data for experiments with NaCl infusion are shown by the *black bar.* Modified from ref. 38.

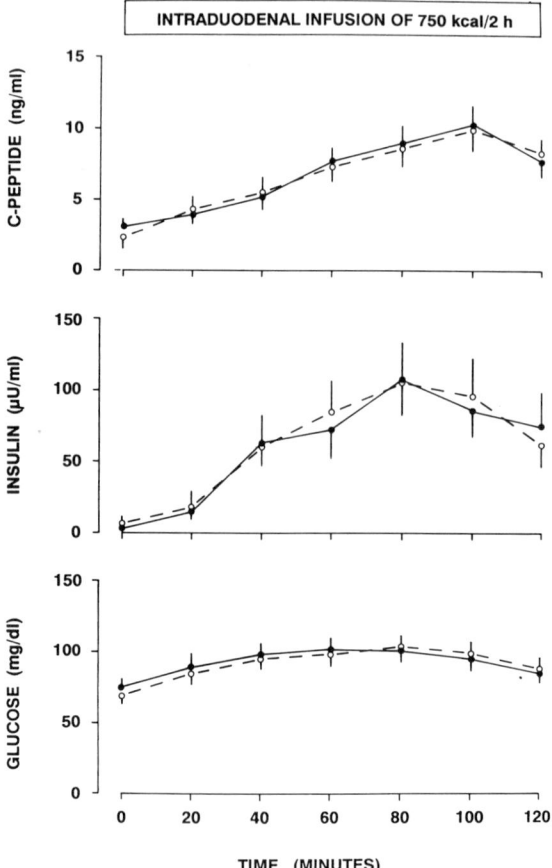

FIGURE 5. Effects of intraduodenal infusion of 750 kcal blenderized liquid test meal on circulating concentrations of glucose, insulin, and C-peptide. All values are given as mean ± SEM from eight subjects. Data from experiments with intravenous infusion of 5 mg/kg · h loxiglumide are shown by *open circles* and *broken line;* data from control experiments with intravenous infusion of NaCl are shown by *closed circles* and *solid line.* Values of glucose, insulin, and C-peptide did not significantly differ between studies with loxiglumide infusion *versus* NaCl infusion at any time point ($p > 0.1$ by analysis of variance). Modified from ref. 68.

physiological and even pharmacological concentrations of CCK and CCK analogs on the gallbladder and exocrine pancreas, did not alter the increase in circulating concentrations of glucose, insulin, and C-peptide after intraduodenal infusion of nutrients[38] (FIG. 5) or after regular oral meals[68] (FIG. 6). Failure of CCK-receptor blockade to alter the meal-induced increase in insulin or C-peptide was true for ingestion of regular meals ranging from 600–1,000 kcal.[68] In the studies with oral meals, we cannot exclude the possibility that the CCK antagonist might also influence gastric emptying and thereby alter the release of insulin due to the nutrients absorbed. The studies with intraduodenal infusion of a test meal avoided the latter problems associated with oral meals, but showed identical results. These results are further supported by recent findings from other investigators.[69,70] Both the nonpeptide antagonist MK-329 as well as loxiglumide failed to alter the meal-stimulated pancreatic endocrine responses to oral and intraduodenal administration of various meals.[69,70] Current studies also showed that administration of the CCK antagonist loxiglumide markedly reduced the increase in plasma pancreatic polypeptide (PP) after a meal, indicating that the antagonist exerted biological actions at the compartments of interest such as the endocrine pancreas.[68]

Results from human studies are in contrast to previous work in the experimental animal. It has been shown that CCK-receptor blockade antagonized the stimulatory effects of CCK on glucose-mediated insulin secretion *in vitro*[8,9,65] and on meal-induced insulin secretion *in vivo*.[64] The discrepancy of the current human studies *versus* the previous animal experiments may be due to species differences. Indeed, a recent study showed that physiologic increases in plasma CCK in humans do not stimulate glucose-mediated insulin secretion; they stimulate only amino acid-mediated insulin secretion.[10] The current study does not exclude the possibility that CCK may increase insulin secretion induced by some amino acids or some mixture of amino acids. However, the results do exclude the possibility that such a mechanism plays a major role in the release of insulin after regular meals in healthy humans.

PHYSIOLOGICAL ACTIONS OF CCK ON PANCREATIC MORPHOLOGY AND GROWTH

It is well established that exogenous CCK and CCK analogs, such as caerulein, stimulate pancreatic growth in the experimental animal.[11,12] The pancreatic acinar

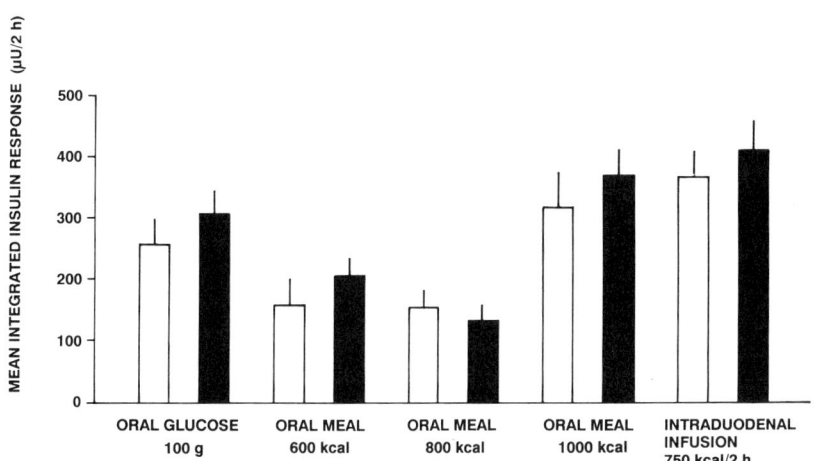

FIGURE 6. Mean integrated insulin response. Mean integrated insulin response to various test meals was calculated by the addition of insulin concentrations at 20–120 minutes after substraction of the corresponding prior basal (fasting) value for each time interval. Data from studies with intravenous infusion of NaCl are indicated by *open bars;* data from studies with intravenous infusion of loxiglumide are indicated by *black bars.* All values are given as mean ± SEM for 8–10 subjects. The various conditions are indicated on the horizontal axis. Mean integrated insulin response did not differ between studies with loxiglumide infusion *versus* NaCl infusion for any condition ($p > 0.1$ by analysis of variance). Modified from ref. 68.

cell is thought to possess two classes of CCK receptors, one with higher affinity and the other with lower affinity for CCK. Recently, a synthetic CCK analog, CCK-JMV-180, has been developed which acts as an agonist at the high-affinity receptor and as an antagonist at the low-affinity receptor.[71] Recent studies show that CCK-JMV-180, similar to CCK-8, is able to stimulate both pancreatic growth as well as enzyme

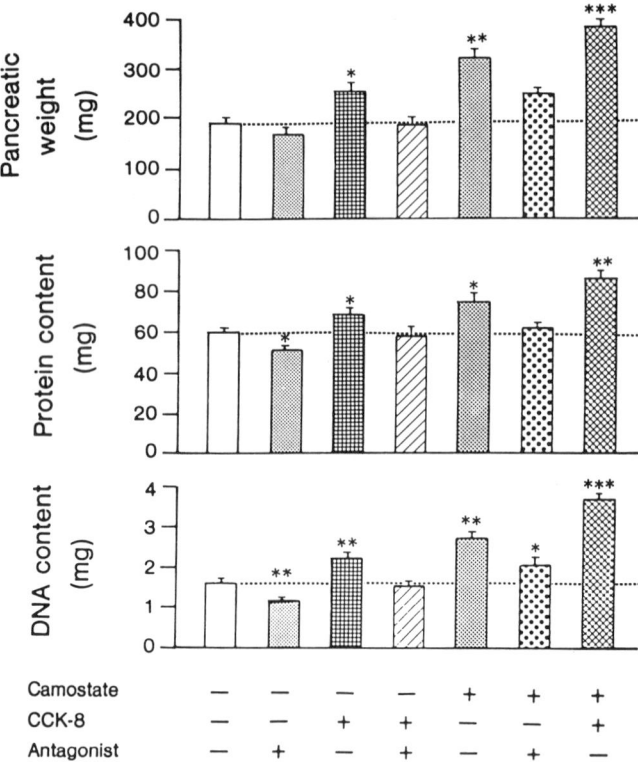

FIGURE 7. Mean ± SE of pancreatic weight ($n = 24$), protein content ($n = 12$), and DNA content ($n = 12$). The different experimental conditions are as indicated: "camostate" was mixed with regular chow and fed to achieve a daily dose of 400 mg/kg for 10 days; no camostate (−) indicates that regular chow was fed *ad libitum;* "CCK-8" was given as subcutaneous injections of 1 μg/kg every 8 hours for 10 days; the CCK receptor "antagonist" was given as subcutaneous injections of 10 mg/kg every 8 hours. In mice that received CCK-8 injections, the antagonist was given 15 minutes before injection of CCK-8. Means of the data for the various conditions in the experimental groups were statistically compared to the corresponding mean data of the group that received no camostate, CCK-8, or antagonist by analysis of variance using Duncan's methods.[26,27] Levels of significance are as indicated: $*p < 0.05$, $**p < 0.01$, $***p < 0.001$. "NS" indicates $p > 0.05$. Modified from ref. 36.

secretion.[71,72] Thus, pancreatic growth and protein secretion are mediated via the high-affinity CCK receptor.

It is also well known that feeding of trypsin inhibitors and pancreaticobiliary diversion stimulate pancreatic growth[16,17] (FIG. 7). Such inhibition or diversion of intraduodenal proteolytic enzymes increases plasma concentration of CCK in rats and mice which is suggested to mediate pancreatic growth under these conditions.[16–18,36] The stimulatory effects of orally administered protease inhibitors and pancreaticobiliary diversion on pancreatic growth can markedly be inhibited by administration of CCK receptor antagonists[36,73] (FIG. 7). Short-term administration of CCK receptor antagonists in the absence of CCK stimulation slightly decreased pancreatic weight and content of DNA and protein[36,73] (FIG. 7). These latter results suggested that CCK may play a physiologic role in the maintenance of pancreatic growth.

Further studies monitored pancreatic growth after long-term feeding of camostate which is a potent inhibitor of serine proteases.[74] The protease inhibitor was fed for 9 months with or without the simultaneous feeding of CR1409 which is a potent and specific CCK receptor antagonist.[74] These experiments also studied pancreatic growth after feeding of the CCK antagonist alone, that is, without camostate.[74] In addition, pancreatic secretory capacity and pancreatic morphology were evaluated, because it had been reported that chronic increases of circulating CCK either by oral administration of a protease inhibitor or by pancreaticobiliary diversion induce formation of hyperplastic or adenomatous nodules in the rat pancreas.[75–77] Similar to previous short-term studies (10 days),[36] long-term feeding of the protease inhibitor camostate for 9 months exerted a stimulatory effect on the growth of the mouse pancreas.[74] In both short- and long-term studies,[36,74] an increase in plasma CCK concentration was probably responsible for the stimulatory effect of camostate on pancreatic growth. Short-term camostate feeding markedly increased plasma CCK concentration to 8 times the control values of chow-fed mice,[36] and simultaneous administration of a CCK inhibitor greatly reduced the stimulatory effect of camostate in both short- and long-term studies[36,74] (FIGS. 7 and 8).

Exogenous CCK-8 had qualitatively similar but quantitatively smaller stimulatory effects on pancreatic growth when compared with camostate feeding[36] (FIG. 7). Injections of the CCK antagonist in addition to (or more precisely shortly before each) injection of CCK-8 completely blocked all stimulatory effects of CCK-8 on pancreatic growth.[36] The CCK antagonist CR 1409, given without exogenous CCK or substances that may release endogenous CCK, exerted antitrophic effects on the pancreas in short-term studies[36] (FIG. 7). This suggests that physiological increases of CCK in response to feeding have trophic effects on the exocrine pancreas. This is in accordance with experimental and clinical observations that long-term parenteral nutrition results in reversible pancreatic atrophy.[79,80] Thus, a lack of physiological postprandial increases in CCK may be one factor responsible for this atrophy. As in previous reports in the rat,[81] both exogenous CCK and even to a greater degree feeding of the protease inhibitor markedly increased the content of the proteolytic enzyme chymotrypsinogen, but left that of the starch-splitting enzyme amylase completely unaffected. This nonparallel effect of CCK on synthesis of different digestive enzymes was seen in both short- and long-term experiments[36,74] (FIGS. 7 and 8).

Long-term release of endogenous CCK greatly increased pancreatic weight by induction of marked pancreatic hypertrophy (increase of protein content) and moderate hyperplasia (increase in DNA content).[74] Compared with previous short-term studies,[36] long-term feeding induced a more pronounced increase in pancreatic growth (compare FIGS. 7 and 8). Long-term feeding of camostate also increased maximal secretory capacity. Long-term blockade of the CCK receptor, however, only slightly inhibited pancreatic growth and secretory capacity. This inhibition was *not* more pronounced than that seen in previous studies using short-term administration of CR1409 or L-364,718[36,73] (compare FIGS. 7 and 8). Thus, CCK is not an essential growth factor for the pancreas, but increases in endogenous and exogenous CCK markedly stimulate pancreatic growth. In long-term experiments, fed animals under

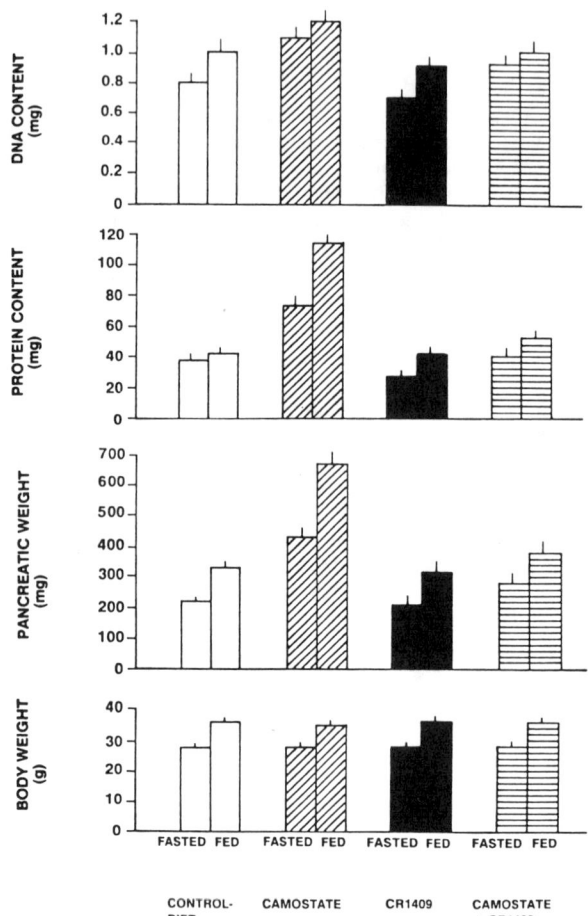

FIGURE 8. Mean ± SE of body weight, pancreatic weight, pancreatic protein content, and pancreatic DNA content (n = 12–24). The different experimental conditions are as indicated: "control diet" indicates mice that received chow without camostate or CR1409. In a second group of mice "camostate" was mixed with regular chow to achieve a daily dose of 100 mg/kg. In a third group the CCK receptor antagonist "CR1409" was mixed with regular chow to achieve a daily dose of 50 mg/kg. A fourth group received chow mixed with "camostate + CR1409" to achieve a daily dose of 100 mg/kg camostate and 50 mg/kg CR1409. "Fed" indicates mice that received the corresponding diets until they were sacrificed (12 mice per group). "Fasted" indicates mice that were fasted for 24 hours before sacrifice (24 mice per group). Mean data for the various conditions were compared to the corresponding control group that received neither camostate nor CR1409 by analysis of variance using Duncan's methods.[26,27] Body weight and pancreatic weight were significantly increased in fed mice compared to fasted mice ($p < 0.01$). Body weights were virtually identical among the four experimental groups ($p > 0.2$). Pancreatic weights were significantly increased in camostate-fed mice compared to the control group under both fed and fasted conditions ($p < 0.01$). Under "fasted" conditions pancreatic weight was slightly but significantly increased in mice that received both camostate and CR1409 when compared to the control group ($p < 0.05$); under "fed" conditions pancreatic weight in mice that received camostate and CR1409 did not differ from control ($p > 0.1$). Pancreatic weight did not differ between mice that received only CR1409 and the control group in both the fasted and the fed state ($p > 0.1$). Modified from ref. 74.

all experimental conditions showed an increase in pancreatic content of protein and DNA compared to animals that had been fasted for 24 hours before the end of the experiments. This increase also occurred in mice that received the CCK antagonist without camostate (FIG. 8). Thus, feeding exerts short-term trophic effects on the pancreas that are not only mediated by CCK.[74]

Despite long-term, marked pancreatic hypertrophy and hyperplasia, formation of hyperplastic or neoplastic nodules could be observed in none of the mice. This is in contrast to previous rat studies in which long-term feeding of protease inhibitors and diversion of pancreaticobiliary juice induced formation of hyperplastic and adenoma-

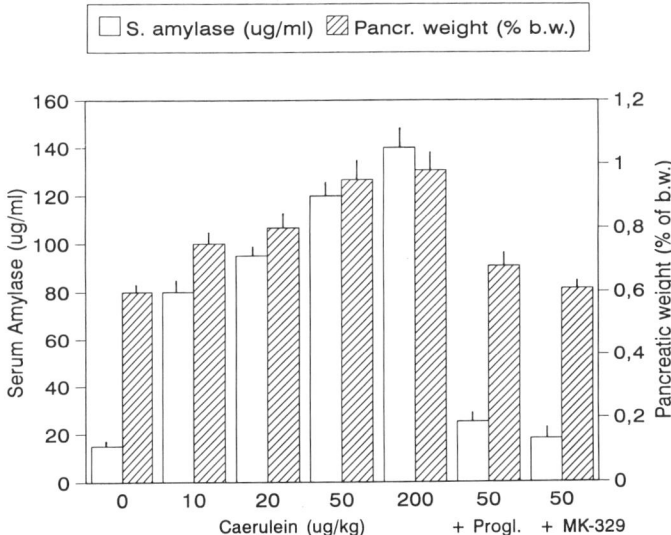

FIGURE 9. Serum amylase concentrations and pancreatic weight after increasing doses of caerulein in the mouse. Caerulein was given as 7 subcutaneous injections at hourly intervals over a 6-hour period. Determinations were made 9 hours after the first caerulein injections from 9–12 animals per group (mean ± SEM). Proglumide (400 mg/kg) and MK-329 (0.1 mg/kg) were given as subcutaneous injections 10 minutes before each of the caerulein injections. Caerulein dose-dependently increased serum amylase and pancreatic weight up to a dose of 50 μg/kg. Both CCK antagonists almost abolished the effects of the 50 μg/kg dose of caerulein. Modified from ref. 30 and from as yet unpublished experiments.

tous nodules.[75-77] The discrepancy between the previous studies in the rat and the present observations in the mouse may be due to a species difference.

PHARMACOLOGICAL ACTIONS OF CCK ON PANCREATIC FUNCTION AND MORPHOLOGY

Infusions and injections of supramaximally stimulating concentrations of CCK or its analog caerulein rapidly induce acute pancreatitis in various species including humans.[30,82-85] Caerulein-hyperstimulation pancreatitis is characterized by hyperamylasemia (FIG. 9), pancreatic edema, and acinar cell vacuolization and necrosis (FIG. 10). Previous experiments using nonselective CCK receptor antagonists have shown

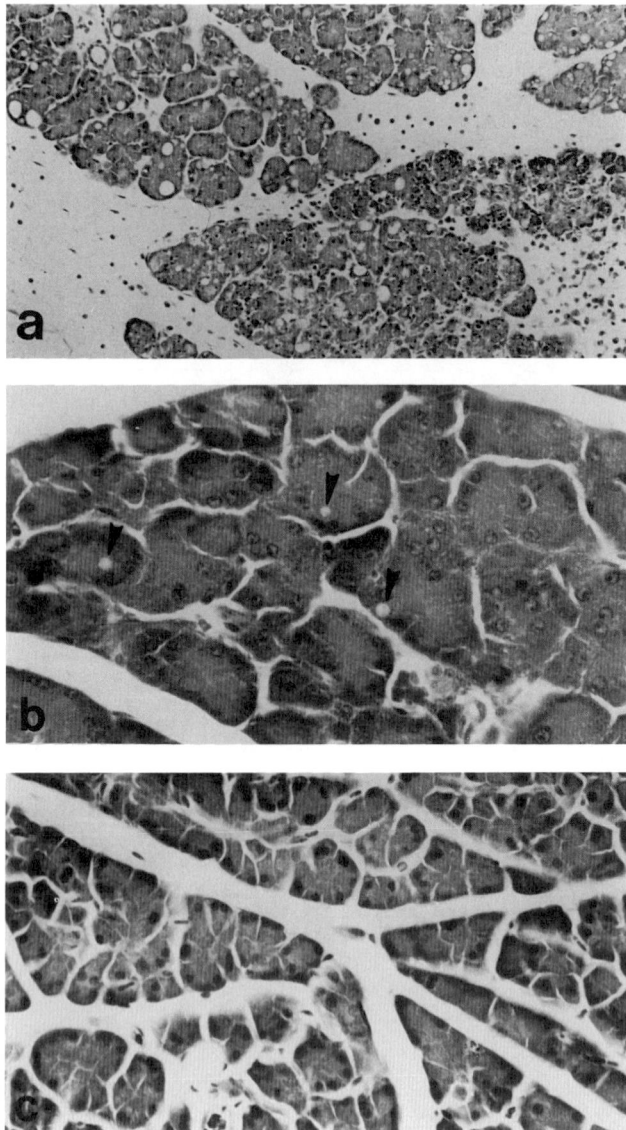

FIGURE 10. (a) Effects of seven repetitive injections of 50 μg/kg caerulein given in hourly intervals on the mouse pancreas. (For details see legend to FIG. 9.) Caerulein hyperstimulation caused interstitial edema and inflammation as well as vacuolization and necrosis of acinar cells. (b) Subcutaneous injections of 400 mg/kg proglumide before caerulein injections markedly reduced pancreatic pathology except for some intracellular vacuoles (*arrows*). (c) Injections of 0.1 mg/kg MK-329 before caerulein injections completely prevented caerulein-induced alterations of pancreatic morphology. Unpublished material.

that caerulein induces pancreatitis by interacting with CCK receptors[30] (FIGS. 9 and 10). The pancreatic acinar cell is thought to possess two classes of CCK receptors, one with higher affinity and the other with lower affinity for CCK. Studies characterizing acinar cell secretion in the presence of increasing CCK concentrations typically reveal a biphasic dose-response relation with stimulation at low CCK concentrations and inhibition at high "supramaximal" concentrations.[30,82,87] Recently, a synthetic CCK analog, CCK-JMV-180, was developed that does not cause inhibition of secretion when the dose that causes maximal stimulation is further increased.[71] On the basis of recently reported binding studies, CCK-JMV-180 probably interacts with both classes of pancreatic CCK receptors; it acts as an agonist at the high-affinity receptor and as an antagonist at the low-affinity receptor. The latter receptor class may mediate inhibition of pancreatic enzyme secretion due to high, supramaximal concentrations of caerulein or CCK-8.[71] The CCK analog CCK-JMV-180 can thus discriminate between high- and low-affinity CCK receptors. These characteristics also allow differentiation of the effects which are mediated by each of the two classes or sites of receptor. It was shown that CCK-JMV-180 even at very high concentrations cannot induce pancreatitis in the rat.[88] Furthermore, it even prevented caerulein-induced pancreatitis. The latter findings suggest that caerulein induces pancreatitis by acting as an agonist at the low-affinity CCK receptor. Little is known about the intracellular events that may be regulated by those receptors.

SUMMARY

This report reviews the effects of CCK on the pancreas and in particular analyzes recent studies in which CCK antagonists were used to evaluate the physiological role of CCK in modulating pancreatic function and morphology. CCK is released from endocrine cells of the small intestine in response to a meal. In various animal species there are CCK receptors on pancreatic acinar cells with two sites; occupation of the high affinity site is thought to mediate pancreatic secretion and growth, whereas occupation of the low affinity site by high CCK concentrations is thought to be responsible for supramaximal inhibition of secretion and pancreatitis. Recently, CCK receptors were also found on postganglionic cholinergic neurons in the gastrointestinal tract. Administration of CCK agonists stimulates pancreatic secretion and growth. Although in some previous studies CCK was given at doses that mimic its postprandial increase in plasma, these studies still did not prove that the actions of exogenous CCK were physiologically important. In addition, it was unclear if CCK primarily acts as a true hormone or as a neurotransmitter. The development of specific CCK receptor antagonists made it possible to better evaluate the physiological role of CCK. In humans, CCK-A antagonists like loxiglumide or L-364,718 at doses that completely inhibited the action of supraphysiological doses of exogenous CCK reduced meal-stimulated pancreatic enzyme secretion only by approximately 50%. On the other hand, atropine abolished the postprandial increase in pancreatic secretion and in addition markedly reduced the increase in pancreatic secretion due to infusion of "physiological" doses of CCK (i.e., CCK doses that mimic its postprandial increase in plasma). The increase in pancreatic bicarbonate secretion was only slightly reduced by CCK blockade. CCK antagonists failed to reduce the postprandial increase in plasma insulin, but markedly reduced the postprandial PP release. CCK-A antagonists caused slight hypotrophy and hypoplasia of the exocrine pancreas. However, even after 9 months of effective blockade of the CCK-A-receptor, mice had normal body weight and an almost normal pancreas. CCK antagonists were unable to alter short-term changes in pancreatic growth due to feeding and fasting. In some species, CCK agonists induced development of pancreatic nodules and increased the growth of malignant tumors. Studies about the effects of CCK antagonists on induction and growth of pancreatic tumors showed controversial results. In conclusion, CCK may act on the pancreas by three pathways: (1) At low doses it serves as a neurotransmitter by acting on cholinergic neurons. (2) At higher doses it may directly act at the high affinity site of the receptor of the acinar cell. (3) At supramaximal doses CCK acts mainly at the low affinity receptor site and may cause pancreatitis. CCK's effects through the cholinergic pathway appear to be more important for the physiology of secretion than the direct receptor-mediated action, at least in humans. CCK is not an insulinotropic factor in humans, but it may be involved in the release of PP. CCK modulates pancreatic growth, but it is not an essential growth factor. Its role in the development of pancreatic malignoma is uncertain.

ACKNOWLEDGMENTS

The authors thank Ms. Oppermann and Ms. Scheil for help in preparation of the manuscript.

REFERENCES

1. WILLIAMS, J. A. 1982. Cholecystokinin: A hormone and a neurotransmitter. Biomed. Res. **3:** 107–115.
2. NIEDERAU, C., T. HEINTGES, L. ROVATI & G. STROHMEYER. 1989. Effects of loxiglumide on gallbladder emptying after a meal or after intravenous infusion of caerulein in healthy human volunteers. Gastroenterology **97:** 1331–1337.
3. BEGLINGER, C., M. FRIED, I. WHITEHOUSE, J. B. JANSEN, C. B. LAMERS & K. GYR. 1985. Pancreatic enzyme response to a liquid meal and to hormonal stimulation. Correlation with plasma secretin and cholecystokinin levels. J. Clin. Invest. **75:** 1471–1476.
4. ANAGNOSTIDES, A. A., V. S. CHADWIK, A. C. SELDEN, J. BARR & P. N. MATON. 1985. Human pancreatic and biliary responses to physiological concentrations of cholecystokinin octapeptide. Clin. Sci. **69:** 259–263.
5. KONTUREK, S. J., J. TASLER, M. CIESZKOWSKI, K. SZEWCZYK & M. HLADIJ. 1988. Effect of cholecystokinin receptor antagonist on pancreatic responses to exogenous gastrin and cholecystokinin and to meal stimuli. Gastroenterology **94:** 1014–1023.
6. UNGER, R. H. & A. H. EISENTRAUD. 1969. Entero-insular axis. Arch. Intern. Med. **123:** 261–266.
7. GOLDFINE, I. D. & J. A. WILLIAMS. 1983. Receptors for insulin and CCK in the acinar pancreas: Relationship to hormone action. Int. Rev. Cytol. **85:** 1–38.
8. VERSPOHL, E. J., H. P. T. AMMON, J. A. WILLIAMS & I. D. GOLDFINE. 1986. Evidence that cholecystokinin interacts with specific receptors and regulates insulin release in isolated rat islets of Langerhans. Diabetes **35:** 38–43.
9. VERSPOHL, E. J., G. WUNDERLE, H. P. T. AMMON, J. A. WILLIAMS & I. D. GOLDFINE. 1986. Proglumide (gastrin and cholecystokinin receptor antagonist) inhibits insulin secretion *in vitro.* Naunyn-Schmiedebergs's Arch. Pharmacol. **332:** 284–287.
10. RUSHAKOFF, R. J., I. D. GOLDFINE, J. C. CARTER & R. A. LIDDLE. 1987. Physiological concentrations of cholecystokinin stimulate amino acid-induced insulin release in humans. J. Clin. Endocrinol. Metab. **65:** 395–401.
11. DEMBINSKI, A. R. & L. R. JOHNSON. 1978. Stimulation of pancreatic growth by secretin, cerulein, and pentagastrin. Endocrinology **106:** 232–328.
12. FÖLSCH, U. R., K. WINCKLER & K. G. WORMSLEY. 1978. Influence of repeated administration of cholecystokinin and secretin on the pancreas of the rat. Scand. J. Gastroenterol. **13:** 663–671.

13. CHERNIK, S. S., S. LEPOWSKI & I. L. CHAIKOFF. 1948. A dietary factor regulating the enzyme content of the pancreas: Changes in size and proteolytic activity of chick pancreas by the ingestion of raw soy bean meal. Am. J. Physiol. **155:** 33–41.
14. FÖLSCH, U. R., K. WINCKLER & K. G. WORMSLEY. 1974. Effect of soybean diet on enzyme content and ultrastructure of the rat exocrine pancreas. Digestion **11:** 161–171.
15. BÜCHLER, M., P. MALFERTHEINER, H. FRIESS, J. SEITZ, K. ROLLE, R. NUSTEDE, A. SCHAF-MAYER & H. G. BEGER. 1989. Pancreatic and GI-hormone adaptation following long-term camostate treatment in man. Pancreas **4:** A612.
16. GREEN, G. M. & R. L. LYMAN. 1972. Feedback regulation of pancreatic enzyme secretion as a mechanism for trypsin inhibitor-induced hypersecretion in the rat. Proc. Soc. Exp. Biol. Med. **140:** 6–12.
17. MIAZZA, B. M., Y. TURBERG, P. GUILLAUME, W. HAHNEN, J. A. CHAYVIALLEE & E. LOIZEAU. 1985. Mechanism of pancreatic growth induced by pancreatico-biliary diversion in the rat. Digestion **20:** 75–83.
18. YONEZAWA, H. 1984. Discrepancy between the potency of various trypsin inhibitors to inhibit trypsin activity and the potency to release biologically active cholecystokinin-pancreozymin. Jpn. J. Physiol. **34:** 849–856.
19. DOWLING, R. H. 1982. Small bowel adaption and its regulation. Scand. J. Gastroenterol. **74:** 53–74.
20. SMITH, J. P., S. T. KRAMER & T. E. SOLOMON. 1991. CCK stimulates growth of six human pancreatic cancer cell lines in serum-free medium. Reg. Pept. **32:** 341–349.
21. POUR, P. M., T. LAWSON, S. HELGESON, T. DONNELLY & K. STEPHAN. 1988. Effect of cholecystokinin on pancreatic carcinogenesis in the hamster model. Carcinogenesis **9:** 597–601.
22. LHOSTE, E. & D. S. LONGNECKER. 1987. Effect of bombesin and caerulein on early stages of carcinogenesis induced by azaserine in the rat pancreas. Cancer Res. **47:** 3273–3277.
23. HARRISON, J. D., J. A. JONES & D. L. MORRIS. 1990. The effect of the gastrin receptor antagonist proglumide on survival in gastric carcinoma. Cancer **66:** 1449–1452.
24. LIDDLE, R. A., I. D. GOLDFINE & J. A. WILLIAMS. 1984. Bioassay of plasma cholecystokinin in rats: Effects of food, trypsin inhibitor, and alcohol. Gastroenterology **87:** 542–549.
25. LIDDLE, R. A., I. D. GOLDFINE, M. S. ROSEN, R. A. TAPLITZ & J. A. WILLIAMS. 1985. Cholecystokinin bioactivity in human plasma: Molecular forms, responses to feeding, and relationship to gallbladder contraction. J. Clin. Invest. **75:** 1140–1142.
26. CHANG, T. M. & W. Y. CHEY. 1983. Radioimmunoassay of cholecystokinin. Dig. Dis. Sci. **28:** 456–468.
27. JANSEN, J. B. M. J. & B. H. H. W. LAMERS. 1983. Radioimmunoassay of cholecystokinin in human tissue and plasma. Clin. Chim. Acta **33:** 2197–2205.
28. WIENER, I., K. INOUE, C. J. FAGAN, P. LILJA, L. C. WATSON & J. C. THOMPSON. 1981. Release of cholecystokinin in man: Correlation of blood levels with gallbladder contraction. Ann. Surg. **194:** 321–327.
29. HAHNE, W. F., R. T. JENSEN, G. F. LEMP & J. D. GARDENER. 1981. Proglumide and benzotript: Members of a different class of cholecystokinin receptor antagonists. Proc. Natl. Acad. Sci. USA **78:** 6304–6310.
30. NIEDERAU, C., L. D. FERRELL & J. H. GRENDELL. 1985. Caerulein-induced acute necrotizing pancreatitis in mice: Protective effects of proglumide, benzotript, and secretin. Gastroenterology **88:** 1192–1204.
31. MAKOVEC, F., R. CHISTE, M. BANI, M. A. PACINI, I. SETNIKAR & L. A. ROVATI. 1985. New glutaramic acid derivatives with potent competitive and specific cholecystokinin-antagonistic activity. Arzneim. Forsch. **35:** 1048–1051.
32. NIEDERAU, M., C. NIEDERAU, G. STROHMEYER & J. H. GRENDELL. 1989. Comparative effects of CCK receptor antagonists on rat pancreatic secretion *in vivo*. Am. J. Physiol. **256:** G150–G157.
33. CHANG, R. S. L., R. L. MONAGHAN, J. BIRNBAUM, E. O. STAPLEY, M. A. GOETZ, G. ALBERS-SCHONBERG, A. A. PATCHETT, J. M. LIESCH, O. D. HENSENS & J. P. SPRINGER. 1985. A potent nonpeptide cholecystokinin antagonist selective for peripheral tissues isolated from Aspergillus aliaceus. Science **230:** 177–179.

34. CHANG, R. S. L. & V. J. LOTTI. 1986. Biochemical and pharmacological characterization of an extremely potent and selective nonpeptide cholecystokinin receptor antagonist. Proc. Natl. Acad. Sci. USA **83:** 4923–4926.
35. NIEDERAU, C., M. NIEDERAU, J. A. WILLIAMS & J. H. GRENDELL. 1986. New proglumide analogue CCK-receptor antagonists: Very potent and selective for peripheral tissues. Am. J. Physiol. **251:** G856–G860.
36. NIEDERAU, C., R. A. LIDDLE, J. A. WILLIAMS & J. H. GRENDELL. 1987. Pancreatic growth: Interaction of exogenous cholecystokinin, a protease inhibitor, and a cholecystokinin receptor antagonist in mice. Gut **28:** 63–69.
37. NIEDERAU, C. & M. KARAUS. 1990. Effects of agonists and antagonists of cholecystokinin on contractile and myoelectric activity of isolated muscle of colon and ileum in the dog and guinea pig. Int. J. Gastrointest. Motil. **2:** 160–175.
38. SCHWARZENDRUBE, J., C. NIEDERAU, R. LÜTHEN & G. STROHMEYER. 1991. Effects of CCK-receptor blockade on endocrine and exocrine pancreatic function in healthy humans. Gastroenterology **100:** 1683–1690.
39. HILDEBRANDT, P., C. BEGLINGER, K. GYR, J. B. JANSEN, L. C. ROVATI, M. ZUERCHER, C. B. LAMERS, I. SETNIKAR & G. A. STALDER. 1990. Effect of a cholecystokinin receptor antagonist on intestinal phase of pancreatic and biliary responses in man. J. Clin. Invest. **85:** 640–646.
40. SCHMIDT, W. E., W. CREUTZFELDT, M. HÖCKER, A. R. CHOUDHURY, R. NUSTEDE, A. SCHLESER, R. NITSCHE, L. C. ROVATI, A. SCHAFMAYER & U. R. FÖLSCH. 1990. Cholecystokinin receptor antagonist loxiglumide: Influence on bilio-pancreatic secretion and gastrointestinal hormones in man. **46:** 232–239.
41. LIDDLE, R. A., B. J. GERTZ, S. KANAYAMA, L. BECCARIA, L. D. COKER, T. A. TURNBULL & E. T. MORITA. 1989. Effects of a novel cholecystokinin receptor antagonist, MK-329, on gallbladder contraction and gastric emptying in humans. Implications for the physiology of CCK. J. Clin. Invest. **84:** 1220–1225.
42. ADLER, G., C. BEGLINGER, U. BRAUN, M. REINSHAGEN, I. KOOP, A. SCHAFMAYER, L. ROVATI & R. ARNOLD. 1991. Interaction of the cholinergic system and cholecystokinin in the regulation of endogenous and exogenous stimulation of pancreatic secretion in humans. Gastroenterology **100:** 537–543.
43. MALAGELADA, J. R., V. L. W. GO & W. H. J. SUMMERSKILL. 1974. Altered pancreatic and biliary function after vagotomy and pyloroplasty. Gastroenterology **66:** 22–27.
44. WORMSLEY, K. G. 1972. The effect of vagotomy on the human pancreatic response to direct and indirect stimulation. Scand. J. Gastroenterol. **7:** 85–91.
45. YOU, C. H., J. M. ROMINGER & W. Y. CHEY. 1982. Effects of atropine on the action and release of secretin in humans. Am. J. Physiol. **242:** G608–611.
46. YOU, C. H. & W. Y. CHEY. 1988. Atropine abolishes the potentiation effect of secretin and cholecystokinin-octapeptide on exocrine pancreatic secretion in humans. Pancreas **3:** 99–104.
47. VALENZUELA, J. E., C. B. LAMERS, I. M. MODLIN & J. H. WALSH. 1983. Cholinergic component in the human pancreatic secretory response to intestinal oleate. Gut **24:** 807–811.
48. SINGER, M. V., W. NIEBEL, K. H. UHDE, D. HOFFMEISTER & H. GOEBELL. 1985. Dose-response effects of atropine on pancreatic response to secretin before and after truncal vagotomy. Am. J. Physiol. **248:** G532–538.
49. SINGER, M. V., W. NIEBEL, J. B. JANSEN, D. HOFFMEISTER, S. GOTTHOLD, H. GOEBELL & C. B. LAMERS. 1989. Pancreatic secretory response to intravenous caerulein and intraduodenal tryptophan studies: Before and after stepwise removal of the extrinsic nerves of the pancreas in dogs. Gastroenterology **96:** 925–934.
50. KÖHLER, H., R. NUSTEDE, M. BARTHEL & A. SCHAFMAYER. 1991. Einfluβ der extrinsischen Denervation des Pankreas auf die nahrungsstimulierte Pankreassekretion und die Freisetzung von Cholezystokinin (CCK) und Neurotensin beim Hund. Z. Gastroenterol. **30:** 125–129.
51. DOCKRAY, G. J. 1989. The integrative functions of CCK in the upper gastrointestinal tract. In The Neuropeptide Cholecystokinin (CCK). J. Hughes et al., eds.: 232–239. Halsted. New York.

52. BEHAR, J. & P. BIANCANI. 1987. Pharmacologic characterization of excitatory and inhibitory cholecystokinin receptors of the cat gallbladder and sphincter of Oddi. Gastroenterology **92:** 764–770.
53. ZARBIN, M. A., J. K. WAMSLEY, R. B. INNIS & M. J. KUHAR. 1981. Cholecystokinin receptors: Presence and axonal flow in the rat vagus nerve. Life. Sci. **29:** 697–705.
54. CREUTZFELDT, W. The incretin concept today. 1979. Diabetologia **16:** 75–85.
55. CREUTZFELDT, W. & R. EBERT. 1985. New developments in the incretin concept. Diabetologia **28:** 565–573.
56. MEADE, R. C., H. A. KNEUBUHLER, W. J. SCHULTE & J. J. BARBOIAK. 1967. Stimulation of insulin secretion by pancreozymin. Diabetes **16:** 141–147.
57. DUPRE, J., S. A. ROSS, D. WATSON & J. D. BROWN. 1973. Stimulation of insulin secretion by gastric inhibitory polypeptide in man. J. Clin. Endocrinol. Metab. **37:** 826–828.
58. FRAME, C. M., M. B. DAVIDSON & R. A. L. STURDEVANT. 1975. Effects of octapeptide of cholecystokinin on insulin and glucagon secretion in dogs. Endocrinology **97:** 549–553.
59. OTSUKI, M., C. SAKAMOTO, H. YUU, M. MAEDA, S. MORITA, A. OHKI, N. KOBAYASHI, K. TERASHI, K. OKANO & S. BABA. 1979. Discrepancies between the doses of cholecystokinin- or caerulein-stimulating exocrine and endocrine responses in perfused isolated rat pancreas. J. Clin. Invest. **63:** 478–484.
60. SAKAMOTO, C., M. OTSUKI, A. OHKI, M. MITSUO, T. YAMASAKI & S. BABA. 1982. Glucose-dependent insulinotropic action of cholecystokinin and caerulein in the isolated perfused rat pancreas. Endocrinology **110:** 398–402.
61. FUJIMOTO, W. Y., R. H. WILLIAMS & J. W. ENSINCK. 1979. Gastric inhibitory polypeptide, cholecystokinin, and secretin effects on insulin and glucagon secretion by islet cell cultures. Proc. Soc. Biol. Med. **160:** 349–353.
62. OTSUKI, M., C. SAKAMOTO, M. MAEDA, H. YUU, S. MORITA & S. BABA. 1979. Effect of caerulein on exocrine and endocrine pancreas in the rat. Endocrinology **105:** 1396–1402.
63. OHNEDA, A., K. HORIGOME, S. ISHII, Y. KAI & M. CHIBA. 1978. Effects of caerulein upon insulin and glucagon secretion in dogs. Hormon. Metab. Res. **10:** 7–14.
64. ROSSETTI, L., G. I. SHULMAN & W. S. ZAWALICH. 1987. Physiologic role of cholecystokinin in meal-induced insulin secretion in conscious rats. Studies with L-364,718, a specific inhibitor of CCK-receptor binding. Diabetes **36:** 1212–1215.
65. ZAWALICH, W. S. & V. D. DIAZ. 1987. Asperlicin antagonizes stimulatory effects of cholecystokinin on isolated islets. Am. J. Physiol. **252:** E370–E374.
66. OKABAYASHI, Y., M. OTSUKI, T. NAKAMURA, M. FUJII, S. TANI, T. FUJISAWA, M. KOIDE, H. HASEGAWA & S. BABA. 1990. Proglumide analogues CR1409 and CR1392 inhibit cholecystokinin-stimulated insulin release more potently than exocrine secretion from the isolated perfused rat pancreas. Pancreas **5:** 291–297.
67. NAKAMURA, T., M. FUJII, Y. OKABAYASHI, T. NAKAMURA, S. TANI, T. FUJISAWA, M. KOIDE, H. HASEGAWA & M. OTSUKI. 1990. Effects of L-364,718 on pancreatic exocrine and endocrine secretion in the rat. Pancreas **5:** 216–221.
68. NIEDERAU, C., J. SCHWARZENDRUBE, R. LÜTHEN & G. STROHMEYER. 1992. The effects of a CCK-receptor blockade on circulating concentrations of glucose, insulin, C-peptide, and pancreatic polypeptide after various meals in healthy human volunteers. Pancreas **7:** 1–10.
69. BONATO, C., A. VALENTINI, M. TACCONI, L. ROVATI & A. MALESCI. 1989. Effect of CCK-receptor blockade on the postprandial release of insulinar hormones (abstr.). Gastroenterology **96:** A51.
70. HILDEBRAND, P., J. W. ENSINCK, S. KETTERER, F. DELCO, S. MOSSI, U. BANGERTER & C. BEGLINGER. 1991. Effect of a cholecystokinin antagonist on meal-stimulated insulin and pancreatic polypeptide release in humans. J. Clin. Endocrinol. & Metab. **72:** 1123–1129.
71. GALAS, M. C., M. F. LIGNON, M. RODRIGUEZ, C. MENDRE, P. FULCRAND, J. LAUR & J. MARTINEZ. 1988. Structure-activity relationship studies on cholecystokinin: Analogues with partial agonist activity. Am. J. Physiol. **88:** G176–G182.
72. DAWRA, R., A. SALUJA, M. M. LERCH, M. SALUJA, A. ZAVERTNIK, D. STEER & M. L.

STEER. 1991. Trophic effect of cholecystokinin (CCK) is mediated by high affinity CCK receptors. Gastroenterology **100:** A270.
73. WISNER, J. R., R. E. MCLAUGHLIN, K. A. RICH, S. OZAWA & I. G. RENNER. 1988. Effects of L-364,718, a new cholecystokinin receptor antagonist, on camostate-induced growth of the rat pancreas. Gastroenterology **94:** 109–113.
74. NIEDERAU, C., R. LÜTHEN, M. NIEDERAU, G. STROHMEYER, L. D. FERRELL & J. H. GRENDELL. 1990. Long-term effects of stimulation and inhibition at the CCK-receptor on morphology, function and growth of pancreas and intestine. Digestion **46:** 217–225.
75. LONGNECKER, L. S. 1987. Interface between adaptive and neoplastic growth in the pancreas. Gut **28:** 253–258.
76. MIAZZA, B. M., S. WIDGREN, J. A. CHAYVIALLEE, T. NICOLET & E. LOIZEAU. 1987. Exocrine pancreatic nodules after longterm pancreaticobiliary diversion in rats. An effect of raised CCK plasma concentrations. Gut **28:** 269–273.
77. STACE, N. H., T. J. PALMER, S. VAJA & R. H. DOWLING. 1987. Longterm pancreaticobiliary diversion stimulates hyperplastic and adenomatous nodules in the rat pancreas: A new model for spontaneous tumor formation. Gut **28:** 265–268.
78. NIEDERAU, C., R. A. LIDDLE, L. D. FERRELL & J. H. GRENDELL. 1986. Beneficial effects of CCK-receptor blockade and inhibition of proteolytic enzyme activity in experimental acute hemorrhagic pancreatitis in mice: Evidence for cholecystokinin as a major factor in the development of acute pancreatitis. J. Clin. Invest. **78:** 1056–1063.
79. JOHNSON, L. R., L. M. SCHANBACHER, S. J. DUDRICK & E. M. COPELAND. 1977. Effect of long-term parenteral feeding on pancreatic secretion and serum secretin. Am. J. Physiol. **233:** E524–E529.
80. KOTLER, D. P. & G. M. LEVINE. 1979. Reversible gastric and pancreatic hyposecretion after long-term parenteral nutrition. N. Engl. J. Med. **300:** 241–242.
81. GÖKE, B. H. PRINTZ, G. RICHTER, G. ADLER & R. ARNOLD. 1986. Beeinflussung der Pankreashypertrophie infolge Camostategabe durch Injektion des CCK-Antagonisten Proglumid. Klin. Wchnschr. **64:** A54.
82. LAMPLE, M. & H. F. KERN. 1977. Acute intestinal pancreatitis in the rat induced by excessive doses of a pancreatic secretagogue. Virchows Arch. **373:** 97–117.
83. ADLER, G., T. HUPP & H. F. KERN. 1979. Course and spontaneous regression of acute pancreatitis in the rat. Virchows Arch. **382:** 32–47.
84. RENNER, I. G., J. R. WISNER & H. RINDERKNECHT. 1983. Protective effects of exogenous secretin on ceruletide-induced acute pancreatitis in the rat. J. Clin. Invest. **72:** 1081–1092.
85. WATANABE, O., F. M. BACCINO, M. L. STEER & J. MELDOLESI. 1984. Supramaximal caerulein stimulation and ultrastructure of rat pancreatitis acinar cell: Early morphological changes during development of experimental pancreatitis. Am. J. Physiol. **246:** G457–G467.
86. NIEDERAU, C., M. NIEDERAU, R. LÜTHEN, G. STROHMEYER, L. D. FERRELL & J. H. GRENDELL. 1990. Pancreatic exocrine secretion in acute experimental pancreatitis. Gastroenterology **99:** 1120–1127.
87. SALUJA, A., I. SAITO, M. SALUJA, M. J. HOULIHAN, R. E. POWERS, J. MELDOLESI & M. L. STEER. 1985. *In vivo* rat pancreatic cell function during supramaximal stimulation with caerulein. Am. J. Physiol. **249:** G702–G710.
88. SALUJA, A. K., M. SALUJA, H. PRINTZ, A. ZAVERTNIK, A. SENGUPTA & M. L. STEER. 1989. Experimental pancreatitis is mediated by low-affinity cholecystokinin receptors that inhibit digestive enzyme secretion. Proc. Natl. Acad. Sci. USA **86:** 8968–8971.

Acid-Base Interactions during Exocrine Pancreatic Secretion

Primary Role for Ductal Bicarbonate in Acinar Lumen Function

STEVEN D. FREEDMAN AND GEORGE A. SCHEELE[a]

Laboratory of Cell and Molecular Biology
Charles A. Dana Research Institute
Thorndike Laboratory, and Department of Medicine (Division of Gastroenterology)
Harvard Medical School and
Beth Israel Hospital
Boston, Massachusetts 02215

Cholecystokinin (CCK) is the major hormone involved in the stimulation of exocytosis within pancreatic acinar cells. In contrast, the primary action of secretin results in the secretion of fluid and bicarbonate from ductal cells. Although pancreatic enzymes are stored as condensed aggregates in secretory granules, it has been assumed that such aggregates dissolve spontaneously during exocytosis and that solubilized (pro)enzymes are conveyed through the duct system by enhanced fluid secretion from duct cells. It is currently believed that bicarbonate secreted from pancreatic duct cells serves solely to neutralize the acidic pH of chyme delivered into the upper intestine from the stomach. According to this view, secretory processes in pancreatic acinar cells function independently of ductal cells, and fluid secretion from ductal cells serves only to transport pancreatic proteins through the ductal system and into the intestinal tract.

However, recent research in our laboratory indicates that acid-base interactions, coordinated within the acinar lumen through the effects of different hormones (CCK and secretin, respectively) on divergent epithelial cells (acinar and duct cells, respectively), play critical roles during pancreatic secretion in response to food ingestion. The importance of acid-base interplay between acinar and duct cells reveals that the initial functions of bicarbonate secreted into the pancreatic duct are served within the acinar lumen.

ROLE OF ACID-BASE INTERACTIONS IN THE REGULATED STORAGE AND RELEASE OF PANCREATIC ENZYMES

It has been known since the early 1980s that a H^+ATPase acidifies the trans-Golgi network (TGN).[1] Studies with DAMP[2,3] and acridine orange[4] indicate that condensing vacuoles and secretory granules are acidified in acinar cells. Available evidence indicates that the lumenal pH within the TGN ranges between 5.5 and 6.5 (discussed in ref. 5). We demonstrated that 14 well-defined canine pancreatic

---

[a]Correspondence to: George Scheele, MD, Dana Research Institute, DA-554, Harvard Medical School and Beth Israel Hospital, 330 Brookline Avenue, Boston, MA 02215.

secretory proteins representing four functional groups of enzymes (endoproteases, exoproteases, glycosidases, and lipases) aggregate under conditions that mimic the acidic environment of the TGN. FIGURE 1 shows the effects of pH and calcium on the aggregation of the mixture of dog pancreatic secretory proteins representing the

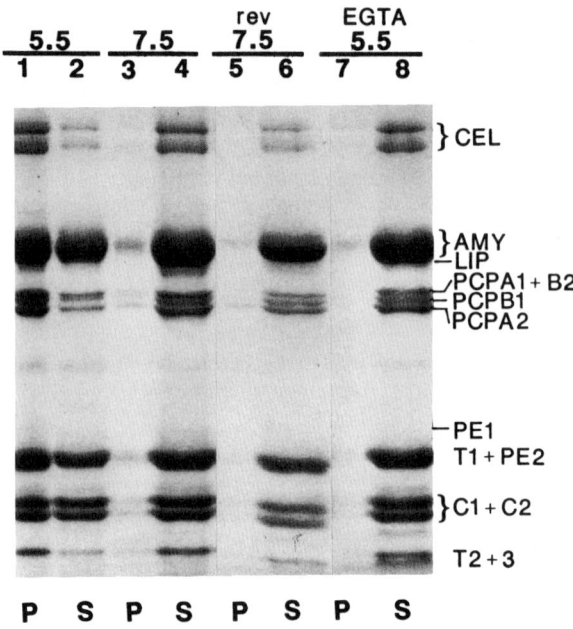

FIGURE 1. Effects of pH and calcium on aggregation of canine pancreatic secretory proteins. Proteins were incubated for 30 minutes at 37°C in the presence of 50 μg/ml FOY-305 under conditions of pH (100 mM Tris-HCl, pH 7.5; 100 mM MES-NaOH, pH 5.5) shown in the figure. pH 7.5 (rev) indicates that after incubation of proteins at pH 5.5 for 30 minutes, pH was increased to 7.5 by the addition of $\frac{1}{10}$th volume of 2M Tris, pH 11.5, for 30 minutes. pH 5.5 (EGTA) indicates that proteins were incubated at pH 5.5 for 30 minutes in the presence of 20 mM EGTA. After the incubation period, reaction mixtures were centrifuged at 220,000 × g and proteins contained in the pellet (P) and supernatant (S) fractions were separated by SDS-PAGE and stained with Coomassie Blue. Potential and actual enzymatic activities shown to the right of the figure were identified after elution of proteins from isoelectric focusing (IEF) gels. Individual bands separated by SDS polyacrylamide gel electrophoresis were then identified by comparison of purified proteins eluted from IEF gels with the complete mixture of secretory proteins. Abbreviations: CEL = putative carboxyl ester lipase; AMY = amylase; LIP = lipase; PCPA = procarboxypeptidase A; PCPB = procarboxypeptidase B; PE = proelastase; T = trypsinogen; C = chymotrypsinogen. Isoenzymic forms are numbered according to isoelectric point as described by the IUPAC-IUB Commission on biochemical nomenclature of multiple forms of enzymes. (Taken from reference 16.)

content fraction of zymogen granules. Under conditions of incubation and sedimentation at neutral pH (7.5), the majority of exocrine proteins remained in the supernatant fraction (compare lanes 3 and 4). Under conditions of incubation and sedimentation at acidic pH (5.5), the majority of all exocrine proteins entered sedimentable complexes that could be recovered in the pellet fraction (compare lanes 1 and 2). On reversal of pH, aggregates were observed to dissociate, as judged by their near-complete recovery in the supernatant fraction (lanes 5 and 6). Zymogen granule content is known to contain millimolar concentrations of calcium. Incubation of exocrine proteins at acidic pH (5.5) in the presence of 20 mM EGTA abolished the aggregation phenomenon (lanes 7 and 8). Prior studies have indicated that constitutively secreted proteins (BSA, IgG) do not aggregate under similar conditions.[5,6] These findings indicate that the mixture of regulated secretory proteins in pancreatic acinar cells aggregate under conditions that mimic the acidic milieu of the TGN. This aggregation process occurs as a function of protein concentration, time, and temperature. Furthermore, reversal of pH results in disruption of protein aggregates. Acid- and calcium-dependent formation of dense aggregates within apical secretory compartments (condensing vacuoles and secretory granules) fulfills the requirement for large scale packaging of secretory products, destined for release at the apical plasma membrane in response to CCK and acetylcholine stimulation. On exocytosis, the acidic pH of released contents must be neutralized before disruption of protein aggregates occurs. Taken together, these data suggest that bicarbonate within the acinar and ductal lumen is required for neutralization of the acidic pH of exocytic contents and solubilization of aggregated proteins.

ROLE OF ACID-BASE INTERACTIONS IN SORTING, ASSEMBLY, AND TRAFFICKING OF ZYMOGEN GRANULE MEMBRANES

GP2, a glycosyl phosphatidylinositol-anchored protein, is the major glycopotein in zymogen granule membranes.[7-11] It colocalizes with the glycolipid-enriched ectoleaflet of apical secretory compartments. GP2 homologs are widely distributed among polarized epithelial cells known to contain highly regulated secretory processes (parotid, submandibular gland, stomach, liver, kidney, and lung).[6] We determined that the COOH-terminal regions (474 amino acids) of rat GP2 and rat THP are highly conserved, demonstrating 53% identity and 86% similarity.[6] Because GP2 is targeted to secretory granules in pancreatic acinar cells and THP is targeted to oblong vesicles in kidney (thick ascending Henle limb) cells, the GP2/THP family appears to represent a new class of GPI-anchored proteins targeted to apical secretory compartments in polarized epithelial cells.[6] Our recent investigations raise the possibility that this family of GPI-anchored proteins, together with proteoglycans, establishes a submembranous matrix in close association with the lumenal surface of apical secretory compartments. The tight association of GP2 and $^{35}SO_4$-labeled proteoglycans (PG) to ZG membranes appears to be mediated, in part, via the GPI anchor of GP2.[12]

We have demonstrated that globular-GP2 released from ZG membranes by PI-PLC enters into tetrameric complexes under conditions that mimic the acidic pH of the TGN.[5] The equilibrium state between GP2 monomers and tetrameric complexes depended on protein concentration, time, temperature, calcium, and pH. It has been hypothesized[12] that tetrameric GP2, tethered to the lumenal leaflet of condensing vacuole membranes via its GPI anchor, organizes a submembranous matrix in association with sulfated proteoglycans. PH-dependent formation of tetrameric GP2 chains would allow for multivalent association of PG chains, resulting in the formation of a fibrillar GP2/PG meshwork. Assembly of a GP2/PG matrix on the lumenal (glycolipid-rich) surface of apical secretory compartments, triggered by the acidic pH of the TGN, may provide the conditions required for inhibition of clathrin-mediated processes on the cytosolic surface and thus prevent vesicular budding activity in these membranes.

Assembly of a submembranous GP2/PG matrix on the lumenal aspect of apical secretory membranes would provide three advantages for membrane microdomains that participate in regulated storage and release of pancreatic enzymes. First, during the process of membrane sorting and ZG assembly within the TGN, polymerization of a submembranous GP2/PG matrix would identify glycolipid-enriched membrane microdomains that remain associated with condensing vacuoles during the granule assembly process. In contrast, phospholipid-rich membrane microdomains (devoid of GP2 and associated PGs) would vesiculate from condensing vacuoles and depart for endolysosomal compartments. Continued remodeling of ZG membranes combined with progressive condensation of secretory products would lead to the formation of mature ZGs. Second, assembly of a GP2/PG submembranous matrix during maturation of condensing vacuoles would result in mature secretory granules with limiting membranes that are quiescent, that is, incapable of further vesiculation activity. Granule membranes that are inactive with regard to vesicular budding provide the optimal conditions for prolonged storage (hours-days) of secretory enzymes. Third, after exocytosis, a submembranous GP2/PG matrix may continue to retard vesicular budding of ZG membranes and therefore inhibit the process of recycling of ZG membranes from apical plasma membranes. Continued association of the GP2/PG matrix with granule membranes after exocytosis would serve to dilate the lumenal membrane and therefore provide increased space for products discharged into the acinar lumen. This relationship is consistent with the well-known observation that acinar lumenae become dilated during CCK-stimulated exocytosis.

Available evidence indicates that GP2 is released from apical plasma membranes by enzymatic cleavage of the GPI anchor.[13] We have proposed that the kinetics of anchor cleavage and release of the GP2/PG matrix from lumenal membranes controls two reciprocal processes: (1) dilatation of the lumenal membrane during exocytosis and (2) retrieval of ZG membranes by vesiculation processes for reuse during the secretory process. We have demonstrated that GP2[13] and $^{35}SO_4$-labeled proteoglycans (S. Freedman and G. Scheele, unpublished results) are released from granule membranes during CCK and secretin stimulation of pancreatic tissue. Alkaline pH may accelerate the enzymatic release of GP2. FIGURE 2 shows the relative efficiencies of GP2 secretion as a function of secretagogue effects that lead to varying rates of exocytosis from acinar cells and fluid/bicarbonate secretion from duct cells. Augmented GP2 secretion, a measure of enzyme-mediated cleavage of the GPI anchor, correlates with those hormones that stimulate fluid and bicarbonate release from ductal cells and correlates most highly with conditions of hormonal stimulation that result in fluid and bicarbonate secretion without enhanced exocytosis, such as low dose secretin stimulation.[13]

The role of bicarbonate-secreting ductal cells in GP2 release from acinar cells has been confirmed by comparative studies on (1) pancreatic lobules, where acinar units comprised of acinar and ductal elements are preserved, and (2) pancreatic acini, where ductal elements are largely removed during the dissociation procedure.[13] High-dose secretin stimulation (10^{-6} M) results in a strong fluid/bicarbonate response from ductal cells and a weak exocytic response in acinar cells. Consistent with the proposed role for bicarbonate in the enzyme-induced release of GP2 from the apical plasma membrane, secretin stimulation of lobules resulted in augmented GP2 secretion. In contrast, secretin stimulation of acini devoid of ductal elements resulted in attenuated GP2 secretion.

MOLECULAR COUPLING FACTORS AND ACID-BASE INTERPLAY BETWEEN ACINAR AND DUCT CELLS DURING COORDINATED PANCREATIC SECRETION

On the basis of the interdependent processes just described, the acinar lumen may be defined as a distinct physiological compartment where molecular coupling interactions between acinar and ductal cells are regulated by acid-base interactions.

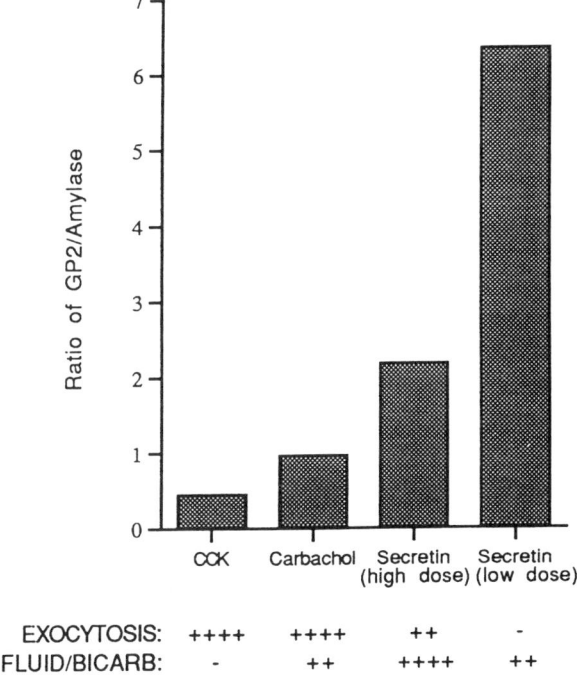

FIGURE 2. Efficiency of GP2 secretion relative to amylase secretion as a function of secretagogue effects on exocytosis in acinar cells and fluid/bicarbonate secretion from ductal elements. Effects of 1 nM CCK, 1 μM carbachol, 1 μM secretin (high dose), and 10 nM secretin (low dose) on GP2 and amylase secretion from rat pancreatic lobules after a 90-minute incubation at 37°C are shown. Basal rates of discharge were subtracted from stimulated rates of secretion for both amylase and GP2. The qualitative effects of each hormone treatment on exocytosis and fluid/bicarbonate secretion are shown below the figure. Symbols are (−), no effect; (++++), maximal stimulation. Taken from ref. 13.

Sequential acid-base interactions during coordinated acinar and duct cell function may be summarized as follows:

1. **Zymogen granule assembly is triggered by the acid milieu within the TGN.** Secretory granules appear to assemble as a result of two acid- and calcium-dependent processes: (1) condensation of pancreatic enzymes into dense aggregates that display nonosmotic characteristics and (2) assembly of a tetrameric GP2/PG matrix associated with the lumenal surface of ZG membranes. This submembranous matrix, formed in close proximity to glycolipid-enriched membranes, identifies these

microdomains for retention in apical secretory compartments and renders these membranes resistant to vesiculation processes in the cell cytosol.[12]

2. **CCK-stimulated exocytosis in acinar cells releases acidic contents of secretory granules into the acinar lumen.** Exocytosis, the last step in the intracellular secretory pathway in acinar cells, exteriorizes the secretory products (digestive enzymes) stored within ZGs and inserts ZG membranes into the apical plasma membrane. The primary secretory product released from acinar cells into the acinar lumen by exocytosis represents secretory enzymes highly aggregated in an acid milieu (pH ~6.2; millimolar calcium).

3. **Secretin-stimulated bicarbonate secretion from ductal cells neutralizes the acidic pH of exocytic contents.** Bicarbonate secreted from ductal elements (ductal cells and probably centroacinar cells) is required to neutralize the pH of exocytic contents. Inasmuch as pH-induced aggregation of secretory proteins is reversible, neutralization of exocytic contents will lead to dissociation of protein aggregates and solubilization of (pro)enzymes within the acinar lumen. The initial phases of dissociation of protein aggregates will greatly increase osmotic forces which, in turn, will enhance the influx of fluid and bicarbonate into these complexes.

4. **Fluid secretion transports solubilized enzymes through the ductal system.** Once aggregated complexes have been converted into solubilized proteins, enhanced fluid secretion from acinar cells (NaCl-rich) and ductal cells (bicarbonate-rich) transports these (pro)enzymes through the ductal system to the intestinal tract.

5. **Alkalinization of the acinar lumen triggers recycling of granule membranes inserted into the apical plasma membrane.** After neutralization of the acidic milieu of exocytic contents and solubilization of secretory proteins in neutral or alkaline medium, increased pH at the apical plasma membrane appears to optimize the conditions for the enzymatic cleavage of the GPI anchor of GP2. The pH-dependent nature of this process would ensure that protein aggregates are dissociated and secretory proteins are solubilized before the GP2/PG matrix is released from the lumenal aspects of ZG membranes inserted into the apical plasma membrane by exocytic processes. Removal of this lumenal matrix may allow vesicular recycling of ZG membranes with concomitant contraction of the apical lumen.[12] Vesicular retrieval, achieved through clathrin-mediated processes, is responsible for recycling granule membranes to the Golgi complex where they may participate in another round of secretion.

Identification of acid-base interactions between acinar and duct cells coupled via the acinar lumen provides a new understanding of the importance of combined CCK and secretin stimulation during pancreatic secretion in response to food ingestion. In addition, an understanding of these interactions provides a new appreciation for cholinergic stimulation which leads to both exocytosis in acinar cells and fluid and bicarbonate secretion from ductal elements. The requirement for coordinated acinar and duct cell secretion in generating optimal acid-base interactions for maximal efficiency in the secretory process provides a rationale for the observed stimulation of cholinergic pathways by low dose CCK stimulation in the dog[14] and human.[15] Because rates of pancreatic fluid secretion are very low under basal conditions in carnivores, immediate stimulation of bicarbonate secretion by ductal cells is required during CCK-induced exocytic release of enzymes from acinar cells. In contrast, rodents demonstrate high rates of fluid and bicarbonate secretion under basal conditions. High constitutive levels of bicarbonate secretion in rodent species ensure initial neutralization of exocytic contents within the acinar lumen.

SUMMARY

The role of acid-base interactions during coordinated acinar and duct cell secretion in the exocrine pancreas is described. The sequence of acid-base events may be summarized as follows: (1) Sorting of secretory proteins and membrane components into the regulated secretory pathway of pancreatic acinar cells is triggered by acid- and calcium-induced aggregation and association mechanisms located in the trans-Golgi network. (2) Cholecystokinin-stimulated exocytosis in acinar cells releases the acidic contents of secretory granules into the acinar lumen. (3) Secretin-stimulated bicarbonate secretion from duct and duct-like cells neutralizes the acidic pH of exocytic contents, which leads to dissociation of protein aggregates and solubilization of (pro)enzymes within the acinar lumen. (4) Stimulated fluid secretion transports solubilized enzymes through the ductal system. (5) Further alkalinization of acinar lumen pH accelerates the enzymatic cleavage of the glycosyl phosphatidyl-inositol anchor associated with GP2 and thus releases the GP2/proteoglycan matrix from lumenal membranes, a process that appears to be required for vesicular retrieval of granule membranes from the apical plasma membrane and their reuse in the secretory process.

We conclude that the central function of bicarbonate secretion by centroacinar and duct cells in the pancreas is to neutralize and then alkalinize the pH of the acinar lumen, sequential processes that are required for (a) solubilization of secreted proteins and (b) cellular retrieval of granule membranes, respectively.

REFERENCES

1. GLICKMAN, J., K. CROEN, S. KELLY & Q. AL-AWQUATI. 1983. Golgi membranes contain an electrogenic hydrogen pump in parallel to a chloride conductance. J. Cell Biol. **97:** 1303–1308.
2. ANDERSON, R. G. W. & R. K. PATHAK. 1985. Vesicles and cisternae in the trans Golgi apparatus of human fibroblasts are acidic compartments. Cell **40:** 635–643.
3. ORCI, L. 1987. The condensing vacuole of exocrine cells is more acidic than the mature secretory vesicle. Nature **326:** 77–79.
4. NIEDERAU, C., R. W. VAN DYKE, B. F. SCHARSCHMIDT & J. H. GRENDELL. 1986. Pancreatic zymogen granules: An actively acidified compartment. Gastroenterology **91:** 1433–1442.
5. FREEDMAN, S. D. & G. A. SCHEELE. 1993. Reversible pH-induced homophilic binding of GP2, a glycosyl phosphatidylinositol-anchored protein in pancreatic zymogen granule membranes. Eur. J. Cell Biol. **61:** 229–238.
6. FUKUOKA, S.-I., S. D. FREEDMAN, H. YU, V. SUKHATME & G. A. SCHEELE. 1992. GP2/THP gene family encodes self-binding GPI-linked proteins in apical vesicular membranes of pancreas and kidney. Proc. Natl. Acad. Sci. USA **89:** 1189–1193.
7. FUKUOKA, S.-I., S. D. FREEDMAN & G. A. SCHEELE. 1991. A single gene encodes membrane bound and free forms of GP-2, the major glycoprotein in pancreatic secretory (zymogen) granule membranes. Proc. Natl. Acad. Sci. USA **88:** 2898–2902.
8. HAVINGA, J. R., J. W. SLOT & G. J. STROUS. 1985. Membrane detachment and release of the major membrane glycoprotein of secretory granules in rat pancreatic exocrine cells. Eur. J. Cell Biol. **39:** 70–76.
9. LEBEL, D. & M. BEATTIE. 1988. The major protein of pancreatic zymogen granule membranes (GP-2) is anchored via covalent bonds to phosphatidylinositol. Biochem. Biophys. Res. Comm. **154:** 818–823.
10. BEAUDOIN, A. R., P. ST-JEAN & G. GRONDIN. 1991. Ultrastructural localization of GP2 in acinar cells of pancreas: Presence of GP2 in endocytic and exocytic compartments. J. Histol. Cytochem. **39:** 575–585.

11. RINDLER, M. J. & T. C. HOOPS. 1990. The pancreatic membrane protein GP2 localizes specifically to secretory granules and is shed into the pancreatic juice as a protein aggregate. Eur. J. Cell Biol. **53:** 154–163.
12. SCHEELE, G. A., S.-I. FUKUOKA & S. D. FREEDMAN. 1994. Role of the GP2/THP family of GPI-anchored proteins in membrane trafficking during regulated exocrine secretion. Pancreas **9:** in press.
13. FREEDMAN, S. D., K. SAKAMOTO & G. A. SCHEELE. 1994. Nonparallel secretion of GP2, a GPI-linked protein in the exocrine pancreas, implies lumenal coupling reactions between acinar and duct cells. Am. J. Physiol., in review.
14. SINGER, M. V. 1993. Neurohormonal control of pancreatic enzyme secretion in animals. *In* The Pancreas, Biology, Pathobiology, and Disease. V. L. W. Go, E. P. DiMagno, J. D. Gardner, E. Lebenthal, H. A. Reber & G. A. Scheele, eds.:425–448. Raven Press. New York.
15. ADLER, G., C. BEGLINGER, U. BROWN, M. REINSHAGEN, I. KOOP, A. SCHAFMAYER, L. ROVATI & R. ARNOLD. 1991. Interaction of the cholinergic system and cholecystokinin in the regulation of endogenous and exogenous stimulation of pancreatic secretion in humans. Gastroenterology **100:** 537–543.
16. FREEDMAN, S. D. & G. A. SCHEELE. 1993. Regulated secretory proteins in the exocrine pancreas aggregate under conditions that mimic the trans-Golgi network. Biochem. Biophys. Res. Comm. **2:** 992–999.

Role of CCK in Gallbladder Function

BIRGIT TER-BORCH GRAM SCHJOLDAGER[a]

Rigshospitalet
University Hospital of Copenhagen
DK-2100 Copenhagen, Denmark

Gallbladder contractility can be regulated by hormones and neurotransmitters and by their antagonists. Gallbladder contractility can be regulated at different levels from the central nervous system to the enteric nervous system, via parasympathetic and sympathetic pathways, through interaction of hormones with their receptors, via coupling of receptors to intracellular effectors, and even to modulation of the contractile apparatus itself. This chapter is concerned with regulation of gallbladder contractility by cholecystokinin (CCK).

THE CHOLECYSTOKININ FAMILY OF PEPTIDES AND RECEPTORS

Cholecystokinin was initially described as a hormonal substance from duodenal mucosa which caused gallbladder contractions in the cat.[1] CCK is mainly produced by the I-cells in the mucosa of the small intestine. Porcine intestinal CCK-33 was isolated and sequenced in 1968 by Mutt and Jorpes.[2] Soon it became apparent that CCK is heterogeneous and constitutes a family of peptides derived from a single gene.[3] The major bioactive forms are CCK-58, CCK-39, CCK-33, CCK-22, and CCK-8, which share the same octapeptide COOH-terminus[4–6] (FIG. 1). CCK circulates in plasma in concentrations of 2 (fasting) to 10 pmol/l (postprandial).[5–9] Gastrin is derived from a gene homologous to the CCK gene.[10] Gastrin is mainly produced in the G-cells of the antroduodenal mucosa. Also, gastrin is heterogeneous and circulates in several bioactive forms, among which are gastrin-71, G-34, G-17, and G-14.[11–14] Gastrin circulates in plasma in concentrations of 10 (fasting) to 100 pmol/l (postprandial).[7,15,16]

Cholecystokinin and gastrin share the same COOH-terminal tetrapeptide, which constitutes "the active site" and exerts full efficacy, but low potency.[17] Whether or not a peptide with this COOH-terminal tetrapeptide behaves like CCK or like gastrin depends on the position of a tyrosine in the immediate NH_2-terminal extension. Cholecystokinin has a sulfated tyrosyl residue in position 7 as counted from the COOH-terminus,[2] whereas gastrin has a tyrosyl residue, sulfated or not, in position 6.[18] The striking homology between CCK and gastrin indicates that they may have developed from a common ancestor.[19] This is also supported through examination of CCK and gastric gene structures.[20] Cionin, newly isolated from the protochordate *Ciona intestinalis*, is suitable as their common ancestor.[21] This peptide has the common CCK/gastrin tetrapeptide COOH-terminus and a sulfated tyrosyl residue in both position 6 and 7 as counted from the COOH-terminus.

Cholecystokinin and gastrin peptides interact with receptors that can be distinguished by their binding affinities. Cholecystokinin peptides display a 1,000-fold higher affinity than gastrin for the CCK_A receptor on gallbladder muscle[22–27] and

---

[a]Address for correspondence: Birgit Schjoldager, MD, Department of Gynecology and Obstetrics, Y 4031, Rigshospitalet, Blegdamsvej 9, DK-2100 Copenhagen Ø, Denmark.

```
Cholecystokinin:
                                SO₃⁻
                                 |
                 -Ser-Asp-Arg-Asp-Tyr-Met-Gly-Trp-Met-Asp-Phe-NH₂

                                 SO₃⁻
                                  |
      Gastrin:    -Glu-Glu-Glu-Glu-Ala-Tyr-Gly-Trp-Met-Asp-Phe-NH₂

                             SO₃⁻ SO₃⁻
                              |    |
      Cionin:         Asn-Tyr-Tyr-Gly-Trp-Met-Asp-Phe-NH₂
```

FIGURE 1. Primary structures of the undecapeptide fragments of mammalian cholecystokinin and gastrin and of the protochordean peptide cionin. These peptides have an identical COOH-terminal tetrapeptide that constitutes the "active" site of the peptides.

pancreatic acinar cells.[28,29] Cholecystokinin and gastrin display almost equal affinity for binding to the CCK_B receptor on gastric parietal cells,[30] gastric smooth muscle cells,[31] fundic somatostatin cells,[26,32,33] pancreatic acinar cells,[34] and brain.[35]

THE GALLBLADDER CCK_A RECEPTOR

In Vivo *Studies*

The gallbladder possesses a resting tone that could be CCK dependent because administration of the CCK antagonists L-364,718 and loxiglumide results in relaxation of the gallbladder.[9,36,37] However, the CCK antagonists may not be strictly specific, because they have been shown to inhibit motilin-induced contractions and to exert nonspecific calcium-antagonistic effects.[38,39] Vagotomy results in gallbladder dilatation, but cholinergic blockade with atropine has no effect on resting tone.[8]

Also, during the interdigestive period, the gallbladder periodically contracts, resulting in emptying of up to 30% of that seen after a meal.[40] This emptying occurs in relation to phase II of the interdigestive motor activity observed in the duodenum[40,41] and correlates with an increase in plasma levels of motilin.[41] Plasma concentrations of CCK remain below 2 pmol/l with no fluctuations.[42] This emptying can be abolished by cholinergic blockade with atropine.[43] Thus, probably cholinergic regulation and maybe motilin, but not CCK, account for the cyclic gallbladder emptying observed.

The digestive period can be divided into a cephalic phase, a gastric phase, and an intestinal phase. During the cephalic phase, with no food yet entering the stomach, gallbladder emptying can amount to 50% of that seen after a meal.[8,44,45] Sham-feeding studies have revealed an atropine-sensitive pathway and unchanged CCK plasma levels of 2 pmol/l.[8,45] Food entering the stomach, or even gastric distention alone, causes the gallbladder to contract.[46] This mechanism is atropine sensitive.[46] Different meal components entering duodenum differently stimulate gallbladder contraction and subsequent emptying. Water instillation stimulates gallbladder emptying with no changes in CCK levels.[45] Carbohydrate in duodenum stimulates gallbladder emptying with little or no increase in plasma CCK levels.[5,47] Protein and fat stimulate gallbladder emptying which correlates well with an increase in plasma CCK levels.[5,7,42,45,58,59] Similarly, exogenous CCK resulting in near postprandial plasma levels stimulates gallbladder emptying.[7,39,48–51] Also, administration of CCK antagonists before a fatty and protein-rich meal or before exogenous CCK results in inhibition of gallbladder emptying.[9,36,37]

Thus, CCK plays a major role in postprandial regulation of gallbladder emptying. CCK plays a minor role, if any, in the early digestive periods and during the interdigestive period.

In vivo studies in different species show that CCK-induced gallbladder emptying partly occurs through interaction with cholinergic nerves, because atropine reduces gallbladder emptying up to 50%[49,55-58] (TABLE 1). Truncated vagotomy has been reported to cause both diminished response to CCK[52] and unchanged[59,60] and enhanced response to CCK.[56,61]

In Vitro *Studies*

Pharmacological Studies. Pharmacological studies were performed on strips of gallbladder or even whole gallbladders connected to strain-gauge transducers to measure force development in response to various hormones and neuropeptides. Cholecystokinin stimulates contractions in all tested species.[22,38,58,62-77] Cholecystokinin and the ancestral peptide cionin induce contractions in a concentration-dependent manner with an efficacy and potency greater than those of other tested agents.[26,27] The ED_{50} (or potency) of CCK and cionin is in the nanomolar range. The potency of CCK is 1,000-fold better than that of gastrin; thus, the receptor type is CCK_A.[22,26,68,78] Most studies show that CCK mainly induces contractions independent of cholinergic blockade with atropine or axonal blockade with tetrodotoxin (TABLE 2). The use of tetrodotoxin, however, does not exclude release of neurotransmitters from the nerve bulb.[65,79] Some studies show significant inhibitory effects of atropine and/or tetrodotoxin (TABLE 2). The presence of CCK receptors on smooth muscle cells has been confirmed using contraction assays on isolated smooth muscle cells from the muscularis layer.[78,80] In contraction assays the potency of CCK-

TABLE 1. Pathways Mediating CCK Effects: *In Vivo* Studies

Species	Atropine Sensitive	TTX Sensitive	Vagotomy Sensitive	Reference
Guinea pig	+			52
	+hexa		+	52
Feline	+	+		51
Canine	+			53
	+			50
Opposum	+(low CCK)			54
	+hexa (low CCK)			54
	−(high CCK)			54
	−hexa (high CCK)			54
Human	+			55
	+		Enhanced	56
	+			57
	+			58
	+			49
			+/−	59
			+/−	60
			Enhanced	61

ABBREVIATIONS: hexa = hexamethonium; low CCK = low dose of CCK; high CCK = high dose of CCK.

induced contractions is in the picomolar range; in contrast to the nanomolar range in strip investigations, this discrepancy is still unclear.

The presence of CCK receptors on neural structures has been confirmed in studies with intracellular recordings from ganglia.[81,82] Here CCK facilitates nicotinic synaptic transmission by enhancing release of acetylcholine from actively transmitting synapses with a potency in the picomolar range.[81,82]

Thus, the majority of CCK functionally interacts with smooth muscle cell CCK_A receptors with a minority interacting with receptors located on cholinergic nerves.

CCK Radioligand Binding Studies. In agreement with this, CCK radioligand binding to histological full wall preparations of gallbladder shows binding limited to the muscularis layer which is devoid of ganglia.[68,74,83]

TABLE 2. Mode of CCK Action: *In Vitro* Studies (Strip Investigations)

Species	Atropine Sensitive	TTX Sensitive	Ach Release	Reference
Guinea pig	−scop	−		62
	−	−	−	63
	−			64
	+scop −hexa	−	+	65
	+			38
			+	66
	−	−		67
	−	−		68
			+	69
	+	+		70
Rabbit	−			71
	−			72
	−			73
Bovine	−	−		74
Feline	−			22
	−	−		75
Canine	−			64
			+	69
	+			76
Human	+			58
	−	−		77

ABBREVIATIONS: scop = scopolamine; hexa = hexamethonium.

Radioligand binding of CCK peptides or CCK analogs to full wall histological preparations or to membrane preparations obtained from muscularis or full wall gallbladders has revealed similar affinity for CCK binding to its receptor independently of the species tested[23–26,68,74,77,84–89] (TABLE 3). K_d values were in the nanomolar range. In human species there was also no difference in affinity of CCK binding to surgically removed gallbladders from healthy persons or from persons with chronic calculus cholecystitis.[25] Also, binding affinity in the human gallbladder was unchanged by age, gender, or weight of the persons.[25] Capacity varies among the different studies (TABLE 3), probably because of the different methods applied and especially because of different degrees of enrichment of membranes before binding. CCK exerts a binding affinity 1,000-fold greater than that of gastrin.[25,26] Only CCK

TABLE 3. Binding Affinity and Capacity

Species	Preparation	K_D (nM)	C (fmol/mg)	Reference
Guinea pig	Full wall			
	Sections	0.3	12	68
	Membranes	<0.1	8–65	84
Bovine	Full wall			
	Sections	1.0		74
	Membranes	0.6	101	85
	Membranes	0.1		86
	Membranes	0.8	4,500	23
	Membranes	0.8–5.2		24
	Membranes	0.5		26
	Membranes	0.4	1,672	87
Porcine	Membranes	0.5		26
Human	Membranes		3–8	88
	Membranes		5–28	89
	Membranes	1.0	230–366	25
	Full wall			
	Sections	6.0	25	77

---

^{125}I-BH-CCK-33:

^{125}I-BH-**Lys**-Ala-Pro-Ser-Gly-Arg-Val-Ser-Met-Ile-**Lys**-

-Asn-Leu-Gln-Ser-Leu-Asp-Pro-Ser-His-Arg-Ile-

$$\overset{SO_3^-}{|}$$
-Ser-Asp-Arg-Asp-Tyr-Met-Gly-Trp-Met-Asp-Phe-NH$_2$

---

^{125}I-D-Tyr-Gly-[(Nle^{28,31})CCK-(26-33)]:

$$\overset{SO_3^-}{|}$$
^{125}I-**D-Tyr**-Gly-Asp-Tyr-Nle-Gly-Trp-Nle-Asp-Phe-NH$_2$

DTP-^{125}I-D-Tyr-Gly-[(Nle^{28,31})CCK-(26-33)]:

$$\overset{SO_3^-}{|}$$
DTP-^{125}I-**D-Tyr**-Gly-Asp-Tyr-Nle-Gly-Trp-Nle-Asp-Phe-NH$_2$

---

^{125}I-D-Tyr-Gly-[Nle^{28,31},pNO$_2$,Phe^{33})CCK-(26-33)]:

$$\overset{SO_3^-}{|} \qquad \overset{NO_2}{|}$$
^{125}I-D-Tyr-Gly-Asp-Tyr-Nle-Gly-Trp-Nle-Asp-**Phe**-NH$_2$

FIGURE 2. Probes for affinity labeling the CCK$_A$ receptor. ^{125}I-BH-CCK-33 is a long probe, chemical cross-linkable through its epsilon amino groups in position 1 and 11. ^{125}I-D-Tyr-Gly-[(Nle^{28,31}) CCK-(26-33)] is a short probe chemical cross-linkable through its alpha amino group on the amino terminal D-tyrosine residue. DTP-^{125}I-D-Tyr-Gly-[(Nle^{28,31})CCK-(26-33)] has its photoactivatable moiety, DTP, at its amino terminus. ^{125}I-D-Tyr-Gly-[(Nle^{28,31},pNO$_2$,Phe^{33}) CCK-(26-33)] has its photoactivatable residue at its carboxyl terminus, within the expected receptor binding region.

peptide family members bind to the CCK_A receptor, not peptides such as vasoactive intestinal peptide, substance P, and glucagon.[25,26]

Affinity Labeling Studies. The biochemistry of the gallbladder CCK_A receptor has been studied in affinity labeling studies[23–26,90] The probes used for affinity labeling the CCK_A gallbladder receptor are shown in FIGURE 2. Both chemical and photochemical cross-linkers were used, extrinsic and intrinsic in nature. All probes labeled the same sized protein in each species tested. The bovine gallbladder CCK_A receptor has an apparent size of $M_r = 70$–85 kD,[23,24,90] different from the human gallbladder CCK_A receptor of apparent size $M_r = 85$–95 kD.[25,90] The human $M_r = 85$–95 kD unit was labeled independent of age, gender, and weight and independent of health or disease of the gallbladder.[25] Use of the bifunctional cross-linker MBS and performance of the experiments in the presence or absence of the reducing reagent dithiothreitol revealed that both the bovine and human gallbladder CCK binding

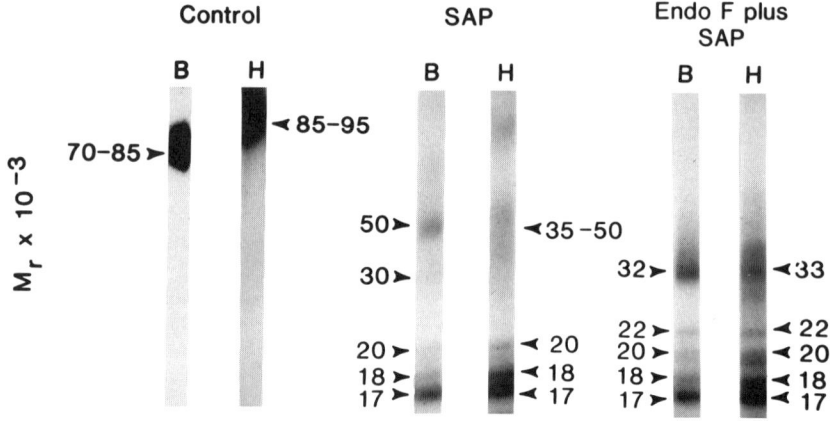

FIGURE 3. *Staphylococcus aureus* V8 protease (SAP) peptide mapping of the bovine (B) and human (H) gallbladder CCK_A binding subunits and their protein cores. Shown is an autoradiograph of an SDS-polyacrylamide gel used to separate affinity-labeled proteins (control) and these treated with SAP or with endoglycosidase F (Endo F, which removes N-linked complex carbohydrates) followed by SAP (Endo F plus SAP). (From reference 90, with permission.)

subunits are likely sulfhydryl-containing glycoproteins that are not disulfide-linked to adjacent proteins.[24,25]

Enzymatic digestion of carbohydrates revealed that both receptors are heavily glycosylated, with different carbohydrate contents.[90] Both receptors contain N-linked, complex carbohydrates with no evidence for existence of O-linked carbohydrate or N-linked simple (mannose-rich) carbohydrates. The presence of sialic acids in the bovine but not the human CCK_A receptor was revealed through neuraminidase treatment of the native CCK-binding subunits.[90]

Enzymatic digestion with endoglycosidase F or chemically deglycosylation with hydrogen fluoride revealed a protein core $M_r = 43$ kD in both CCK_A receptors.[90] Further enzymatic digestion of the proteins with *Staphylococcus aureus* protease revealed almost identically sized fragments[90] (FIG. 3). Probably the protein core contains the CCK binding region, which seems to be phylogenetically well preserved. Data are consistent with the newly generated data on purification and cloning of the rat pancreatic CCK_A receptor,[91] which was found to be a heavily glycosylated glycoprotein of apparent size M_r = 85–95 kD with N-linked, complex carbohydrates and sialic acids and a protein core of M_r = 42 kD.

SUMMARY AND CONCLUSION

Cholecystokinin may play a role in regulation of interdigestive motility, but this still remains to be investigated. CCK constitutes the major hormonal stimulus for postprandial gallbladder emptying. CCK exerts its contractile effects mainly through interaction directly with receptors on the gallbladder smooth muscle cells in the muscle layer, but also through interaction with cholinergic nerves extrinsic and/or intrinsic in nature. Furthermore, CCK can enhance ongoing nicotinic ganglionic transmission occurring in the serosal layer by release of acetylcholine. CCK interaction with the gallbladder smooth muscle CCK_A receptor was studied in further detail. CCK contracts strips of gallbladder muscle in a concentration-dependent way with a potency in the nanomolar range in all tested species. The potency is 1,000-fold better than that of gastrin; thus, the receptor is of type CCK_A. CCK binding to this receptor is specific and of high affinity, 1,000-fold better than that of gastrin with no differences between the tested species including bovine, porcine, and human. Also, CCK binding affinity was independent of age, gender, or weight of the person and pathology of the human gallbladder. The biochemistry of the CCK_A receptor varies between the tested species (bovine and human). Both CCK_A receptors are heavily glycosylated, but of different size and carbohydrate content. The bovine CCK_A receptor is of apparent size M_r = 70–85 kD with N-linked complex carbohydrates and sialic acids. The human CCK_A receptor is of M_r = 85–95 kD, with N-linked complex carbohydrates, but no sialic acids. They both have a protein core of apparent size M_r = 43 kD, with almost identically sized fragments after enzymatic cleavage. Probably the protein cores contain the receptor binding region, which seems well preserved between species.

CCK and the CCK_A gallbladder muscularis receptor are main regulators of postprandial gallbladder emptying. The biochemistry of the CCK_A gallbladder smooth muscle receptor is in accord with newly generated data of purification and cloning of the rat pancreatic CCK_A receptor.

REFERENCES

1. IVY, A. C. & E. A. OLDBERG. 1928. A hormone mechanism for gallbladder contraction and evacuation. Am. J. Physiol. **86**: 599–613.
2. MUTT, V. & J. E. JORPES. 1968. Structure of porcine cholecystokinin-pancreozymin. Eur. J. Biochem. **6**: 156–162.
3. DESCHENES, R. J., R. S. HAUN, C. L. FUNCKES & J. E. DIXON. 1985. A gene encoding rat cholecystokinin. Isolation, nucleotide sequence, and promoter activity. J. Biol. Chem. **260**: 1280–1286.
4. EYSSELEIN, V. E., C. W. DEVENEY, H. SANKARAN, J. R. REEVE & J. H. WALSH. 1983. Biological activity of canine intestinal cholecystokinin-58. Am. J. Physiol. **245**: G313–G320.
5. LIDDLE, R. A., I. D. GOLDFINE, M. S. ROSEN, R. A. TAPLITZ & J. A. WILLIAMS. 1985. Cholecystokinin bioactivity in human plasma. J. Clin. Invest. **75**: 1144–1152.
6. REHFELD, J. F. 1989. Cholecystokinin. *In* Handbook of Physiology. The Gastrointestinal System. G. M. Makhlouf & S. G. Schultz, eds. Vol **2**: 337–358. American Physiology Society. Bethesda, Maryland.

7. CANTOR, P., L. PETRONIJEVIC, J. F. PEDERSEN & H. WORNING. 1986. Cholecystokinetic and pancreozymic effect of O-sulfated gastrin compared with nonsulfated gastrin and cholecystokinin. Gastroenterology **91:** 1154–1163.
8. HOPMAN, W. P. M., J. B. M. J. JANSEN, G. ROSENBUSCH & C. B. H. W. LAMERS. 1987. Cephalic stimulation of gallbladder contraction in humans: Role of cholecystokinin and the cholinergic system. Digestion **38:** 197–203.
9. LIDDLE, R. A., B. J. GERTZ, S. KANAYAMA, L. BECCARIA, L. D. COKER, T. A. TURNBULL & E. T. MORITA. 1989. Effects of a novel cholecystokinin (CCK) receptor antagonist, MK-329, on gallbladder contraction and gastric emptying in humans. J. Clin. Invest. **84:** 1220–1225.
10. WIBORG, O., L. BERGLUND, E. BOEL, F. NORRIS, K. NORRIS, J. F. REHFELD, K. A. MARCKER & J. VUUST. 1984. The structure of a human gastrin gene. Proc. Natl. Acad. Sci. USA **81:** 1067–1069.
11. REHFELD, J. F. 1972. Three components of gastrin in human serum. Gel filtration studies on the molecular size of immunoreactive serum gastrin. Biochim. Biophys. Acta **285:** 364–372.
12. GREGORY, R. A. & H. J. TRACY. 1972. Isolation of two "big gastrins" from Zollinger-Ellison tumour tissue. Lancet **ii:** 797–799.
13. REHFELD, J. F. & F. STADIL. 1973. Gel filtration studies on immunoreactive gastrin in serum from Zollinger-Ellison patients. Gut **14:** 369–373.
14. GREGORY, R. A. & H. J. TRACY. 1974. Isolation of two minigastrins from Zollinger-Ellison tumour tissue. Gut **15:** 683–685.
15. SCHILLER, L. R., J. H. WALSH & M. FELDMAN. 1982. Effect of atropine on gastrin release stimulated by an amino acid meal in humans. Gastroenterology **83:** 267–272.
16. ANDERSEN, B. N., L. D. MAGISTRIS & J. F. REHFELD. 1983. Radioimmunochemical quantitation of sulfated and nonsulfated gastrins in serum. Clin. Chim. Acta **127:** 29–39.
17. MORLEY, J. S., H. J. TRACY & R. A. GREGORY. 1965. Structure-function relationships in the active C-terminal tetrapeptide sequence of gastrin. Nature **207:** 1356–1359.
18. GREGORY, H., P. M. HARDY, D. S. JONES, G. W. KENNER & R. C. SHEPPARD. 1964. The antral hormone gastrin. Nature **204:** 931–933.
19. LARSSON, L.-I. & R. F. REHFELD. 1977. Evidence for a common evolutionary origin of gastrin and cholecystokinin. Nature **269:** 335–338.
20. DESCHENES, R. J., S. V. L. NARAYANA, P. ARGOS & J. E. DIXON. 1985. Primary structural comparison of the preprohormones cholecystokinin and gastrin. FEBS Lett. **182:** 135–138.
21. JOHNSEN, A. H. & J. F. REHFELD. 1990. Cionin: A disulfotyrosyl hybrid of cholecystokinin and gastrin from the neural ganglion of the protochordate Ciona Intestinalis. J. Biol. Chem. **265:** 3054–3058.
22. CHOWDHURY, J. R., J. M. BERKOWITZ, M. PRAISSMAN & J. W. FARA. 1975. Interaction between octapeptide-cholecystokinin, gastrin, and secretin on cat gallbladder in vitro. Am. J. Physiol. **229:** 1311–1315.
23. SHAW, M. J., E. M. HADAC & L. J. MILLER. 1987. Preparation of enriched plasma membranes from bovine gallbladder muscularis for characterization of cholecystokinin receptors. J. Biol. Chem. **262:** 14313–14318.
24. SCHJOLDAGER, B., S. P. POWERS & L. J. MILLER. 1988. Affinity labeling of the bovine gallbladder cholecystokinin receptor using a battery of probes. Am. J. Physiol. **255:** G579–G586.
25. SCHJOLDAGER, B., X. MOLERO & L. J. MILLER. 1989. Functional and biochemical characterization of the human gallbladder muscularis cholecystokinin receptor. Gastroenterology **96:** 1119–1125.
26. SCHJOLDAGER, B., J. PARK, A. H. JOHNSEN AH, T. YAMADA & J. F. REHFELD. 1991. Cionin, a protochordean hybrid of cholecystokinin and gastrin: Biological activity in mammalian systems. Am. J. Physiol. **260:** G977–G982.
27. SCHJOLDAGER, B., S. S. POULSEN, P. SCHMIDT, D. H. COY & J. J. HOLST. 1991. Gastrin-releasing peptide is a transmitter mediating porcine gallbladder contraction. Am. J. Physiol. **260:** G577–G585.

28. JENSEN, R. T., G. F. LEMP & J. D. GARDNER. 1980. Interaction of cholecystokinin with specific membrane receptors on pancreatic acinar cells. Proc. Natl. Acad. Sci. USA **77:** 2079–2083.
29. SANKARAN, H., I. D. GOLDFINE, W. C. DEVENEY, K.-Y. WONG & J. A. WILLIAMS. 1980. Binding of cholecystokinin to high affinity receptors on isolated rat pancreatic acini. J. Biol. Chem. **255:** 1849–1853.
30. SOLL, A. H., D. A. AMIRIAN, L. P. THOMAS, T. J. REEDY & J. D. ELASHOFF. 1984. Gastrin receptors on isolated canine parietal cells. J. Clin. Invest. **73:** 1434–1447.
31. MENOZZI, D., J. D. GARDNER, R. T. JENSEN & P. N. MATON. 1989. Properties of receptors for gastrin and CCK on gastric smooth muscle cells. Am. J. Physiol. **257:** G73–G79.
32. SOLL, A. H., D. A. AMIRIAN, J. PARK, J. D. ELASHOFF & T. YAMADA. 1985. Cholecystokinin potently releases somatostatin from canine fundic mucosal cells in short-term culture. Am. J. Physiol. **248:** G569–G573.
33. PARK, J., T. CHIBA, K. YAKABI & T. YAMADA. 1987. Cholecystokinin (CCK) stimulates somatostatin release from isolated canine gastric D-cells via both gastrin and CCK-selective receptors (Abstr.). Gastroenterology **92:** 1566.
34. YU, D.-H., M. NOGUCHI, Z.-C. ZHOU, M. L. VILLANUEVA, J. D. GARDNER & R. T. JENSEN. 1987. Characterization of gastrin receptors on guinea pig pancreatic acini. Am. J. Physiol. **253:** G793–G801.
35. SAITO, A., I. D. GOLDFINE & J. A. WILLIAMS. 1981. Characterization of receptors for cholecystokinin and related peptides in mouse cerebral cortex. J. Neurochem. **37:** 483–490.
36. MEYER, B. M., C. BEGLINGER, J. B. M. J. JANSEN, L. C. ROVATI, B. A. WERTH, P. HILDEBRAND, D. ZACH & G. A. STALDER. 1989. Role of cholecystokinin in regulation of gastrointestinal motor functions. Lancet **ii:** 12–15.
37. SCHMIDT, W. E., W. CREUTZFELDT, A. SCHLESER, A. J. CHOUDHURY, R. NUSTEDE, M. HÖCKER, R. NITSCHE, H. SOSTMANN, L. C. ROVATI & U. R. FÖLSCH. 1991. Role of CCK in regulation of pancreaticobiliary functions and GI motility in humans: Effects of loxiglumide. Am J. Physiol. **260:** G197–G206.
38. KUBOTA, K., K. SUGAYA, N. SUNAGANE, I. MATSUDA & T. URUNO. 1985. Cholecystokinin antagonism by benzodiazepines in the contractile response of the isolated guinea-pig gallbladder. Eur. J. Pharmacol. **110:** 225–231.
39. HANYU, N., W. J. DODDS, R. D. LAYMAN, W. J. HOGAN & D. G. COLTON. 1991. Effect of two new cholecystokinin antagonists on gallbladder emptying in opossums. Am. J. Physiol. **260:** G258–G264.
40. MARZIO, L., M. NERI, F. CAPONE, F. DI FELICE, C. DE ANGELIS, A. MEZZETTI & F. CUCCURULLO. 1988. Gallbladder contraction and its relationship to interdigestive duodenal motor activity in normal human subjects. Dig. Dis. Sci. **33:** 540–544.
41. ITOH, Z. & I. TAKAHASHI. 1981. Periodic contractions of the canine gallbladder during the interdigestive state. Am. J. Physiol. **240:** G183–G189.
42. DALE, W. E., C. M. TURKELSON & T. E. SOLOMON. 1989. Role of cholecystokinin in intestinal phase and meal-induced pancreatic secretion. Am. J. Physiol. **257:** G782–G790.
43. SVENBERG, T., N. D. CHRISTOFIDES, M. L. FITZPATRICK, F. AREOLA-ORTIZ, S. R. BLOOM & R. B. WELBOURN. 1982. Interdigestive biliary output in man: Relationship to fluctuations in plasma motilin and effect of atropine. Gut **23:** 1024–1028.
44. FISHER, R. S., E. ROCK & L. S. MALMUD. 1986. Gallbladder emptying response to sham feeding in humans. Gastroenterology **90:** 1854–1857.
45. YAMAMURA, T., T. TAKAHASHI, M. KUSUNOKI, M. KANTOH, Y. SEINO & J. UTSUNOMIYA. 1988. Gallbladder dynamics and plasma cholecystokinin responses after meals, oral water, or sham feeding in healthy subjects. Am. J. Med. Sci. **295:** 102–107.
46. DEBAS, H. T. & T. YAMAGISHI. 1979. Evidence for a pylorocholecystic reflex for gallbladder contraction. Ann. Surg. **190:** 170–175.
47. FISHER, R. S., E. ROCK & L. S. MALMUD. 1987. Effects of meal composition on gallbladder and gastric emptying in man. Dig. Dis. Sci. **32:** 1337–1344.

48. HOPMAN, W. P. M., P. J. S. M. KERSTENS, J. B. M. J. JANSEN, G. ROSENBUSCH & C. B. H. W. LAMERS. 1985. Effect of graded physiologic doses of cholecystokinin on gallbladder contraction measured by ultrasonography. Gastroenterology **89:** 1242–1247.
49. HOPMAN, W. P. M., J. B. M. J. JANSEN, G. ROSENBUSCH & C. B. H. W. LAMERS. 1990. Role of cholecystokinin and the cholinergic system in intestinal stimulation of gallbladder contraction in man. Hepatology **11:** 261–265.
50. STRAH, K. M., R. L. MELENDEZ, T. N. PAPPAS & H. T. DEBAS. 1986. Interactions of vasoactive intestinal polypeptide and cholecystokinin octapeptide on the control of gallbladder contraction. Surgery **99:** 469–473.
51. BEHAR, J. & P. BIANCANI. 1987. Pharmacologic characterization of excitatory and inhibitory cholecystokinin receptors on the cat gallbladder and sphincter of oddi. Gastroenterology **92:** 764–770.
52. TAKAHASHI, T., D. MAY & C. OWYANG. 1991. Cholinergic dependence of gallbladder response to cholecystokinin in the guinea pig in vivo. Am. J. Physiol. **261:** G565–G569.
53. TAKAHASHI, I., T. SUZUKI, I. AIZAWA & Z. ITOH. 1982. Comparison of gallbladder contractions induced by motilin and cholecystokinin in dogs. Gastroenterology **82:** 419–424.
54. HANYU, N., W. J. DODDS, R. D. LAYMAN, W. J. HOGAN, W. Y. CHEY & I. TAKAHASHI. 1990. Mechanism of cholecystokinin-induced contraction of the opossum gallbladder. Gastroenterology **98:** 1299–1306.
55. GULLO, L., L. BOLONDI, P. PRIORI, P. CASANOVA & G. LABÒ. 1984. Inhibitory effect of atropine on cholecystokinin-induced gallbladder contraction in man. Digestion **29:** 209–213.
56. FISHER, R. S., E. ROCK & L. S. MALMUD. 1985. Cholinergic effects on gallbladder emptying in humans. Gastroenterology **89:** 716–722.
57. MARZIO, L., A. M. DI GIAMMARCO, M. NERI, F. CUCCURULLO & P. MALFERTHEINER. 1985. Atropine antagonizes cholecystokinin and cerulein-induced gallbladder evacuation in man: A real-time ultrasonographic study. Am. J. Gastroenterol. **80:** 1–4.
58. TAKAHASHI, T., T. YAMAMURA, Y. ISHIKAWA, M. KANTOH & J. UTSUNOMIYA. 1986. Effects of cholecystokinin-octapeptide on the human gallbladder both in vivo and in vitro. Gastroenterol. Jpn. **21:** 49–54.
59. SHAFFER, E. A. 1982. The effect of vagotomy on gallbladder function and bile composition in man. Ann. Surg. **195:** 413–418.
60. PELLEGRINI, C. A., M. LEWIN, M. G. PATTI, M. J. THOMAS, T. RYAN & L. W. WAY. 1985. Gallbladder filling and response to cholecystokinin are not affected by vagotomy. Surgery **98:** 452–458.
61. MASCLEE, A. A. M., J. B. M. J. JANSEN, W. M. M. DRIESSEN, L. M. GEUSKENS & C. B. H. W. LAMERS. 1990. Effect of truncal vagotomy on cholecystokinin release, gallbladder contraction, and gallbladder sensitivity to cholecystokinin in humans. Gastroenterology **98:** 1338–1344.
62. YAU, W. M., G. M. MAKHLOUF, L. E. EDWARDS & J. T. FARRAR. 1973. Mode of action of cholecystokinin and related peptides on gallbladder muscle. Gastroenterology **65:** 451–456.
63. YAU, W. M. & M. L. YOUTHER. 1984. Modulation of gallbladder motility by intrinsic cholinergic neurons. Am. J. Physiol. **247:** G662–G666.
64. RAKOVSKA, A., K. MILENOV & S. YANEV. 1986. Mode of action of cholecystokinin octapeptide on smooth muscles of stomach, ileum and gall bladder. Meth. Find. Exp. Clin. Pharmacol. **8:** 697–703.
65. YAMAMURA, T., T. TAKAHASHI, M. KUSUNOKI, M. KANTOH, Y. ISHIKAWA & J. UTSUNOMIYA. 1986. Cholecystokinin octapeptide-evoked [^{3}H]acetylcholine release from guinea pig gallbladder. Neurosci. Lett. **65:** 167–170.
66. TAKAHASHI, T., T. YAMAMURA, M. KUSUNOKI, M. KANTOH, Y. ISHIKAWA & J. UTSUNOMIYA. 1987. Differences between muscular receptors and neural receptors for cholecystokinin-octapeptide in the guinea-pig gallbladder. Eur. J. Pharmacol. **136:** 255–258.

67. GRIDER, J. R. & G. M. MAKHLOUF. 1987. Regional and cellular heterogeneity of cholecystokinin receptors mediating muscle contraction in the gut. Gastroenterology **92:** 175–180.
68. VON SCHRENCK, T., T. H. MORAN, P. HEINZ-ERIAN, J. D. GARDNER & R. T. JENSEN. 1988. Cholecystokinin receptors on gallbladder muscle and pancreatic acinar cells: A comparative study. Am. J. Physiol. **255:** G512–G521.
69. RAKOVSKA, A., K. MILENOV & A. BOCHEVA. 1989. Effect of cholecystokinin octapeptide and somatostatin on the motility of guinea pig and canine gallbladder. Comp. Biochem. Physiol. **94C:** 649–653.
70. BROTSCHI, E. A., J. PATTAVINO & L. F. WILLIAMS. 1990. Intrinsic nerves affect gallbladder contraction in the guinea pig. Gastroenterology **99:** 826–830.
71. AMER, M. S. & W. E. BECVAR. 1969. A sensitive in-vitro method for the assay of cholecystokinin. J. Endocrinol. **43:** 637–642.
72. AMER, M. S. 1972. Studies with cholecystokinin in vitro. III. Mechanism of the effect on the isolated rabbit gall bladder strips. J. Pharmacol. Exp. Ther. **183:** 527–534.
73. JOHNSON, A. G., C. E. MARSHALL & I. A. I. WILSON. 1982. Effects of some drugs and peptide hormones on the responsiveness of the rabbit isolated gall-bladder to cholecystokinin. J. Physiol. **332:** 415–425.
74. SCHJOLDAGER, B., M. J. SHAW, S. P. POWERS, P. F. SCHMALZ, J. SZURZEWSKI J. & L. J. MILLER. 1988. Bovine gallbladder muscularis: Source of a myogenic receptor for cholecystokinin. Am. J. Physiol. **254:** G294–G299.
75. LEE, K. Y., P. BIANCANI & J. BEHAR. 1989. Calcium sources utilized by cholecystokinin and acetylcholine in the cat gallbladder muscle. Am. J. Physiol. **256:** G785–G788.
76. POZO, M. J., M. D. SALIDO, J. A. MADRID & G. M. SALIDO. 1990. In-vitro effect of pirenzepine on motility of canine gall-bladder. J. Pharm. Pharmacol. **42:** 89–93.
77. TOKUNAGA, Y., K. L. COX, R. COLEMAN, W. CONCEPCION, P. NAKAZATO & C. O. ESQUIVEL. 1993. Characterization of cholecystokinin receptors on the human gallbladder. Surgery **113:** 155–162.
78. GRIDER, J. R. & G. M. MAKHLOUF. 1990. Distinct receptors for cholecystokinin and gastrin on muscle cells of stomach and gallbladder. Am. J. Physiol. **259:** G184–G190.
79. KANTOH, M., T. TAKAHASHI, M. KUSUNOKI, T. YAMAMURA & J. UTSUNOMIYA. 1987. Dual action of cholecystokinin-octapeptide on the guinea pig antrum. Gastroenterology **92:** 376–382.
80. SEVERI, C., J. R. GRIDER & G. M. MAKHLOUF. 1988. Functional gradients in muscle cells isolated from gallbladder, cystic duct, and common bile duct. Am. J. Physiol. **255:** G647–G652.
81. MAWE, G. M. 1991. The role of cholecystokinin in ganglionic transmission in the guinea-pig gall-bladder. J. Physiol. **439:** 89–102.
82. BAUER, A. J., M. HANANI, T. C. MUIR & J. H. SZURZEWSKI. 1991. Intracellular recordings from gallbladder ganglia of opossums. Am. J. Physiol. **260:** G299–G306.
83. AOKI, T., T. UENO, A. TOYONAGA, R. SAKATA, Y. KIMURA, K. GONDO, S. INUZUKA, T. TORIMURA, H. YOSHIDA, E. SASAKI & K. TANIKAWA. 1991. Radiographic evidence of cholecystokinin octapeptide receptors in the hamster gallbladder. Scand. J. Gastroenterol. **26:** 1165–1172.
84. POSTON, G. J., P. SINGH, D. G. MACLELLAN, C. Z. YAO, T. UCHIDA, C. M. TOWNSEND & J. C. THOMPSON. 1988. Age-related changes in gallbladder contractility and gallbladder cholecystokinin receptor population in the guinea pig. Mech. Ageing Dev. **46:** 225–236.
85. STEIGERWALT, R. W., I. D. GOLDFINE & J. A. WILLIAMS. 1984. Characterization of cholecystokinin receptors on bovine gallbladder membranes. Am. J. Physiol. **247:** G709–G714.
86. CHANG, R. S. L. & V. J. LOTTI. 1986. Biochemical and pharmacological characterization of an extremely potent and selective nonpeptide cholecystokinin antagonist. Proc. Natl. Acad. Sci. USA **83:** 4923–4926.
87. MOLERO, X. & L. J. MILLER. 1991. The gall bladder cholecystokinin receptor exists in two guanine nucleotide-binding protein-regulated affinity states. Mol. Pharmacol. **39:** 150–156.

88. PORTINCASA, P., A. HOWARD, G. M. MURPHY & R. H. DOWLING. 1986. Cholecystokinin receptor binding by human gall bladder myocyte membranes (Abstr.). Gut **27:** A1261.
89. UPP, J. R., W. H. NEALON, P. SINGH, C. J. FAGAN, A. S. JONAS, G. H. GREELEY & J. C. THOMPSON. 1987. Correlation of cholecystokinin receptors with gallbladder contractility in patients with gallstones. Ann. Surg. **205:** 641–647.
90. SCHJOLDAGER, B., X. MOLERO & L. J. MILLER. 1990. Gallbladder CCK receptors: Species differences in glycosylation of similar protein cores. Regul. Pept. **28:** 265–272.
91. WANK, S. A., R. HARKINS, R. T. JENSEN, H. SHAPIRA, A. DE WERTH & T. SLATTERY. 1992. Purification, molecular cloning, and functional expression of the cholecystokinin receptor from rat pancreas. Proc. Natl. Acad. Sci. USA **89:** 3125–3129.

Effect of Cholecystokinin on Gastric Motility in Humans[a]

CHRISTOPH BEGLINGER

Division of Gastroenterology
University Hospital
CH-4031 Basel, Switzerland

Cholecystokinin (CCK) was first described over 60 years ago as a putative hormone that caused gallbladder contraction in response to fat in the small intestine.[1] Three decades later, Jorpes and Mutt[2] showed that CCK was chemically identical to the peptide pancreozymin, another candidate hormone that caused pancreatic enzyme secretion in response to intestinal fat or protein.[3] Since that time the gallbladder and pancreas have been the principal target organs of CCK. However, CCK receptors are located throughout the entire gut, having been identified on smooth muscle cells of the esophagus, stomach, small intestine, and colon.[4] A number of physiologic actions have been proposed for CCK including the classic effects on gallbladder contraction and pancreatic enzyme secretion, but also regulation of gastric emptying, stimulation of intestinal and colonic motility, stimulation of hormone release, and induction of satiety. TABLE 1 summarizes many of the reported actions of exogenous CCK in man.

The recent elaboration of peptide hormone antagonists with CCK as a model has opened the way to defining the quantitative role of CCK in gastrointestinal functions. Studies with CCK receptor antagonists provide strong evidence for a physiologic role of CCK as a major regulator of gallbladder contraction, exocrine pancreatic secretion, postprandial pancreatic polypeptide, and gastrin release.[6-9] It is still controversial whether CCK plays a major role in gastric motility. The present work summarizes all available evidence obtained in human studies focusing on studies with physiologic doses of exogenous CCK and studies with specific CCK-A receptor antagonists.

EFFECTS OF INTRAVENOUS INFUSION OF CCK ON GASTRIC EMPTYING

Digestive products of fat and protein are potent stimulants of CCK release.[10] Inasmuch as these nutrients are also potent inhibitors of gastric emptying, the hypothesis was formulated that CCK has a role in the regulation of gastric motility.[11] It has long been well established that exogenous infusion of pharmacologic doses of CCK inhibit gastric emptying in humans.[12] Whether this action represents a physiologic action of CCK is controversial.[13,14] Recently, two groups found that CCK in doses imitating postprandial plasma concentrations strongly inhibited gastric emptying rates of liquid and semisolid meals.[15,16] The effect of CCK was suggested to constitute a feedback system whereby CCK would regulate its own release; whenever food would enter the duodenum, CCK would be released; the released CCK would stimulate gallbladder contraction and pancreatic enzyme secretion and at the same time inhibit gastric emptying. As a consequence, less food is delivered to the duodenum which in turn reduces the stimulus to further CCK release. In this hypothesis, CCK would play a role as an integrator of postprandial digestive

[a] The study was supported by the Swiss National Science Foundation (grant 32–31336.91).

TABLE 1. Actions of Exogenous CCK-Like Peptides on Gastrointestinal Functions of Humans

Target Organ or Function	Effect
1. *Biliary tract*	
Gallbladder contraction	+
Bile secretion	+
Sphincter of Oddi motility	−
2. *Exocrine pancreas*	
Enzyme secretion	+
Bicarbonate secretion	+
3. *Endocrine pancreas*	
Insulin secretion	no effect
Pancreatic polypeptide secretion	+
4. *Stomach*	
Acid secretion	±
Somatostatin-14 secretion	+
Gastrin secretion	−
Gastric emptying	−
Gastric motility	−
5. *Esophagus*	
Lower esophageal sphincter pressure	−
6. *Gut motility*	
Small intestinal transit	+
Colonic transit	−

NOTE: + indicates stimulation; − indicates inhibition or relaxation. Adapted from Solomon.[5]

functions. It is still controversial whether this concept is correct. The main problem arises from the finding that multiple molecular forms of CCK circulate in human plasma, making it difficult to simulate postprandial CCK concentrations through infusion of one molecular form. Caution must therefore be exercised in the interpretation of these previous gastric emptying studies. Recent work with specific CCK-A receptor antagonists provide some answers, but also cause some further controversy (to be discussed).

Information on the effects of exogenous CCK on gastric motility in humans is scarce. Intraduodenal perfusion of fat or intravenous infusion of CCK8 caused suppression of antral contractile activity and induction of isolated pyloric contractions, but the effect was partially blocked by atropine and occurred at supraphysiologic doses of CCK8,[17,18] suggesting that CCK is not the major mediator of these effects. Furthermore, relaxation of the gastric corpus has been demonstrated with the CCK analog caerulein.[19] All these phenomena could be associated with delayed gastric emptying, but experimental support for the concept is still insufficient.

EFFECT OF CCK RECEPTOR ANTAGONISTS ON GASTRIC EMPTYING

Several studies have investigated the effect of CCK-A receptor blockade on gastric emptying of nutrient meals in humans, with divergent results. Some of these discrepancies are probably related to methodologic problems, as different CCK receptor antagonists have been employed. In addition, different techniques have been used to assess gastric emptying. A summary of the various studies is given in TABLE 2.

Thorough investigation of the effect of CCK-A receptor blockade was reported by Fried and coworkers.[20] First, the effect of a physiologic dose of CCK8 (20 pmol/kg per hour) on gastric emptying rates (measured by the double indicator technique) of a 500 ml saline meal was investigated. CCK8 significantly retarded the gastric emptying rate of the saline solution compared to that in the control experiment. This inhibitory effect was completely abolished by the administration of the specific CCK-A antagonist loxiglumide. In further experiments, it was shown that loxiglumide significantly accelerated by about 40% the gastric emptying rates of both a liquid mixed meal and a pure (20%) glucose meal. Additional experiments using gamma-scintigraphy confirmed the accelerating effect of loxiglumide on gastric emptying rate of the liquid mixed meal. In all these experimental conditions, significant CCK release occurred after test meal intake. However, the gastric emptying rate of a guar meal which did not stimulate endogenous CCK release was not affected by the administration of the CCK antagonist.

Liddle and coworkers,[21] however, failed to show an effect of the CCK antagonist MK329 (also called devazepide) on gastric emptying rates (measured by scintigraphy) of either the liquid or the solid phase of a mixed meal. Moreover, no effect after administration of loxiglumide was shown in a study in which ultrasonography was used to quantify gastric emptying rates of a meal in humans.[22] This latter technique, however, is not a validated method to assess gastric emptying, and the results are therefore not reliable. Finally, we showed that loxiglumide significantly accelerated gastric clearance of radiopaque markers provided the markers were given with a liquid mixed meal.[6] No acceleration was observed when the markers were given with a solid mixed meal or a guar meal, and no intrinsic effect of loxiglumide on gastric emptying was observed. Gastric clearance of radiopaque markers, however, is an indirect assessment of gastric emptying of a meal as the markers can only be cleared from the stomach when all the food has been emptied into the duodenum. This latter study would therefore favor the hypothesis that CCK-A receptor blockade induces early phase III patterns of the migrating motor complex.

In summary, the effect of CCK-A receptor blockade on gastric emptying rates of liquid and/or solid meals in humans is not clear yet. The available evidence supports the concept that postprandially released CCK exerts a regulatory function on gastric liquid emptying in humans. Thus, CCK may act as a coordinating and synchronizing factor of postprandial upper digestive functions by adjusting the ratio of nutrients to digestive juices (pancreatic enzymes, bile acids) in the duodenum (FIG. 1).

TABLE 2. Effect of CCK Receptor Blockade on Gastric Emptying in Humans: Comparison of Different Techniques and Meals

Antagonist	Technique of Gastric Emptying Measurement	Meal Type	Effect
Loxiglumide			
Fried et al.[20]	Double indicator perfusion technique	Liquid meal	+
	Scintigraphy	Liquid meal	+
Meyer et al.[6]	Gastric clearance of radiopaque markers	Liquid meal	+
Corazziari et al.[22]	Real-time ultrasonography	Yolk meal	−
Niederau et al.[24]	Scintigraphy	Solid/liquid meal	−
MK329			
Liddle et al.[21]	Scintigraphy	Solid/liquid meal	−

NOTE: + indicates acceleration of gastric emptying; − indicates no effect.

EFFECT OF CCK-A BLOCKADE ON ANTRODUODENAL MOTILITY

Katschinski and coworkers[23] investigated the effect of loxiglumide on antroduodenal motility after sham feeding experiments. They showed that antroduodenal motility is primarily under cholinergic control. CCK blockade, however, induced distinct effects; endogenous CCK seems to prolong the reappearance of phase III following sham feeding and increases antral contractile activity and antroduodenal coordination; loxiglumide reduced the contraction frequency and motility index in the antrum by 70 and 75%, respectively, and suppressed the probability of coordinated antroduodenal contractions by 85–90%. No CCK release in the circulation was detectable under these experimental conditions, supporting the hypothesis that neuronally released CCK acts as a local regulator under this experimental setting.

GASTROILEAL AND GASTROCOLONIC RESPONSES

Eating a meal can increase motor activity in the ileum, and this response could be mediated by CCK. Kellow and Phillips[25] demonstrated that patients with irritable

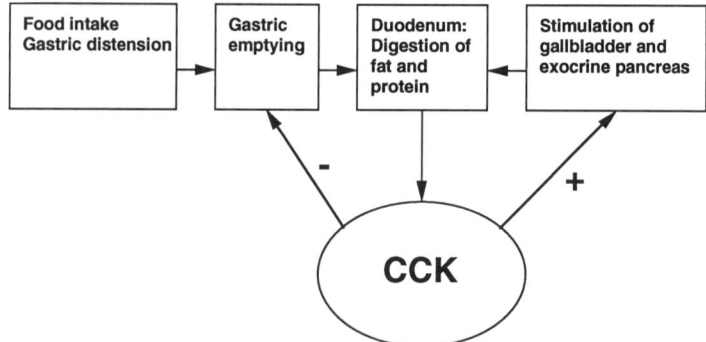

FIGURE 1. Schematic representation of the role of CCK in controlling postprandial upper digestive functions.

bowel syndrome (IBS) show an exaggerated response to food intake. Using an intravenous dose of CCK that caused 50% contraction of the gallbladder as measured by real-time ultrasonography, they showed that ileal motility to this stimulation was greater in patients with IBS than in healthy controls.[26]

The first indication that CCK may be involved in the pathophysiology of the IBS came with the pioneering work of Harvey and Read.[27] Infusion of CCK caused an abnormal increase in colonic motility in IBS patients. Further support for involvement of CCK in the gastrocolonic response comes from the observation that the CCK receptor antagonist loxiglumide abolished the response in normal volunteers without affecting basal colonic motility.[28,29]

SUMMARY

Gastric emptying after food ingestion is regulated by neural and hormonal factors. However, the relative contributions of each pathway is not yet clearly defined. The classic gut hormone CCK seems to be involved in the regulation of gastric emptying in humans. Experimental evidence is best for gastric emptying of liquid meals that release CCK from the duodenum: (1) CCK infused at postprandial plasma concentrations inhibits gastric emptying of a liquid and a semisolid meal.[15,16] (2) Administration of the CCK antagonist loxiglumide significantly accelerated gastric emptying of a liquid mixed meal and a glucose meal.[20]

Discrepant results with the antagonist MK329[21] are difficult to explain considering the marked acceleration of gastric emptying rates by the specific and potent antagonist MK329 shown in several animal studies.[30–32] Taken together, current information favors the conclusion, however, that CCK mainly controls gastric emptying of the liquid but not the solid components.

Thus, CCK is involved in the physiologic regulation of gastric emptying and gastric motility in man. Blocking CCK-A receptors accelerates gastric emptying of liquid meals and abolishes the gastrocolonic reflex. Therefore, CCK may play a role as a common regulator of postprandial gallbladder contraction and pancreatic enzyme secretion as well as of gastric emptying rates under certain conditions. Such common control would optimize the nutrient-to-digestive juices concentration ratio. The importance of endogenous CCK on gastric emptying of solid meals, however, is poorly understood and remains to be defined. Only very limited information is available on gastric motility. Much more work has to be done before a clear concept can be developed.

ACKNOWLEDGMENTS

I would like to thank Carita Frei for editorial help in the preparation of this manuscript.

REFERENCES

1. Ivy, A. C. & E. Oldberg. 1928. A hormone mechanism for gallbladder contraction and evacuation. Am. J. Physiol. **86:** 599–613.
2. Jorpes, E. & V. Mutt. 1966. Cholecystokinin and pancreozymin, one single hormone? Acta Physiol. Scand. **66:** 196–202.
3. Harper, A. A. & H. S. Raper. 1943. Pancreozymin, a stimulant of the secretion of pancreatic enzymes in extracts of the small intestine. J. Physiol. (Lond.) **102:** 115–125.
4. Bishop, A. E., Y. D. Zhao, D. R. Springall & J. M. Polak. 1991. The morphological localization of cholecystokinin and its binding sites in the diffuse neuroendocrine system. *In* Cholecystokinin Antagonists in Gastroenterology. Basic and Clinical Status. G. Adler & C. Beglinger, eds.:10–26. Springer. Berlin-Heidelberg-New York.
5. Solomon, T. E. 1991. Biological actions of CCK in the gastrointestinal tract. *In* Cholecystokinin Antagonists in Gastroenterology. Basic and Clinical Status. G. Adler & C. Beglinger, eds: 35–43. Springer. Berlin-Heidelberg-New York.
6. Meyer, B. M., B. A. Werth, C. Beglinger, P. Hildebrand, J. B. M. J. Jansen, D. Zach, L. C. Rovati & G. A. Stalder. 1989. Role of cholecystokinin in regulation of gastrointestinal motor functions. Lancet **II:** 12–15.
7. Hildebrand, P., C. Beglinger, K. Gyr, J. B. M. J. Jansen, L. C. Rovati, M. Zuercher, C. B. H. W. Lamers, I. Setnikar & G. A. Stalder. 1990. Effects of a cholecystokinin receptor antagonist on intestinal phase of pancreatic and biliary responses in man. J. Clin. Invest. **85:** 640–646.
8. Meier, R., P. Hildebrand, M. Thumshirn, C. Albrecht, B. Studer, K. Gyr & C. Beglinger. 1990. Effect of loxiglumide, a cholecystokinin antagonist, on pancreatic polypeptide release in humans. Gastroenterology **99:** 1757–1762.

9. BEGLINGER, C., P. HILDEBRAND, R. MEIER, P. BAUERFEIND, H. HASSLOCHER, N. URSCHELER, F. DELCO, A. EBERLE & K. GYR. 1992. A physiological role for cholecystokinin as a regulator of gastrin secretion. Gastroenterology **103:** 490–495.
10. LIDDLE, R. A., I. D. GOLDFINE, M. S. ROSEN, R. A. TAPLITZ & J. A. WILLIAMS. 1985. Cholecystokinin bioactivity in human plasma. Molecular forms, responses to feeding, and relationship to gallbladder contraction. J. Clin. Invest. **75:** 1144–1152.
11. MEYER, J. H. 1987. Motility of the stomach and gastroduodenal junction. *In* Physiology of the Gastrointestinal Tract. L. R. Johnson, ed.: 613–629. Raven. New York.
12. CHEY, W. Y., S. HITANANT, J. HENDRICKS & S. H. LORBER. 1970. Effect of secretin and cholecystokinin on gastric emptying and gastric secretion in man. Gastroenterology **58:** 820–827.
13. VALENZUELA, J. E. & C. DEFILIPPI. 1981. Inhibition of gastric emptying in humans by secretin, the octapeptide of cholecystokinin, and intraduodenal fat. Gastroenterology **81:** 898–902.
14. KONTUREK, S. J., N. KWIECIEN, W. OBTULOWICZ, B. KOPP, J. OLEKSY & L. ROVATI. 1990. Cholecystokinin in the inhibition of gastric secretion and gastric emptying in humans. Digestion **45:** 1–8.
15. LIDDLE, R. A., E. T. MORITA, C. K. CONRAD & J. A. WILLIAMS. 1986. Regulation of gastric emptying in humans by cholecystokinin. J. Clin. Invest. **77:** 992–996.
16. KLEIBEUKER, J. H., H. BEEKHUIS, J. B. M. J. JANSEN, D. A. PIERS & C. B. H. W. LAMERS. 1988. Cholecystokinin is a physiological hormonal mediator of fat-inhibition of gastric emptying in man. Eur. J. Clin. Invest. **18:** 173–177.
17. HASLER, W., B. BOWLING & C. OWYANG. 1989. Intraduodenal lipids induce pyloric contractions: Role of cholecystokinin and the cholinergic and opiate pathways. Gastroenterology **96:** A200.
18. FRASER, R., D. FONE, M. HOROWITZ & J. DENT. 1990. Dose related stimulation of pyloric motility in humans by cholecystokinin octapeptide. Gastroenterology **98:** A351.
19. SCARPIGNATO, C., G. ZIMBARO, F. VITULO & G. BERTACCINI. 1981. Caerulein delays gastric emptying of solids in man. Arch. Int. Pharmacodyn. Ther. **249:** 98–105.
20. FRIED, M., U. ERLACHER, W. SCHWIZER, C. LÖCHNER, J. KOERFER, C. BEGLINGER, J. B. JANSEN, C. B. LAMERS, F. HARDER, A. BISCHOF-DELALOYE, G. A. STALDER & L. ROVATI. 1991. Role of cholecystokinin in the regulation of gastric emptying and pancreatic enzyme secretion in humans. Gastroenterology **101:** 503–511.
21. LIDDLE, R. A., B. J. GERTZ, S. KANAYAMA, L. BECCARIA, L. D. COKER, T. A. TURNBULL & E. T. MORITA. Effects of a novel cholecystokinin (CCK) receptor antagonist, MK-329, on gallbladder contraction and gastric emptying in humans. Implications for the physiology of CCK. J. Clin. Invest. **84:** 1220–1225.
22. CORAZZIARI, E., R. RICCI, D. BILIOTTI, I. BONTEMPO, N. PALLOTTA & A. TORSOLI. 1990. Oral administration of CCK antagonist loxiglumide inhibits postprandial gallbladder contraction without affecting gastric emptying. Dig. Dis. Sci. **35:** 50–54.
23. KATSCHINSKI, M., G. DAHMEN, M. REINSHAGEN, C. BEGLINGER, H. KOOP, R. NUSTEDE & G. ADLER. 1992. Cephalic stimulation of gastrointestinal secretory and motor responses in humans. Gastroenterology **103:** 383–391.
24. NIEDERAU, C., W. MECKLENBECK, T. HEINDGES & R. LÜTHEN. 1990. CCK hemmt die Magenentleerung einer regulären Mahlzeit unter physiologischen Bedingungen beim Menschen nicht. Z. Gastroenterol. **28:** 510.
25. KELLOW, J. E. & S. F. PHILLIPS. 1987. Altered small bowel motility in the irritable bowel syndrome is correlated with symptoms. Gastroenterology **92:** 1885–1893.
26. KELLOW, J. E., L. J. MILLAR & S. F. PHILLIPS. 1988. Dysmotility of the small intestine is provoked by stimuli in the irritable bowel syndrome. Gut **29:** 1236–1243.
27. HARVEY, R. F. & A. E. READ. 1973. Effect of cholecystokinin on colonic motility and symptoms in patients with the irritable bowel syndrome. Lancet **I:** 1–3.
28. JEHLE, E. C. & A. L. BLUM. 1990. The role of cholecystokinin in the regulation of basal colonic motility in the gastrocolonic response. Gastroenterology **98:** A361.
29. READ, N. W. 1991. The rational use of CCK antagonists in irritable bowel syndrome. *In* Cholecystokinin Antagonists in Gastroenterology. Basic and Clinical Status. G. Adler & C. Beglinger, eds.: 214–219. Springer. Berlin-Heidelberg-New York.

30. LOTTI, V. J., R. G. PENDLETON, R. J. GOULD, H. M. HANSON, R. S. L. CHANG & B. V. CLINESCHMIDT. 1987. In vivo pharmacology of L-364,718, a new potent nonpeptide peripheral cholecystokinin antagonist. J. Pharmacol. Exp. Ther. **241:** 103–109.
31. GREEN, T., R. DIMALINE, S. PEIKIN & G. J. DOCKRAY. 1988. Action of the cholecystokinin antagonist L364,718 on gastric emptying in the rat. Am. J. Physiol. **255:** G685–G689.
32. KONTUREK, S. J., J. TASLER, M. CIESZKOWSKI, K. SZEWCZY & M. HLADJI. 1988. Effect of cholecystokinin receptor antagonist on pancreatic responses to exogenous gastrin and cholecystokinin and to meal stimuli. Gastroenterology **94:** 1014–1023.

Effects of Dietary Fat on Postprandial Gastrointestinal Motility Are Inhibited by a Cholecystokinin Type A Receptor Antagonist

R. DE GIORGIO,[a] V. STANGHELLINI,[a,b]
M. RICCI MACCARINI,[a] A. M. MORSELLI-LABATE,[a]
G. BARBARA,[a] L. FRANZOSO,[a] L. C. ROVATI,[c]
R. CORINALDESI,[a] L. BARBARA,[a] AND V. L. W. GO[d]

[a]Institute of Internal Medicine & Gastroenterology
S. Orsola-Malpighi Hospital
University of Bologna
Bologna, Italy

[c]Department of Clinical Pharmacology
Rotta Research Laboratorium
Monza, Italy

[d]Brain Research Institute
UCLA School of Medicine
Los Angeles, California

Ingestion of a fat, overly rich meal delays gastric emptying and frequently results in the onset of dyspeptic symptoms in patients as well as in healthy subjects.[1] Ever since Farrel and Ivy[2] in 1926 observed that the introduction of fats into the duodenum inhibited the motility of a transplanted fundic pouch, it has generally been thought that endocrine mediators are responsible for this inhibitory effect. In the large number of studies that have since investigated the effects of a variety of humoral factors on gastrointestinal motility and in the comprehensive reviews that have been published,[3,4] such peptides as gastrin, cholecystokinin, somatostatin, secretin, endogenous opioids, neurotensin, and peptide YY have all been credited with delaying gastric emptying.[4-6] However, the various mechanisms by which transit is impaired still remain unclear.

Cholecystokinin (CCK) is a brain-gut peptide that can act as either a neurotransmitter/neuromodulator in enteric neurons or a hormone/paracrine substance, being released from endocrine cells of the intestinal mucosa.[7,8] Among nutrients, dietary fats are strong stimulants of CCK release in both experimental animals and humans.[9,10] The functions served by CCK are mediated by two different types of receptors: type A is mainly, but not exclusively, present in peripheral tissues (i.e., stomach, gut, pancreas, and gallbladder); type B is prominent in the central nervous system.[11]

Loxiglumide (D, L-4-(3,4 dichlorobenzoylamono)-5-(n-3-methoxy-propyl-penty-alamino)-5-oxo-pentanoic acid) (or CR-1505) is a new, potent, selective, and competi-

---

[b]Address for correspondence: Vincenzo Stanghellini, MD, Institute of Internal Medicine & Gastroenterology, S. Orsola-Malpighi Hospital, Via Massarenti, 9, 40138 - Bologna, Italy.

tive CCK-A receptor antagonist.[11-14] This CCK antagonist, therefore, has been used effectively to investigate the possible physiological role played by meal-stimulated CCK release on gastrointestinal functions.

In a study of healthy volunteers, loxiglumide dose-dependently inhibited pancreatic enzyme secretion stimulated by graded doses of CCK-8; it also inhibited the potentiating effect of CCK-8 on the bicarbonate response to secretin, as well as CCK-8-induced pancreatic polypeptide release.[15] Selectivity of action was demonstrated by the lack of activity on bombesin-stimulated pancreatic enzyme and bicarbonate secretion, by the secretin-induced increase in fluid and bicarbonate secretion, and by pentagastrin-stimulated gastric acid secretion.[15] Recently, Meyer et al.[16] showed that loxiglumide exerts a potent prokinetic effect on the gastrointestinal tract, accelerating colonic transit time and, particularly, gastric emptying of liquid meals in healthy volunteers. These observations were confirmed further by Fried et al.[17]

The present study was undertaken to test the hypothesis that loxiglumide can affect the response of gastrointestinal motility to fat during the postprandial period.

MATERIALS AND METHODS

Participants

Four healthy subjects (2 women, 2 men; age range 19–25 years) without gastrointestinal symptoms entered the study after giving their written informed consent.

Gastrointestinal Manometry

Continuous recording of gastrointestinal contractile activity was carried out by a low-compliance perfusion system (Arndorfer Medical Specialties, Inc., Greendale, Wisconsin), connected to a 9-channel polyvinyl chloride (PVC) (Dural Plastic, NSW, Australia; internal diameter [ID]: 0.96 mm; outer diameter [OD]: 0.5 cm). The side openings of the manometric probe were located under manometric control across the antroduodenal junction (5 and 1 cm apart) and in the proximal small bowel (3 and 10 cm apart). The ninth lumen was used to inflate a balloon located at the tip of the probe to allow more rapid positioning of the manometric tube. The balloon was then deflated during the test. Strain-gauge transducers (Sensormedics, 4-327-1, SM, Anaheim, California) were used to transform intraluminal pressure changes into electrical signals that were directly printed on a multichannel paper chart recording (Dynograph R 611, Beckman Instruments, Inc., Anaheim, California). Another PVC tube (ID: 0.59 mm; OD: 0.98 mm) was glued by tetrahydrofuran to the manometric tube, with the end opening 10 cm proximal to the upper recording site. This larger channel was used for intragastric infusion of fat emulsion. The maximal external diameter of the complete manometric assembly was approximately 6 mm. Motility was recorded for 3 hours during both fasting and postprandial periods.

Test Meal and Intragastric Infusions

Each subject ate a low-fat solid-liquid meal consisting of chicken breast (120 g), boiled rice (60 g), tomato juice (40 g), white bread (25 g), and a glass of water (200 ml) (total KCal = 513; protein 24%; carbohydrate 66%; fat 9%).

Fifteen minutes before ingestion of the meal, the tube was advanced 5–8 cm to correct changes in its position due to postcibal accommodation of the stomach. The meal was cooked in real-time to improve the palatability while keeping fat concentration as low as possible.

Two different emulsions were infused into the stomach during the studies: either bovine albumin 3 g + saline 0.9% 150 cc (control emulsion, CE) or albumin (3 g), saline (70 cc) + corn oil 80 g (fat infusion, FE).

Loxiglumide Administration

A 180-minute intravenous infusion of either saline (S), as placebo, or loxiglumide (Rotta Research Laboratorium, Monza, Italy) was started in each study day 20 minutes before beginning the meal ingestion. Loxiglumide was administered as bolus (5 mg/kg infused in 10 minutes) followed by infusion of 10 mg/kg per hour for 170 minutes.

Experimental Procedure

Every subject was studied on four separate occasions, each a week apart. After an overnight fast, the probe was introduced transnasally and positioned under manometric control. The probe reached the correct location in 40–90 minutes. During each test, healthy volunteers laid supine on a hospital bed, in a single quiet room, with the head end of the bed elevated 30 degrees from the horizontal. After 3 hours of interdigestive recording, subjects ate the test meal in 10–30 minutes. Twenty minutes before meal ingestion, each volunteer started an intravenous infusion of either S (placebo) or loxiglumide. Ten minutes after the beginning of meal ingestion, one of the two emulsions was infused intragastrically by a perfusion pump (Mini plus 2, Gilson, Villiers Le Bell, France) over a period of 20 minutes. Both intragastric emulsions and infusions were blindly administered according to a randomized scheme.

Analysis of Manometric Tracings

Manometric tracings were visually analyzed. We first identified the interdigestive migrating motor complex (IDMMC), but only the contractile response of both the distal antrum and descending duodenum to food ingestion was analyzed. The distal antrum was defined as the most distal recording site not exhibiting tonic increases of the baseline and registering a maximum contraction frequency of 3 per minute.[18] The number (N) and the sum of the amplitudes of waves (SAW) were computed at 10-minute intervals over 180 minutes of the postprandial period, and the result was expressed as mean ($\pm$ SD) motility index (MI) (MI = [N $\times$ SAW\10 min] $\times$ 10-3 at 180 min).

RESULTS

A summary of the results obtained in this study is shown in TABLE 1. Ingestion of the meal invariably converted fasting into fed motility. Antral motility was significantly decreased by the intragastric infusion of FE (MI = 20.3 ± 20.1; m ± SD) as compared to CE (MI = 39.9 ± 18.9; p <0.001; ANOVA). Intravenous infusion of loxiglumide did not modify the antral response to a low fat meal during intragastric infusion of CE (31.6 ± 20.8), but completely prevented the inhibitory effect exerted by FE (32.5 ± 13.4; p <0.001; ANOVA vs FE + S). Loxiglumide induced a marked decrease in the duodenal motor response to meal ingestion during intragastric infusion of both CE (32.4 ± 31.8) and FE (30.9 ± 47.9) (p <0.001 vs CE + S and FE + S; ANOVA).

DISCUSSION

The present study demonstrates that dietary fats induce inhibition of the antral response to meal ingestion mediated by CCK, probably through its type A receptor. It also shows that CCK markedly stimulates duodenal contractility induced by caloric meals regardless of their fat content.

In man as well as in many mammalian species, ingestion of a meal abruptly

TABLE 1. Effect of Loxiglumide on Antroduodenal Motility after Fat Infusion

	FE+L	CE+S	FE+S	CE+L
A MI	32.5 ± 13.4[a]	39.1 ± 18.9	20.3 ± 20.1	31.6 ± 20.8
D MI	30.9 ± 47.9[b]	131.2 ± 87.7	186.0 ± 85.0	32.4 ± 31.8[b]

ABBREVIATIONS: MI = motility index (number of waves × sum of amplitudes × 10−3 at 180 min); CE+S = control emulsion with saline; FE+S = fat emulsion with saline; CE+L = control emulsion with loxiglumide; FE+L = fat emulsion with loxiglumide; A MI = antral motility index: p <0.001 vs CE+S.
[a] p <0.001 vs FE+S. D MI = descending duodenum motility index.
[b] p <0.001 vs CE+S and FE+S.

interrupts the cyclic occurrence of the interdigestive migrating motor complex. At the same time, food present in the stomach triggers a more repetitive type of motility which, in the gastric antrum, is represented by frequent, intense contractions capable of breaking down digestible solids and, in the duodenum, by weaker contractions that are apparently uncoordinated and favor absorption and transport of the chyme. The hormonal and neural control mechanisms of this complex motor pattern and of the integrated secretory functions are still largely unknown. CCK is released by meal ingestion and is known to act as both a circulating hormone[19] and a putative neurotransmitter in intrinsic, enteric neurons.[7] Several other peptides, however, are potentially involved in the modulation of postprandial motility, and specific antagonists are crucial for understanding their actual physiological role. Loxiglumide is a new, potent, CCK-A receptor antagonist that makes it possible to evaluate the effects of the peptide on different gastrointestinal functions while avoiding the pitfalls of previous studies in which pharmacological doses of CCK were administered. We are not aware of any study targeted at investigating the effects of loxiglumide on antral contractility. On the other hand, several reports have indicated that loxiglumide markedly increases gastric emptying.[16,17] Studies in experimental animals showed that this CCK-A receptor antagonist, at doses that abolish the effects of endogenous

CCK, is capable of decreasing the intestinal motor response to feeding.[20] Our study used doses of loxiglumide that have previously been shown to abolish the effects exerted by caerulein-induced CCK plasma levels (similar to those detectable postprandially),[21] as well as to inhibit the changes in gallbladder contractions and tone evoked by meal ingestion.[22]

Little is known about the mechanisms by which CCK regulates gastrointestinal motility after feeding. This peptide may act either directly through specific receptors on smooth muscle cells or, alternatively, through the release of other substances (i.e., different transmitters or paracrine/endocrine molecules). The latter hypothesis is supported by an *in vitro* study indicating that CCK is not able to induce any inhibitory effects on isolated smooth muscle cells.[23] In addition, Soll *et al.*[24] reported that CCK is a potent releaser of somatostatin (from canine antral mucosa), a peptide whose inhibitory actions on the gastrointestinal tract are well known. It is therefore possible that CCK *in vivo* may act indirectly by releasing different humoral mediators; it has been shown that CCK antagonist loxiglumide reduces the postprandial rise of pancreatic polypeptide,[25] suggesting that this peptide also can mediate the effects of CCK on gastrointestinal tract.

In conclusion, the results of the present study indicate that dietary fats inhibit meal-stimulated antral motor activity through a CCK-A receptor mechanism.

REFERENCES

1. TALLEY, J. N. & S. F. PHILLIPS. 1988. Non-ulcer dyspepsia: Potential causes and pathophysiology. Ann. Int. Med. **108:** 865–879.
2. FARREL, J. I. & A. C. IVY. 1926. Studies on the motility of the transplanted gastric pouch. Am. J. Physiol. **76:** 227–228.
3. RUPPIN, H. & W. DOMSCHKE. 1980. Gastrointestinal hormones and motor function of the gastrointestinal tract. *In* Gastrointestinal Hormones. G. B. J. Glass, ed.:587–612. Raven Press. New York, NY.
4. WIENBECK, M. & J. ERCKENBRECHT. 1982. The control of gastrointestinal motility by GI hormones. Clin. Gastroenterol. **11:** 523–543.
5. BLACKBURN, A. M., S. R. BLOOM, R. G. LONG, N. CHRISTOFIDES, M. FITZPATRICK & J. BARON. 1980. Effect of neurotensin on gastric function in man. Lancet **I:** 987–989.
6. HILL, F. L. C., T. ZHANG, G. GOMEZ & G. H. GREELEY. 1991. Peptide YY, a new gut hormone (a mini-review). Steroids **56:** 77–82.
7. SCHMID, R., V. SCHUSDZIARRA, H. BUTSCHER & M. CLASSEN. 1990. Composition of amino acids infusions and effect of cholecystokinin on insulin release in dogs. Clin. Physiol. Biochem. **8:** 244–249.
8. NIEDERAU, C., T. HEINDGES, L. ROVATI & G. STROHMEYER. 1989. Effects of loxiglumide on gallbladder emptying in healthy volunteers. Gastroenterology **97:** 1331–1336.
9. GREEN, G. M., S. TAGUCHI, J. FRIESTMAN, W. Y. CHEY & R. A. LIDDLE. 1989. Plasma secretin, CCK, and pancreatic secretion in response to dietary fat in the rat. Am. J. Physiol. **256:** G1016–G1021.
10. LIDDLE, R. A., I. D. GOLDFINE, M. S. ROSEN, R. A. TAPLITZ & J. A. WILLIAMS. 1985. Cholecystokinin bioactivity in human plasma: Molecular forms, responses to feeding, and relationship to gallbladder contraction. J. Clin. Invest. **75:** 1144–1152.
11. WOODRUF, G. N. & J. HUGHES. 1991. Cholecystokinin antagonists. Ann. Rev. Pharmacol. Toxicol. **31:** 469–501.
12. SETNIKAR, I., M. BANI, R. CEREDA, R. CHISTE', F. MAKOVEC, M. A. PACINI, L. REVEL, L. C. ROVATI & L. A. ROVATI. 1987. Pharmacological characterization of a new potent and specific nonpolypeptidic cholecystokinin antagonist. Arzneim. Forsch. Drug Res. **37:** 703–707.
13. SETNIKAR, I., M. BANI, R. CEREDA, R. CHISTE', F. MAKOVEC, M. A. PACINI & L. REVEL. 1987. Anticholecystokinin activities of loxiglumide. Arzneim. Forsch. Drug Res. **37:** 1168–1171.

14. SETNIKAR, I., M. BANI, R. CEREDA, R. CHISTE', F. MAKOVEC, M. A. PACINI & L. REVEL. 1987. Loxiglumide protects against experimental pancreatitis. Arzneim. Forsch. Drug Res. **37**: 1172–1174.
15. BEGLINGER, C., M. FRIED, I. WHITEHOUSE, J. B. JANSEN, C. B. H. W. LAMERS & K. GYR. 1985. Pancreatic enzyme response to a liquid meal and to hormonal stimulation. Correlation with plasma secretin and cholecystokinin levels. J. Clin. Invest. **75**: 1471–1475.
16. MEYER, B. M., B. A. WERTH, C. BEGLINGER, P. HILDEBRAND, J. B. M. J. JANSEN, D. ZACH, L. C. ROVATI & G. A. STADLER. 1989. Role of cholecystokinin in regulation of gastrointestinal motor function. Lancet **II**: 12–15.
17. FRIED, M., U. ERLACHER, W. SCHWIZER, C. LOCHNER, J. KOERFER, C. BEGLINGER, J. B. JANSEN, F. HARDER, A. BISCHOF-DELALOYE, G. A. STALDER & L. C. ROVATI. 1991. Role of CCK in the regulation of gastric emptying and pancreatic enzyme secretion in man. Studies with the CCK receptor antagonist loxiglumide. Gastroenterology **101**: 503–511.
18. CAMILLERI, M., J. R. MALAGELADA, V. STANGHELLINI, A. R. ZINSMEISTER, P. C. KAO & C. H. LI. 1986. Dose-related effect of synthetic human b-endorphin and naloxone on fed gastrointestinal motility. Am. J. Physiol. **251**: G147–G154.
19. DI MAGNO, E. P., J. C. HENDRICKS, V. L. W. GO & R. R. DOZOIS. 1979. Relationship among canine fasting pancreatic and biliary secretions, pancreatic duct pressure and duodenal phase III motor activity-Boldyreff revisted. Dig. Dis. Sci. **24**: 689–693.
20. NIEDERAU, C. & M. KARAUS. 1991. Effects of CCK receptor blockade on intestinal motor activity in conscious dogs. Am. J. Physiol. **260**: G315–G324.
21. SCHMIDT, W. E., W. CREUTZFELDT, A. SCHLESER, A. R. CHOUDHURY, R. NUSTEDE, M. HOCKNER, R. NITSCHE, H. SOSTMANN, L. C. ROVATI & U. R. FOLSCH. 1991. Role of CCK in regulation of pancreaticobiliary functions and GI motility in humans: Effects of loxiglumide. Am. J. Physiol. **260**: G197–206.
22. KONTUREK, S. J., N. KWIECIEN, B. OBTULOWICZ, B. KOPP, J. OLESKY & L. ROVATI. 1990. Cholecystokinin in the inhibition of gastric secretion and gastric emptying in humans. Digestion **45**: 1–8.
23. SOLL, A., D. AMIRIAN, L. P. THOMAS, T. J. REEDY & J. D. ELASHOFF. 1984. Gastrin receptors on isolated canine parietal cells. J. Clin Invest. **73**: 1434–1447.
24. SOLL, A., D. AMIRIAN, J. PARK, J. D. ELASHOFF & T. YAMADA. 1985. Cholecystokinin potently releases somatostatin from canine fundic mucosal cells in short-term culture. Am. J. Physiol. **248**: G569–G573.
25. THOR, P., J. LASKIEWICZ, P. KONTUREK & S. J. KONTUREK. 1988. Cholecystokinin in the regulation of intestinal motility and pancreatic secretion in dogs. Am. J. Physiol. **255**: G498–G504.

Cholecystokinin and Satiety: A Time Line

GREGORY N. ERVIN

Glaxo Inc. Research Institute
Five Moore Drive
P.O. Box 13358
Research Triangle Park, North Carolina 27709

"The feeling of satiation is little understood, but it is important and deserves further attention."

Walter B. Cannon, *The Wisdom of the Body*, 1932

Satiety may still be little understood, but because of the recent study of cholecystokinin (CCK), it is better understood today than it was in 1932. For reasons that are obvious in TABLE 1, space limitations do not permit a review of the most important literature on CCK, feeding, and satiety. Instead of reviewing a few salient papers (and ignoring their controversy), I will review the literature in a different way, by presenting estimates of total citation counts for these various topics over time.

Citation counts were summoned from two databases, Scisearch and Medline. The Medline database for human and animal studies takes us back to 1966 and Scisearch to 1974. Over that period, the citation count for Feeding (or Eating) was enormous (TABLE 1). (Duplicate counts for all topics in TABLE 1 were deleted except for the Feeding topic, because of its size. Based on other topics, total Feeding citations are probably overestimated by about 25%.) The total number of citations for CCK was also large, but only a fraction of these dealt specifically with both CCK and either feeding or satiety.

Total citation counts for CCK and Feeding, Satiety, and CCK and Satiety are presented as time lines: 1966–1969, 1970–1979, 1980–1989, and 1990–1993 (FIGS. 1, 2, and 3, respectively). Citations for all three of these topics was very low in the first epoch (1966–1969). This is not surprising. Studies in the CCK and Feeding area include investigations on some effect of CCK in either the fasted or the fed state. The first attempt specifically to relate CCK and satiety came in 1971 when Glick *et al.*[1] reported that intraperitoneal or intraaortic administration of 12–30 Crick, Harper, and Raper units had no significant effect on the feeding of fasted or fed rats. (Their doses were very low and, in retrospect, undoubtedly subthreshold for marked anorexia.) In 1973 Gibbs *et al.*[2,3] of the Bourne Lab (Cornell University Medical Center/The New York Hospital, White Plains, NY) reported that CCK (either synthetic or partially purified) reduced the food intake (liquid or solid), but not water intake, of intact rats[2] or the liquid diet intake of sham-feeding rats, in which food was diverted with a gastric fistula before entering the intestine.[3] This definitely got research on CCK and feeding and CCK and satiety rolling, but the publication output did not show prolific growth till the 1980s (FIGS. 1 and 3). The Bourne Lab has endured in its study of CCK-induced anorexia, and a summary report will be given by Gerry Smith (this volume).

The novel finding of CCK-induced anorexia attracted attempts at both replication and alternate explanations. For example, it was reported in a letter[4] (not a refereed manuscript) to *Nature* that CCK-8 could induce mild to moderate taste aversion conditioning in rats; these investigators suggested that CCK-8-induced anorexia might reflect "some form of sickness" rather than satiation. Of course, the relation between anorexia and the induction of taste aversions is neither straightforward nor well understood (see ref. 5). Just because CCK induces effects in addition

TABLE 1. Estimated Total Citation Counts for Human and Animal Studies from 1966 to the Present

Topic	Counts
Cholecystokinin (CCK)	13,918
Feeding or eating	119,334[a]
CCK and feeding	1,987
Satiety	1,664
CCK and satiety	536

[a]For all topics except Feeding, the computer was able to delete duplicate citations. Citation counts before deletions were overestimates of about 25%. Citation counts for Feeding are probably an overestimate of about 25%.

to anorexia, such as altered duodenal activity,[6] "defensive burying",[7] or even enhanced memory retention,[8] does not mean that such effects account for the anorexia. Are we throwing the baby out with the bathwater?

Also in the mid-1970s, CCK was shown to be present in the CNS.[9] One of the contributors to this volume, Rafael Schick, has been a pioneer in the study of central CCK and satiety.

In the early 1980s evidence also emerged that vagal innervation of the gut was critical for the peripheral CCK anorectic effect. This topic is discussed by both Gerry Smith and Bob Ritter (this volume). Both Smith and Ritter will also discuss their results pertaining to the possible paracrine or neurotransmitter roles of CCK in inducing anorexia.

In the early 1980s the work of Kissileff et al.,[10] Pi-Sunyer et al.,[11] and Stacher et al.[12] demonstrated that in humans infusions of CCK-8 could decrease test meal size without reported side effects. This pattern of results has continued,[13,14] and Lamers

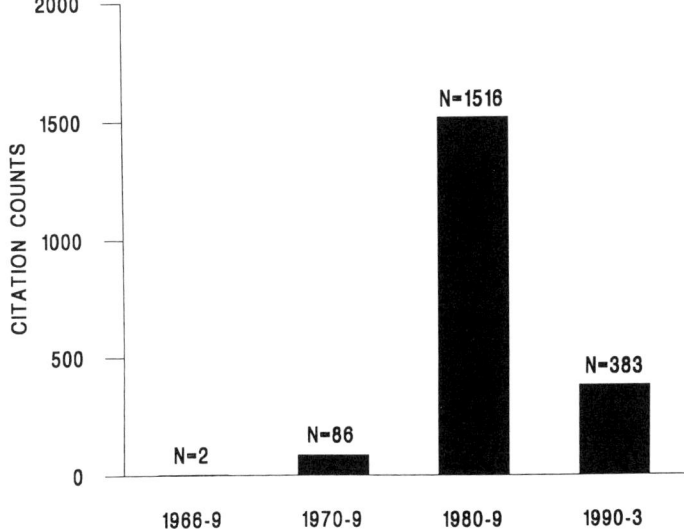

FIGURE 1. Citation counts for cholecystokinin and feeding (or eating) from 1966 to the present.

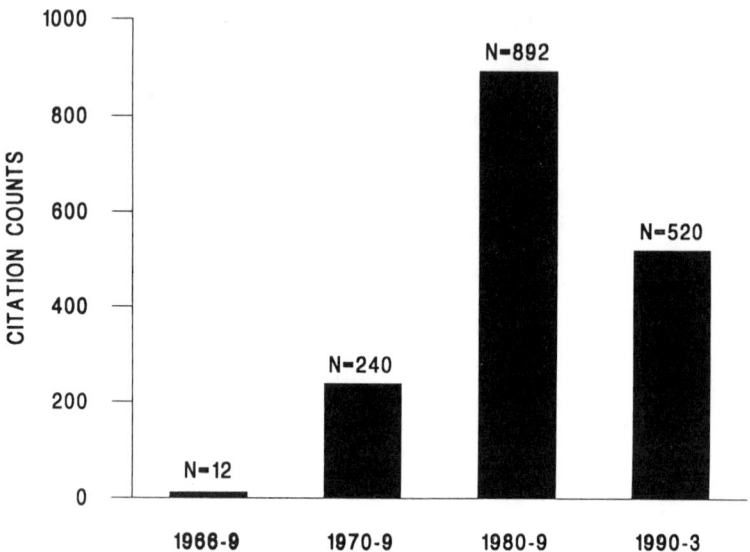

FIGURE 2. Citation counts for satiety from 1966 to the present.

(this volume) will present his data on the satiety and anorectic effects of CCK-33 in humans.

The study of satiety has grown enormously since 1980 (FIG. 2), and studies of CCK and satiety (FIG. 3) have in parallel made a relatively large contribution.

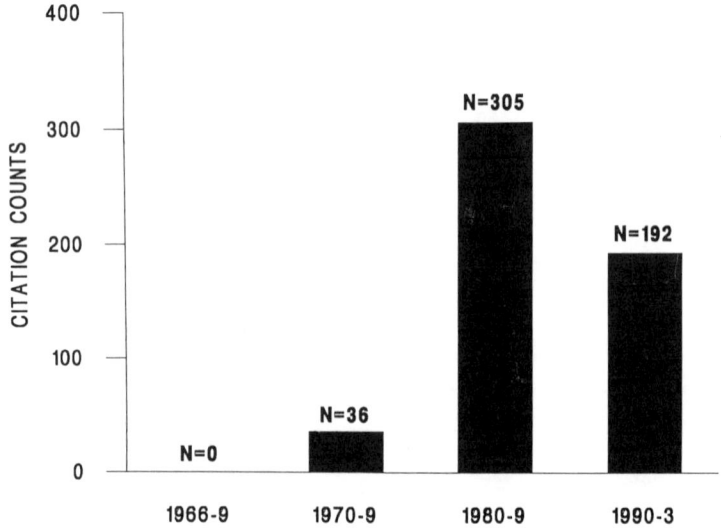

FIGURE 3. Citation counts for cholecystokinin and satiety from 1966 to the present.

ACKNOWLEDGMENTS

The author wishes to thank his colleagues, Barbara B. Bertram and Larry S. Birkemo, for their help, respectively, in collecting citation counts and in expressing them graphically.

REFERENCES

1. GLICK, Z., D. W. THOMAS & J. MAYER. 1971. Absence of effect of injections of the intestinal hormones secretin and cholecystokinin-pancreozymin upon feeding behavior. Physiol. Behav. **6:** 5–8.
2. GIBBS, J., R. C. YOUNG & G. P. SMITH. 1973. Cholecystokinin decreases food intake in rats. J. Comp. Physiol. Psychol. **44:** 488–495.
3. GIBBS, J., R. C. YOUNG & G. P. SMITH. 1973. Cholecystokinin elicits satiety in rats with open gastric fistulas. Nature **245:** 323–325.
4. DEUTSCH, J. A. & W. T. HARDY. 1977. Cholecystokinin produces bait shyness in rats. Nature **266:** 196.
5. ERVIN, G. N. & M. N. TEETER. 1986. Cholecystokinin octapeptide and lithium produce different effects on feeding and taste aversion learning. Physiol. Behav. **36:** 507–512.
6. DEUTSCH, J. A., T. R. THIEL & L. H. GREENBERG. 1978. Duodenal motility after cholecystokinin injection or satiety. Behav. Biol. **24:** 393–399.
7. BOWERS, R. L., C. D. HERZOG, E. H. STONE & T. J. DIONNE. 1992. Defensive burying following injections of cholecystokinin, bombesin, and LiCl in rats. Physiol. Behav. **51:** 969–072.
8. FLOOD, J. & J. E. MORLEY. 1989. Cholecystokinin receptors mediate enhanced memory retention produced by feeding or gastrointestinal peptides. Peptides **10:** 809–813.
9. VANDERHAEGHEN, J. J., F. LOTSTRA, J. DEMEY & C. GILLES. 1980. Immunohistochemical localization of cholecystokinin- and gastrin-like peptides in the brain and hypophysis of the rat. Proc. Natl. Acad. Sci. USA **77:** 1190–1198.
10. KISSILEFF, H. R., F. X. PI-SUNYER, J. THORNTON & G. P. SMITH. 1981. C-terminal octapeptide of cholecystokinin decreases food intake in man. Am J. Clin. Nutr. **34:** 154–160.
11. PI-SUNYER, F. X., H. R. KISSILEFF, J. THORNTON & G. P. SMITH. 1982. C-terminal octapeptide of cholecystokinin decreases food intake. Physiol. Behav. **29:** 627–630.
12. STACHER, G., H. STEINRINGER, G. SCHMIERER, C. SCHNEIDER & S. WINKLEHNER. 1982. Cholecystokinin octapeptide decreases intake of solid food in man. Peptides **1:** 133–136.
13. GEARY, N., H. R. KISSILEFF, F. X. PI-SUNYER & V. HINTON. 1992. Individual, but not simultaneous, glucagon and cholecystokinin infusions inhibit feeding in men. Am. J. Physiol. **262:** R975–R980.
14. LIEVERSE, R., J. JANSEN, A. MASCLEE & C. LAMERS. 1993. Satiety effects of a physiological dose of cholecystokinin in man. Gastroenterology **104:** A632.

Satiating Effect of Cholecystokinin[a]

G. P. SMITH AND J. GIBBS

Department of Psychiatry
Cornell University Medical College
and
E. W. Bourne Behavioral Research Laboratory
The New York Hospital–Cornell Medical Center
White Plains, New York 10605

In 1937, MacLagan[1] reported that a duodenal extract obtained from Lim inhibited food intake in rabbits. The inhibitory effect was achieved after subcutaneous or intravenous administration and lasted 1 hour. This extract was obtained after the duodenum had been exposed to olive oil. Kosaka and Lim[2] had named the active principle in the extract enterogastrone, because it inhibited gastric acid secretion. Because Kosaka and Lim[2] found that another extract (gift of A. C. Ivy) that had cholecystokinetic activity also inhibited gastric acid secretion under their conditions, it is probable that they thought their preparation of enterogastrone also had cholecystokinetic activity. (See Gregory[3] for discussion of the history of enterogastrone preparations.) MacLagan's observation was not followed up until 1960 when Ugolev[4] reported that extracts of rat duodenum decreased food intake in mildly deprived rats. This effect was limited to the first 30 minutes after intraperitoneal administration. Ugolev's extract was specific in the sense that similarly prepared extracts of stomach and spleen did not inhibit intake.

It was the purification of cholecystokinin (CCK) from duodenal and upper jejunal porcine extracts by Jorpes et al.[5] and the synthesis of the carboxy-terminal octapeptide of CCK (CCK-8) by Ondetti et al.,[6] however, that made the modern attack on the problem of the satiating effect of CCK possible. This began with the 1973 paper of Gibbs et al.[7] which showed that intraperitoneal administration of an impure extract of cholecystokinin, synthetic CCK-8, or ceruletide (an amphibian peptide of similar structure and with potent cholecystokinetic activity) produced inhibition of food intake in rats. The effect was dose-related and lasted 15–30 minutes. The effect was behaviorally specific because doses that inhibited food intake in food-deprived rats did not inhibit water intake in water-deprived rats. Furthermore, there were no signs of toxicity.

Because the inhibitory effect was apparently specific and did not occur in the initial phase of the test meals, we interpreted the inhibition of food intake as a satiating effect of CCK and hypothesized that endogenous CCK released by ingested nutrients entering the duodenum and upper jejunum during a meal participated in the satiating process that terminated eating. In this review, we describe the current status of the hypothesis and indicate the important problems associated with it that require further investigation.

TYPE OF RECEPTOR MEDIATION

The initial structure-activity relationships of CCK-8 and related agonists indicated that sulfated CCK-8 was at least 100-fold more potent for inhibiting food

[a] This work was supported by research grants DK33248, MH40010, and MH00149 from the National Institutes of Health.

intake than was desulfated CCK-8, gastrin I, or gastrin II.[7,8] This profile of agonist potency was consistent with an action mediated by CCK_A receptors. This interpretation was confirmed when specific antagonists became available, because antagonists of CCK_A receptors blocked the satiating effect of peripherally administered CCK-8, but a CCK_B antagonist did not.[9-11] Recent evidence has shown that the CCK_A receptors are of the low-affinity type.[12]

USE OF ANTAGONISTS TO TEST THE HYPOTHESIS

Because CCK_A antagonists, such as devazepide and loxiglumide, were potent and specific antagonists of the satiating effect of exogenous CCK-8, they could be used to test the hypothesized satiating effect of endogenous CCK released from the small intestine by ingested nutrients. The hypothesis predicted that administration of a CCK_A antagonist before a meal would increase the size of the meal because it would eliminate the usual satiating effect of endogenous CCK. This prediction has been fulfilled in more than 20 experiments under a variety of conditions in rats, mice, pigs, and monkeys.

The strongest evidence for the satiating effect of endogenous CCK from the small intestine comes from experiments in which the inhibitory effect on meal size of specific stimuli for the release of CCK from the small intestine was blocked by prior administration of a CCK_A antagonist. These stimuli include sodium oleate,[13,14] Intralipid,[14] and soybean trypsin inhibitor.[15,16]

On the basis of the reliable and reproducible effect of CCK_A antagonists to increase meal size, we conclude that the hypothesis is proven. This is a significant advance in understanding the control of meal size, because CCK is the first physiological satiating signal to be identified. Other putative control mechanisms, such as peripheral peptides like pancreatic glucagon, insulin, or bombesin-like peptides, central peptides like corticotropin-releasing factor or oxytocin, or vagally mediated gastric distention lack a similar body of supporting evidence.

Although CCK is the first physiological control of satiation that has been identified, it is clearly not the only satiating mechanism. This follows from the fact that pretreatment with CCK_A antagonists does not always increase meal size[17] and from the observation that CCK_A antagonists do not prevent the termination of eating, they simply delay it.

Even though we consider the hypothesis to be proven in rodents, its role in the control of eating in humans is not clear yet (see Lamers, this volume). Furthermore, many important problems remain to be solved before this behavioral function of CCK can be considered to be understood in a scientific sense. These are the site of the necessary CCK_A receptors, the mode of action, the site and mechanisms of central processing of the vagal afferent signal produced by peripheral CCK, and synergistic interactions with pancreatic glucagon, insulin, and estrogen.

SITE OF CCK_A RECEPTORS

The necessary CCK_A receptors are in the abdomen, because abdominal vagotomy abolished the satiating effect of low doses of CCK-8 (less than 8 µg/kg intraperitoneally) and markedly reduced the effect of larger doses.[18] The critical lesion was of the afferent fibers,[19] some of which are capsaicin-sensitive (see Raybould, this volume).

There is autoradiographic evidence of CCK_A receptors in the circular muscles of the pyloric sphincter[20] and in all the afferent, abdominal vagal branches.[21] Pylorectomy decreases the satiating potency of doses of CCK-8 larger than 2 μg/kg intraperitoneally, but not of lower doses.[22] This has been interpreted as evidence that part of the satiating effect of doses of CCK-8 larger than 2 μg/kg is mediated by CCK-8 binding to CCK_A receptors on smooth muscle cells in the circular muscle of the sphincter. The contractile effect produced by CCK-8 would then be detected by the mechanoreceptors of vagal afferent fibers, and the resultant afferent activity would be relayed to the nucleus tractus solitarius. Before this interpretation can be accepted, however, the possibility that the effect of pylorectomy depends on removal of CCK_A receptors on vagal afferent fibers in the pylorus must be experimentally excluded.

Whatever the eventual interpretation of the effect of pylorectomy, it is clear that low doses of CCK-8 decrease meal size significantly in the pylorectomized rat. Because total abdominal vagotomy abolishes the inhibitory effect of those doses of CCK-8, it is reasonable to conclude that CCK_A receptors on abdominal vagal afferent fibers mediate the decrease of meal size in the pylorectomized rat. Direct evidence for this conclusion, however, is not available yet.

MODE OF ACTION

In our 1973 paper, we proposed that the satiating effect of CCK was a hormonal function of the peptide similar to its classical action on the gallbladder and pancreas. This appears to be wrong, at least in the rat, because when CCK-8 was infused into the portal vein, its satiating potency was 4–8-fold less than that of intraperitoneally administered CCK-8.[23] It was possible that intraperitoneal CCK-8 was more potent because it was absorbed into the systemic circulation. This possibility was rejected, however, when we recently demonstrated that injections of CCK-8 (2–8 μg/kg) into the inferior vena cava had no significant effect on food intake.[24]

These results and those from R. Ritter's laboratory (see Ritter, this volume) are strong evidence that the mode of CCK-8's satiating effect is local (neurocrine or paracrine) rather than hormonal. The mode of action of CCK-8 in other animals and in humans remains to be determined, but available evidence from subhuman primates[25–27] and human studies is consistent with a hormonal mode of action (see Lamers, this volume).

SITE AND MECHANISMS OF CENTRAL PROCESSING

Knowledge of the sites and mechanisms of central processing of vagal afferent information produced by peripheral CCK-8 beyond the vagal afferent terminal projections in the nucleus tractus solitarius is fragmentary. Lesions of the hypothalamus, particularly those involving the paraventricular nuclei,[28] have been reported to block the satiating effect of peripherally administered CCK-8, but larger lesions involving the paraventricular and ventromedial nuclei had no effect.[18] Administration of a CCK_A antagonist into the paraventricular nucleus decreased the satiating effect of peripheral CCK-8,[29] suggesting that CCK released from central neurons could participate in the processing of the information produced by peripheral CCK-8.

Note that the possible role of centrally released CCK in the processing of satiating information produced by peripheral CCK-8 is different from the problem of the analysis of the direct inhibitory effect on food intake produced by central administration of CCK-8 in various brain sites (see Schick, this volume). Although the pharmacology of the inhibitory effect of central CCK-8 demonstrates that this effect is mediated by CCK_A receptors, the behavioral specificity and physiological relevance of these central effects remain to be demonstrated.

Although processing of the information provided by CCK-8 is likely to occur at hypothalamic and other forebrain sites, forebrain processing is not necessary for the satiating effect of CCK-8 on the ingestion of 0.1 M sucrose, because peripherally administered CCK-8 decreased the intake of 0.1 M sucrose in chronic decerebrate rats.[30] Thus, the caudal brainstem has sufficient neural complexity to process the peripheral stimulus produced by CCK-8 into a central command to stop eating.

Recent work suggests that central serotonergic (5-HT) mechanisms are involved in central processing. Poeschla *et al.*[31] reported that systemic administration of 8-hydroxy-2-(di-n-propylamino) tetralin (8-OH-DPAT) significantly attenuated the satiating action of CCK-8. This result complements those from experiments showing that systemic administration of 5-HT antagonists, particularly those that act at $5-HT_{2C}$ receptors,[32,33] also decreases the satiating effect of CCK-8. Further work with central injections of 8-OH-DPAT and of specific antagonists is necessary to clarify the proposed role of central 5-HT in processing the peripheral CCK-8 signal.

The only other specific interactive central mechanism that has been identified is insulin. Intraventricular administration of a low dose of insulin increases the satiating potency of peripherally administered CCK-8 in the baboon.[34] This result is interesting because it suggests that insulin, a central long-term stimulus for the inhibition of food intake and body weight, affects food intake by enhancing the potency of CCK-8, a short-term mechanism for the control of meal size.

Although current information about the sites and mechanisms of central processing is fragmentary and preliminary, the problem seems accessible to analysis with currently available techniques and deserves more attention than it has received.

INTERACTIONS WITH GLUCAGON AND ESTROGEN

Most of the literature concerned with the satiating effect of peripheral CCK-8 has been interpreted as if CCK-8 acted alone. This has been a useful simplification, but recent work suggests that synergistic interactions between CCK-8 and other peptides or steroids known to inhibit food intake will begin to put CCK into its physiological context.

For example, although pancreatic glucagon produces a potent, specific, and dose-related inhibition of food intake, glucagon has no significant inhibitory effect on intake when the postingestive effects of food are eliminated by sham feeding. But when as little as 150 ng/kg of CCK-8 is administered with glucagon to sham-feeding rats, intake is markedly inhibited.[35]

The inhibition of food intake by estrogen is well known, but poorly understood. The possibility that this effect involves a synergistic interaction with peripheral CCK-8 has been investigated recently. Ovariectomy decreased the satiating potency of CCK-8 and estrogen replacement increased the satiating potency.[36] Further work is required to determine if the site of this effect of estrogen is central or peripheral.

The decreased satiating potency of CCK-8 in ovariectomized rats suggests that women with abnormally low concentrations of estrogen may have a tendency to eat larger meals than normal because the satiating potency of CCK-8 has been reduced. Given our ignorance of the pathophysiology of clinical hyperphagia, such speculation may be heuristic.

CONCLUSION

Twenty years after the hypothesis was proposed, the satiating effect of endogenous CCK released from the small intestine during a meal is proven in rodents. Its status in other animals and humans is still uncertain. The knowledge that CCK-8 acts initially on CCK_A receptors in the abdomen and that this action is mediated by vagal afferent fibers to the nucleus tractus solitarius can now be used to investigate the major problems associated with the satiating effect of CCK. These include the site of the necessary peripheral CCK_A receptors, the mode of action, the sites and mechanisms of central processing, and synergistic interactions with other controls of intake such as pancreatic glucagon and estrogen.

ACKNOWLEDGMENT

We thank Jane Magnetti for processing the manuscript.

REFERENCES

1. MacLagan, N. F. 1937. The role of appetite in the control of body weight. J. Physiol. **90:** 385–394.
2. Kosaka, T. & R. K. S. Lim. 1930. Demonstration of the humoral agent in fat inhibition of gastric secretion. Proc. Soc. Exp. Biol. & Med. **27:** 890–891.
3. Gregory, R. A. 1962. Secretory Mechanisms of the Gastro-Intestinal Tract. Edward Arnold Ltd. London.
4. Ugolev, A. M. 1960. The influence of duodenal extracts on general appetite. Doklady Akademii Nauk SSSR **133:** 1251–1254.
5. Jorpes, J. E., V. Mutt & K. Toczko. 1964. Further purification of cholecystokinin and pancreozymin. Acta Chem. Scand. **18:** 2408–2410.
6. Ondetti, M. A., J. Pluscec, E. F. Sabo, J. T. Sheehan & N. Williams. 1970. Synthesis of cholecystokinin-pancreozymin. I. The C-terminal dodecapeptide. J. Am. Chem. Soc. **92:** 195–216.
7. Gibbs, J., R. C. Young & G. P. Smith. 1973. Cholecystokinin decreases food intake in rats. J. Comp. Physiol. Psychol. **84:** 488–495.
8. Lorenz, D. N., G. Kreielsheimer & G. P. Smith. 1979. Effect of cholecystokinin, gastrin, secretin and GIP on sham feeding in the rat. Physiol. Behav. **23:** 1065–1072.
9. Dourish, C. T., A. C. Ruckert, F. D. Tattersall & S. D. Iversen. 1989. Evidence that decreased feeding induced by systemic injection of cholecystokinin is mediated by CCK-A receptors. Eur. J. Pharmacol. **173:** 233–234.
10. Moran, T. H., P. J. Ameglio, G. J. Schwartz & P. R. McHugh. 1991. Blockade of type A, not type B, CCK receptors attenuates satiety actions of exogenous and endogenous CCK. Am. J. Physiol. **262:** R46–R50.
11. Smith, G. P., A. Tyrka & J. Gibbs. 1991. Type-A CCK receptors mediate the inhibition of food intake and activity by CCK-8 in 9- to 12-day old rat pups. Pharmacol. Biochem. Behav. **38:** 207–210.
12. Weatherford, S. C., W. B. Laughton, J. Salabarria, W. Danho, J. W. Tilley, L. A. Netterville, G. J. Schwartz & T. H. Moran. 1993. CCK satiety is differentially mediated by high- and low-affinity CCK receptors in the mice and rats. Am. J. Physiol. **264:** R244–R249.
13. Yox, D. P., L. Brenner & R. C. Ritter. 1992. CCK-receptor antagonists attenuate suppression of sham feeding by intestinal nutrients. Am. J. Physiol. **262:** R554–R561.
14. Greenberg, D., N. I. Torres, G. P. Smith & J. Gibbs. 1989. The satiating effects of fats is attenuated by the cholecystokinin antagonist lorglumide. Ann. N. Y. Acad. Sci. **575:** 517–520.

15. WELLER, A., G. P. SMITH & J. GIBBS. 1990. Endogenous cholecystokinin reduces feeding in young rats. Science **247:** 1589–1591.
16. GARLICKI, J., P. K. KONTUREK, J. MAJKA, N. KWIECIEN & S. J. KONTUREK. 1990. Cholecystokinin receptors and vagal nerves in control of food intake in rats. Am. J. Physiol. **258:** E40–E45.
17. SCHNEIDER, L. H., R. B. MURPHY, J. GIBBS & G. P. SMITH. 1988. Comparative potencies of CCK antagonists for the reversal of the satiating effect of cholecystokinin. *In* Cholecystokinin Antagonists. R. Y. Wang & R. Schoenfeld, eds.: 263–284. Alan R. Liss, Inc. New York, NY.
18. SMITH, G. P., C. JEROME, B. J. CUSHIN, R. ETERNO & K. J. SIMANSKY. 1981. Abdominal vagotomy blocks the satiety effect of cholecystokinin in the rat. Science **213:** 1036–1037.
19. SMITH, G. P., C. JEROME & R. NORGREN. 1985. Afferent axons in abdominal vagus mediate satiety effect of cholecystokinin in rats. Am. J. Physiol. **249:** R638–R641.
20. SMITH, G. T., T. H. MORAN, J. T. COYLE, M. KUHAR, T. L. O'DONOHUE & P. R. MCHUGH. 1984. Anatomical localization of cholecystokinin receptors to the pyloric sphincter. Am. J. Physiol. **246:** R127–R130.
21. MORAN, T. H., G. P. SMITH & A. M. HOSTETLER. 1987. Transport of cholecystokinin (CCK) binding sites in subdiaphragmatic vagal branches. Brain Res. **415:** 149–152.
22. MORAN, T. H., L. SHNAYDER, A. M. HOSTETLER & P. R. MCHUGH. 1988. Pylorectomy reduces the satiety action of cholecystokinin. Am. J. Physiol. **255:** R1059–R1063.
23. GREENBERG, D., G. P. SMITH & J. GIBBS. 1987. Infusion of CCK-8 into the hepatic-portal vein fails to reduce food intake in rats. Am. J. Physiol. **252:** 1015–1018.
24. MELVILLE, L. D., D. GREENBERG, G. P. SMITH, J. GIBBS & M. J. RUSS. 1993. Intraperitoneally administered CCK-8 acts locally, not hormonally, to inhibit food intake. Soc. Neurosci. Abstr. **19:** 816.
25. STEIN, L., S. C. WOODS, D. P. FIGLEWICZ & D. PORTE, JR. 1986. The effect of fasting interval on CCK-8 suppression of food intake in the baboon. Am. J. Physiol. **250:** R851–R855.
26. GIBBS, J., J. D. FALASCO & P. R. MCHUGH. 1976. Cholecystokinin-decreased food intake in rhesus monkeys. Am. J. Physiol. **230:** 15–18.
27. MORAN, T. H. & P. R. MCHUGH. 1982. Cholecystokinin suppresses food intake by inhibiting gastric emptying. Am. J. Physiol. **242:** R491–R497.
28. CRAWLEY, J. N. & J. Z. KISS. 1985. Paraventricular nucleus lesions abolish the inhibition of feeding induced by systemic cholecystokinin. Peptides **6:** 927–935.
29. SCHWARTZ, D. H., D. B. DORFMAN, L. HERNANDEZ & B. G. HOEBEL. 1988. Cholecystokinin. 1. CCK antagonists in the PVN induce feeding 2. Effects of CCK in the nucleus accumbens on extracellular dopamine turnover. *In* Cholecystokinin Antagonists. R. Y. Wang & R. Schoenfeld, eds.: 285–305. Alan R. Liss, Inc. New York, NY.
30. GRILL, H. J. & G. P. SMITH. 1988. Cholecystokinin decreases sucrose intake in chronic decerebrate rats. Am. J. Physiol. **254:** R853–R856.
31. POESCHLA, B., J. GIBBS, K. J. SIMANSKY & G. P. SMITH. 1992. The 5-HT$_{1A}$ agonist 8-OH-DPAT attenuates the satiating action of cholecystokinin. Pharmacol. Biochem. Behav. **42:** 541–543.
32. POESCHLA, B. D., J. GIBBS, K. J. SIMANSKY, D. GREENBERG & G. P. SMITH. 1992. Cholecystokinin-induced satiety depends upon activation of 5-HT$_{1C}$ receptors. Am. J. Physiol. **264:** R62–R64.
33. STALLONE, D., S. NICOLAÏDIS & J. GIBBS. 1989. Cholecystokinin-induced anorexia depends on serotoninergic function. Am. J. Physiol. **256:** R1138–R1141.
34. FIGLEWICZ, D. P., D. B. WEST, L. J. STERN, S. C. WOODS & D. PORTE, JR. 1986. Insulin alters the sensitivity of baboons to CCK-induced single meal suppression. Am. J. Physiol. **250:** R856–R860.
35. LE SAUTER, J. & N. GEARY. 1987. Pancreatic glucagon and cholecystokinin synergistically inhibit sham feeding in rats. Am. J. Physiol. **253:** R719–R725.
36. LINDEN, A., K. UVNAS-MOBERG, G. FORSBERG, I. BEDNAR & P. SODERSTEN. 1990. Involvement of cholecystokinin in food intake. III. Oestradiol potentiates the inhibitory effect of cholecystokinin octapeptide on food intake in ovariectomized rats. J. Neuroendocrinol. **2:** 979–801.

Brain Regions Where Cholecystokinin Exerts Its Effect on Satiety[a]

RAFAEL R. SCHICK,[b,c] VOLKER SCHUSDZIARRA,[b]
TONY L. YAKSH,[d] AND VAY LIANG W. GO[e]

[b]Department of Internal Medicine II
Technical University of Munich D-81664
Munich, Germany

[d]Department of Anesthesiology
University of California
San Diego, California

[e]Department of Medicine
University of California
Los Angeles, California

Regulation of feeding termination and satiety is complex and involves both gastrointestinal and brain mechanisms.[1] The arrival of food in the gastrointestinal tract results in the activation of satiety signals which are determined by the volume of the meal as well as by the nutrient composition. Thus, gastric distention is an important factor that regulates the termination of food intake.[2-4] In addition, the nutrient content of the meal can also contribute to the reduction of food consumption and may further potentiate the distention-induced satiety stimulus.[5,6] Gastrointestinal satiety signals are subsequently transmitted to integration areas within the central nervous system, which are believed to predominantly lie within the hypothalamus.[7] As mediators for this information transmission, we have to consider both circulating gastrointestinal hormones[8] and afferent neuronal pathways.[9] Most likely candidates for an afferent neuronal connection from the gut to the brain are the vagus nerves which, at the diaphragmatic level, consist of more than 90% afferent fibers.[10]

It is currently not fully understood how peripherally induced satiety signals are conveyed to the brain under physiological conditions. On the basis of the pioneering work of Gibbs and associates, the classical gut hormone cholecystokinin (CCK)[11] has been suggested to act as an intestinal mediator of satiety[12] and has since been the most extensively studied candidate for a peripheral satiety signal. It now appears that peripheral CCK does act not as a hormonal factor, but rather as a locally acting neuropeptide.[13-15] The anorexigenic action of CCK, induced in the periphery, however, appears to be of value in establishing the pathway by which gastrointestinal satiety signals might be relayed to the brain. Thus, the satiety effect of peripherally injected CCK is critically dependent on gastric vagal afferent fibers[16,17] as well as on the integrity of the nucleus tractus solitarii (NTS) and neuronal connections from the NTS to the hypothalamus.[18-20]

The hypothalamus itself represents a brain area at which various signals involved

---

[a]These studies were supported by DFG (Schi 237/1-1, 237/2-1, 237/2-2: R.R.S.) and by NIH (AM-34988-P3 and AM-34988-CD: T.L.Y. and V.L.W.G.).
[c]Address for correspondence: Priv. Doz. Dr. Rafael R. Schick, II. Medizinische Klinik und Poliklinik der Technischen Universität München, Klinikum rechts der Isar, D-81664 Munich, Germany.

in the control of feeding behavior are likely integrated. This assumption is based on a series of classical experiments which have demonstrated that the destruction of the ventromedial hypothalamus results in hyperphagia,[21] whereas electrical stimulation of the same locus inhibits ongoing feeding behavior.[22] Moreover, comparative manipulations carried out in the lateral hypothalamus will generally produce a reciprocal behavioral syndrome.[22,23] Although many classical neurotransmitters and neuropeptides have been identified within the hypothalamus, their individual relevance for satiety is not yet well defined. Recently, a large body of evidence was obtained which suggests that the brain neuropeptide cholecystokinin (CCK) may play a physiological role in the central control of food intake and satiety.

CCK, A CENTRAL SUPPRESSOR OF FOOD INTAKE

Cholecystokinin, first described by Ivy and Oldberg[11] in 1928 as a hormonal factor stimulating gallbladder contraction, has also been identified within the central nervous system.[24] In the brain, CCK may act as a neurotransmitter and/or neuromodulator, based on the findings that it (1) is localized to synaptic vesicles of nerve terminals,[25] (2) possesses specific high-affinity binding sites on neuronal elements,[26] (3) is released from synaptosomal preparations by depolarizing stimuli in a calcium-dependent fashion *in vitro* and *in vivo*,[27,28] (4) depolarizes neurons after iontophoretic administration,[29] and (5) is degraded by a selective brain enzyme.[30]

In addition, evidence has accumulated that indicates the potential relevance of centrally acting CCK for the regulation of feeding termination and satiety. Della-Fera and Baile[31] first reported that continuous injections of CCK octapeptide (CCK-8) into the lateral ventricles of sheep can suppress food intake. These findings have subsequently been extended to numerous species, such as pigs,[32] chicks,[33] hamsters,[34] dogs,[35] baboons,[36] and rats.[37-39] In rats, however, the doses of CCK-8 required for suppression of food intake appear to be clearly higher[37] than those effective in sheep,[31] which may reflect a species-dependent different sensitivity to intracerebroventricularly administered CCK-8. Nevertheless, intracerebroventricular CCK effectively suppresses food intake in rats not only when given acutely,[37-39] but also when infused continuously[40] for 7 days at a rate of 75 pmol/min (FIG. 1).

Therefore, it is conceivable that the effects of intracerebrally administered CCK are mediated by local populations of CCK receptors associated with brain structures that modulate ingestive behaviors. It must be ruled out, however, that centrally injected CCK is redistributed to the periphery via the blood circulation and that the feeding suppressive effects of centrally applied CCK are mediated at peripheral rather than at central sites. This issue was addressed in rats by simultaneous assessment of food consumption and CCK plasma levels following intracerebroventricular or intravenous injection of CCK-8 (FIG. 2). Intracerebroventricular CCK-8 at a dose of 10 nmol significantly prolongs the onset of feeding in 24-hour fasted rats by a median of 6 minutes[37] and significantly inhibits food consumption recorded after initiation of feeding by 45%, whereas circulating plasma CCK levels are not significantly affected (FIG. 2). After an intravenous bolus injection of 1 nmol CCK-8, however, which causes a significant increase in circulating plasma CCK levels by 55 pg/ml above basal (122 pg/ml), no inhibition of rat feeding behavior occurs (FIG. 2). A feeding suppressive effect of intravenous CCK-8 is observed only when an even higher intravenous dose of 10 nmol CCK-8 is injected, resulting in circulating CCK plasma levels about 10-fold above baseline (1,400 pg/ml).[37]

It therefore appears that centrally injected CCK indeed acts at central but not at peripheral sites to suppress food intake in fasted rats. Therefore, it was the aim of

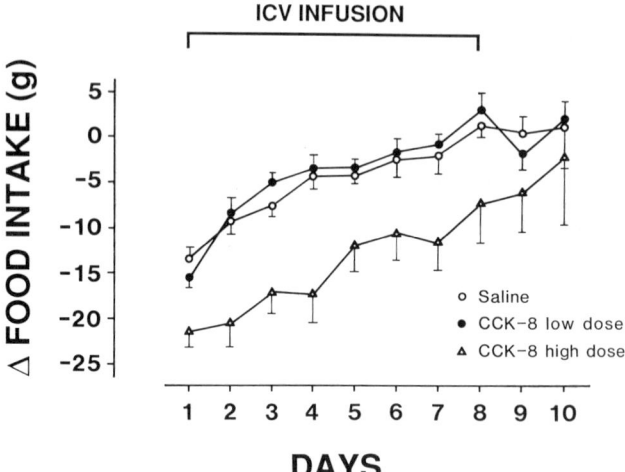

FIGURE 1. Effect of intracerebroventricular (ICV) infusions of saline solution or CCK-8 at a low dose (7.5 pmol/min) or a high dose (75 pmol/min) on daily food intake expressed as the difference between baseline (i.e., before implantation of ventricular cannulas and osmotic mini-pumps) and the postimplantation period during 8 postoperative days.

subsequent studies to identify brain regions likely involved in CCK-mediated central control of satiety.

ROLE OF HYPOTHALAMIC CCK IN THE REGULATION OF SATIETY

Effect of Exogenously Injected CCK on Food Intake

In an attempt to determine brain regions that are sensitive to the feeding suppressive effect of centrally injected CCK, both the central distribution of CCK and its receptors as well as the relevance of specific brain areas for feeding regulation have to be considered. Previous localization studies have clearly demonstrated the presence of both CCK-like immunoreactivity (CCK-LI) and CCK receptors in the hypothalamus.[24,26,41]

In addition, depolarization-evoked release of CCK from the hypothalamus is much greater in genetically obese Zucker (fa/fa) rats than in lean littermates, whereas no such difference exists in the releasability from frontal cortex.[42] Furthermore, hypothalamic CCK concentrations in rats are increased immediately after a meal compared with those in fasted rats. Also, hypothalamic CCK levels are higher in obese rats than in lean rats.[43] These data demonstrate that levels of endogenous CCK peptides are altered in various states of nutrition and satiation and thus provide further evidence that central CCK may play a role in the regulation of feeding and satiety.

In view of the likely involvement of the lateral and ventromedial hypothalamus in the central control of food intake,[21-23] we tested whether these two hypothalamic regions were sensitive to the feeding suppressive action of exogenously injected CCK. Under ketamine anesthesia, rats were equipped with stainless steel cannulas aimed at the lateral or ventromedial hypothalamus according to stereotaxic coordinates as taken from the atlas by Pellegrino et al.[44] After 1 week of recovery, animals received microinjections of either 1 nmol CCK-8 or 0.5 µl saline solution, and feeding behavior was subsequently assessed by recording latency to feed and by measuring net food consumption following the initiation of feeding, as previously described.[37]

Although latency to feed was not significantly altered by injection of CCK-8 into the lateral hypothalamus, the amount of food consumed was significantly reduced.[45] Thus, lateral hypothalamic injection of CCK-8 significantly inhibited food intake during the first 20 minutes after initiation of feeding by 25% compared to saline solution (= vehicle) injection (1.9 vs 2.5 g; FIG. 3). After 1 hour, CCK injected 24-hour fasted rats had consumed significantly less (1.0 g) than saline-injected animals (FIG. 3). When CCK-8 was injected into the ventromedial hypothalamus, no alteration in feeding behavior of 24-hour fasted rats was observed in our experiments,[45] whereas others previously reported that the ventromedial hypothalamus also represents a brain area sensitive to the feeding-suppressive action of centrally injected CCK. In those experiments, however, bilateral injections of CCK had been performed, while we injected CCK unilaterally. Compared to the lateral hypothalamus, the ventromedial hypothalamus may thus possess a reduced sensitivity for the anorexigenic effect of CCK, possibly requiring bilateral activation.

In our experiments, the lateral hypothalamus clearly represents a brain region that is sensitive to the satiating action of centrally acting CCK. To determine the physiological significance of this feeding-suppressive action, however, one has to

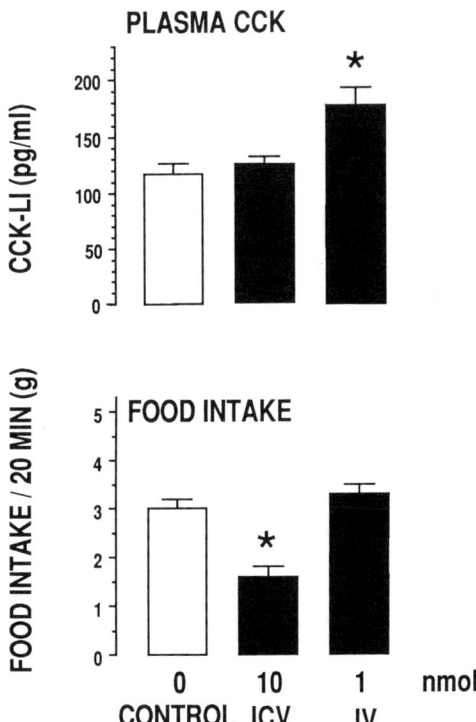

FIGURE 2. Plasma levels of CCK-like immunoreactivity (CCK-LI; pg/ml) and feeding response in 24-hour fasted rats, measured as food consumption during the first 20 minutes after initiation of feeding following intracerebroventricular (ICV) or intravenous (IV) injections of CCK-8 at the doses given. Control: no injection was performed; CCK levels are preprandial baseline levels.

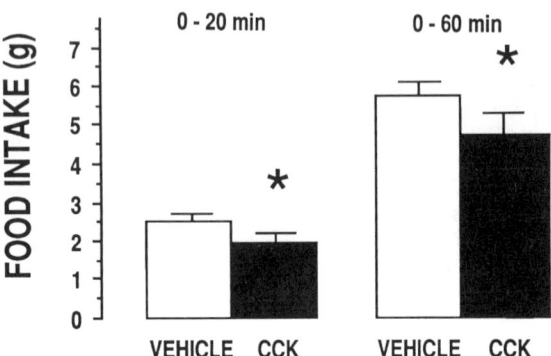

FIGURE 3. Effect of lateral hypothalamic (LH) microinjections of 1 nmol CCK-8 or saline (= vehicle) on cumulative food intake, measured 20 or 60 minutes after the initiation of feeding in 24-hour fasted rats. (*$p < 0.05$ vs vehicle.)

examine (1) if endogenous CCK is released from hypothalamic neurons by stimuli that physiologically are associated with satiety (e.g., a meal load) and, if so, (2) if the endogenously released CCK acts similar to exogenously injected CCK to inhibit ongoing feeding behavior.

Release of Endogenous Hypothalamic CCK during Meal Intake

Evidence for the hypothesis that in a state of food satiation a biological factor is present in the hypothalamus that serves to inhibit further food intake was previously obtained by Yaksh and Myers[46] in conscious monkeys. By use of the push-pull perfusion technique, hypothalamic perfusate was collected from satiated donor monkeys and reperfused into homologous hypothalamic sites of food-deprived recipient monkeys. In these experiments the effluent obtained from a satiated primate did, in fact, suppress the spontaneous feeding behavior of a food-deprived recipient monkey, suggesting that following food intake locally active factors are released within the hypothalamus that actively suppress the ongoing feeding behavior.

Although a putative central satiety factor, however, remained unidentified in those studies, we hypothesized that among others CCK may be a good candidate for such a hypothalamic satiety factor and therefore attempted to determine in cats if CCK-like material could be released from hypothalamic neurons (1) by activation of vagal afferent fibers that are known to participate in the conduction of satiety messages and (2) secondary to intragastric meal loads (with or without nutrients) that are physiological stimuli leading to satiety.

Release of hypothalamic CCK-LI was assessed by collecting push-pull perfusate from the hypothalamic extracellular space as previously described.[47] Perfusion experiments were performed in halothane-anesthetized cats in which the perfusion cannulas were stereotaxically aimed at the lateral hypothalamus and artificial cerebrospinal fluid was perfused at 25 µl/min. Hypothalamic perfusion samples were obtained in 30-minute intervals, and at the end of each experiment 40 mM potassium chloride was added to the artificial cerebrospinal fluid to cause neuronal depolarization and nonspecific neurotransmitter release from local nerve terminals (FIG. 4).

This paradigm allowed us to determine, at any given perfusion site, if CCK-releasing terminals were present or not. Concentrations of CCK-LI in hypothalamic push-pull perfusate were determined by radioimmunoassay.[48-50]

To determine hypothalamic release of CCK during activation of vagal afferents, we electrically stimulated the afferent cervical vagus nerves bilaterally at 10 or 100 Hz and assayed the collected hypothalamic perfusate for CCK-LI. Although release of CCK-LI during baseline perfusion was near the detection limit of the radioimmunoassay employed, a significant and frequency-dependent increase in hypothalamic CCK-LI release was noted during electrical stimulation at 10 Hz (9-fold) or 100 Hz (16-fold).[48] This indicates that activation of a neuronal pathway (i.e., vagal afferent fibers) that has been shown to conduct satiety messages from the gastrointestinal tract to the brain[17] causes local release of the hypothalamic neuropeptide CCK, suggesting that hypothalamic CCK may play a correlated role in the central regulation of satiety.

We further examined this issue by measuring local hypothalamic CCK release secondary to an intragastric load of either a protein/carbohydrate meal (4 g of each) in 30 ml of water or a nutrient-free water load only.[49,50] Similar to the effect observed during electrical vagal afferent stimulation, the intragastric administration of both the nutrient meal and the volume load resulted in a significant increase in hypothalamic CCK-LI release (FIG. 4), suggesting that the effective stimulus was gastrointestinal volumetric distention and was not related to the nutrient content of the meal.[50] This phenomenon, however, was dependent on the integrity of the vagus nerves and

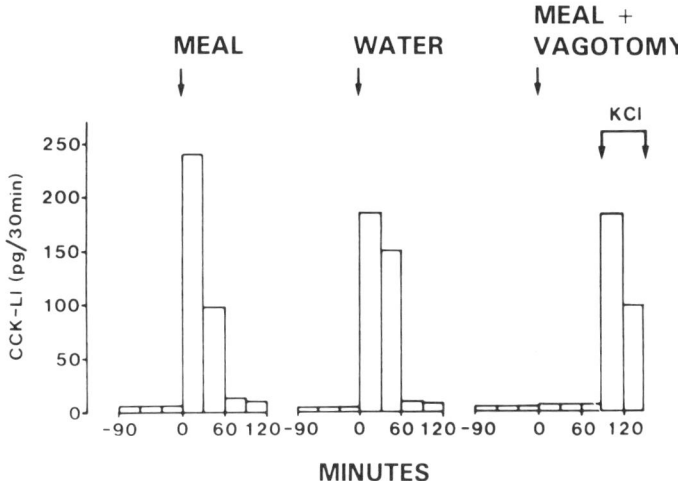

FIGURE 4. Effect of an intragastric nutrient meal (*left panel*) or water load (*middle panel*) on lateral hypothalamic (LH) CCK-LI release, illustrated by single representative push-pull perfusion experiments in the feline lateral hypothalamus of normal cats or of a vagotomized cat (*right panel*). Secondary to both the nutrient and the water load, CCK-LI in hypothalamic perfusate collected from normal cats rises from below the detection limit of the assay in the basal state (-90 to 0 min) to a maximum of 240 pg/30 min (*left panel*) or 180 pg/30 min (*middle panel*), respectively, whereas no such increase is observed after vagotomy (*right panel*). To demonstrate the presence of CCK-releasing terminals in the vagotomy experiment, the depolarizing chemical potassium chloride (40 mM) was added to the perfusion solution, which resulted in release of CCK-LI (*right panel*).

was abolished after bilateral cervical vagotomy (FIG. 4). In addition, such postprandial hypothalamic CCK release was also observed in a primate species.[51]

Subsequent experiments revealed that the molecular form of the released hypothalamic CCK-LI was the octapeptide of CCK[49,50] which is the most abundant form in the brain.[52] No gastrin was detected. Moreover, CCK-LI collected from hypothalamic perfusate did indeed originate from hypothalamic sources and not from the periphery,[49] which is important to note, because the arrival of food in the gastrointestinal tract additionally causes release of intestinal CCK into the blood circulation.[53] Although there are brain regions that lack a blood-brain barrier for CCK (such as the area postrema), we did not observe penetration of circulating CCK into the hypothalamic extracellular space in our experiments[49] which is in agreement with findings by others.[54]

In summary, these data indicate that stimuli that are associated with satiety, such as filling of the stomach or activation of afferent "satiety pathways" (i.e., vagal afferents), can induce release of the hypothalamic neuropeptide CCK, further supporting a physiologically correlated role for CCK in the hypothalamic regulation of food intake and satiety.

Contribution of Endogenously Released Hypothalamic CCK to Feeding Inhibition

After it was demonstrated that the exogenous administration of CCK suppresses feeding behavior at the level of the lateral hypothalamus where endogenous CCK can be released following a meal load, it was of particular interest to determine if the endogenously released hypothalamic CCK also acts to inhibit ongoing feeding behavior. This issue can be addressed by blockade of endogenous CCK receptors by specific CCK receptor antagonists. On the basis of receptor binding and functional studies, CCK receptors are now classified into two subtypes, which have been termed CCK-A (alimentary) or CCK-B (brain) receptors according to their predominant localization.[55,56] In addition, it is well known that CCK-A receptors are also present in some areas of the brain and CCK-B receptors can also be found in the periphery.[57]

For both CCK receptor subtypes, selective antagonists, such as devazepide (formerly MK-329; CCK-A) or L-365,260 (CCK-B/gastrin), have been described and characterized.[58,59] Previously, it was reported that both devazepide and L-365,260 can increase food intake and postpone the onset of satiety in rats following peripheral injection.[60-62] This led to the conclusion that endogenous CCK acts to inhibit feeding behavior similar to exogenously applied CCK. In those studies, however, it could not be conclusively determined at which sites of action the effects of endogenous CCK were blocked, because the peripheral route of administration enabled the CCK receptor antagonists to uniformly block both peripheral and central CCK receptor sites.

We therefore examined whether endogenous CCK in the lateral hypothalamus does contribute to meal satiety.[63] For this purpose, the specific CCK-B receptor antagonist L-365,260 (generously provided by Merck Sharp & Dohme Research Laboratories, Rahway, NJ) or dimethylsulfoxide (= vehicle) was microinjected into the lateral hypothalamus of 24-hour fasted rats, and feeding behavior was subsequently recorded.[63] Following injection of 10 μg L-365,260, food intake during the first 20 minutes after initiation of feeding was significantly increased by 30% compared to vehicle injection (2.7 g vs 2.1 g; $p < 0.05$).[63] This increase in food intake was paralleled by a significant increase in feeding duration, assessed as the percentage of time spent with feeding which after 60 minutes was still significantly enhanced (83% vs 74%; $p < 0.05$).[63] The limited duration of action (approximately 60 minutes) of L-365,260 when injected into the lateral hypothalamus is in agreement with the time course of the CCK release in the lateral hypothalamus secondary to stomach loading which is also confined to 1 hour postprandially.[49,50] Thus, evidence that meal-induced release of CCK in the lateral hypothalamus occurs only during a restricted period of time is thereby further supported.

These data indicate that the lateral hypothalamus represents at least one brain locus at which central CCK released by meal intake may act to suppress ongoing feeding behavior. This further supports the notion that CCK released from hypothalamic neurons during feeding may play a role in the termination of feeding and satiety.

INVOLVEMENT OF EXTRAHYPOTHALAMIC BRAIN REGIONS IN CCK-INDUCED SUPPRESSION OF FOOD INTAKE

In view of the wide distribution of CCK throughout the central nervous system,[24,41,64-66] it is conceivable that brain areas other than the hypothalamus may also contribute to feeding suppression observed after intraventricular administration of CCK. Particularly the feeding-suppressive effect observed after fourth ventricular injection of CCK argues in favor of this hypothesis. Thus, injection of CCK-8 into the fourth ventricle results in a significant increase in latency to feed by 5 minutes compared to saline injection. Subsequent food intake during the first 20 minutes after initiation of feeding is also significantly reduced by 25%.[45] When india ink is injected into the fourth ventricle as opposed to injection of india ink into the lateral ventricles, no staining of the rostral parts of the ventricular system is observed as opposed to injection of India ink into the lateral ventricle which stains the entire ventricular system.[45] This suggests that more caudally located brain loci may also be involved in CCK-induced satiety. We therefore attempted to determine which extrahypothalamic brain areas might participate in the feeding suppression induced by exogenously injected CCK.

For this purpose, rats were chronically equipped with unilateral stainless steel microinjection cannulas aimed at the lateral thalamus, medial amygdala, medial pons, and lateral or medial medulla.[45] No alteration of feeding behavior of 24-hour fasted rats was observed when CCK-8 at a dose of 1 nmol was injected into thalamic sites, ranging from the rostral to the caudal pole, medial aspects of the amygdala (FIG. 5), or medial medulla (not depicted). However, when 1 nmol CCK-8 was injected into the medial pons or lateral medulla, latency to feed was significantly increased by 13.5 minutes (pons) or 6 minutes (medulla), respectively (FIG. 5) compared to saline injection. Food consumption during the first 20 minutes after initiation of feeding was significantly reduced by 0.6 g in both groups (FIG. 5).

The differential sensitivity of various brain loci to the feeding-suppressive effect of centrally injected CCK further supports the concept that centrally applied CCK acts in the brain and not in the periphery. Based on the assumption that the integrity of the blood-brain barrier will be affected similarly at various injection sites, it could be expected that after injection into tissue, CCK would be as readily cleared from all sites in the brain examined, but in fact there were clear differences in activity.

Thus, mapping of CCK-sensitive brain sites revealed that active sites, where CCK significantly suppresses food intake, lie not only in the lateral hypothalamus (see above), but also in the medial pons and lateral medulla in the vicinity of the nucleus tractus solitarius, where vagal afferent fibers terminate. The overall feeding-suppressive effect of CCK (reflecting both the increase in latency to feed and the reduction of subsequent food intake) is summarized in FIGURE 6 for the three

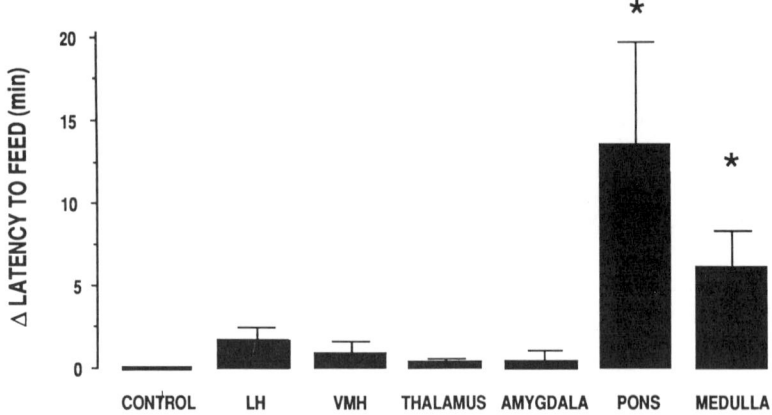
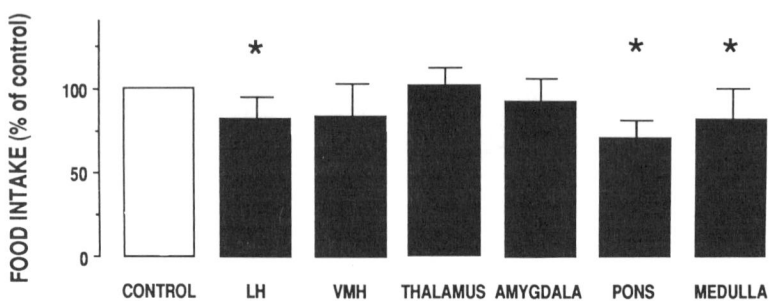

FIGURE 5. Effect of 1 nmol CCK-8 or saline on feeding behavior of 24-hour fasted rats after microinjection into different brain regions. Latency to feed (min) is expressed as difference between latencies observed after injection of CCK-8 or saline solution. Food intake during the first 20 minutes after initiation of feeding is expressed as percentage of control (= vehicle injection). (*$p < 0.05$ vs control.)

CCK-sensitive brain areas tested. Although injections of CCK into the nucleus tractus solitarius have previously failed to show suppression of feeding in rats,[67] the wider distribution of sites in the vicinity of the nucleus tractus solitarius suggests that neurons outside its borders may participate in the CCK-induced suppression of feeding.[45]

This is of particular interest, inasmuch as electrical stimulation in the vicinity of the nucleus tractus solitarii can also evoke CCK release in the lateral hypothalamus, similar to the release observed during vagal stimulation and following stomach loading. These findings support the concept that neuronal elements in the vicinity of the nucleus tractus solitarii may be a relay station in the afferent "satiety pathway" between stomach distention and hypothalamic CCK-LI release.

Furthermore, the brain loci that were clearly sensitive to CCK-induced feeding

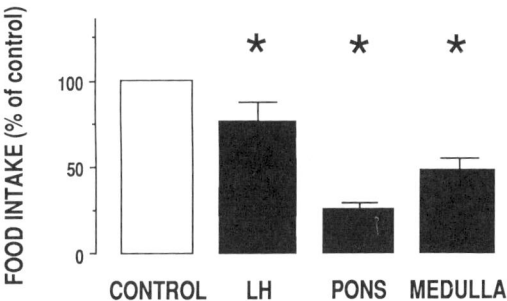

FIGURE 6. Effect of 1 nmol CCK-8 or saline solution on food intake of 24-hour fasted rats after microinjections into brain regions which appeared to be sensitive to the feeding-suppressive effect of CCK. Food intake during the first 20 minutes after injection is expressed as percentage of control (= vehicle injection) and reflects both the increase in latency to feed and the reduction in subsequent food intake, that is, after initiation of feeding. CCK-sensitive loci include the lateral hypothalamus (LH), medial pons, and lateral medulla in the vicinity of the nucleus of the solitary tract. ($^*p < 0.05$ vs control.)

suppression appear to reflect locations in brain which have previously been suggested to participate in the transmission of peripheral "satiety" signals.[18-20] Thus, sites in the medial pontine area may be part of the pathway ascending from the nucleus tractus solitarius to the parabrachial area and sites within the lateral hypothalamus are likely part of an integrative locus for feeding behavior.

SUMMARY

The neuropeptide cholecystokinin (CCK), which is localized within the hypothalamus in integrative centers of feeding regulation, can suppress feeding behavior when exogenously applied into the lateral hypothalamus. Moreover, the endogenous peptide can be released from the same brain locus by stimuli that physiologically are associated with satiety (i.e., gastric meal loads). This endogenously released CCK contributes to the inhibition of feeding behavior during meal intake. These data strongly suggest that hypothalamic CCK may play a physiological role in the termination of feeding behavior.

The presence of additional sites sensitive to CCK in extrahypothalamic regions (e.g., medial pons and lateral medulla) argue that the CCK receptor systems may functionally (1) have several links in a linear chain or (2) exist as several parallel systems. The relevance of these extrahypothalamic loci for feeding regulation will require further studies which need to be directed towards the physiological role of the endogenously released CCK in these particular areas, by use of selective CCK antagonists.

ACKNOWLEDGMENTS

The authors wish to thank Sylvia J. Casey, Gail J. Harty, Sandy Michener, Diane R. Roddy, and Jens P. Zimmermann for expert technical assistance.

REFERENCES

1. MORLEY, J. E. 1987. Neuropeptide regulation of appetite and weight. Endocr. Rev. **8:** 256–287.
2. ROBINSON, P. H., P. R. MCHUGH, T. H. MORAN & J. D. STEPHENSON. 1988. Gastric control of food intake. J. Psychosom. Res. **32:** 593–606.
3. JANOWITZ, H. D. & M. I. GROSSMAN. 1949. Some factors affecting the food intake of normal dogs and dogs with esophagostomy and gastric fistula. Am. J. Physiol. **159:** 143–148.
4. GELIEBTER, A., S. WESTREICH & D. GAGE. 1988. Gastric distention by balloon and test-meal intake in obese and lean subjects. Am. J. Clin. Nutr. **48:** 592–594.
5. SCHICK, R. R., V. SCHUSDZIARRA, B. SCHRÖDER & M. CLASSEN. 1991. Effect of intraduodenal or intragastric nutrient infusion on food intake in man. Z. Gastroenterol. **29:** 637–641.
6. SCHICK, R. R., B. REGENSBURGER, B. SCHRÖDER & M. CLASSEN. 1991. Role of gastric distention and nutrient content for satiety in humans. Gastroenterology **100:** A546.
7. GROSSMAN, S. P. 1975. Role of the hypothalamus in the regulation of food and water intake. Psychol. Rev. **82:** 200–224.
8. KOOPMANS, H. S. 1983. A stomach hormone that inhibits food intake. J. Auton. Nerv. Syst. **9:** 157–171.
9. EWART, W. R. & D. L. WINGATE. 1983. Central representation and opioid modulation of gastric mechanoreceptor activity in the rat. Am. J. Physiol. **244:** G27–G32.
10. HOFFMAN, H. H. & H. SCHNITZLEIN. 1969. The number of vagus nerves in man. Anat. Rec. **139:** 429–435.
11. IVY, A. C. & E. OLDBERG. 1928. A hormone mechanism for gallbladder contraction and evacuation. Am. J. Physiol. **86:** 599–613.
12. GIBBS, J., R. YOUNG & G. P. SMITH. 1973. Cholecystokinin decreases food intake in rats. J. Comp. Physiol. Psychol. **84:** 488–495.
13. PAPPAS, T. N., R. L. MELENDEZ, K. M. STRAH & H. T. DEBAS. 1985. Cholecystokinin is not a peripheral satiety signal in the dog. Am. J. Physiol. **249:** G733–G738.
14. REIDELBERGER, R. D. & T. E. SOLOMON. 1986. Comparative effects of CCK-8 on feeding, sham feeding and exocrine pancreatic secretion in rats. Am. J. Physiol. **251:** R97–R105.
15. SCHICK, R. R., V. SCHUSDZIARRA, J. MÖSSNER, J. NEUBERGER, B. SCHRÖDER, R. SEGMÜLLER, V. MAIER & M. CLASSEN. 1991. Effect of CCK on food intake in man: Physiological or pharmacological effect? Z. Gastroenterol. **29:** 53–58.
16. SMITH, G. P., C. JEROME, J. CUSHIN, R. ETERNO & K. J. SIMANSKY. 1981. Abdominal vagotomy blocks the satiety effect of cholecystokinin in the rat. Science **213:** 1036–1037.
17. SMITH, P. G., E. JEROME & R. NORGREN. 1985. Afferent axons in abdominal vagus mediate the satiety effect of cholecystokinin in rats. Am. J. Physiol. **249:** R638–R641.
18. CRAWLEY, J. N. & J. S. SCHWABER. 1984. Abolition of the behavioral effects of cholecystokinin following bilateral radiofrequency lesions of the parvocellular subdivision of the nucleus tractus solitarius. Brain Res. **295:** 289–299.
19. CRAWLEY, J. N., J. Z. KISS & E. MEZEY. 1984. Bilateral midbrain transections block the behavioral effects of cholecystokinin on feeding and exploration in rats. Brain Res. **322:** 316–321.
20. CRAWLEY, J. N. & J. Z. KISS. 1985. Paraventricular nucleus lesions abolish the inhibition of feeding induced by systemic cholecystokinin. Peptides **6:** 927–935.
21. HETHERINGTON, A. W. & S. W. RANSON. 1940. Hypothalamic lesions and adiposity in the rat. Anat. Rec. **78:** 149–172.
22. LE MAGNEN, J. 1983. Body energy balance and food intake: A neuroendocrine regulatory mechanism. Physiol. Rev. **63:** 314–386.
23. ANAND, B. K. & J. R. BROBECK. 1951. Hypothalamic control of food intake in rats and cats. Yale J. Biol. Med. **24:** 123–140.
24. VANDERHAEGHEN, J. J., F. LOTSTRA, J. DEMEY & C. GILLES. 1980. Immunohistochemical localization of cholecystokinin- and gastrin-like peptides in the brain and hypophysis of the rat. Proc. Natl. Acad. Sci. USA **77:** 1190–1194.

25. REHFELD, J. F., N. GOTTERMANN, L.-I. LARSSON, P. M. EMSON & C. M. LEE. 1979. Gastrin and cholecystokinin in central and peripheral neurons. Fed. Proc. **38**: 2325–2329.
26. SAITO, A., H. SANKARAN, I. D. GOLDFINE & J. A. WILLIAMS. 1980. Cholecystokinin receptors in the brain: Characterization and distribution. Science **208**: 1155–1156.
27. PINGET, M., E. STRAUS & R. S. YALOW. 1979. Release of cholecystokinin peptides from a synaptosome-enriched fraction of rat cerebral cortex. Life Sci. **25**: 339–342.
28. WANG, J.-Y., T. L. YAKSH & V. L. W. GO. 1983. In vivo studies on the basal and evoked release of cholecystokinin and vasoactive intestinal polypeptide from cat cerebral cortex and periventricular structures. Brain Res. **280**: 105–117.
29. DODD, J. & J. S. KELLY. 1979. Excitation of CA1 pyramidal neurons of the hippocampus by the tetra- and octapeptide C-terminal fragments of cholecystokinin. J. Physiol. (Lond.) **295**: 61–62.
30. STRAUS, E., A. MALESCI & R. S. YALOW. 1978. Characterization of a nontrypsin cholecystokinin converting enzyme in mammalian brain. Proc. Natl. Acad. Sci. USA **75**: 5711–5714.
31. DELLA-FERA, M. A. & C. A. BAILE. 1979. Cholecystokinin octapeptide–continuous picomole injections into the cerebral ventricles of sheep suppress feeding. Science **206**: 471–473.
32. PARROTT, R. F. & B. A. BALDWIN. 1981. Operant feeding and drinking in pigs following intracerebroventricular injection of synthetic cholecystokinin octapeptide. Physiol. Behav. **26**: 419–422.
33. DENBOW, D. M. & R. D. MYERS. 1982. Eating, drinking and temperature responses to intracerebroventricular cholecystokinin in the chick. Peptides **3**: 739–743.
34. MICELI, M. O. & C. W. MALSBURY. 1983. Feeding and drinking responses in the golden hamster following treatment with cholecystokinin and angiotensin II. Peptides **4**: 103–106.
35. SAKATANI, N., A. INUI, T. INOUE, M. OYA, H. MORIOKA & S. BABA. 1987. The role of cholecystokinin octapeptide in the central control of food intake in the dog. Peptides **8**: 651–656.
36. FIGLEWICZ, D. P., A. J. SIPOLS, P. GREEN, D. PORTE JR. & S. C. WOODS. 1989. IVT CCK-8 is more effective than IV CCK-8 at decreasing meal size in the baboon. Brain Res. Bull. **22**: 849–852.
37. SCHICK, R. R., T. L. YAKSH & V. L. W. GO. 1986. Intracerebroventricular injections of cholecystokinin octapeptide suppress feeding in rats: Pharmacological characterization of this action. Reg. Peptides **14**: 277–291.
38. STERN, J. J., C. A. CUDILLO & J. KRUPER. 1976. Ventromedial hypothalamus and short-term feeding suppression by caerulein in male rats. J. Comp. Physiol. Psychol. **90**: 484–490.
39. MADDISON, S. 1977. Intraperitoneal and intracranial cholecystokinin depress operant responding for food. Physiol. Behav. **19**: 819–824.
40. SCHICK, R. R., C. W. STEVENS, T. L. YAKSH & V. L. W. GO. 1988. Chronic intraventricular administration of cholecystokinin octapeptide (CCK-8) suppresses feeding in rats. Brain Res. **448**: 294–298.
41. BEINFELD, M. C. & M. PALKOVITS. 1981. Distribution of cholecystokinin (CCK) in the hypothalamus and limbic system of the rat. Neuropeptides **2**: 123–129.
42. MICEVYCH, P. E., V. L. W. GO & T. L. YAKSH. 1984. In vitro release of cholecystokinin from hypothalamus and frontal cortex of Sprague-Dawley, Zucker lean (Fa/−) and obese (fa/fa) rats. Peptides **5**: 73–80.
43. MCLAUGHLIN, C. L., C. A. BAILE, M. A. DELLA-FERA & T. G. KASSER. 1985. Meal-stimulated increased concentration of CCK in the hypothalamus of Zucker obese and lean rats. Physiol. Behav. **35**: 215–220.
44. PELLEGRINO, L. J., A. S. PELLEGRINO & A. CUSHMAN. 1979. A Stereotaxic Atlas of the Rat Brain. Plenum Press. New York, NY.
45. SCHICK, R. R., G. J. HARTY, T. L. YAKSH & V. L. W. GO. 1990. Sites in the brain at which cholecystokinin octapeptide (CCK-8) acts to suppress feeding in rats: A mapping study. Neuropharmacology **29**: 109–118.

46. YAKSH, T. L. & R. D. MYERS. 1972. Neurohumoral substances released from hypothalamus of the monkey during hunger and satiety. Am. J. Physiol. **222:** 503–515.
47. YAKSH, T. L. & H. I. YAMAMURA. 1974. Factors affecting performance of the push-pull cannula in brain. J. Appl. Physiol. **37:** 428–434.
48. SCHICK, R. R., T. L. YAKSH & V. L. W. GO. 1991. Postprandial release of hypothalamic cholecystokinin (CCK). *In* Brain-Gut Interactions. Y. Taché & D. Wingate, eds.: 267–278. CRC Press. Boca Raton, FL.
49. SCHICK, R. R., T. L. YAKSH & V. L. W. GO. 1986. An intragastric meal releases the putative satiety factor cholecystokinin from hypothalamic neurons in cats. Brain Res. **370:** 349–353.
50. SCHICK, R. R., T. L. YAKSH, D. R. RODDY & V. L. W. GO. 1989. Release of hypothalamic cholecystokinin in cats: Effects of nutrient and volume loading. Am. J. Physiol. **256:** R248–R254.
51. SCHICK, R. R., W. M. REILLY, D. R. RODDY, T. L. YAKSH & V. L. W. GO. 1987. Neuronal cholecystokinin-like immunoreactivity is postprandially released from primate hypothalamus. Brain Res. **418:** 20–26.
52. REHFELD, J. F. 1978. Immunochemical studies on cholecystokinin. II. Distribution and molecular heterogeneity in the central nervous system and small intestine of man and hog. J. Biol. Chem. **253:** 4022–4030.
53. WALSH, J. H., C. B. LAMERS & J. E. VALENZUELA. 1982. Cholecystokinin octapeptide-like immunoreactivity in human plasma. Gastroenterology **82:** 438–444.
54. OLDENDORF, W. H. 1981. Blood-brain barrier permeability to peptides: Pitfalls in measurement. Peptides **2** (Suppl. 2): 109–111.
55. MORAN, T. H., P. H. ROBINSON, M. S. GOLDRICH & P. R. MCHUGH. 1986. Two brain cholecystokinin receptors: Implications for behavioral actions. Brain Res. **362:** 175–179.
56. DOURISH, C. T. & D. R. HILL. 1987. Classification and function of CCK receptors. Trends Pharmacol. Sci. **8:** 207–208.
57. HILL, D. R. & T. M. SHAW. 1988. *In* Cholecystokinin Antagonists. R. Y. Wang & R. Schoenfeld, eds.: 133–148. Alan R. Liss. New York, NY.
58. LOTTI, V. J. & R. S. L. CHANG. 1989. A new potent and selective non-peptide gastrin antagonist and brain cholecystokinin receptor (CCK-B) ligand: L-365,260. Eur. J. Pharmacol. **162:** 273–280.
59. LOTTI, V. J., R. G. PENDLETON, R. J. GOULD, H. M. HANSON, R. S. L. CHANG & B. V. CLINESCHMIDT. 1987. *In vivo* pharmacology of L-364,718, a new potent nonpeptide peripheral cholecystokinin antagonist. J. Pharmacol. Exp. Ther. **241:** 103–109.
60. DOURISH, C. T., W. RYCROFT & S. D. IVERSEN. 1989. Postponement of satiety by blockade of brain cholecystokinin (CCK-B) receptors. Science **245:** 1509–1511.
61. WELLER, A., G. P. SMITH & J. GIBBS. 1990. Endogenous cholecystokinin reduces feeding in young rats. Science **247:** 1589–1591.
62. REIDELBERGER, R., G. VARGA & T. E. SOLOMON. 1991. Effects of selective cholecystokinin antagonists L364,718 and L365,260 on food intake in rats. Peptides **12:** 1215–1221.
63. SCHICK, R. R., V. SCHUSDZIARRA, C. ENDRES, T. EBERL & M. CLASSEN. 1991. Putative sleep factors and satiety in rats: Role of cholecystokinin (CCK) and delta sleep inducing peptide (DSIP). Neuropeptides (Life Sci. Adv.) **10:** 41–48.
64. ZARBIN, M. S., J. K. WAMSLEY, R. B. INNIS & M. J. KUHAR. 1981. Cholecystokinin receptors: Presence and axonal flow in the rat vagus nerve. Life Sci. **29:** 697–705.
65. PALKOVITS, M., J. Z. KISS, M. C. BEINFELD & T. H. WILLIAMS. 1982. Cholecystokinin in the nucleus of the solitary tract of the rat: Evidence for its vagal origin. Brain Res. **252:** 386–390.
66. INAGAKI, S., Y. SHIOTANI, M. YAMANO, S. SHIOSAKA, H. TAKAGI, K. TATEISHI, E. HASHIMURA, T. HAMAOKA & M. TOHYAMA. 1984. Distribution, origin, and fine structures of cholecystokinin-8-like immunoreactive terminals in the nucleus ventromedialis hypothalami of the rat. J. Neurosci. **4:** 1289–1299.
67. CRAWLEY, J. 1985. Neurochemical investigation of the afferent pathway from the vagus nerve to the nucleus tractus solitarius in mediating the "satiety syndrome" induced by systemic cholecystokinin. Peptides **6** (Suppl. 1): 133–137.

Endogenous CCK and the Peripheral Neural Substrates of Intestinal Satiety

ROBERT C. RITTER,[a] LYNNE A. BRENNER, AND
CONNIE S. TAMURA

Department of V.C.A.P.P.
College of Veterinary Medicine
Washington State University
Pullman, Washington 99164

Participation of cholecystokinin (CCK) in control of food intake is supported by three types of observations: (1) exogenous CCK reduces food intake and elicits other behavioral concomitants of satiation[1,2] (See also Smith in this volume), (2) CCK is released prandially by "I cells" of the intestinal mucosa in response to chemical constituents of intestinal chyme,[3,4] and (3) food intake is increased by systemic administration of nonpeptide[5-8] as well as peptidyl[9] CCK_A receptor antagonists (FIG. 1). The observation that CCK receptor antagonism increases food intake is the most compelling evidence in support of a role for endogenous CCK in the control of food intake.

The source(s) of endogenous CCK and the site(s) of its participation in control of feeding remains uncertain. However, Smith *et al.*[10] demonstrated that reduction of food intake by injection of exogenous CCK depends on the vagus nerve, a finding that many other groups have independently replicated. Furthermore, reduction of intake by exogenous CCK is mediated by a capsaicin-sensitive[11-13] neuronal population in the sensory component of the vagus. Finally, the vagus nerve transports CCK binding sites,[14] and we recently found that many vagal sensory neurons express CCK_A receptor mRNA[15] (FIG. 2). All of these results suggest that CCK of peripheral origin could exert control on food intake through actions on vagal sensory neurons.

CCK's history as a hormone, together with evidence for vagal receptor mechanisms responsive to exogenous CCK, have fostered the view that CCK of intestinal mucosal origin controls food intake by endocrine action on vagal sensory neurons. This "endocrine hypothesis" (FIG. 3) has guided research into the ingestive effects of CCK for nearly two decades. However, tests of the hypothesis that circulating CCK is a physiological participant in the control of ingestion have yielded mostly negative results. (See for example refs. 16 and 17.) Furthermore, we now know that both CCK[18-22] and its receptors[14,15,23-27] are expressed by many neurons in the central and peripheral nervous systems. Consequently, it is possible that the source of endogenous CCK involved in control of food intake is neuronal ("neuronal hypothesis"), not endocrine, and that the CCK control of ingestion could be by actions at central as well as peripheral CCK receptive neurons (FIG. 3). In accordance with the possibility of multiple sites for CCK participation in control of food intake, it is interesting that electrophysiological data support the existence of a peripheral vagal site for some actions of CCK. For example, exogenous CCK is reported to modulate the activity of gastric mechanoreceptive neurons[28-31] and to activate intestinal mucosal neurons that may be chemoreceptive.[32] Furthermore, work we did in collaboration with Ewart

---

[a] Address for correspondence: Dr. Robert C. Ritter, Dept. of VCAPP, Washington State University, Pullman, WA 99164–6520.

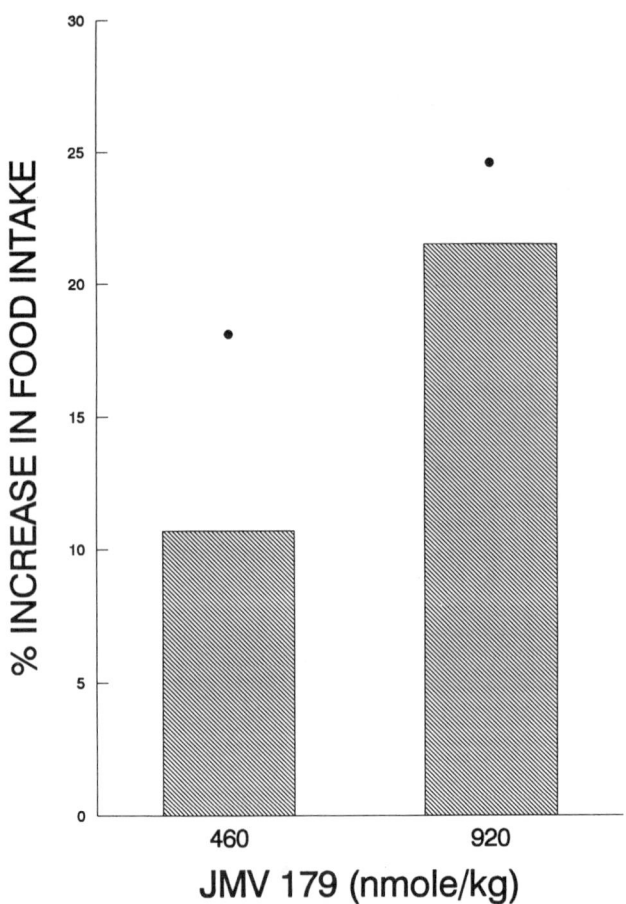

FIGURE 1. Dose-related increase in liquid food intake in rats elicited by the heptapeptide CCK receptor antagonist JMV 179. Animals were food deprived for 18 hours before introduction of a 15% sucrose solution. Intraperitoneal JMV 179 injections were given 5 minutes before sucrose. Data are expressed as percentage intake above that which occurred after intraperitoneal injection of the vehicle solution. For review of JMV 179 and other peptoid CCK antagonists, see Martinez in this volume.

and Wingate[30] indicates that cells of the dorsal vagal complex receive input from capsaicin-sensitive, CCK-responsive neurons and also from non-capsaicin-sensitive afferents, responding to gastric distention but not to CCK. These results all support some form of participation of CCK, outside the CNS, in vagal sensory signals, some of which may control food intake. On the other hand, there have been reports of alterations of food intake produced by intracerebral applications of CCK agonists[33] and antisera.[34] Also, Schick and coworkers[35] reported release of CCK-like immunoreactivity from some brain areas following gastrointestinal stimulation. Thus, central CCK circuits may control feeding and, even with regard to the site of action of peripheral CCK, there are multiple candidates, which are not mutually exclusive.

Our approach to analyzing the role of CCK in the control of food intake has been one of "behavioral reductionism." We feel that the nature and sites of this peptide's contributions to control of food intake may vary, depending on the control inputs. In other words, CCK might participate in altering feeding behavior in response to gastric, intestinal, metabolic, or environmental signals. But there is no reason to assume that the CCK-releasing or CCK-receptive cells are the same for all signals. Therefore, it seems appropriate to us to study the role of CCK in changes in feeding

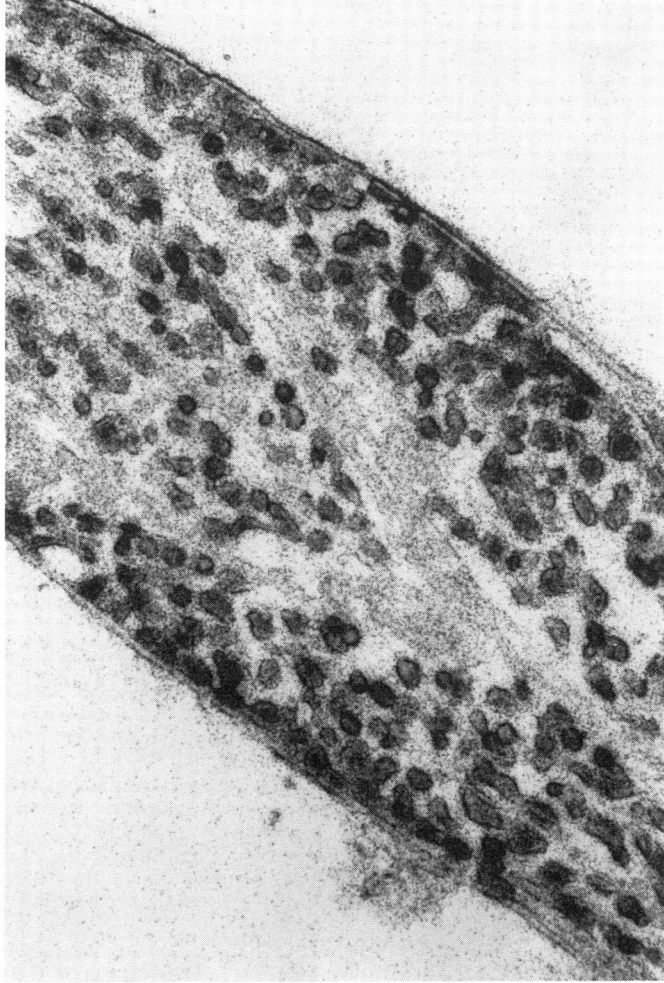

FIGURE 2. CCK_A receptor mRNA localized to neuronal cell bodies of the vagal nodose ganglion of the rat demonstrated using *in situ* hybridization. *In situ* hybridization was performed on 15 μm longitudinal sections, using an antisense, [^{35}S]-UTP-labeled riboprobe, transcribed from cDNA (pCDNA-1 vector, gift of Stephen Wank). (Photograph was made using 10X objective.)

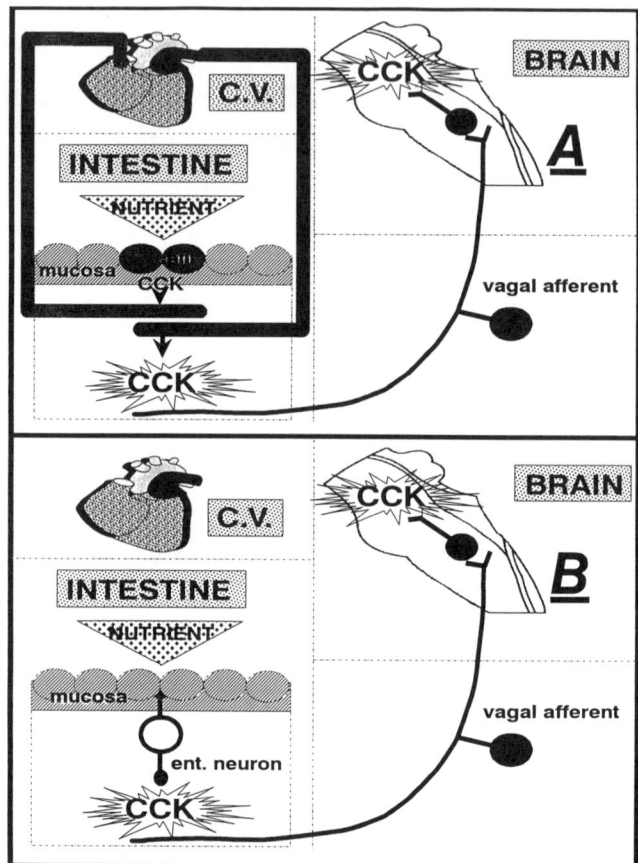

FIGURE 3. Two hypotheses regarding the source(s) and site(s) of action of endogenous CCK participating in control of food intake by intestinal nutrient stimulation. The *upper panel* (**A**) depicts an endocrine hypothesis. According to this scheme, CCK released by intestinal mucosal "I" cells enters the venous drainage of the intestine and is carried to the heart. Hormonal CCK is returned to the abdominal viscera via the arterial circulation and activates target receptors on vagal sensory neurons. Vagal sensory input to the brain results in a behavioral response—termination of eating. The *lower panel* (**B**) depicts a neural hypothesis of endogenous CCK participation in control of food intake by intestinal nutrient stimulation. According to this hypothesis, intestinal mucosal CCK secretion is not involved in reduction of food intake by intestinal nutrients. Rather, CCK participates as a neurotransmitter, acting at peripheral and/or brain CCK receptors.

elicited by specific stimuli, acting at known locations, over a restricted time period. Reduction of food intake by intestinal infusions of liquid diets and some nutrient solutions has been reported in a variety of species, including rats, monkeys, and humans.[36–41] Inasmuch as CCK is released from the small intestine in response to nutrients, we have focused much of our effort on reduction of food intake produced by intestinal infusion of specific nutrients into the intestine of sham-feeding rats.

This preparation has the following advantages: (1) it prevents intestinal and postabsorptive influences of nutrients in the ingesta itself, (2) it obviates the influence of gastric distention as a control of intake, and (3) it eliminates possible variation of gastric and postgastric stimulation by reflex changes in gastric emptying.

We find that some, but not all, nutrients produce reliable reductions of sham feeding when they are infused in isotonic, pH 7 solutions, at infusion rates approximating gastric emptying during a liquid meal. For example, the long chain fatty acid, oleic acid, reliably reduces sham feeding, while the medium chain fatty acid, octanoic, does not.[39] L-phenylalanine reduces sham intake, while D-phenylalanine, hydrolyzed or unhydrolyzed casein have little or no effect.[18,39] Sham feeding is also reduced more by a variety of oligosaccharides than by their constituent monosaccharides.[42] Thus, intestinal stimulation by specific nutrients does influence food intake and could play a role in its physiological control.

If endogenous CCK participates in the control of food intake by intestinal nutrients, then the following conditions should pertain: (1) Both exogenous CCK and nutrients should act via the same peripheral neurons to reduce food intake; (2) CCK receptor antagonists should attenuate reduction of intake produced by intestinal nutrient; and (3) Nutrient-induced reduction of intake should be accompanied by CCK release. With regard to the first condition, we previously demonstrated that the vagus nerve is necessary for reduction of sham feeding by some intestinal nutrients[43] (FIG. 4). In addition, we demonstrated that reduction of sham feeding by exogenous CCK and some intestinal nutrients is mediated by capsaicin-sensitive fibers of the vagus.[39,44] Therefore, control of food intake by both exogenous CCK and intestinal nutrients appears to be dependent on similar, if not identical, capsaicin-sensitive, vagal sensory neurons. These findings support condition number 1. We also found that reduction of sham intake by some, but not all, intestinal nutrients is abolished by systemic pretreatment with CCK_A receptor antagonists[45,46] (FIG. 5). A CCK_B antagonist[46] was not effective in antagonism of reduction of intake by intestinal nutrients (data not shown). These results suggest that reduction of sham intake, at least by some intestinal nutrients, depends on occupation of CCK_A receptors. The results appear to satisfy condition 2, because they indicate possible congruency of the CCK receptor mechanisms mediating reduction of sham intake by some nutrients with an established CCK_A receptor mechanism for exogenous CCK's action on food intake. (For review, see Smith in this volume.)

The fact that CCK is released prandially into the circulation by cells in the intestinal mucosa makes endocrine CCK secretion the prime candidate for mediator of nutrient-induced reduction of sham feeding. To examine this possibility, we compared CCK bioactivity in plasma following intestinal infusion of various nutrients with the ability of these same nutrients to reduce sham feeding.[18] We found that there is no apparent correlation between elevation of plasma CCK by a nutrient and its ability to reduce sham intake (FIG. 6). For example, the disaccharide, maltose, reduces sham intake, and this reduction is abolished by CCK_A receptor antagonists. However, maltose does not elevate plasma CCK concentrations. Furthermore, unhydrolyzed casein causes marked elevation of plasma CCK. Yet under identical infusion conditions, it fails to reduce sham feeding. Hence, we must conclude that under conditions in which alterations of gastric filling and emptying are obviated, release of circulating CCK does not participate in reduction of sham feeding by intestinal nutrients. As work with receptor antagonists indicates that CCK is important for control of food intake by intestinal nutrients, even in the absence of elevated levels of circulating CCK, the source of CCK involved is likely to be nonendocrine cells, that is, neurons.

CCK-like immunoreactivity exists in neurons and terminals of the brain, spinal

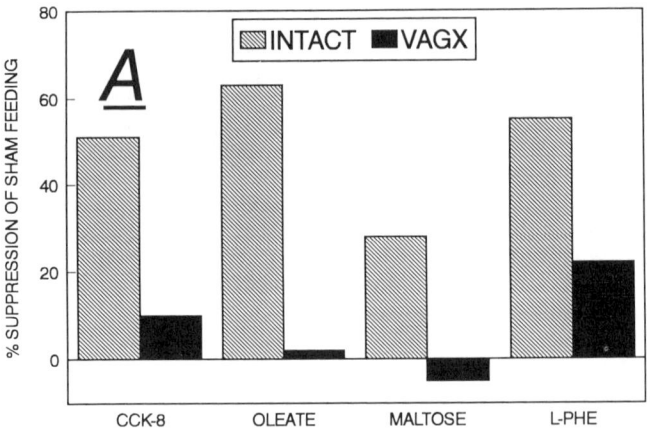

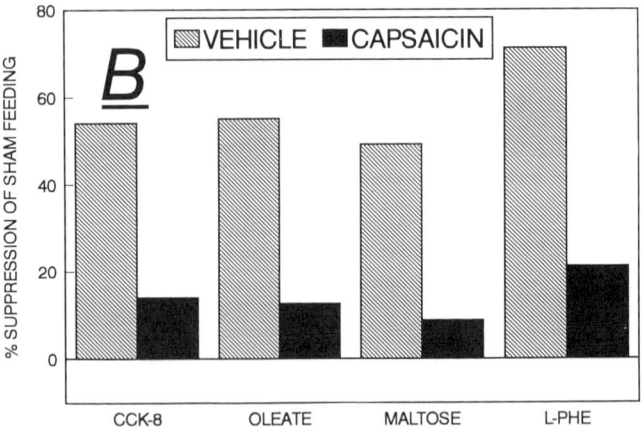

FIGURE 4. Reduction of sham feeding by both exogenous CCK and intestinal nutrients depends on capsaicin-sensitive neural substrate(s). **(A)** Reductions of sham intake by exogenous CCK-8, oleate, maltose, and L-phenylalanine (L-PHE) are attenuated in rats with total subdiaphragmatic vagotomies. **(B)** Reductions of sham intake by exogenous CCK-8, oleate, maltose, and (L-PHE) are attenuated in rats pretreated as adults with intraperitoneal capsaicin 2 weeks to 3 months before behavioral testing. Results are depicted as % suppression. % suppression = 100 × (intake after vehicle infusion or injection − intake after nutrient infusion or CCK injection)/(intake after vehicle infusion or injection).

cord, and autonomic ganglia and in the enteric nervous system.[20–23,47,48] Furthermore, preproCCK mRNA has been localized in the neuronal perikarya of the central nervous system.[49,50] Ligand binding studies indicate that CCK_A receptors are found in the brain as well as on peripheral neural structures.[14,16,25,26] Furthermore, as reviewed by other authors in this volume, electrophysiological work indicates that CCK_A receptors mediate neural responses at central and peripheral synapses. Thus, it is possible that CCK's involvement in reduction of food intake by intestinal nutrients could result from the release of central and/or peripheral neuronal CCK.

As a preliminary test of the possibility that activation of brain CCK receptors is necessary for reduction of sham feeding by intestinal nutrients, we compared reduction of sham feeding by intestinal oleate infusion after intraperitoneal and intracerebroventricular administration of the CCK_A receptor antagonist MK329.[51] We found that intraperitoneal MK329, at doses of 75–300 µg/rat, attenuated or abolished reduction of sham feeding by intestinal oleate. However, when injected intracerebroventricularly, the antagonist failed to attenuate reduction of intake by oleate, even at doses four times higher than those that abolished oleate-induced reduction of sham feeding when injected intraperitoneally (FIG. 7). Assuming that high doses of intracerebroventricular MK329 produce central antagonist concentrations at least as high as those achieved after intraperitoneal administration, then these results argue against the role of brain CCK in reducing sham feeding by intestinal nutrient infusion. Consequently, these findings suggest that CCK released in small amounts, at high concentration, close to its site of action, by peripheral neurons, may mediate reduction of sham feeding by intestinal nutrient stimulation.

As mentioned earlier, vagal sensory neurons transcribe CCK_A receptor mRNA[15] and transport CCK_A ligand binding sites.[14] Furthermore, CCK-like immunoreactivity is expressed in a small but significant population of neurons of both the myenteric and submucous plexes of the enteric nervous system.[47,48] Therefore, elements of a system exist by which enteric neuronal CCK could mediate or modulate vagal sensory responses to intestinal nutrient stimulation. Our attempts to analyze this possibility are in their early stages. However, one potentially illuminating avenue of investigation is examination of nutrient-induced reduction of sham feeding in rats pretreated with low doses of capsaicin intraintestinally. Intraintestinal infusion of 5 mg of capsaicin reduces sham feeding, but does not cause degeneration of vagal sensory

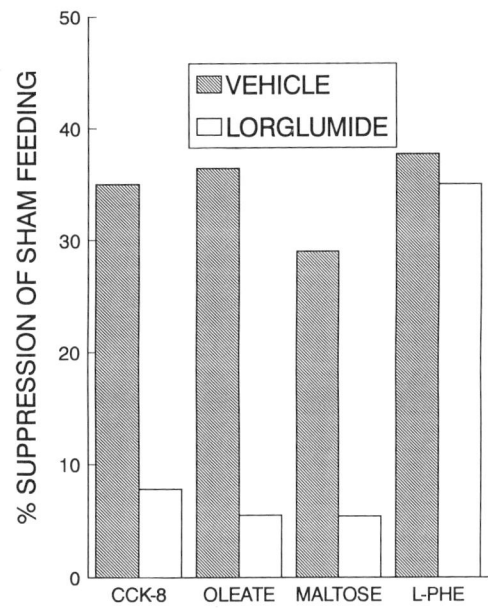

FIGURE 5. CCK_A receptor antagonist attenuates reduction of sham feeding by exogenous CCK-8 or intraintestinal infusion of some nutrients. In this experiment the CCK_A receptor antagonist lorglumide (CR1409), 300 µg/kg, was injected intraperitoneally 5 minutes before CCK injection or the start of intestinal infusion. Note that the antagonist virtually abolished reduction of sham feeding by exogenous CCK, oleate, or maltose, but it did not attenuate reduction of sham intake by L-PHE. Comparable results were obtained using MK329, another CCK_A receptor antagonist. Results suggest that endogenous CCK participates in reduction of food intake by some, but not all, intestinal nutrients. Results are expressed as % suppression of sham feeding. (See FIGURE 4 caption for details.)

neurons or functional signs of systemic neurotoxicity.[12,52] Nonetheless, 24 hours after intestinal capsaicin infusion, rats fail to reduce sham intake in response to intestinal infusion of oleate[53,54] (FIG. 8). They do, however, reduce their intake in response to exogenous CCK. By 48 hours after capsaicin infusion, reduction of sham feeding by

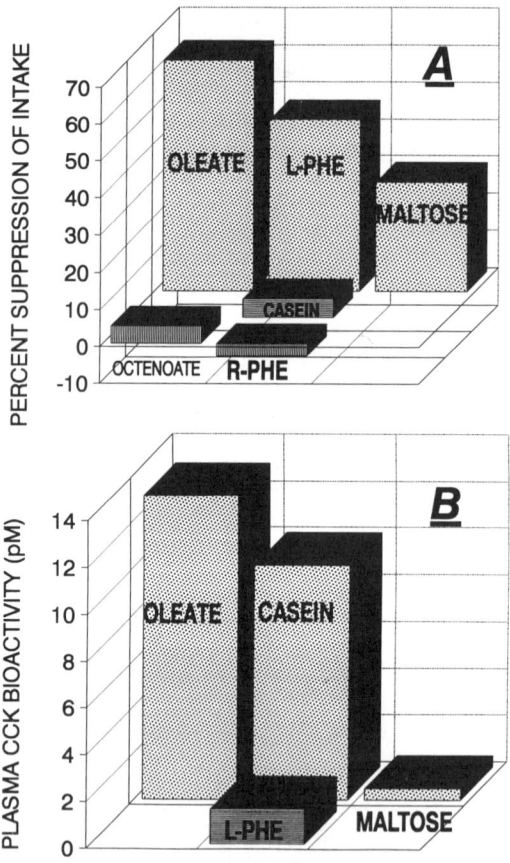

FIGURE 6. Comparison of reduction of sham feeding and elevation of plasma CCK concentrations by intestinal nutrient infusions. (**A**) Intestinal infusion of oleate, L-PHE, or maltose all significantly reduce sham feeding; octenoate, R-PHE, or unhydrolyzed casein has little or no effect. (**B**) Only oleate and casein cause significant elevations of plasma CCK. Note that although intestinal casein infusion elevates plasma CCK, it does not cause reduction of sham feeding. On the other hand, maltose does not elevate plasma CCK, but it does reduce sham feeding. These results do not support participation of circulating CCK in control of food intake by intestinal nutrients.

intestinal oleate infusion is no longer attenuated. Thus, intestinal capsaicin transiently attenuates reduction of intake by nutrient stimulation, but not by exogenous CCK. There are several tenable interpretations of these results. First, it is possible that intestinal capsaicin desensitizes mucosal, intestinal, vagal afferents that are not

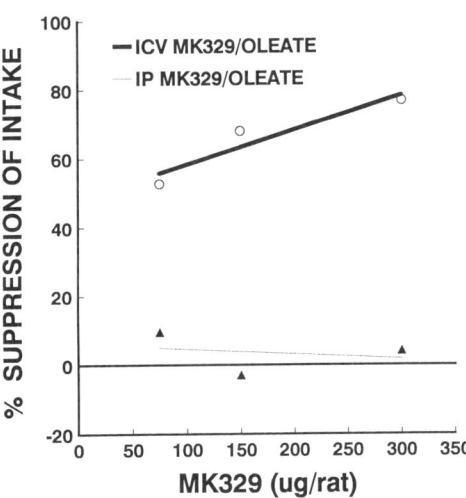

FIGURE 7. Reduction of sham feeding by intestinal oleate is attenuated by intraperitoneal but not intracerebroventricular injections of MK329, a CCK_A receptor antagonist. Note that while intraperitoneal MK329 abolished reduction of sham feeding by intestinal oleate at a dose as low as 75 μg/rat, even 300 μg/rat given intracerebroventricularly did not attenuate reduction of sham feeding by intestinal oleate infusion. Neither intraperitoneal nor intracerebroventricular MK329 altered sham feeding when given alone or in association with vehicle injection or infusion.

CCK sensitive, leaving capsaicin-insensitive or capsaicin-inaccessible afferents responsive to CCK. Nonintestinal (gastric) vagal afferents may not be accessible to intestinal, neuronal CCK or intestinal capsaicin. The finding that at least some gastric vagal afferents are responsive to systemic CCK also is compatible with this

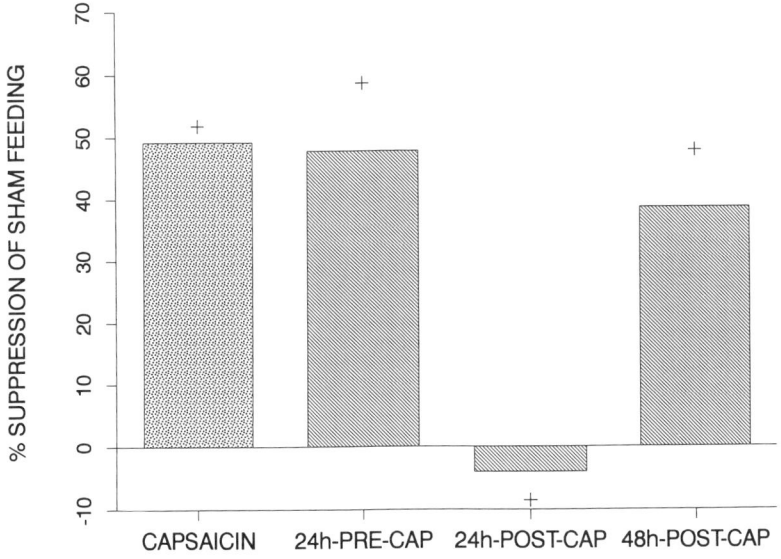

FIGURE 8. Reduction of sham feeding by intestinal oleate infusion is transiently lost after intestinal capsaicin infusion. Oleate-induced reduction of sham feeding returns to precapsaicin levels by 48 hours after capsaicin infusion. The capsaicin dose used (5 mg/rat) does not produce systemic neurotoxicity when infused into the intestine. Also, intestinal oleate absorption is not impaired 24 hours after intestinal capsaicin. See text for additional details.

hypothesis. A second possibility, however, is that intestinal capsaicin desensitizes enteric neurons that are presynaptic to the vagal sensory innervation of the intestine. Such a presynaptic desensitization would not alter CCK responsiveness of vagal sensory fibers themselves. In support of this latter hypothesis, it is noteworthy that MK329 attenuates suppression of sham feeding by intestinal capsaicin infusion,[53] suggesting that capsaicin might deplete neuronal CCK. Capsaicin is reported to release several peptides from the enteric plexes *in vitro*,[55-60] elevating the possibility that release of enteric neuropeptides, perhaps including CCK, may activate vagal sensory neurons in response to intestinal stimulation (FIG. 3).

In summary, our results indicate that intestinal nutrient infusions reduce food intake by acting on capsaicin-sensitive vagal neurons similar to those that mediate suppression of feeding by exogenous CCK. The fact that reduction of intake by some, but not all, intestinal nutrients is attenuated by CCK_A antagonists suggests that endogenous CCK mediates reduction of food intake by some intestinal stimuli. At the same time, it is clear that CCK released into the circulation (endocrine CCK) is not responsible for reductions of sham feeding by nutrients. Therefore, our results suggest that reduction of food intake by intestinal nutrients is mediated by CCK of neural origin. The source of neuronal CCK is not known but could be the enteric plexus, the brain, or both (FIG. 3).

REFERENCES

1. ANTIN, J., J. GIBBS, J. HOLT, R. C. YOUNG & G. P. SMITH. 1975. Cholecystokinin elicits complete behavioral satiety sequence in rats. J. Comp. Physiol. Psychol. **89:** 784–790.
2. GIBBS, J., R. C. YOUNG & G. P. SMITH. 1973. Cholecystokinin decreases food intake in rats. J. Comp. Physiol. Psychol. **84:** 488–495.
3. IVY, A. C. & E. OLDENBERG. 1928. A hormone mechanism for gallbladder contraction and evacuation. Am. J. Physiol. **86:** 599–613.
4. LIDDLE, R. A., I. D. GOLDFINE & J. A. WILLIAMS. 1984. Bioassay of plasma cholecystokinin in rats: effects of food, trypsin inhibitor, and alcohol. Gastroenterology **87**(3): 542–549.
5. SCHILLABEER, G. & J. S. DAVISON. 1984. The cholecystokinin antagonist proglumide, increases food intake in the rat. Regul. Pept. **8:** 171–176.
6. SILVERMAN, M., S. BANK & S. LENDVAI. 1987. The cholecystokinin antagonist, L-364,718, increases food consumption. Dig. Dis. Sci. **32:** 1188.
7. MORAN, T. H., P. J. AMEGLIO, G. J. SCHWARTZ & P. R. MCHUGH. 1992. Blockade of type A, not type B, CCK receptors attenuates satiety action of exogenous and endogenous CCK. Am. J. Physiol. **262:** R46–R50.
8. REIDELBERGER, R. D. & M. F. O'ROURKE. 1989. Potent cholecystokinin antagonist L 364718 stimulates food intake in rats. Am. J. Physiol. **257:** R1512–R1518.
9. BRENNER, L. A. & R. C. RITTER. 1992. Peptide CCK receptor antagonist increases real feeding and attenuates suppression of sham feeding by exogenous CCK-8 in rats. Soc. Neurosci. Abstr. **18:** 1428.
10. SMITH, G. P., C. JEROME, B. CUSHIN, R. ETERNO & K. SIMANSKY. 1981. Abdominal vagotomy blocks the satiety effect of cholecystokinin in the rat. Science **213:** 1036–1037.
11. SMITH, G. P., C. JEROME & R. NORGREN. 1985. Afferent axons in abdominal vagus mediate satiety effect of cholecystokinin in rats. Am. J. Physiol. **249:** R638–R641.
12. RITTER, R. C. & E. E. LADENHEIM. 1985. Capsaicin pretreatment attenuates suppression of food intake by cholecystokinin. Am. J. Physiol. **248:** R501–R504.
13. SOUTH, E. H. & R. C. RITTER. 1988. Capsaicin application to central or peripheral vagal fibers attenuates CCK satiety. Peptides **9:** 601–612.
14. MORAN, T. H., G. P. SMITH, A. M. HOSTETLER & P. R. MCHUGH. 1987. Transport of cholecystokinin (CCK) binding sites in subdiaphragmatic vagal branches. Brain Res. **415:** 149–152.

15. BRENNER, L. A., K. ULIBARRI & R. C. RITTER. 1993. Sensory neurons of the nodose ganglion contain mRNA for CCKA receptor protein. Soc. Neurosci. Abstr. **19:** 730.
16. BRENNER, L. A., D. P. YOX & R. C. RITTER. 1993. Suppression of sham feeding by intestinal nutrients is not correlated with plasma cholecystokinin elevation. Am. J. Physiol. **264:** R972–R976.
17. SMITH, G. P., D. GREENBERG, J. D. FALSCO, A. A. AVILION, J. GIBBS, R. A. LIDDLE & J. A. WILLIAMS. 1989. Endogenous cholecystokinin does not decrease food intake or gastric emptying in fasted rats. Am. J. Physiol. **257:** R1462–R1466.
18. BEINFELD, M. G., D. K. MEYER, R. L. ESKAY, R. T. JENSEN & M. BROWNSTEIN. 1981. The distribution of cholecystokinin immunoreactivity in the central nervous system of the rat as determined by radioimmunoassay. Brain Res. **212:** 51–57.
19. HOKFELT, T., M. HERRERA-MARSCHUTZ, M. SCHALLING, K. SEROOGY, M. SCHALLING, U. UNGERSTEDT, C. POST, J. REHFELD, P. FREY, J. FISCHER, G. DOCKRAY, T. HAMAOKA, J. WALSH & M. GOLDSTEIN. 1988. Immunohistochemical studies on cholecystokinin (CCK)-immunoreactive neurons in the rat using sequence specific antisera and with special reference to the caudate nucleus and primary sensory neurons. J. Chem. Neuroanat. **1:** 11–52.
20. LARSSON, L. I. & J. F. REHFELD. 1979. Localization and molecular heterogeneity of cholecystokinin in the central and peripheral nervous systems. Brain Res. **165:** 201–218.
21. REHFELD, J. F. 1978. Immunohistochemical studies of cholecystokinin. II. Distribution and molecular heterogeneity in the central nervous system and the small intestine of man and hog. J. Biol. Chem. **253:** 4022–4030.
22. INGRAM, S. M., R. G. KRAUSE II, F. BALDINO, JR., L. C. SKEEN & M. E. LEWIS. 1989. Neuronal localization of cholecystokinin mRNA in the rat brain by *in situ* hybridization histochemistry. J. Comp. Neurol. **287:** 260–272.
23. HILL, D. R. & G. N. WOODRUFF. 1990. Differentiation of central cholecystokinin receptor binding sites using the non-peptide antagonists MK-329 and L-365,260. Brain Res. **526:** 276–283.
24. LIN, C. W. & T. R. MILLER. 1992. Both CCKA and CCKB/gastrin receptors are present on rabbit vagus nerve. Am. J. Physiol. **263:** R591–R595.
25. GHILARDI, J. R., C. J. ALLEN, S. R. VIGNA, D. C. MCVEY & P. W. MANTYH. 1992. Trigeminal and dorsal root ganglion neurons express CCK receptor binding sites in the rat, rabbit, and monkey: Possible site of opiate-CCK analgesic interactions. J. Neurosci. **12:** 4854–4866.
26. MANTYH, P. W., M. D. CATTON, C. J. ALLEN, M. E. LABENSKI, J. E. MAGGIO & S. R. VIGNA. 1992. Receptor binding sites for cholecystokinin, galanin, somatostatin, substance P and vasoactive intestinal polypeptide in sympathetic ganglia. Neuroscience **46:** 739–754.
27. WANK, S. A., J. R. PISEGNA & A. DE-WEERTH. 1992. Brain and gastrointestinal cholecystokinin receptor family: Structure and functional expression. Proc. Natl. Acad. Sci. USA **89:** 8691–8695.
28. DAVISON, J. S. & G. D. CLARKE. 1988. Mechanical properties and sensitivity to CCK of vagal gastric slowly adapting mechanoreceptors. Am. J. Physiol. **255:** G55–G61.
29. RAYBOULD, H. E., R. J. GAYTON & G. J. DOCKRAY. 1985. CNS effects of circulating CCK-8: Involvement of brainstem neurones responding to gastric distension. Brain Res. **342:** 187–190.
30. RITTER, R. C., S. RITTER, W. R. EWART & D. L. WINGATE. 1989. Capsaicin attenuates hindbrain neuron responses to circulating cholecystokinin. Am. J. Physiol. **257:** R1162–R1168.
31. SCHWARTZ, G. J., P. R. MCHUGH & T. H. MORAN. 1991. Integration of vagal afferent responses to gastric loads and cholecystokinin in rats. Am. J. Physiol. **261:** R64–R69.
32. BLACKSHAW, L. A. & D. GRUNDY. 1990. Effects of cholecystokinin (CCK-8) on two classes of gastroduodenal vagal afferent fibre. J. Auton. Nerv. Syst. **31:** 191–201.
33. FIGLEWICZ, D. P., A. J. SIPOLS, D. PORTE, S. C. WOODS & R. A. LIDDLE. 1989. Intraventricular CCK inhibits food intake and gastric emptying in baboons. Am. J. Physiol. **256:** R1313–R1317.
34. DELLA-FERA, M. A., C. A. BAILE, B. S. SHNEIDER & J. A. GRINKER. 1981. Cholecystokinin

antibody injected in cerebral-ventricles stimulates feeding in sheep. Science **212:** 687–689.
35. SCHICK, R. R., T. L. TAKSH, D. R. RODDY & V. L. W. GO. 1989. Release of hypothalamic cholecystokinin in cats: Effects of nutrient and volume loading. Am. J. Physiol. **256:** R248–R254.
36. GREENBERG, D., J. GIBBS & G. P. SMITH. 1986. Intraduodenal infusions of fat inhibit sham feeding in Zucker rats. Brain Res. Bull. **17:** 599–604.
37. MCHUGH, P. R. & T. H. MORAN. 1986. The inhibition of feeding produced by direct intraintestinal infusion of glucose: Is this satiety? Brain Res. Bull. **17:** 415–418.
38. REIDELBERGER, R. D., T. J. KALOGERIS, P. M. LEUNG & V. E. MENDEL. 1983. Postgastric satiety in the sham feeding rat. Am. J. Physiol. **244:** R872–R881.
39. YOX, D. P. & R. C. RITTER. 1988. Capsaicin attenuates suppression of sham feeding induced by intestinal nutrients. Am. J. Physiol. **255:** R569–R574.
40. GIBBS, J., S. P. MADDISON & E. T. ROLLS. 1981. Satiety role of the small intestine examined in sham-feeding rhesus monkeys. J. Comp. Physiol. Psychol. **95:** 1003–1015.
41. WELCH, I. M., C. P. SEPPLE & N. W. READ. 1988. Comparisons of the effects on satiety and eating behavior of infusion of lipid into the different regions of the small intestine. Gut **29:** 306–311.
42. RITTER, R. C. & E. SIMON. 1989. Suppression of feeding by intraintestinal maltose is mediated by phloridzin-sensitive mechanism. Soc. Neurosci. Abstr. **16:** 646.
43. YOX, D. P., H. STOKESBERRY & R. C. RITTER. 1991. Vagotomy attenuates suppression of sham feeding induced by intestinal nutrients. Am. J. Physiol. **260:** R503–508.
44. YOX, D. P., H. STOKESBERRY & R. C. RITTER. 1991. Fourth ventricular capsaicin attenuates suppression of sham feeding induced by intestinal nutrients. Am. J. Physiol. **260:** R681–R687.
45. YOX, D. P., L. BRENNER & R. C. RITTER. 1992. CCK-receptor antagonists attenuate suppression of sham feeding by intestinal nutrients. Am. J. Physiol. **262:** R554–R561.
46. BRENNER, L. A. & R. C. RITTER. 1990. CCK-A but not CCK-B antagonist attenuates suppression of food intake by exogenous CCK or intraintestinal oleate. Soc. Neurosci. Abstr. **16:** 978.
47. SCHULTZBERG, M., T. HOKFELT, G. NILSSON, L. TERENIUS, J. F. REHFELD, M. BROWN, R. ELDE, M. GOLDSTEIN & S. SAID. 1980. Distribution of peptide- and catecholamine-containing neurons in the gastro-intestinal tract of rat and guinea-pig: Immunohistochemical studies with antisera to substance P, vasoactive intestinal polypeptide, enkephalins, somatostatin, gastrin/cholecystokinin, neurotensin and dopamine B-hydroxylase. Neuroscience **5:** 689–744.
48. FURNESS, J. B., M. COSTA, I. L. GIBBINS & I. J. LLEWELLYN-SMITH. 1985. Neurochemically similar myenteric and submucous neurons directly traced to the mucosa of the small intestine. Cell Tissue Res. **241:** 155–163.
49. INGRAM, S. M., R. G. KRAUSE II, F. BALDINO, JR., L. C. SKEEN & M. E. LEWIS. 1989. Neuronal localization of cholecystokinin mRNA in the rat brain by *in situ* hybridization histochemistry. J. Comp. Neural. **287:** 260–272.
50. HOKFELT, T., R. CORTES, M. SCHALLING, S. CECCATELLI, M. PELTO-HUIKKO, H. PERSSON & M. J. VILLAR. 1991. Distribution of patterns of CCK and CCK mRNA in some neuronal and non-neuronal tissues. Neuropeptides **19**(Suppl.): 31–43.
51. BRENNER, L. A. & R. C. RITTER. 1991. CCK-A receptor antagonist is more effective peripherally than centrally for attenuation of suppression of sham feeding by intestinal oleate. Soc. Neurosci. Abstr. **17:** 490.
52. RITTER, S. & T. T. DINH. 1988. Capsaicin-induced neuronal degeneration: silver impregnation of cell bodies, axons, and terminals in the central nervous system of the adult rat. J. Comp. Neurol. **271:** 79–90.
53. TAMURA, C. S. & R. C. RITTER. 1991. Transient, selective attenuation of oleate and CCK-induced suppression of sham feeding by intra-intestinal capsaicin. Soc. Neurosci. Abstr. **17:** 542.
54. TAMURA, C. S. & R. C. RITTER. 1992. Intestinal capsaicin attenuates oleate-induced suppression of food intake without causing anatomically detectable neuronal damage or impaired oleate absorption. Soc. Neurosci. Abstr. **18:** 1232.

55. Donnerer, J., L. Bartho, P. Holzer & F. Lembeck. 1984. Intestinal peristalsis associated with release of immunoreactive substance P. Neuroscience **11:** 913–918.
56. Holzer, P. 1988. Local effector functions of capsaicin-sensitive sensory nerve endings: Involvement of tachykinin, calcitonin gene-related peptide and other neuropeptides. Neuroscience **24:** 739–768.
57. Mayer, E. A., C. B. M. Koelbel, W. J. Snape, Jr., V. Eysselein, H. Ennes & A. Kodner. 1990. Substance P and CGRP mediate motor response of rabbit colon to capsaicin. Am. J. Physiol. **259:** G889–G897.
58. Renzi, D., S. Evangelista, P. Mantellini, P. Santicioli, C. A. Maggi, P. Geppetti & C. Surrenti. 1991. Capsaicin-induced release of neurokinin A from muscle and mucosa and gastric corpus: Correlation with capsaicin-evoked release of calcitonin gene-related peptide. Neuropeptides **19:** 137–145.
59. Hottenstein, O. D., W. W. Pawlik, G. Remak & E. D. Jacobson. 1991. Capsaicin-sensitive nerves modulate resting blood flow and vascular tone in rat gut. Naunyn-Schmiedeberg's Arch. Pharmacol. **343:** 179–184.
60. Bartho, L. & J. Szolesanyi. 1978. The site of action of capsaicin on the guinea-pig isolated ileum. Naunyn-Schmiedeberg's Arch. Pharmacol. **305:** 75–81.

# Role of Cholecystokinin in the Regulation of Satiation and Satiety in Humans

R. J. LIEVERSE,[a] J. B. M. J. JANSEN,[b] A. A. M. MASCLEE,[a] AND C. B. H. W. LAMERS[a,c]

Department of Gastroenterology and Hepatology
University Hospitals of Leiden[a] and Nijmegen[b]
Leiden, the Netherlands

In 1928 cholecystokinin (CCK) was identified from preparations of intestinal extracts by its ability to stimulate gallbladder contraction.[1] Later, other biological actions of CCK, such as stimulation of pancreatic exocrine secretion, delayed gastric emptying, stimulation of intestinal motility, and stimulation of insulin secretion, were identified.[1]

From 1973 a number of reports have demonstrated that CCK induces satiety in several species.[2-36] There are central and peripheral satiation signals. Feeding depression was caused by CCK injected intraperitoneally in rats,[2,9,11,30,32] intraarterially in pigs,[5] intravenously in cats and pigs,[4,6] into the cerebral ventricles in monkeys, rats, dogs, and sheep,[2,10,13,16,34] and intravenously in obese[21] and nonobese humans.[24,35] Inasmuch as plasma CCK was not measured in these studies, it is not clear if this satiation-inducing effect of the administered doses of CCK represented a physiologic or a pharmacologic effect of the peptide.

To elucidate the physiologic role of CCK in the regulation of satiation and satiety in humans, we measured food intake and preprandial and postprandial satiety parameters during the following experiments: (1) infusion of the CCK-receptor antagonist loxiglumide; (2) infusion of a physiologic dose of CCK without and with a preload; and (3) stimulation of endogenous CCK by a low dose of intraduodenal fat. To determine possible differences between lean and obese subjects, we performed the first two studies in both lean and obese persons.

SATIETY EFFECTS OF THE CCK RECEPTOR ANTAGONIST LOXIGLUMIDE

We gave the CCK-A receptor antagonist loxiglumide to 14 healthy (7 lean, 7 obese) women and compared the effects on food intake and hunger feelings with a control saline infusion in a randomized double-blind protocol. The dose of loxiglumide given (10 mg/kg/h) is known to completely inhibit pancreatic enzyme secretion, gallbladder contraction, and bilirubin output in response to exogenous CCK-8 administered in a dose that produced plasma CCK concentrations higher than those observed after a meal.[37]

Loxiglumide did not significantly influence intake of the carbohydrate-rich meal or affect pre- and postprandial hunger feelings. Thus, this study does not support an important role of CCK in the regulation of satiation or satiety.[38]

[c]Address for correspondence: Prof. Dr. C. B. H. W. Lamers, Dept. of Gastroenterology and Hepatology, University Hospital, Building 1, C4-P, Rijnsburgerweg 10, 2333 AA Leiden, the Netherlands.

INFUSION OF CCK LEADING TO PHYSIOLOGIC PLASMA LEVELS

Because in previous studies in humans the doses of CCK that induced satiety might well have led to supraphysiologic plasma levels, we studied the effect of infusion of a physiologic dose of CCK-33 on food intake and hunger feelings. One IDU/kg ideal weight/h CCK-33 was infused, which led to similar plasma CCK levels as found after a large mixed meal. In the first studies the amount of banana slices eaten 60 minutes after the start of CCK infusion and the pre- and postprandial hunger feelings were compared with those of a control saline infusion in a double-blind randomized experiment.[39] We chose bananas because most people like them, and as a carbohydrate-rich meal they do not induce endogenous CCK release. Otherwise the endogenously released CCK added to the CCK infusion might have led to supraphysiologic plasma levels.

In the 18 subjects (9 lean, 9 obese) studied food intake during saline (553 ± 55 g) was somewhat higher than that during CCK infusion (486 ± 52 g), but the difference just failed to reach statistical significance.

Because in human studies by Pi-Sunyer et al.[21] and Kissileff et al.[24] in which CCK decreased food intake after a preload was given, we repeated our experiment on 18 other women (10 lean, 8 obese). In this experiment 60 minutes after the start of the infusion a preload, consisting of 100 g of bananas supplemented with 300 ml of water and mixed, was ingested 15 minutes before the banana slice meal. In this experiment the same dose of CCK induced significant feeding suppression from 346 ± 31 to 282 ± 29 g ($p < 0.05$).[40]

Hunger feelings tended to be decreased by CCK in this experiment. After the preload, CCK induced also a satiety effect specific for fatty items. No significant differences were noted between lean and obese subjects. CCK plasma levels were measured by a sensitive and specific radioimmunoassay.[41] Infusion of CCK resulted in significant increases in plasma CCK concentrations, stabilizing within 60 minutes of infusion at values fluctuating around 12 pM in both lean and obese subjects.[39,40] After a large mixed meal, similar plasma CCK concentrations were found in healthy volunteers using the same assay.[42] In conclusion, a physiologic dose of CCK influences food intake and satiety parameters especially after a preload meal.

SATIETY EFFECTS OF ENDOGENOUS CCK

In 10 healthy lean volunteers we studied the satiety effect of endogenous CCK. A low dose of intraduodenal fat (6 g intralipid 20%/h) was given to stimulate endogenous CCK release, and the effect of food intake and hunger feelings was compared with a control experiment in which saline solution was given intraduodenally.[43] To determine if CCK was responsible for satiety effects if present, we also gave intraduodenal fat combined with the CCK-A receptor antagonist loxiglumide (10 mg/kg/h). In that experiment intraduodenal fat had only a weak effect on food intake (269 ± 37 vs 206 ± 36 g; $p = 0.09$) and satiety. This effect was specific for fatty items and largely prevented by loxiglumide, which increased food intake to 245 ± 30 g and significantly reversed satiety parameters.

The only other study on the effect of intraduodenal fat on plasma CCK and satiety employed a much larger amount of fat.[44] In that study Drewe et al.[44] demonstrated that an intraduodenal infusion of 36 g of lipid per hour induced significant satiation compared to saline solution which could not be blocked by loxiglumide.[44] The discrepancy between both studies may be due to differences in the amounts of fat administered intraduodenally. It is possible that disturbed gastrointestinal motility after the high caloric load by the high fat dose may have overruled the satiety effect of CCK.[45] In our studies, using a much smaller dose of intraduodenal fat, we found evidence that endogenous CCK does exert satiety effects in humans. The effects, however, were rather weak.

CONCLUSION

Our experiments demonstrate that CCK in physiologic plasma concentrations inhibits food intake and increases satiety in both lean and obese humans. The effect, however, is weak and depends on the experimental protocol. It is possible that interaction with other mechanisms, such as the serotonergic system, is necessary for full expression of CCK's action on satiety.[46-48]

REFERENCES

1. LIDDLE, R. A. 1989. Integrated actions of cholecystokinin on the gastrointestinal tract: Use of the cholecystokinin bioassay. Gastroenterol. Clin. North Am. **18:** 735–756.
2. LINDEN, A. 1989. Role of cholecystokinin in feeding and lactation. Acta Physiol. Scand. Suppl. **585:** 1–49.
3. GIBBS, J., R. C. YOUNG & G. P. SMITH. 1973. Cholecystokinin decreases food intake in rats. J. Comp. Physiol. Psychol. **84:** 488–495.
4. BADO, A., M. RODRIGUEZ, M. J. M. LEWIN, J. MARTINEZ & M. DUBRASQUET. 1988. Cholecystokinin suppresses food intake in cats: Structure-activity characterization. Pharmacol. Biochem. Behav. **31:** 297–303.
5. GREGORY, P. C., M. MCFADYEN & D. V. RAYNER. 1989. Duodenal infusion of fat, cholecystokinin secretion and satiety in the pig. Physiol. Behav. **45:** 1021–1024.
6. EBENEZER, I. S., C. DE LA RIVA & B. A. BALDWIN. 1990. Effects of the CCK receptor antagonist MK-329 on food intake in pigs. Physiol. Behav. **47:** 145–148.
7. WELLER, A., G. P. SMITH & J. GIBBS. 1989. Endogenous cholecystokinin reduces feeding in young rats. Science **247:** 1589–1591.
8. HEWSON, G., G. E. LEIGHTON, R. G. HILL & J. HUGHES. 1988. The cholecystokinin receptor antagonist L 364,718 increases food intake in the rat by attenuation of the action of endogenous cholecystokinin. Br. J. Pharmacol. **93:** 79–84.
9. MCCOY, J. G., F. STUMP & D. D. AVERY. 1990. Intake of individual macronutrients following ip injections of BBS and CCK in rats. Peptides **11:** 221–225.
10. DELLA-FERA, M. A. & C. A. BAILE. 1979. Cholecystokinin octapeptide: Continuous picomole injections into the cerebral ventricles of sheep suppress feeding. Science **206:** 471–473.
11. GOURCH, A., M. OROSCO, M. RODRIGUEZ, J. MARTINEZ, Y. COHEN & C. JACQUET. 1990. Effects of a new cholecystokinin analogue (JMV236) on food intake and brain monoamines in the rat. Neuropeptides **15:** 37–41.
12. SMITH, G. P. 1984. The therapeutic potential of cholecystokinin. Int. J. Obes. **8** suppl 1: 35–38.
13. FIGLEWICZ, D. P., A. SIPOLS, D. PORTE, JR. & S. C. WOODS. 1986. Intraventricular bombesin can decrease single meal size in the baboon. Brain. Res. Bull. **17:** 535–537.
14. SILVER, A. J., J. FLOOD, A. M. SONG & J. E. MORLEY. 1989. Evidence for a physiological role for CCK in the regulation of food intake in mice. Am. J. Physiol. **256:** R646–R652.
15. REIDELBERGER, R. D. & M. F. O'ROURKE. 1989. Potent cholecystokinin antagonist L 364718 stimulates food intake in rats. Am. J. Physiol. **257:** R1512–R1518.
16. INUI, A., M. OKITA, T. INOUE, O. SAKATANI, M. OYA, H. MORIOKA, M. OIMOMI & S. BABA. 1989. Effect of cholecystokinin octapeptide analogues on food intake in the dog. Am. J. Physiol. **257:** R949–R951.

17. STACHER, G. 1986. Effects of cholecystokinin and caerulein on human eating behavior and pain sensation: A review. Psychoneuroendocrinology **11:** 39–48.
18. MCHUGH, P. R. & T. H. MORAN. 1986. The stomach, cholecystokinin and satiety. Fed. Proc. **45:** 1384–1390.
19. MORLEY, J. E. 1987. Neuropeptide regulation of appetite and weight. Endocr. Rev. **8:** 256–287.
20. STALLONE, D., S. NICOLAIDIS & J. GIBBS. 1989. Cholecystokinin-induced anorexia depends on serotoninergic function. Am. J. Physiol. **256:** R1138–R1141.
21. PI-SUNYER, X., H. R. KISSILEFF, J. THOMTON & G. P. SMITH. 1982. C-Terminal octapeptide of cholecystokinin decreases food intake in obese man. Physiol. Behav. **29:** 627–630.
22. PIETROWSKY, R., S. PREUSS, J. BORN, et al. 1989. Effects of cholecystokinin and calcitonin on evoked brain potentials and satiety in man. Physiol. Behav. **46:** 513–519.
23. BAILE, C. A., C. L. MCLAUGHLIN & M. A. DELLA-FERA. 1986. Role of cholecystokinin and opioid peptides in control of food intake. Physiol. Rev. **66:** 172–234.
24. KISSILEFF, H. R., X. PI-SUNYER, J. THORNTON & G. P. SMITH. 1981. C-terminal octapeptide of cholecystokinin decreases food intake in man. Am. J. Clin. Nutr. **34:** 154–160.
25. MORAN, T. H. & P. R. MCHUGH. 1988. Gastric and nongastric mechanisms for satiety action of cholecystokinin. Am. J. Physiol. **254:** R628–R632.
26. WEST, D. B., D. FEY & S. C. WOODS. 1984. Cholecystokinin persistently suppresses meal size but not food intake in free-feeding rats. Am. J. Physiol. **246:** R776–R787.
27. MINEKA, S. & C. T. SNOWDON. 1987. Inconsistency and possible habituation of CCK-induced satiety. Physiol. Behav. **21:** 65–72.
28. MCLAUGHLIN, C. L. & C. A. BAILE. 1980. Decreased sensitivity of Zucker obese rats to the putative satiety agent cholecystokinin. Physiol. Behav. **25:** 543–548.
29. LE SAUTER, J. & N. GEARY. 1990. Redundant vagal mediation of the synergistic satiety effect of pancreatic glucagon and cholecystokinin in sham feeding rats. J. Auton. Nerv. Syst. **30:** 13–22.
30. MCLAUGHLIN, C. L., S. R. PEIKIN & C. A. BAILE. 1983. Food intake response to modulation of secretion of cholecystokinin in Zucker rats. Am. J. Physiol. **244:** R676–R685.
31. MCLAUGHLIN, C. L., S. R. PEIKIN & C. A. BAILE. 1983. Trypsin inhibitor effects on food intake and weight gain in Zucker rats. Physiol. Behav. **31:** 487–491.
32. MCLAUGHLIN, C. L., C. A. BAILE & F. C. BUONOMO. 1985. Effect of CCK antibodies on food intake and weight gain in Zucker rats. Physiol. Behav. **34:** 277–282.
33. MCLAUGHLIN, C. L. & C. A. BAILE. 1980. Feeding and drinking behavior response of adult Zucker obese rats to cholecystokinin. Physiol. Behav. **25:** 535–541.
34. DELLA-FERA, M. A. & C. A. BAILE. 1979. Cholecystokinin octapeptide: Continuous picomole injections into the cerebral ventricles of sheep suppress feeding. Science **206:** 471–473.
35. STACHER, G., H. STEINRINGER, G. SCHMIERER, C. SCHNEIDER & S. WINKLEHNER. 1982. Cholecystokinin octapeptide decreases intake of solid food in man. Peptides **1:** 133–136.
36. SILVER, A. J. & J. E. MORLEY. 1991. Role of CCK in regulation of food intake. Prog. Neurobiol. **36:** 23–34.
37. SCHMIDT, W. E., W. CREUTZFELDT, A. SCHLESER, A. R. CHOUDHURY, R. NASTEDE, M. HÖCKER, R. NIHDRE, H. SOSTMANN, L. C. ROVATI & U. R. FÖLSCH. 1991. Role of CCK in regulation of pancreaticobiliary functions and GI motility in humans: Effects of loxiglumide. Am. J. Physiol. **260:** G197–G206.
38. LIEVERSE, R. J. 1993. Peripheral Regulation of Satiety in Humans. I.C.G. Printing. Dordrecht, The Netherlands.
39. LIEVERSE, R. J., J. B. M. J. JANSEN, A. VD ZWAN, L. SAMSON, A. A. M. MASCLEE & C. B. H. W. LAMERS. 1993. Effects of a physiological dose of cholecystokinin on food intake and postprandial satiation in man. Regul. Pept. **43:** 83–89.
40. LIEVERSE, R. J., J. B. M. J. JANSEN, A. A. M. MASCLEE & C. B. H. W. LAMERS. 1993. Satiety effects of a physiologic dose of cholecystokinin in man. Gastroenterology **104:** A632.

41. JANSEN, J. B. M. J. & C. B. H. W. LAMERS. 1983. Radioimmunoassay of cholecystokinin in human tissue and plasma. Clin. Chim. Acta **131:** 305–316.
42. FRIED, M., E. A. MAYER, J. B. M. J. JANSEN, C. B. H. W. LAMERS, I. L. TAYLOR, S. R. BLOOM & J. H. MEYER. 1988. Temporal relationships of cholecystokinin release, pancreatobiliary secretion, and gastric emptying of a mixed meal. Gastroenterology **95:** 1344–1350.
43. LIEVERSE, R. J., J. B. M. J. JANSEN, A. A. M. MASCLEE & C. B. H. W. LAMERS. 1993. Satiety and satiation effects of endogenous cholecystokinin in humans. Gastroenterology **104:** A632.
44. DREWE, J., A. GADIENT, L. C. ROVATI & C. BEGLINER. 1992. Role of circulating cholecystokinin in control of fat-induced inhibition of food intake in humans. Gastroenterology **102:** 1654–1659.
45. EHRLEIN, H. J. 1992. Recording of intestinal motility is a useful control of enteral nutrition. Clin. Nutr. **11**(Suppl. 62).
46. COOPER, S. J. & C. T. DOURISH. 1990. Multiple cholecystokinin (CCK) receptors and CCK-monoamine interactions are instrumental in the control of feeding. Physiol. Behav. **48:** 849–857.
47. COOPER, S. J., C. T. DOURISH & D. J. BARBER. 1990. Reversal of the anorectic effect of (+)-fenfluramine in the rat by the selective cholecystokinin receptor antagonist MK-329. Br. J. Pharmacol. **99:** 65–70.
48. POESCHLA, B., J. GIBBS, K. J. SIMANSKY, D. GREENBERG & G. P. SMITH. 1993. Cholecystokinin-induced satiety depends on activation of 5-HT_{1C} receptors. Am. J. Physiol. **264:** R62–R64.

The Cholecystokinin Hypothesis of Anxiety and Panic Disorder[a]

JACQUES BRADWEJN AND DIANA KOSZYCKI

Department of Psychiatry
McGill University
St Mary's Hospital
3830 Lacombe Ave.
Montreal, Quebec, Canada H3T 1M5

Panic disorder is one of the more incapacitating anxiety disorders that afflicts approximately 2% of the general population. The hallmark of panic disorder is the repeated occurrence of discrete episodes of intense anxiety that appear to occur spontaneously, are perceived to be uncontrollable, and are accompanied by unpleasant physical sensations such as palpitations, chest pain, dyspnea, choking, sweating, tremors, faintness and paraesthesia, psychosensory symptoms such as depersonalization, and cognitive symptoms such as fear of losing control, going crazy, or dying.[1] A panic attack can last from a few minutes to more than an hour, and intense fatigue is frequently reported at the conclusion of the episode. Outbursts of dramatic behavior, other than appearing ill at ease, seldom occur during an attack. Stress or aversive life events may precipitate panic attacks in vulnerable individuals; however, many individuals experience recurrent attacks of panic anxiety during nonstressful periods.[2] Panic disorder typically emerges in young adults and is reduced after age 65.[3]

Panic disorder invariably imparts anticipatory fear that these attacks of panic anxiety will recur unexpectedly.[4] In many individuals, agoraphobia develops as a consequence of panic experiences and anticipatory anxiety. Typically, the agoraphobic person exhibits marked fear of a constellation of situations in which escape might be difficult or help not available in the event of a panic attack. These situations include unfamiliar places, crowds, public places, tunnels and bridges, traveling in a car, bus, or train, and being alone. In its extreme form the individual becomes completely housebound. Although the prevalence of panic disorder is evenly distributed between males and females in the absence of agoraphobia, panic disorder with agoraphobia affects twice as many women as men. In any event, panic disorder with or without agoraphobia is chronic, punctuated by pervasive social alterations,[5,6] health risks[7-9] and comorbid psychiatric disturbances, particularly depression,[6] increased risk for suicide,[10] and substance abuse.[11] Panic disorder appears to be familial,[12,13] and data derived from twin studies are compatible with a genetic transmission hypothesis for the disorder.[14]

During the last decade studies investigating the neurobiology of panic disorder have proliferated. Some of the research strategies that have been adopted have involved analysis of (1) plasma and urinary metabolite concentrations associated with some behavioral concomitants of the disorder, (2) hormonal release profiles accompanying pharmacological challenges as an indicant of hypothalamic pituitary

---

[a]The clinical studies reviewed in this paper received financial support from the Fonds de la Recherche en Santé du Québec, the Medical Research Council of Canada, St Mary's Hospital Foundation, and Psychopharmacology Fund.

dysfunction and central noradrenergic and/or serotonergic receptor alteration, (3) peripheral receptor alterations associated with the disorder, (4) pharmacological interventions that are effective in blocking panic attacks, (5) cerebral blood flow profiles, and (6) induction of panic with various panicogenic challenges.

These studies have generated theoretical constructs concerning the etiology of panic disorder. In particular, it has been hypothesized that central noradrenaline (NE), serotonin (5-HT), adenosine, and GABA activity play a significant role in mediating symptoms of panic. Recent work primarily conducted in our laboratory has led to speculation that alterations of cholecystokinin (CCK) activity contribute to the pathophysiology of panic disorder. Clinical evidence in support of the CCK hypothesis of panic is described in this report. It is important to emphasize that any unitary neurochemical hypothesis of panic disorder is overly simplistic and potentially counterproductive. The diverse behavioral and neurochemical profile associated with this disorder and the considerable interindividual variability that has been described in the clinical literature suggest that panic attacks may well follow from the interactive and cascading influence of various neuronal systems that vary as a function of the duration and severity of the illness, the influence of comorbidity, as well as genetic and organismic variables. Moreover, the recent demonstration of colocalization mosaics in the central nervous system and the neuromodulatory role of various neuropeptides[15] suggest a complex neurochemical interaction in promoting symptoms of panic.

CCK HYPOTHESIS OF PANIC DISORDER: HISTORICAL PERSPECTIVE

The hypothesis that CCK may be a mediator of anxiety originated from electrophysiological experiments by Bradwejn and de Montigny[16] which demonstrated that benzodiazepine receptor agonists (flurazepam, chlordiazepoxide, lorazepam, or diazepam) selectively and specifically antagonized CCK-8S–induced excitation of hippocampal pyramidal neurons in rats and that this effect was reversed by pretreatment with the benzodiazepine receptor antagonist flumazenil. Additional experiments with PK 8165, a partial benzodiazepine receptor agonist with anxiolytic but no demonstrable sedative, anticonvulsant, or myorelaxant effects, revealed that the antagonism by benzodiazepines of CCK-8S–induced excitation was specifically related to their anxiolytic action.[17] Dose response curves of the intravenous effect of lorazepam or diazepam on excitations produced by CCK-8S revealed ED_{50} (effective dose for 50% inhibition) values of 32 and 106 µg per kilo, respectively. These values fall within the range of clinically used doses for these medications.

These studies provided the first evidence that anxiolytic benzodiazepines could antagonize the central action of a neuropeptide, and it was proposed that benzodiazepine-mediated antagonism of CCK-induced excitation might be an important mechanism by which benzodiazepines exert their clinically relevant action. More importantly, the observation that an anxiolytic could block the excitatory action of CCK raised questions about whether CCK might be an endogenous anxiogen. Two pilot studies, one in patients with panic disorder and the other in healthy subjects with no personal or family history of panic attacks, were conducted using the tetrapeptide form of CCK (CCK-4) to address this question. The decision to administer the tetrapeptide form to patients with panic disorder was based on anecdotal data presented at a CCK conference in 1984 by the biochemist Jens Rehfeld. In the course of investigating the neuroendocrine effects of CCK-4 in healthy human subjects, he noted that CCK-4 produced a number of "side effects" such as anxiety, dyspnea, and depersonalization.[18,19] In our assessment, these side effects were strikingly similar to symptoms experienced by panic patients during their spontaneous panic attacks.

Bradwejn and colleagues first administered CCK-4 to patients with a current-point diagnosis of panic disorder using a double-blind placebo control methodology. Bolus injections of CCK-4 (50 μg) precipitated a panic attack, as defined by DSM-III criteria and patient self-report, within 1 minute after administration in 11 trial patients studied, whereas none of the patients panicked after placebo.[20] In addition, CCK-4 elicited an average of 12 symptoms per patient, the most common symptoms being dyspnea, palpitations/rapid heart, chest pain/discomfort, faintness, dizziness, paraesthesia, hot flushes/cold chills, nausea/abdominal distress, anxiety/fear/apprehension, and fear of losing control. De Montigny first reported that exogenous CCK-4 produced "panic-like" attacks in healthy volunteers and that these effects could be attenuated by pretreatment with lorazepam.[21]

Taken together, these preliminary data suggested a potential link between CCK activity and panic disorder.

VALIDATION OF CCK-4 AS A PANICOGENIC AGENT

Our finding of a close analogy between symptoms produced by CCK-4 and those reported to occur during patients' spontaneous panic attacks was intriguing and suggested that CCK-4 might be a suitable paradigm for studying the neurobiology of panic disorder and for anxiety research in general. An important task we set for ourselves was to systematically evaluate the validity of CCK-4 as a model of panic using the seven criteria for an "ideal" panicogenic agent described by Guttmacher *et al.*[22] and Gorman *et al.*[23] The seven criteria are as follows:

1. *The agent should be safe.* CCK-4 is safe to administer to human subjects. We injected CCK-4 in over 200 subjects, and except for a brief vasovagal reaction occurring in less than 5% of subjects, no significant adverse effects were observed.

2. *The agent should induce affective as well as somatic symptoms of a panic attack.* CCK-4 generates both emotional (e.g., anxiety, fear, and apprehension) and somatic symptoms (e.g., dyspnea, palpitations, choking, sweating, and faintness) that typically occur during a panic attack.[24] In our studies, a subjective sense of anxiety, fear and/or apprehension as well as at least four DSM-III-R somatic symptoms are important criteria for judging the occurrence of a panic attack.

3. *The agent should provoke attacks that resemble the patient's clinical panic attacks.* The panic attacks induced by CCK-4 have been appraised by patients as identical or very similar to their spontaneous panic attacks in terms of the type and quality of symptoms.[20,25] This has been important criterion of panic attack in our studies with patients. Moreover, CCK-4 does not induce a stereotyped response in patients. Rather it mimics the individual symptom profile usually experienced by each patient. Most patients reported that the main difference between the CCK-4–induced panic attack and their clinical attacks is that the symptoms induced with CCK-4 occur more abruptly and are generally of shorter duration.

4. *The effects of the agent should be specific for patients with a history of panic attacks.* We found that the response to CCK-4 reliably differentiates panic disorder patients from healthy controls with no personal or family history of panic attacks. In a double-blind placebo control study we noted that patients with panic disorder experienced more symptoms and more intense symptoms after challenge with two doses of CCK-4 (25 and 50 μg).[25] In addition, the incidence of panic attacks was markedly higher in patients than controls after injection of 25 μg (91% *versus* 17%) and 50 μg (100% *versus* 47%) of the peptide. Interestingly, we noted that the number

and intensity of symptoms as well as the symptom profile were remarkably similar in both patients and normal subjects who panicked with the 50 µg dose of CCK-4, suggesting that the enhanced response to CCK in patients could not readily be attributed to a tendency to overendorse symptoms. Our results are corroborated by a study by Abelson and Nesse[26] using pentagastrin, a CCK agonist that incorporates the identical 4-amino acid sequence of CCK-4. These investigators found that pentagastrin provoked panic attacks at a higher frequency in patients with panic disorder than in healthy subjects. Further studies are required to determine if the effects of CCK-4 can differentiate patients with panic disorder from those with other psychiatric syndromes.

5. *The effects of the agent should be reliable.* To determine if the behavioral effects of CCK-4 could be replicated in the same individual, we administered 25 µg of CCK-4 to 11 panic patients on two separate occasions in the absence of intervening treatment.[27] Although the latency to effect symptoms with CCK-4 was significantly shorter on the second challenge day, the vulnerability of patients to the panicogenic properties of CCK-4 was undiminished with repeated challenge. Panic attack frequency after the initial and subsequent challenge was 82% and 73%, respectively. In addition, the number and intensity of symptoms remained constant with rechallenge.

The effectiveness of CCK-4 in provoking panic responses also appears to be dose dependent. In a double-blind dose response study of CCK-4 (0, 10, 15, 20, and 25 µg) in patients with panic disorder, a significant linear relation was found for the number and sum intensity of symptoms evoked with CCK-4.[28] All doses of CCK-4 produced a significantly greater number of symptoms than did the placebo, whereas the sum intensity scores were significantly higher with the 15, 20, and 25 µg dose of CCK-4 than with placebo. The panic attack rate was 17% (10 µg), 64% (15 µg), 75% (20 µg), and 75% (25 µg). None of the patients panicked with placebo (0 µg). The difference between treatments in panic frequency was significant, and there was a significant linear dose-response effect. Paralleling the behavioral changes induced with CCK-4, a marked and dose-related increase in heart rate and blood pressure was evident. In another double-blind study with 36 healthy volunteers, CCK-4 (0, 9, 25, and 50 µg) was also found to induce panic attacks in a dose-dependent manner; the panic rate was 11% (9 µg), 17% (25 µg), and 47% (50 µg).[29] No panic attacks occurred with placebo injections.

6. *Antipanic agents should block the effects of the agent.* Recently, we demonstrated that the panicogenic effects of CCK-4 can be antagonized by chronic treatment with imipramine.[30] Specifically, 11 patients with panic disorder who displayed a positive panicogenic response to CCK-4 (20 µg) were treated with imipramine on a chronic basis and rechallenged with CCK-4 (20 µg) after being free of both panic and agoraphobic symptoms for at least 8 weeks. With rechallenge, patients displayed a marked reduction in the number and sum intensity of symptoms, duration of symptoms, and cardiovascular responsiveness. Moreover, only 2 of the 11 patients who previously panicked with CCK-4 experienced a panic attack when rechallenged. Also, patients who ingested higher doses of imipramine experienced fewer and less intense panic symptoms at rechallenge, suggesting that the decreased sensitivity to CCK-4 after chronic imipramine therapy was most likely attributed to a drug effect rather than to other factors such as spontaneous remission of symptoms.

7. *The effects of the agent are not antagonized by drugs without antipanic effects.* Indirect evidence indicates that CCK-4 also satisfies this criterion. In the context of investigating the effects of CCK-B receptor antagonists on CCK-4–induced panic symptoms, we observed that pretreatment with placebo failed to antagonize CCK-4–induced panic symptoms in patients with panic disorder.[24] In another study which

investigated the possible mediating role of benzodiazepine receptors in CCK-4–induced panic symptoms, pretreatment with the benzodiazepine receptor antagonist flumazenil, a compound without any known antipanic activity, failed to diminish the response to CCK-4 challenge in healthy volunteers.[31]

Another research approach we employed in evaluating whether CCK-4 is a valid panicogen was to compare its effects with those produced by other valid pharmacological models of panic. So far, we compared the response to a 25-µg dose of CCK-4 and a single inhalation of 35% CO_2 in patients with panic disorder[32] and healthy volunteers.[33] In the study with patients, CCK-4 produced more symptoms and symptoms of more intensity than did 35% CO_2. CCK-4 was also more effective than CO_2 in inducing panic attacks (91% *versus* 45%), but the profile of symptoms that emerged in response to either agent was similar in patients who experienced a panic attack. Although CCK-4 produced more intense panic symptoms than did CO_2 in healthy volunteers, these concentrations of CCK-4 and CO_2 were equipotent in promoting panic attacks (17% *versus* 21%). It will be interesting in future studies to compare CCK-4 with other panicogenic challenges, particularly the frequently employed sodium lactate infusion.

Overall, the data just summarized demonstrate that CCK-4 satisfies previously established criteria for an ideal panicogenic agent and it compares well to at least one widely accepted pharmacological model of panic. It is also important to mention that of all the pharmacological agents known to provoke panic attacks in humans, including sodium lactate, CO_2, caffeine, yohimbine, isoproterenol, and mCPP, CCK-4 is the only one that fulfills criteria for a neurotransmitter. Cholecystokinin is well characterized in the CNS and is abundant in brain regions implicated in the promotion of panic attacks including the brainstem, hippocampus, amygdala, and cerebral cortex.[34] Moreover, biochemical and electrophysiological data suggest interactions between CCK and multiple neurotransmitter systems, including serotonin, noradrenaline, GABA, and dopamine. As a panicogenic agent, therefore, CCK-4 provides an important opportunity to identify an endogenous anomaly associated with panic disorder and to enhance our understanding of the multiple neurotransmitter systems that potentially contribute to the generation of panic attacks.

Another important feature of CCK-4 is that it is simple to administer in a low volume intravenous bolus infusion (in less than 5 seconds). This method of administration has considerable advantages over the slow infusion procedures required to induce symptoms of panic with other panicogens, particularly sodium lactate. The relatively protracted infusion interval has been associated with physiological alterations, such as volume overload, and metabolic changes that can introduce nonspecific psychological effects.[35] Another technical advantage is that the latency to effect symptoms of panic with CCK-4 is rapid and predictable, permitting measurement of central and peripheral nervous system activity during the interval associated with peak panic symptoms. Considered together, the technical advantage of CCK-4 administration, coupled with its presence in the CNS, commends its use for research into the pathophysiology of panic disorder.

The data generated from our validation studies also highlight the usefulness of CCK-4 as a panicogenic challenge for research in anxiety. For instance, demonstration that the effects of CCK-4 are reproducible in the same patient has important implications in testing the effectiveness of antipanic drugs in blocking CCK-4–induced panic symptoms. In addition, the dose-response study in patients indicated that a 20-µg dose of CCK-4, which produced panic attacks in 75% of patients, might be suitable for efficacy studies. In particular, this dose promotes noticeable changes in behavior and other indices of anxiety without being so potent as to mask the effectiveness of potential antipanic drugs to block the effects of CCK-4. We successfully used this dose to evaluate the effects of a CCK-B receptor antagonist and imipramine on CCK-4–induced panic symptoms.

Finally, the behavioral effects of exogenous CCK-4 in clinical paradigms are paralleled by data describing the effects of exogenous CCK-4 in nonhuman primates. Ervin et al.[36] reported that intravenous CCK-4 administration in the unrestrained green vervet monkey produced behavioral activation reminiscent of fear and defense posturing. The emergence of these behaviors was dose-related and largely influenced by the baseline behavioral profile of the individual animal in its social environment. For example, high CCK-4 doses produced immobilization and freezing in ordinarily anxious and fidgety monkeys, but it actually promoted mild restlessness and activation in naturally calm monkeys. Immobilization and freezing have been observed in monkeys in response to social stress or threat, and they are thought to be behavioral equivalents of human fear and panic.[37] CCK agonists, such as CCK-4, pentagastrin, and CCK-8, are also reported to have potent anxiogenic effects in rodent models of anxiety.[38]

MECHANISM OF ANXIOGENIC ACTION OF CCK-4

The mechanism and localization of CCK-4–induced panic symptoms are still largely unknown. Several investigations using animal models of anxiety revealed that the anxiogenic effects of CCK-4 are blocked by selective CCK-B receptor antagonists, suggesting that CCK-B receptors are an important site of anxiogenic action of exogenous CCK-4. We recently completed a study which suggests that CCK-B receptors are also important mediators of the behavioral and cardiovascular changes during CCK-4 challenge in humans.[39] Patients with panic disorder were pretreated with L-365,260 (10 or 50 mg po) or placebo 90 minutes before challenge with CCK-4. Analysis of the data indicated that the 50-mg dose of L-365,260 was superior to placebo in reducing the number of symptoms induced with CCK-4, the sum intensity of symptoms, and the panic attack frequency. Moreover, when compared with placebo, both the 10- and 50-mg dose of the antagonist dramatically decreased CCK-4–evoked increases in heart rate. It will be important to determine in future studies if other CCK-B receptor antagonists are equally effective in attenuating the effects of CCK-4 in humans and if these compounds have therapeutic value in the treatment of clinical panic attacks.

In addition to investigating the involvement of CCK-B receptors, we evaluated if benzodiazepine receptors contribute to the behavioral effects of CCK-4. As indicated earlier, benzodiazepine receptor agonists selectively and specifically antagonized CCK-8S–induced excitation of rat hippocampal neurons. It was subsequently demonstrated that neuronal responsiveness to CCK-8 in rats decreases after long-term administration of benzodiazepine agonists.[40] Evidence also exists that benzodiazepine receptor agonists attenuate the anxiogenic effects of exogenous CCK-4 in nonhuman primates[41] and healthy volunteers;[21] however, such data to not establish that benzodiazepine receptor activity invariably contribute to the panicogenic effects of CCK-4.

To further explore the role of benzodiazepine receptors in CCK-4–induced panic symptoms, we determined if pretreatment with the benzodiazepine receptor antagonist flumazenil could influence response to CCK-4 in healthy volunteers using a double-blind placebo control cross-over design. In investigating the potential interaction between CCK and benzodiazepine receptors in CCK-4–induced panic response, we proposed a model that was based on the premise that exogenous CCK-4, through actions on CCK-B receptors, interacts with benzodiazepine receptors in eliciting symptoms by indirectly acting as a benzodiazepine receptor inverse agonist. In other words, we postulated that CCK-4 might act as an endogenous "virtual" inverse agonist of benzodiazepine receptors. To support this hypothesis, it was necessary to determine if flumazenil could antagonize the panicogenic effects of CCK-4. Our findings indicate that benzodiazepine receptors are not mediators of CCK-4–induced panic symptoms in normal subjects. We found no discernible difference between flumazenil and placebo pretreatment in the number of symptoms induced with CCK-4, sum intensity of symptoms, and panic attack frequency.[31]

The mechanism by which the NE, 5-HT, and adenosine systems participate in CCK-4–induced anxiety has yet to be investigated. Our study which showed that chronic treatment with imipramine, which inhibits NE and 5-HT reuptake, could antagonize the panicogenic effects of CCK-4 in patients with panic disorder argues that these monoamines may be instrumental in interacting with CCK in promoting symptoms of panic. Also, some interesting data suggest that 5-HT_3 receptors are mediators of CCK-induced anxiety. In this respect, Vasar and his associates[42] reported that the anxiogenic effect of caerulein, a CCK agonist, was prevented by prior treatment with the 5-HT_3 receptor antagonist ondansetron. The possible interaction between CCK and adenosine receptors is supported by the finding that NECA (N-ethylcarboxamido-adenosine), an agonist of adenosine A_2 receptors, antagonized the anxiogenic effects of CCK-4 in nonhuman primates.[41]

Another question of central importance concerns the site(s) of action of this peptide in humans. Currently, there is no available evidence that CCK-4 crosses the blood-brain barrier, but the possibility exists that CCK-4 affects CCK-B receptors in brain regions that are not fully protected by the blood-brain barrier. Knowledge of cardiovascular neurophysiology as well as studies of the behavioral and cardiovascular effects of CCK-4 permits speculation as to the possible site of action of CCK-4. Some investigators have suggested that brainstem regions ordinarily function to monitor sympathetic nerve discharge and vasomotor tone. Increases in blood pressure and heart rate have been observed after electrical or pharmacological stimulation of the nucleus tractus solitarius (NTS),[43] the medullary nuclei,[44,45] and the parabrachial nucleus.[46] These brainstem regions are interrelated by diverse neuronal projections and are connected to adrenergic structures,[47,48] such as the locus coeruleus, which are postulated to play a role in panic attacks.[49] Furthermore, experimental data indicate that CCK interacts with these brainstem mechanisms in modulating respiratory and cardiovascular functions. Microiontophoretic application of CCK-8S to neurons of the NTS decreased both neuronal firing and respiratory frequency in cats, effects that were reversed by the administration of CCK-4.[50]

Our clinical investigations have demonstrated that exogenous CCK-4 produces robust and dose-dependent increases in heart rate and blood pressure.[28] Moreover, pretreatment with the CCK-B antagonist L-365,260 significantly decreased CCK-4–induced increases in heart rate.[39] It might be argued that increases in cardiovascular activity in response to CCK-4 challenge may be the result of direct or indirect stimulation of CCK receptors in brainstem structures such as the NTS. It is also conceivable that the evocation of emotional and psychosensorial symptoms after CCK-4 challenge results from an action of CCK-4 on brainstem structures and subsequent activation or inhibition of higher CNS regions mediated by neuronal projections. As these brainstem structures are not fully shielded by the blood-brain barrier, CNS penetration by CCK-4 might not even be necessary for this action. This might also explain the rapid (in less than 1 minute) appearance of symptoms observed in both patients with panic disorder and normal control subjects after a CCK-4 challenge.

CONCLUSION

Data supporting the validity of CCK-4 as a panicogenic agent and the hypothesis that alterations in cholecystokinin activity might be involved in the pathogenesis of panic disorder are summarized. It remains to be determined if the experience of panic anxiety is related to an endogenous malfunction of the CCK system. Conventional approaches, such as measurement of body fluid concentrations of metabolites, might be helpful in answering this question. Lydiard and his colleagues[51] reported that cerebrospinal fluid concentrations of CCK-8S were markedly decreased in panic patients than in control subjects. These results suggest that panic disorder might be due to an abnormal production or turnover of CCK-8S or CCK-4. This hypothesis can be systematically tested once more sensitive analytical techniques that permit measurement of shorter CCK fragments, such as CCK-4, are available. Nevertheless, the finding that panic patients, relative to control subjects, have decreased concentrations of CCK-8S, a mixed CCK-A/CCK-B receptor agonist, and a more severe panic response to CCK-4, a selective CCK-B receptor agonist, suggests that panic attacks may result from an imbalance between CCK-A and CCK-B receptor systems. Admittedly speculative, such a hypothesis deserves further consideration particularly in view of recent findings that CCK-A and CCK-B agonists have opposite effects on NTS neurons.[52]

An important step in testing the hypothesis that panic disorder is the result of an endogenous anomaly of the CCK-B system will be pharmacological validation. If spontaneous panic attacks are the result of enhanced activity of the CCK-B system, then CCK-B antagonists should have antipanic effects. Fortunately, clinical research with CCK-4 has received considerable attention from industry. Several pharmaceutical companies recently developed CCK-B receptor antagonists and put these agents on fast-track drug development programs with the intention of testing their efficacy in panic and other anxiety disorders. It should be emphasized that even if studies on the pharmacological validation of the CCK hypothesis of panic yield negative results, the CCK-4 challenge paradigm could nevertheless remain a practical research tool that can enhance our knowledge of the neurobiological mechanisms subserving panic attacks and lead to the development of novel antipanic drugs.

REFERENCES

1. American Psychiatric Association. 1987. Diagnostic and Statistical Manual for Mental Disorders. 3rd Ed., revised. American Psychiatric Association Press. Washington, DC.
2. FARAVELLI, C. 1985. Life events preceding the onset of panic disorder. J. Affect. Dis. **9:** 103–105.
3. ROBINS, L. N. & D. A. REIGER. 1990. Psychiatric Disorders in America.: 155–179. The Free Press. New York, NY.
4. KLEIN, D. & H. KLEIN. 1989. The nosology, genetics and theory of spontaneous panic attacks and phobia. *In* Psychopharmacology of Anxiety. P. Tyrer, ed.: 163–179. Oxford University Press. Oxford, UK.
5. MARKOWITZ, J. F., M. M. WEISSMAN, R. OUELLETE, J. D. LISH & G. L. KLERMAN. 1989. Quality of life in panic disorder. Arch. Gen. Psychiat. **46:** 984–992.
6. WITTCHEN, H.-U. 1990. The natural course and spontaneous remissions of untreated anxiety disorders: Results from the Munich follow-up study (MFS). *In* Panic and Phobia 2: Treatment and Variables Affecting Course and Outcome. I. Hand & H.-U. Wittchen, eds.: 3–17. Springer-Verlag. Berlin.
7. BOWEN, R. C., C. D'ARCY & R. C. ORCHARD. 1991. The prevalence of anxiety disorders among patients with mitral valve prolapse syndrome and chest pain. Psychosomatics **4:** 400–406.

8. WALKER, E. A., P. P. ROY-BYRNE & W. J. KATON. 1990. Irritable bowel syndrome and psychiatric illness. Am. J. Psychiatry **147:** 565–572.
9. STEWART, W. F., M. S. LINET & D. D. CELENTANO. 1989. Migraine headaches and panic attacks. Psychosom. Med. **51:** 559–569.
10. JOHNSON, J., M. M. WEISSMANN & G. L. KLERMAN. 1990. Panic disorder, comorbidity and suicide attempts. Arch. Gen. Psychiatry **47:** 805–808.
11. COX, B. J., G. R. NORTON, R. P. SWINSON & N. S. ENDLER. 1990. Substance abuse and panic-related anxiety: A critical review. Behav. Res. Ther. **28:** 385–393.
12. NOYES, R., R. S. CROWE, R. L. HARRIS, B. J. HAMRA, C. H. MCCHESNEY & D. R. CHAUDHRY. 1986. Relationship between panic disorder and agoraphobia. Arch. Gen. Psychiatry **43:** 227–232.
13. CROWE, R. R. 1990. Panic disorder: Genetic considerations. J. Psychiat. Res. **24**(Suppl. 2): 129–134.
14. TORGERSON, S. 1983. Genetic factors in anxiety disorders. Arch. Gen. Psychiatry **40:** 1085–1092.
15. HOKFELT, T., O. JOHANSSON & M. GOLDSTEIN. 1984. Chemical anatomy of the brain. Science **225:** 1326–1329.
16. BRADWEJN, J. & C. DE MONTIGNY. 1984. Benzodiazepines antagonize cholecystokinin-induced activation of rat hippocampal neurons. Nature **312:** 363–364.
17. BRADWEJN, J. & C. DE MONTIGNY. 1985. Effects of PK 8165, a partial benzodiazepine receptor agonist, on cholecystokinin-induced activation of hippocampal pyramidal neurons: A microiontophoretic study in the rat. Eur. J. Pharmacol. **112:** 415–418.
18. REHFELD, J. F. 1992. CCK and anxiety: Introduction. In Multiple Cholecystokinin Receptors in Man. S. Iversen, C. Dourish & F. Cooper, eds.: 117–120. Oxford University Press. Oxford, England.
19. VANDERHAEGHEN, J. & J. CRAWLEY. 1985. Neuronal cholecystokinin. Ann. N.Y. Acad. Sci. **448:** 1–697.
20. BRADWEJN, J., D. KOSZYCKI & G. METERISSIAN. 1990. Cholecystokinin-tetrapeptide induced panic attacks in patients with panic disorder. Canad. J. Psychiatry **35:** 83–85.
21. DE MONTIGNY, C. 1989. Cholecystokinin tetrapeptide induces panic-like attacks in healthy volunteers: Preliminary findings. Arch. Gen. Psychiatry **46:** 511–517.
22. GUTTMACHER, L. B., D. L. MURPHY & T. R. INSEL. 1983. Pharmacologic models of anxiety. Compr. Psychiatry **24:** 312–326.
23. GORMAN, J. M., M. R. FYER, M. R. LIEBOWITZ & D. F. KLEIN. 1987. Pharmacologic provocation of panic attacks. In Psychopharmacology: A Third Generation of Progress. H. Y. Meltzer, ed.: 980–983. Raven Press. New York, NY.
24. BRADWEJN, J. & D. KOSZYCKI. 1992. CCK-4 and panic attacks in man. In Multiple Cholecystokinin Receptors in Man. S. Iversen, C. Dourish & F. Cooper, eds.: 121–131. Oxford University Press. Oxford, England.
25. BRADWEJN, J., D. KOSZYCKI & C. SHRIQUI. 1991. Enhanced sensitivity to cholecystokinin-tetrapeptide in PD: Clinical and behavioral findings. Arch. Gen. Psychiatry **48:** 603–607.
26. ABELSON, J. L. & R. M. NESSE. 1990. Cholecystokinin-4 and panic. Arch. Gen. Psychiatry **47:** 395.
27. BRADWEJN, J., D. KOSZYCKI, R. PAYEUR, M. BOURIN & H. BORTHWICK. 1992. Study of the replication of action of cholecystokinin in panic disorders. Am. J. Psychiatry **149:** 962–964.
28. BRADWEJN, J., D. KOSZYCKI, L. ANNABLE, A. COUETOUX DU TERTRE, S. REINES & C. KARKANIAS. 1992. A dose-ranging study of the behavioral and cardiovascular effects of CCK-tetrapeptide in PD. Biol. Psychiatry **32:** 903–912.
29. BRADWEJN, J., D. KOSZYCKI & M. BOURIN. 1991. Dose ranging study of the effect of CCK_4 in healthy volunteers. J. Psychiatry Neurosci. **16:** 260–264.
30. BRADWEJN, J. & D. KOSZYCKI. 1994. Imipramine antagonism of the panicogenic effects of cholecystokinin tetrapeptide in panic disorder patients. Am. J. Psychiatry, in press.
31. BRADWEJN, J., D. KOSZYCKI, A. COUETOUX-DU-TERTRE, M. PARADIS & M. BOURIN. 1993. Lack of effect of flumazenil on CCK-4-panic. Psychopharmacology, in press.
32. BRADWEJN, J. & D. KOSZYCKI. 1991. Comparison of CO_2-induced panic attacks with cholecystokinin-induced panic attacks in PD. Prog. Neuro-Psychopharmacol. Biol. Psychiat. **15:** 237–239.

33. KOSZYCKI, D., J. BRADWEJN & M. BOURIN. 1991. Comparison of the effects of cholecystokinin and carbon dioxide in healthy volunteers. Eur. Neuropharmacol. **1:** 137–141.
34. KARKANIAS, C. D., G. A. BLOCK, S. REINES & J. BRADWEJN. 1989. Neurobiology of panic disorder. Letter. Am. J. Psychiatry **146:** 1357.
35. MARGRAF, J., A. EHLERS & W. T. ROTH. 1986. Sodium lactate infusions and panic attacks: A review and critique. Psychosom. Med. **48:** 23–51.
36. ERVIN, F., R. PALMOUR & J. BRADWEJN. 1991. A new primate model for PD. New Research Program and Abstracts, 144rd Meeting of the American Psychiatric Association. New Orleans, NR 216: 100.
37. FRIEDMAN, S., G. S. SUNDERLAND & L. A. ROSENBLAUM. 1987. A non-human model or PD. Psychiatry Res. **23:** 65–75.
38. HARRO, J., E. VASAR & J. BRADWEJN. 1993. Cholecystokinin in animal and human research on anxiety. Trends Pharmacol. Sci. (TIPS) **14:** 244–249.
39. BRADWEJN, J., D. KOSZYCKI, A. COUETOUX-DU-TERTRE, H. VAN MEGEN, J. DEN BOER, H. WESTENBERG, C. KARKANIAS & J. HAIGH. 1992. L-365,260: A CCK-B antagonist blocks CCK_4-panic in panic disorder. Clin. Neuropharmacol. **15**(Suppl. 1): 59B.
40. BOUTHILLIER, A. & C. DE MONTIGNY. 1988. Long term benzodiazepine treatment reduces neuronal responsiveness to cholecystokinin: An electrophysiological study in the rat. Eur. J. Pharmacol. **115:** 135–138.
41. PALMOUR, R., J. BRADWEJN & F. ERVIN. 1992. The anxiogenic effects of CCK_4 in monkeys are reduced by CCK-B antagonists, benzodiazepines or adenosine A2 agonists. Clin. Neuropharmacol. **15**(Suppl. 1): 489B.
42. VASAR, E., E. PEURANEN, T. ÖÖPIK, J. HARRO & P. MÄNNISTÖ. 1993. Ondansetron, and antagonist of 5HT3 receptors, antagonizes the anti-exploratory effect of caerulein, an agonist of CCK receptors, in the elevated plus maze. Psychopharmacology **110:** 213–218.
43. JORDAN, D. & K. M. SPYER. 1986. Brainstem integration of cardiovascular and pulmonary afferent activity. Prog. Brain Res. **67:** 295–314.
44. DAMPNEY, R. A. L., A. K. GOODCHILD, L. G. ROBERTSON & W. MONTGOMERY. 1982. Role of ventrolateral medulla in vasomotor regulation: A correlative anatomical and physiological study. Brain Res. **249:** 223–235.
45. PILOWSKY, R., M. WEST & J. CHALMERS. 1985. Renal sympathetic nerve responses to stimulation, inhibition and destruction of the ventrolateral medulla in the rabbit. Neurosci. Lett. **60:** 51–55.
46. MAROVITCH, S., M. KUMADA & D. J. REIS. 1982. Role of parabrachialis in cardiovascular regulation in the cat. Brain Res. **232:** 57–75.
47. DAMPNEY, R. A. L., J. CZACHURSKI, K. DEMBOWSKY, A. K. GOODCHILD & H. SELLER. 1977. Afferent connections and spinal projections of the pressor region in the rostral ventrolateral medulla of the cat. J. Auton. Nerv. Syst. **20:** 73–86.
48. ROSS, C. A., D. A. RUGGIERO, D. H. PARK, T. H. JOH, A. F. SVED, J. FERNANDEZ-PARDAL, J. M. SAAVERDA & D. J. REIS. 1984. Tonic vasomotor control by the rostral ventrolateral medulla: Effect of electrical or chemical stimulation of the area containing C1 adrenaline neurons on arterial pressure, heart rate, and plasma catecholamines and vasopressin. J. Neurosci. **4:** 474–494.
49. GORMAN, J. M., M. R. LIEBOWITZ, A. J. FYER & J. STEIN. 1989. Neuro-anatomical hypothesis for panic disorder. Am. J. Psychiatry **146:** 148–161.
50. DENAVIT-SAUBIÉ, M., M. A. HURLÉ, M. P. MORIN-SURUN, A. S. FOUTZ & J. CHAMPAGNAT. 1985. The effects of cholecystokinin-8 in the nucleus tractus solitarius. *In* Neuronal Cholecystokinin, J. J. Vanderhaeghen & J. N. Crawley, eds. Ann. N. Y. Acad. Sci. **448:** 375–384.
51. LYDIARD, B., J. BALLENGER, M. LARAIA, R. PAYEUR & M. BEINFELD. 1992. CCK-8 concentrations in CSF of panic disorder and normal controls. Am. J. Psychiatry **149:** 691–693.
52. BRANCHEREAU, P., G. A. BÖHME, J. CHAMPAGNAT, M. P. MORIN-SURUN, C. DURIEUX, J. C. BLANCHARD, B. P. ROQUES & M. DENAVIT-SAUBIE. 1992. Cholecystokinin$_A$ and cholecystokinin$_B$ receptors in neurons of the brainstem solitary complex of the rat: Pharmacological identification. J. Pharmacol. Exp. Ther. **260:** 1433–1440.

Cholecystokinin Stimulates Ca^{2+} Mobilization and Clonal Growth in Small Cell Lung Cancer through CCK_A and CCK_B/Gastrin Receptors[a]

THOMAS HERGET,[b] TARIQ SETHI,[b] S. VINCENT WU,[c]
JOHN H. WALSH,[c] AND ENRIQUE ROZENGURT[b]

[b]Imperial Cancer Research Fund
PO Box 123
Lincoln's Inn Fields
London WC2A 3PX, UK

[c]Department of Medicine
University of California
Los Angeles, California 90024

The incidence of carcinoma of the lung in the western world has been increasing at a dramatic rate during the last 50 years and it has become the principal cause of cancer deaths. Small cell lung cancer (SCLC), which constitutes 25% of all pulmonary cancers, follows a very aggressive clinical course despite initial sensitivity to chemotherapy and radiotherapy.[1] Novel therapeutic approaches are needed and they will arise, most likely, from a better understanding of the factors and intracellular events that are responsible for stimulating the rapid growth of SCLC cells.

Small cell lung cancer is characterized by the presence of intracytoplasmic neurosecretory granules and by its ability to secrete many hormones and neuropeptides, including bombesin, neurotensin, vasopressin, and cholecystokinin (CCK).[2-7] These neuroendocrine properties, which are prominent but not exclusive for SCLC, attracted clinical interest because they provide useful markers for the pathologic diagnosis of SCLC and also can cause endocrine abnormalities, that is, syndrome of inappropriate secretion of antidiuretic hormone. Recent studies demonstrated that small cell lung cancers not only produce neuropeptides but also express receptors for multiple Ca^{2+}-mobilizing neuropeptides.[8-12] Moreover, these peptides are recognized to act as potent growth factors for a variety of cell types including SCLC.[10-12] These findings support the hypothesis that SCLC growth is regulated and sustained by an extensive network of multiple autocrine and paracrine circuits.

The present article summarizes studies in which CCK and gastrin are shown to initiate signal transduction and colony growth in SCLC cell lines. We describe the cloning of the human CCK_B/gastrin receptor and provide direct evidence demonstrating its expression in SCLC cell lines, as shown by Northern blot analysis and by polymerase chain reaction (PCR) methodology. Our findings also show that certain SCLC cell lines express CCK_A rather than CCK_B/gastrin receptors. CCK-8 acting through either CCK_B or CCK_A receptors promotes rapid Ca^{2+} mobilization and stimulates clonal growth of several SCLC cell lines.

---

[a]This work was supported in part by NIH grants DK 17294 and DK 41301 (CURE) and by Veterans Administration Research Funding.

DIFFERENTIAL EXPRESSION OF THE CCK_B/GASTRIN RECEPTOR IN SCLC

Receptors within the cholecystokinin/gastrin family are divided into CCK_A, CCK_B, and gastrin subtypes based on different binding affinities to agonists and antagonists.[13,14] Recent pharmacological and molecular biological data confirmed the difference between the gastrin and CCK_A receptors, but also suggested that the gastrin and CCK_B receptors are identical.[15,16] We therefore refer to the receptor for CCK_B and gastrin as CCK_B/gastrin receptor.

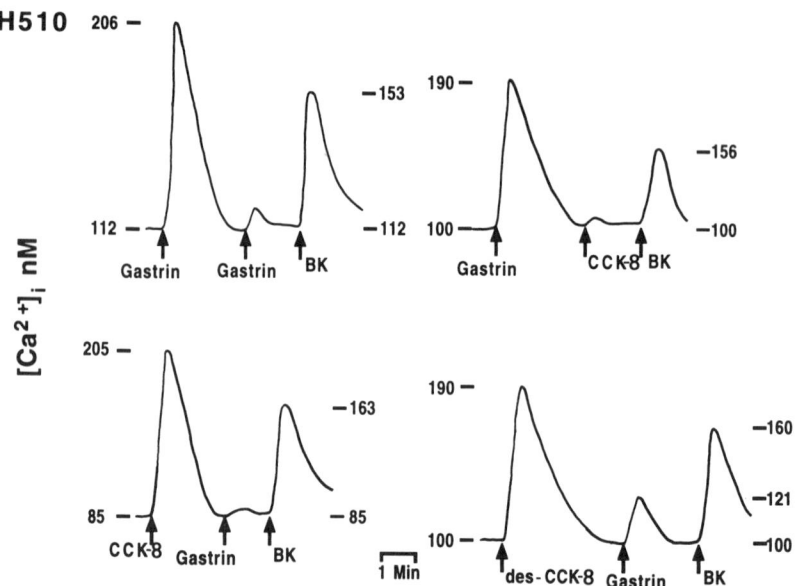

FIGURE 1. Effect of sequential additions of gastrin, CCK-8, and des-CCK-8 on $[Ca^{2+}]_i$ in SCLC cell line H 510. H 510 cells, cultured, washed, and loaded with fura-2/AME were resuspended in electrolyte solution and placed in a quartz cuvette. Fluorescence was monitored and basal and peak $[Ca^{2+}]_i$ calculated as described previously.[41] Agonists were added sequentially at the following final concentrations: gastrin = 100 nM gastrin; CCK-8 = 100 nM cholecystokinin-8; des-CCK-8 = 100 nM des(SO_3)cholecystokinin-8; BK = 5 nM bradykinin.

CCK_B-Stimulated Ca^{2+} Mobilization

Mobilization of calcium from internal stores leading to a rapid increase in the cytoplasmic concentration of Ca^{2+} ($[Ca^{2+}]_i$) has provided a useful assay to study the effects of agonists and antagonists in SCLC cell lines. The addition of gastrin or CCK-8 induced a prominent Ca^{2+} mobilization in the SCLC line H 510 loaded with the fluorescent Ca^{2+} indicator fura-2 (FIG. 1). The magnitude of the increase in $[Ca^{2+}]_i$ induced by gastrin in this cell line ($\Delta[Ca^{2+}]_i$ = 150 nM) was greater than the response induced by other Ca^{2+}-mobilizing neuropeptides including bradykinin, vasopressin, or galanin ($\Delta[Ca^{2+}]_i$ = 100, 70, and 50 nM, respectively). The increase in $[Ca^{2+}]_i$ induced by gastrin in H 510 cells resulted from the release of Ca^{2+} from internal stores because it still occurred after the addition of EGTA to chelate extracellular Ca^{2+}, just prior to the addition of gastrin.[12]

Repeated additions of gastrin caused homologous desensitization of Ca^{2+} mobilization (FIG. 1). Furthermore, the addition of gastrin attenuated the increase in $[Ca^{2+}]_i$ induced by CCK-8 and, reciprocally, brief exposure to CCK-8 prevented the Ca^{2+} response induced by gastrin. Neither gastrin nor CCK-8 prevented the increase in $[Ca^{2+}]_i$ through a distinct neuropeptide receptor such as bradykinin (FIG. 1). Similar results were obtained in the SCLC cell lines H 345 and H 69. These data suggest that gastrin and CCK-8 induce Ca^{2+} mobilization in H 510 cells through a common receptor.

Gastrin and CCK share a common COOH-terminal pentapeptide and bind to at least two different receptor subtypes. The CCK_B/gastrin receptors bind both CCK and gastrin with approximately equal affinities, whereas the CCK_A receptors exhibit a 500-fold higher affinity for CCK than for gastrin.[13,14] In H 510 cells, gastrin17-I (unsulfated), gastrin17-II (sulfated on position 6 from the COOH-terminus), CCK-8 (sulfated on position 7 from the COOH-terminus), and des(SO_3)CCK-8 (desulfated CCK-8) increased the peak level of $[Ca^{2+}]_i$ in a concentration-dependent manner. The concentrations required to induce half-maximum stimulation (EC_{50}) by these agonists were 7, 2.5, 5, and 2.5 nM, respectively.[12] Thus, the receptors expressed by H 510 cells recognized gastrin and CCK agonists with approximately equal apparent affinities.

Effect of Various CCK_B/Gastrin Antagonists

To gain further insight into the receptors that mediate the increase in $[Ca^{2+}]_i$ in response to gastrin and CCK-8 in H 510 cells, we tested the effect of various receptor antagonists. The addition of the specific CCK_B/gastrin receptor antagonist L-365.260[17,18] inhibited the Ca^{2+} response induced by CCK-8 (IC_{50} = 1 nM) in H 510 cells (FIG. 2). In contrast, the CCK_A-preferring antagonist L-364.718 (15 nM) had little effect on the increase in $[Ca^{2+}]_i$ induced by 5 nM gastrin in this cell line.[12] The selective CCK_B/gastrin antagonist CAM-2200[19] profoundly inhibited the increase in $[Ca^{2+}]_i$ induced by 10 nM CCK-8 (IC_{50} = 80 pM). In contrast, the novel selective CCK_A antagonist CAM-1481[20] at 10 nM did not prevent the increase in $[Ca^{2+}]_i$ induced by CCK-8 (10 nM) in H 510 cells (FIG. 2). Taken together, these results indicate that the Ca^{2+}-mobilizing effects of CCK-8 are mediated through a CCK_B/gastrin receptor in H 510 cells (Sethi, Herget, Wu, Walsh, and Rozengurt, manuscript in preparation).

Cloning of the Human CCK_B/Gastrin Receptor

Although cDNAs encoding the CCK_B/gastrin receptors from different species have been cloned and sequenced,[15,16,21–23] direct evidence demonstrating the expression of CCK_B/gastrin receptor in SCLC is, as yet, not available. At the start of this study there was no specific probe for the human CCK_B/gastrin receptor available to analyze its expression at the mRNA level in SCLC cells. Therefore, we attempted to clone part of the coding region of the human CCK_B/gastrin receptor and designed primers to amplify the region between the second and third intracellular loops. The primer sequences were deduced according to the nucleotide sequences of the recently cloned cDNAs encoding the canine CCK_B/gastrin[15] and the rat CCK_A receptor.[22] Polymerase chain reaction using primer No. 2 (5'-GAG C/AGA TAC/T

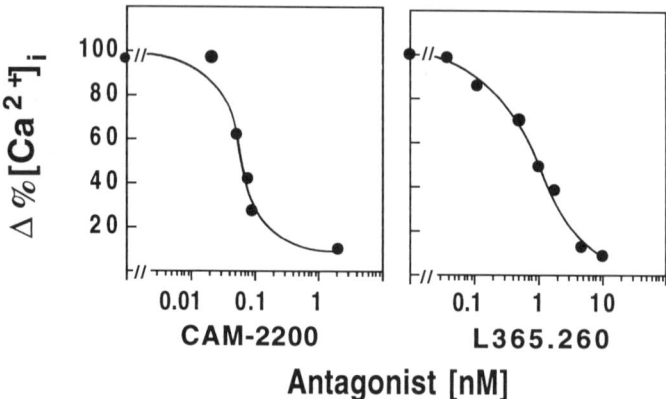

FIGURE 2. Effect of CCK_B/gastrin receptor antagonists CAM-2200 and L 365.260 on CCK-8 induced Ca^{2+} mobilization in the SCLC cell line H 510. H 510 cells loaded with fura-2/AME were resuspended in electrolyte solution and placed in a quartz cuvette. Fluorescence was monitored and basal and peak $[Ca^{2+}]_i$ calculated. Dose-dependent inhibition of Ca^{2+} mobilization induced by 10 nM CCK-8 in the H 510 SCLC cell line by the CCK_B/gastrin receptor antagonists CAM-2200 and L 365.260 was measured. $\Delta[Ca^{2+}]_i$, i.e., peak $[Ca^{2+}]_i$—basal $[Ca^{2+}]_i$ was calculated at each antagonist concentration. $\Delta[Ca^{2+}]_i$ induced by 10 nM CCK-8 was taken as 100%.

A/GGC GCC ATC TGC-3') and primer No. 4 (5'-CGC TTC TTG GCC/T AA/TC AGG/C TTG G-3') and a human fetal brain cDNA library cloned in λZAP-II as a template resulted in the amplification of a single DNA fragment of the expected size of about 550 bp. The PCR product was cloned and the nucleotide sequence was determined as described previously.[24] The corresponding peptide sequence showed homology with the rat and canine receptor sequence, but it also revealed a surprising difference. Specifically, the pentapeptide Ala/Thr-Ala/Gly-Pro-Gly-Pro (residues 272–276) of the canine/rat gastrin receptor corresponding to the third cytosolic loop (FIG. 3C), a region thought to play a critical role in signal transduction, was absent in the amplified human sequence.

FIGURE 3. (A) $HuCCK_B$ receptor intron sequence. The sequence of the intron found in $HuCCK_B$ receptor cDNAs is printed in *small letters,* of the coding region in *capital letters.* **Bold numbers** indicate the position of the amino acids of the coding region; *small numbers* mark the start and the end of the intron. Bases corresponding to splice signals are *underlined;* the *Eco*RI site is written in italic. (B) Nucleotide and deduced protein sequences of the CCK_B receptor cDNA. Two cDNA libraries were synthesized from human fetal brain mRNA and cloned in λgt11 and λZAP-II. They were screened under standard conditions[44] with a 550-bp radiolabeled polymerase chain reaction probe from the third cytoplasmic domain of the CCK_B/gastrin receptor. (See text for details.) Inserts of positive cDNA clones were subcloned into pBluescript-II and sequenced.[45] *Lines* above the nucleotide sequence indicate the seven putative transmembrane spanning regions (I–VII). The AATAAA RNA cleavage and polyadenylation signal is *underlined.* *Triangle* marks the location of the intron shown in **A**. Positions for the nucleotide sequence are given on the *left side,* for the amino acid sequence on the *right side.* (C) Alignment of the third cytoplasmic domain of the human (this study), rat,[22] *Mastomys,*[23] and dog[15] CCK_B/gastrin receptor.

A

```
              1
    ACC TG gtgagcttgcccataaaggctatcctaggaattcctttctcaccccctattagatg
217 T  W
    cttacgaccattgcccagaatcttcctccagcttcccggagaattaccacgccaactcctat
    tctgcatccaccaccctggagttccagtttggggcccctccccagttctctctcccttccca
                              210
    gcggcaccccaaatcctactcctacttcag G TCC GTA
                                   S   V  220
```

B

```
   1 CCAGGCGGGGCGAGCCGCGGGAGAGTGGAGGGCAGGCGCCTGGGCTGGGGGCGGGGACCA
  61 GGCGGGGCAGGGGGCAGGGAGAGGAGGGCGGCGGGAGGCCTGAGCCGGAATCGCAGCGTGA
 121 GCAGGTGGAGCCGCGGTGGGAGCCGCCGGGTCGAGCTGAGTAAGGCGGCGGGCTCGGCGG
 181 GGGCCATGGAGCTGCTAAAGCTGAACCGGAGCGTGCAGGGAACCGGACCCGGGCCGGGGG
       M  E  L  L  K  L  N  R  S  V  Q  G  T  G  P  G  P  G  A       19
 241 CTTCCCTGTGCCGCCCGGGGGCGCCTCTCCTCAACAGCAGCAGTGTGGGCAACCTCAGCT
       S  L  C  R  P  G  A  P  L  L  N  S  S  S  V  G  N  L  S  C    39
 301 GCGAGCCCCCTCGCATTCGCGGAGCCGGGACACGAGAATTGGAGCTGGCCATTAGAATCA
       E  P  P  R  I  R  G  A  G  T  R  E  L  E  L  A  I  R  I  T    59
                                   I
 361 CTCTTTTACGCAGTGATCTTTCCTGATGAGCGTTGGAGGAAATATGCTCATCATCGTGGTCC
       L  Y  A  V  I  F  L  M  S  V  G  G  N  M  L  I  I  V  V  L    79
 421 TGGGACTGAGCCGCCGCCTGAGGACTGTCACCAATGCCTTCCTCCTCTCACTGGCAGTCA
       G  L  S  R  R  L  R  T  V  T  N  A  F  L  L  S  L  A  V  S    99
                                      II
 481 GCGACCTCCTGCTGGCTGTGGCTTGCATGCCCTTCACCCTCCTGCCCAATCTCATGGGCA
       D  L  L  L  A  V  A  C  M  P  F  T  L  L  P  N  L  M  G  T   119
 541 CATTCATCTTTTGGCACCGTCATCTGCAAGGCGGTTTCTACCTCATGGGGGTGTCTGTGA
       F  I  F  G  T  V  I  C  K  A  V  S  Y  L  M  G  V  S  V  S   139
                                  III
 601 GTGTGTCCACGCTAAGCCTCGTGGCCATCGCACTGGAGCGATATAGCGCCATCTGCCGAC
       V  S  T  L  S  L  V  A  I  A  L  E  R  Y  S  A  I  C  R  P   159
 661 CACTGCAGGCACGAGTGTGGCAGACAGCGCGCTCCCACGCGGCTCGCGTGATTGTAGCCACGT
       L  Q  A  R  V  W  Q  T  R  S  H  A  A  R  V  I  V  A  T  W   179
                                      IV
 721 GGCTGCTGTCCGGACTACTCATGGTGCCCTACCCCGTGTACACTGTCGTGCAACCAGTGG
       L  L  S  G  L  L  M  V  P  Y  P  V  Y  T  V  V  Q  P  V  G   199
                                                      Δ
 781 GGCCTCGTGTGCTGCAGTGCGTGCATCGCTGGCCCAGTGCGCGGGTCCGCCAGACCTGGT
       P  R  V  L  Q  C  V  H  R  W  P  S  A  R  V  R  Q  T  W  S   219
                                         V
 841 CCGTACTGCTGCTTCTGCTCTTGTTCTTCATCCCAGGTGTTGTTATGGCCGTGGCCTACG
       V  L  L  L  L  L  L  F  F  I  P  G  V  V  M  A  V  A  Y  G   239
 901 GGCTTATCTCTCGCGAGCTCTACTTAGGGCTTCGCTTTGACGGCGACAGTGACAGCGACA
       L  I  S  R  E  L  Y  L  G  L  R  F  D  G  D  S  D  S  D  S   259
 961 GCCAAAGCAGGGTCCGAAACCAAGGCGGGCTGCCAGGGGCTGTTCACCAGAACGGGCGTT
       Q  S  R  V  R  N  Q  G  G  L  P  G  A  V  H  Q  N  G  R  C   279
1021 GCCGGCCTGAGACTGGCGCGGTTGGCAAAGACAGCGATGGCTGCTACGTGCAACTTCCAC
       R  P  E  T  G  A  V  G  K  D  S  D  G  C  Y  V  Q  L  P  R   299
1081 GTTCCCGGCCTGCCCTGGAGCTGACGGCGCTGACGGCTCCTGGGCCGGGATCCGGCTCCC
       S  R  P  A  L  E  L  T  A  L  T  A  P  G  P  G  S  G  S  R   319
1141 GGCCCACCCAGGCCAAGCTGCTGGCTAAGAAGCGCGTTGGTGCGAATGTTGCTGGTGATCG
       P  T  Q  A  K  L  L  A  K  K  R  V  V  R  A  L  L  V  I  V   339
                                     VI
1201 TTGTGCTTTTTTTTCTGTGTTGGTTGCCAGTTTATAGTGGCAACACGTGGCGCGCCTTTG
       V  L  F  F  L  C  W  L  P  V  Y  S  A  N  T  W  R  A  F  D   359
1261 ATGGCCCGGGTGCACACCGAGCACTCTCGGGTGCTCCTATCTCCTTCATTCACTTGCTGA
       G  P  G  A  H  R  A  L  S  V  A  P  I  S  F  I  H  L  L  S   379
                                        VII
1321 GCTACGCCTCGGCCTGTGTCAACCCCCTGGTCTACTGCTTCATGCACCGTCGCTTTCGCC
       Y  A  S  A  C  V  N  P  L  V  Y  C  F  M  H  R  R  F  R  Q   399
1381 AGGCTGCCTGGAAACTTGCGCTCGCTGCTGCCCCCGGCCTCCACGAGCTCGCCCCCAGGG
       A  C  L  E  T  C  A  R  C  C  P  R  P  R  A  R  P  R  A     419
1441 CTCTTCCCGATGAGGACCCCTCCCACTCCCTCCATTGCTTTGCTGTCCAGGCTTAGCTACA
       L  P  D  E  D  P  P  T  P  S  I  A  S  L  S  R  L  S  Y  T   439
1501 CCACCATCAGCACACTGGGCCCTGGCTGAGGAGTAGAGGGGCCGTGGGGGTTGAGGCAGG
       T  I  S  T  L  G  P  G  *                                    447
1561 GCAAATGACATGCACtGACCCTTCCAGACATAGAAAACACAAACCACAACTGACACAGGA
1621 AACCAACACCCAAAGCATGGACTAACCCCAAGCACAGGAAAAAGGTAGCTTACCTGACTCA
1681 GAGGAATAAGAATGGAGCAGTACATGGGAAAGGAGGCATGCCTCTGATATGGGACTGAGC
1741 CTGGCCCATAGAAACATGACACTGACCTTGAGAGACACAGCGTCCCTAGCAGTGAACTA
1801 TTTCTACACAGTGGGAACTCTGACAAGGGCTGACCTGCCTCTCACACACATAGATTAATG
1861 GCACTGATTGTTTTAGAGACTTATGAGCCTGGCACAGGACTGACTCTGGGATGCTCCTAG
1921 TTGACCTCACAGTGACCTTTCCCAATCAGTCACTGAAAATACCGTCAGGCCTAATCTCATA
1981 CCTCTGACCAACAGGCTGTTCGCACTGAAAAGGTTCTTCATCCCTTTCCAGTTAAGGACC
2041 GTGGCCCTGCCCTCTCCTTCCTTACCCAAACTGTTCAAGAAATAATAAATTGTTTGGCTT
2101 CCTCCTGAAAAAAAAAAAAAAAAAAAAAAAAAAAAAAAAAAAAAAAA             2152
```

C

```
         244
HumCCKB: ELYLGLRFDG DSDSDSQSRV RNQGGLPGA- ----VHQNGR CRPETGAVGE
RatCCKB: ELYLGLRHFDG ENDSETQSRA RNQGGLPGGA APGPVHQNGG CRPVTSVAGE
MasCCKB: ELYLGLRFDG DNDSDTQSRV RNQGGLPGGT APGPVHQNGG CRHVT-VAGE
DogCCKB: ELYLGLRFDE DSDSE--SRV RSQGGLRGGA GPGPAPPNGS CRPEGGLAGE

                                                              323
HumCCKB: DSDGCYVQLP RSRPALELTA LTAPGPG--S GSRPTQAKLL AKKRVVR
RatCCKB: DSDGCCVQLP RSR--LEMTT LTTPTPGPVP GPRPNQAKLL AKKRVVR
MasCCKB: DNDGCYVQLP RSR--LEMTT LTTPTPGPGL ASA-NQAKLL AKKRVVR
DogCCKB: DGDGCYVQLP RSRQTLELSA LTAPTPGPGG GPRPYQAKLL AKKRVVR
```

FIGURE 3. See legend on facing page.

This observation prompted us to confirm the difference in sequence by isolating cDNA clones encoding the human CCK_B/gastrin receptor. Therefore, we screened two independent cDNA libraries synthesized from mRNA isolated from human fetal brain, one constructed in the λZapII vector (2×10^6 plaques) and the other in λgt11 (10^6 plaques) using the cloned PCR fragment as a probe. We isolated in total 10 independent clones from the λZapII library, all of which were subcloned into the pBluescript phagemid by *in vivo* excision. Their sequences revealed that these clones were derived from three independent clones with insert sizes of 1.0, 1.8, and 2.1 kb.

The largest clone was isolated four times and contained an intron of 210 bases (FIG. 3A) including an *Eco*RI restriction site and all splice signals,[25] but it showed no significant homology to any other known sequence. The *Eco*RI site was experimentally confirmed in Southern blot experiments with human genomic DNA.[16] The position of the intron in the complete CCK_B receptor cDNA is denoted by a triangle in FIGURE 3B.

All clones from the cDNA library confirmed the differences between the human and the dog and rat receptors noted previously by PCR, but they did not provide a complete sequence. The screening of the λgt11 library yielded four clones, one of which with an insert-size of 1.7 kb ($HuCCK_B$) contained the complete coding region. The final cDNA sequence (FIG. 3B) of overlapping clones is 2152 bp in length including a poly(A)-tail of 45 bases. At the 5' end, 185 nucleotides precede an ATG codon, which is present in the consensus sequence for translation initiation.[26] After the translation start site there is a single open reading frame, which predicts a protein of 447 amino acid residues (calculated molecular mass of 48.5 kD) including seven putative transmembrane spanning regions. At the 3' end the termination codon (TGA) is followed by 578 bp of untranslated sequence containing a typical polyadenylation signal. The complete nucleotide and the deduced amino acid sequence are shown in FIGURE 3B.

Alignment of the human CCK_B/gastrin receptor (this study) shows a high degree of overall similarity of about 90% with the one from canine parietal cells,[15] rat brain[22] and *Mastomys* enterochromaffin-like carcinoid tumor cells.[23] However, the sequence comparison also emphasizes the important difference in the region corresponding to the less conserved third cytosolic domain (FIG. 3C). Interestingly, two potential sites for protein kinase C phosphorylation on serines (S 82 and S 300) and the two potential sites for protein kinase A phosphorylation (S 154 and S 437) are conserved among the CCK_B receptors of all four species. The role of these potential phosphorylation sites in receptor function and signal transduction remains to be elucidated.

During the course of this work Pisegna *et al.*[21] and Lee *et al.*[16] published the cloning and sequencing of the human CCK_B/gastrin receptor from brain and stomach. Their sequences are in good agreement with the human fetal brain sequence presented here. However, residue 288, which in the PCR fragment and in one of our four cDNAs is a lysine (K) residue, is a glutamate (E) in the three other cDNAs and in the sequence reported by Pisegna *et al.*[21] and Lee *et al.*[16] In addition to the two already published sequences, our sequence covers the complete coding region as cDNA and provides additional 5' untranslated sequences (FIG. 3B). To confirm that $HuCCK_B$ codes for a functional CCK_B/gastrin receptor, we cloned the 1.7-kb insert containing the complete coding region into a mammalian expression vector and transfected COS-1 cells for 48 hours. The addition of 100 nM gastrin to such $HuCCK_B$-transfected cells induced a significant ($p < 0.03$) increase in the production of total inositol phosphates (FIG. 4). In contrast, no change in production of total inositol phosphates occurred in cells transfected with the empty expression vector (pcDNAI-Neo) with or without the addition of gastrin, indicating that these cells do not express endogenous CCK_B/gastrin receptors (FIG. 4). These results confirm that the isolated cDNA clone encodes a functional CCK_B/gastrin receptor and that this receptor type triggers intracellular signaling through activation of phospholipase C.

Expression of CCK_B/Gastrin Receptor in SCLC Cell Lines

Using the sequence of the human CCK_B/gastrin receptor determined in this study (FIG. 3B), we analyzed the expression of its corresponding mRNA in SCLC by

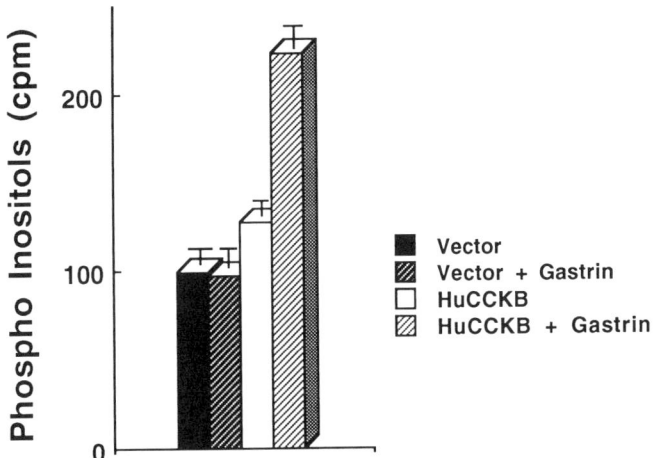

FIGURE 4. Analysis of total inositol phosphate production in COS-1 cells expressing the recombinant human CCK_B receptor. The cDNA clone $HuCCK_B$ containing the complete coding region was cloned into the mammalian expression vector pcDNAI-Neo (Stratagene). After transfection of 10^6 COS-1 cells in 33-mm dishes with 5 μg DNA using Lipofectin reagent (GibcoBRL), cells were grown for 24 hours. Then, cultures were labeled for 16–18 hours in 1 ml of medium containing 5 μCi of [2-^{3}H]inositol, stimulated for 20 minutes with 100 nM gastrin, and the production of total inositol phosphates was analyzed.[46] No change was noted in the production of inositol phosphates in cells transfected with the empty expression vector (pcDNAI-Neo) with or without the addition of gastrin (99 cpm ± 5 SEM), indicating that these cells do not express endogenous CCK_B/gastrin receptors. Gastrin induced a twofold increase in production of total inositol phosphates in $HuCCK_B$ transfected cells (from 125 cpm ± 5 SEM to 245 cpm ± 10 SEM). Each bar represents the mean ± SEM of six replicates each. Similar results were obtained in four independent experiments.

Northern blot hybridization. We used PCR methodology to obtain a probe from the beginning of the coding region to the third cytoplasmic domain. Using the upstream primer No. 38 covering the start codon (5'-GCC *ATG* GAG CTG CTA AAG CTG AAC-3') in combination with primer No. 4 and the full-length CCK_B/gastrin receptor cDNA ($HuCCK_B$) as a template resulted in the amplification of a DNA fragment of about 1 kb as expected.

The SCLC lines H 510, H 345, H 69, GLC 28, and GLC 19 were grown in serum-free HITESA medium[27] for 3 days, their total RNA isolated, gel-fractionated, and hybridized with the radiolabeled 1-kb human CCK_B receptor probe. The

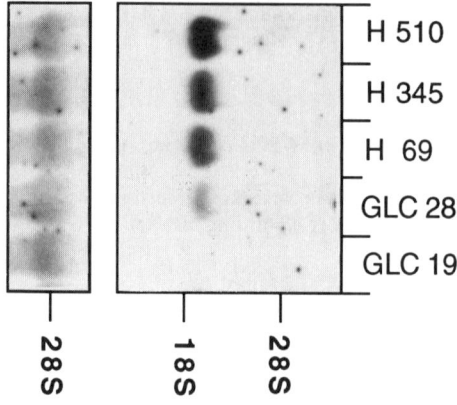

FIGURE 5. Northern blot analyses of different human SCLC lines. Thirty micrograms of total RNA isolated from SCLC lines H 510, H 345, H 69, GLC 28, and GLC 19[47] were separated on a 1% agarose/2.2 M formaldehyde gel, blotted, then hybridized with a radiolabeled[48] 1-kb human CCK_B receptor cDNA probe (see text for details), and washed under high stringent conditions as described in Herget et al.[24] (*upper panel*). Exposure time was 3 days. Migration positions of 28S and 18S rRNA are indicated on the *right*. The blot was re-probed with a 28S rRNA[24] probe to demonstrate equal loading of all lanes of the gel (*lower panel*).

autoradiogram (FIG. 5) shows a single hybridizing transcript of about 2.4 kb. The intensity varies greatly with the cell line. The strongest signal was detected in H 510. Intermediate signals were observed in H 345 and H 69, whereas only a faint band was visible in GLC 28. However, GLC19 had no detectable CCK_B/gastrin receptor mRNA levels at all. Accordingly, treatment of the GLC19 SCLC cell line with gastrin, at nanomolar concentrations, did not cause any increase in $[Ca^{2+}]_i$. In summary, expression of the CCK_B/gastrin receptor mRNA correlates extremely well with the responsiveness of different SCLC lines for this hormone (Sethi, Herget, Wu, Walsh, and Rozengurt, manuscript in preparation).

To provide direct evidence that SCLC cell lines express CCK_B/gastrin receptors, mRNAs isolated from H 510 and H 345 cells were primed by oligo-dT and reverse transcribed. Using these cDNAs as templates together with various primers deduced from the $HuCCK_B$ coding sequence resulted in the amplification of overlapping PCR fragments which were subcloned and sequenced. These sequences of the CCK_B/gastrin receptor from SCLC cells were identical to the CCK_B/gastrin receptor shown in FIGURE 3 and previously reported from human brain.[16,21] In particular, the nucleotide sequence of the third cytoplasmic loop of the CCK_B/gastrin receptors in both SCLC cell lines lacks residues 272–276 present in canine/rat CCK_B/gastrin receptors (FIG. 3C). Hence, we provide direct evidence that CCK_B/gastrin receptors are expressed in SCLC cells and that these receptors are identical to those in human brain.

EXPRESSION OF CCK_A RECEPTORS IN SCLC

CCK and Gastrin $[Ca^{2+}]_i$ Mobilization in H 510 and GLC 19 SCLC Cell Lines

As described in the preceding sections, expression of the CCK_B/gastrin receptor in SCLC cell lines H 510, H 345, and H 69 can account for the responsiveness of these cell lines to both gastrin and CCK-8. In contrast to the results obtained with H 510, H 345, and H 69, the addition of gastrin (100 nM) to the SCLC cell line GLC 19 did not stimulate Ca^{2+} mobilization, whereas the addition of 100 nM CCK-8 caused a rapid and transient increase in $[Ca^{2+}]_i$ (FIG. 6). Furthermore, prior addition of gastrin did not attenuate the increase in $[Ca^{2+}]_i$ induced by CCK-8 in this cell line. These results suggest that the GLC 19 SCLC cell line expresses CCK_A rather than CCK_B/gastrin receptors.

This conclusion was further substantiated by the dose responses of CCK-8 and gastrin on $[Ca^{2+}]_i$ in H 510 and GLC 19 cells (data not shown). CCK-8 and gastrin increased $[Ca^{2+}]_i$ in H 510 cells at identical concentrations (EC_{50} = 5 nM). In contrast, CCK-8 caused a dose-dependent increase in $[Ca^{2+}]_i$ in the GLC 19 cell line (EC_{50} = 15 nM), whereas gastrin, over the concentration range of 1–100 nM, had no effect.

Effect of Specific CCK_A and CCK_B/Gastrin Antagonists

Next, we attempted to distinguish the CCK receptors expressed by SCLC cell lines H 510 and GLC 19 by using selective antagonists. As shown in FIGURE 2 the specific CCK_B/gastrin antagonist CAM-2200 profoundly inhibited the increase in $[Ca^{2+}]_i$ stimulated by 10 nM CCK-8 (IC_{50} = 80 pM) in H 510. In contrast, this antagonist had little effect on the Ca^{2+} mobilization mediated by 10 nM CCK-8 in

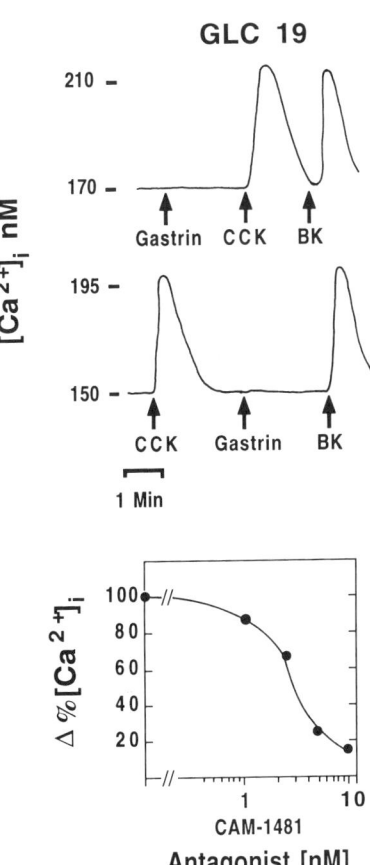

FIGURE 6. (**Upper Panel**) Effect of sequential additions of gastrin and CCK-8 on $[Ca^{2+}]_i$ in SCLC cell line GLC 19. Cells loaded with fura-2/AME were resuspended in electrolyte solution and placed in a quartz cuvette. Fluorescence was monitored and basal and peak $[Ca^{2+}]_i$ calculated as described.[41] Gastrin, CCK-8 (CCK), and bradykinin (BK) were added sequentially at the following final concentrations: 100 nM, and 5 nM, respectively. (**Lower Panel**) Effect of CCK_A receptor antagonist CAM-1481 on the increase in $[Ca^{2+}]_i$ induced by CCK-8 in the GLC 19 SCLC cell line. GLC 19 cells loaded with fura-2/AME were resuspended in electrolyte solution and placed in a quartz cuvette. Fluorescence was monitored and basal and peak $[Ca^{2+}]_i$ calculated. Dose-dependent inhibition of Ca^{2+} mobilization induced by 10 nM CCK-8 in GLC 19 SCLC cell line by the CCK_A receptor antagonist CAM-1481 was measured. $\Delta[Ca^{2+}]_i$, that is, peak $[Ca^{2+}]_i$ – basal $[Ca^{2+}]_i$, was calculated at each antagonist concentration. $\Delta[Ca^{2+}]_i$ induced by 10 nM CCK-8 was taken as 100%.

GLC 19. Conversely, the CCK_A antagonist CAM-1481 profoundly inhibited the increase in $[Ca^{2+}]_i$ induced by 10 nM CCK-8 in GLC 19 (IC_{50} = 3 nM) (FIG. 6, lower panel), but it had little effect on the Ca^{2+} mobilization stimulated by 10 nM CCK-8 in H 510 cells.

GLC 28 SCLC Cells Express CCK_B/Gastrin and CCK_A Receptors

In addition to cell lines that express either CCK_B/gastrin (H 510) or CCK_A receptors (GLC 19), we found that SCLC cell line GLC 28 expresses both CCK_A and CCK_B/gastrin receptors. Several lines of evidence support this conclusion: (1) GLC 28 cells show a low level of expression of the CCK_B/gastrin receptor mRNA (FIG. 5); (2) CCK-8 induced an increase in $[Ca^{2+}]_i$ of higher magnitude than that stimulated by gastrin in these cells; (3) prior exposure to gastrin did not prevent CCK-8 increasing $[Ca^{2+}]_i$, whereas CCK-8 completely prevented the response to a subsequent addition of gastrin; and (4) CCK_A and CCK_B/gastrin selective antagonists were effective in preventing the increase in $[Ca^{2+}]_i$ induced by CCK-8 and gastrin, respectively (Sethi, Herget, Wu, Walsh, and Rozengurt, manuscript in preparation). These results show that SCLC cell lines can express the two distinct CCK receptor subtypes, CCK_A and CCK_B/gastrin, either independently or coexisting in the same cell.

STIMULATION OF CLONAL GROWTH THROUGH CCK_B/GASTRIN AND CCK_A RECEPTORS

The possibility that gastrin and CCK could act as growth factors has attracted considerable interest. The administration of gastrin induces growth-promoting effects in the mucosa of the digestive tract especially the enterochromaffin-like endocrine cells[28] and exocrine pancreas.[29] The nonselective receptor antagonists proglumide and benzotript were shown to prevent the trophic effect of gastrin.[30] Furthermore, a decrease in the levels of circulating gastrin induced by antrectomy resulted in atrophy of colonic mucosa in the rat, an effect reversed by administration of pentagastrin.[31] Gastrin appears to be a growth-promoting hormone for malignant cells grown as xenografts in nude mice.[32] Cholecystokinin was reported to exert trophic effects on normal pancreas and to stimulate the growth of rat stomach *in vivo* and has also been implicated in the growth of gut tumors.[33,34] Taken together, these observations strongly suggest that gastrin and CCK are potent growth factors. However, it is difficult to obtain unambiguous evidence for a direct mitogenic effect of these hormones *in vivo*. Their administration could stimulate the release of other biologically active peptides or growth factors that could act as proximal effectors of the action of gastrin or CCK.

Cultured cells have provided useful model systems for elucidating the extracellular factors that promote cell growth without the interpretative complexities of experiments in whole animals. Nevertheless, compelling evidence that gastrin and CCK act as cellular growth factors or as autocrine factors in tumors has not been obtained using cell cultures. Indeed, studies with gastrin receptor antagonists and colon carcinoma cells lines produced controversial results. Experiments with the antagonists benzotript and proglumide suggested that gastrin plays a role as an autocrine growth factor for colon carcinoma cells.[35,36] However, another study using the specific CCK_B/gastrin receptor antagonist L-365.260 led to the opposite conclusion.[37] The lack of a convincing model system has impeded the elucidation of whether gastrin can act as a direct growth factor *in vitro*.

A possible role of gastrin and CCK in the control of cell proliferation of lung cancer is also of considerable interest, because gastrin and its precursor progastrin and CCK are synthesized by bronchogenic carcinomas and specifically by small cell carcinomas.[6,7] Therefore, we explored whether SCLC lines can respond to gastrin and CCK through specific receptors and whether these hormonal peptides can act as direct growth factors for SCLC cells.

Tumor and transformed cells are able to form colonies in agarose medium. A positive correlation exists between cloning efficiency of the cells and the histological involvement and invasiveness of the tumor in specimens taken from SCLC.[38] We determined the effect of CCK_A and CCK_B/gastrin receptor occupancy on the ability of GLC 19 and H 510 cells to form colonies in agarose-containing medium. We found that CCK-8 markedly stimulates colony formation in both cells. In contrast, gastrin promoted colony formation only in the H 510, but not in the GLC 19 cell line (FIG. 7). The selective CCK_A antagonist CAM-1481 inhibited the CCK-stimulated colony

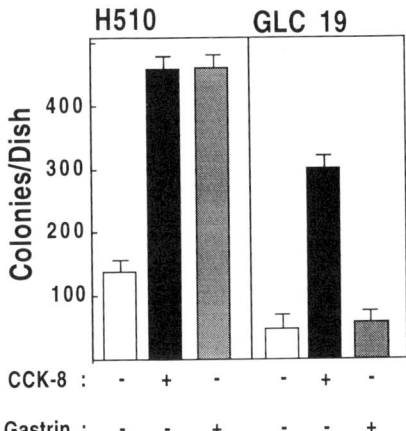

FIGURE 7. Effect of CCK-8 and gastrin on colony formation in H 510 and GLC 19 SCLC cell lines. H 510 and GLC 19 cell cultures, 3–5 days postpassage in HITESA,[41] were washed, and 10^4 viable cells per milliliter were plated in HITESA medium containing 0.3% agarose on top of a base of 0.5% agarose in culture medium. Both layers contained no additions, 100 nM gastrin, or 100 nM CCK-8, as indicated. Cultures were incubated at 37°C in a humidified atmosphere at 10% CO_2: 90% air for 21 days and then stained with nitrotetrazolium blue. Colonies were aggregates of cells >16 cells (120-μm diameter) and were counted under a microscope. Each column shows the mean of two independent experiments each with five replicates ± SEM.

formation in GLC 19 but not in H 510 cells, whereas the selective CCK_B/gastrin antagonist CAM-2200 inhibited the CCK-stimulated colony formation in H 510 but not in GLC 19 cells (Sethi, Herget, Wu, Walsh, and Rozengurt, manuscript in preparation). These results demonstrate that gastrin and CCK-8 acting through the CCK_B/gastrin receptor in the H 510 SCLC cell line and CCK-8 acting through the CCK_A receptor in the GLC 19 SCLC cell line can stimulate colony growth. Thus, gastrin and CCK act as direct growth factors for human cultured cells, and both hormones can stimulate growth of cells outside the gastrointestinal tract.

CONCLUDING REMARKS

Neuropeptides are increasingly recognized to act as cellular growth factors, and their mechanisms of action are attracting considerable attention. Many studies to identify the molecular pathways by which neuropeptide mitogens elicit cellular growth have used cultured murine 3T3 cells as a model system. Binding of several neuropeptides including bombesin, vasopressin, bradykinin, vasoactive intestinal peptide, endothelin, and vasoactive intestinal contractor to their specific receptors initiate a cascade of intracellular signals in these cells.[39,40] One of the earliest events to occur after receptor binding is a rapid mobilization of Ca^{2+} from internal stores, which leads to a transient increase in the $[Ca^{2+}]_i$ and subsequently to Ca^{2+} efflux and decreased Ca^{2+} content of the cell. A rapid increase in $[Ca^{2+}]_i$ should be regarded as an indicator of a productive ligand–receptor interaction. Ca^{2+} mobilization is, however, only one of the components of a complex array of signaling events rather than the signal that promotes cell growth.

In the present study we analyzed gastrin and CCK for their ability to induce a transient increase in $[Ca^{2+}]_i$ in SCLC cell lines (TABLE 1). We established that expression of mRNA coding for CCK_B/gastrin receptors correlates extremely well with the responsiveness in Ca^{2+} mobilization of SCLC cell lines for gastrin. Signal transduction and growth stimulation by gastrin are mediated by the CCK_B/gastrin receptor whose complete sequence is presented in FIGURE 3. Further studies have demonstrated that certain SCLC cell lines also express the CCK_A receptor either independently or coexisting with the CCK_B/gastrin receptor. The identification of human cell lines expressing either CCK_B/gastrin or CCK_A receptors (summarized in

TABLE 1. CCK_A and CCK_B/Gastrin Receptors in SCLC Cell Lines

SCLC Cell Line	Increase in $[Ca^{2+}]_i$ by:		Inhibition by:		Expression of $HuCCK_B$ mRNA	Receptor Subtype
	Gastrin	CCK	CAM-2200	CAM-1481		
H 510	++++	++++	Yes	No	+++	CCK_B
H 345	++	++	ND	ND	++	CCK_B
H 69	++	++	ND	ND	++	CCK_B
GLC 28	+	++	Partial	Partial	+	CCK_A and CCK_B
GLC 19	−	+++	No	Yes	−	CCK_A

Abbreviation: ND = not done.

TABLE 1) should facilitate the screening for novel antagonists that may be useful in the treatment of SCLC as well as in other areas of clinical pharmacology.

Recent results from our laboratory show that at optimal concentrations, neurotensin, vasopressin, gastrin-releasing peptide, galanin, and bradykinin induce comparable increases in SCLC clonal growth of responsive cell lines in soft agar.[10,11] Consequently, it was hypothesized that SCLC growth is regulated by multiple autocrine and/or paracrine circuits involving Ca^{2+}-mobilizing neuropeptides.[8–12,41] Interestingly, SCLC cells have also been shown to express gastrin and CCK peptides.[6,7] Thus, the findings that SCLC expresses two distinct functional CCK receptors, namely, CCK_B/gastrin and CCK_A receptor, both of which can mediate Ca^{2+} mobilization and growth of SCLC cell lines (TABLE 1), further extend the hypothesis that SCLC growth may be regulated by multiple autocrine and paracrine loops involving neuropeptides, including CCK and gastrin. Indeed, an autocrine loop involving CCK constitutes a unique case in which a single peptide can induce signal transduction and clonal growth through two different receptor subtypes (i.e., CCK_A and CCK_B/gastrin) with equal potency. Broad spectrum neuropeptide antagonists[42,43] provide a strategy to block SCLC growth which takes into account the mitogenic complexity of these tumors.

REFERENCES

1. SMYTH, J. F., S. M. FOWLIE, A. GREGOR, G. K. CROMPTON, A. BUSUTTIL, R. C. LEONARD & I. W. GRANT. 1986. The impact of chemotherapy on small cell carcinoma of the bronchus. Quart. J. Med. **61:** 969–973.
2. MAURER, L. H. 1985. Ectopic hormone syndrome in small cell carcinoma of the lung. Clin. Oncol. **4:** 1289–1296.
3. CUTTITTA, F., D. N. CARNEY, J. MULSHINE, T. W. MOODY, J. FEDORKO, A. FISCHLER & J. D. MINNA. 1985. Bombesin-like peptides can function as autocrine growth factors in human small-cell lung cancer. Nature **316:** 823–826.
4. GOEDERT, M., J. G. REEVE, P. C. EMSON & N. M. BLEEHEN. 1984. Neurotensin in human small cell lung carcinoma. Br. J. Cancer **50:** 179–183.
5. SAUSVILLE, E., D. CARNEY & J. BATTEY. 1985. The human vasopressin gene is linked to the oxytocin gene and is selectively expressed in a cultured lung cancer cell line. J. Biol. Chem. **260:** 10236–10241.
6. REHFELD, J. F., L. BARDRUM & L. HILSTED. 1989. Gastrin in human bronchogenic carcinomas: Constant expression but variable processing of progastrin. Cancer Res. **49:** 2840–2843.
7. GEIJER, T., R. FOLKESSON, J. F. REHFELD & H.-J. MONSTEIN. 1990. Expression of the cholecystokinin gene in a human (small-cell) lung carcinoma cell-line. FEBS Lett. **270:** 30–32.
8. WOLL, P. J. & E. ROZENGURT. 1989. Multiple neuropeptides mobilize Ca^{2+} in small cell lung cancer: Effects of vasopressin, bradykinin, cholecystokinin, galanin and neurotensin. Biochem. Biophys. Res. Commun. **164:** 66–73.
9. BUNN, P. A., D. G. DIENHART, D. CHAN, T. T. PUCK, M. TAGAWA, P. B. JEWETT & E. BRAUNSCHWEIGER. 1990. Neuropeptide stimulation of calcium flux in human lung cancer cells: Delineation of alternative pathways. Proc. Natl. Acad. Sci. USA **87:** 2162–2166.
10. SETHI, T., S. LANGDON, J. SMYTH & E. ROZENGURT. 1992. Growth of small cell lung cancer cells: Stimulation by multiple neuropeptides and inhibition by broad spectrum antagonists *in vitro* and *in vivo*. Cancer Res. **52** (9 Suppl.): 2737s–2742s.
11. SETHI, T. & E. ROZENGURT. 1991. Multiple neuropeptides stimulate clonal growth of small cell lung cancer: Effects of bradykinin, vasopressin, cholecystokinin, galanin and neurotensin. Cancer Res. **51:** 3621–3623.
12. SETHI, T. & E. ROZENGURT. 1992. Gastrin stimulates Ca^{2+} mobilization and clonal growth in small cell lung cancer cells. Cancer Res. **52:** 6031–6035.
13. JENSEN, R. T., S. A. WANK, W. H. ROWLEY, S. SATO & J. D. GARDNER. 1989. Interaction of CCK with pancreatic acinar cells. Trends Pharmacol. Sci. **10:** 418–423.
14. LIN, C. W., M. W. HOLLADAY, R. W. BARRETT, C. A. WOLFRAM, T. R. MILLER, D. WITTE, J. F. KERWIN, F. WAGENAAR & A. M. NADZAN. 1989. Distinct requirements for activation at CCK-A and CCK-B/gastrin receptors: Studies with a C-terminal hydrazide analogue of cholecystokinin tetrapeptide (30–33). Mol. Pharmacol. **36:** 881–886.
15. KOPIN, A. S., Y.-M. LEE, E. W. MCBRIDE, L. J. MILLER, M. LU, H. LIN, L. F. KALOWSKI & M. BEINBORN. 1992. Expression cloning and characterization of the canine parietal cell gastrin receptor. Proc. Natl. Acad. Sci. USA **89:** 3605–3609.
16. LEE, Y.-L., M. BEINBORN, E. W. MCBRIDE, M. LU, L. F. KOLAKOWSKI & A. S. KOPIN. 1993. The human brain cholecystokinin-B/gastrin receptor: Cloning and characterization. J. Biol. Chem. **268:** 8164–8169.
17. LOTTI, V. J. & R. L. CHANG. 1984. A new potent and selective nonpeptide gastrin antagonist and brain cholecystokinin receptor ligand 365,260. Eur. J. Pharmacol. **162:** 273–280.
18. BOCK, M. G., R. M. DIPARDO, B. E. EVANS, K. E. RITTLE, W. L. WHITTER, D. E. VEBER, P. S. ANDERSON & R. M. FREIDINGER. 1989. Benzodiazepine gastrin and brain cholecystokinin receptor ligands: L-365,260. J. Med. Chem. **32:** 13–16.
19. HIGGINBOTTOM, M., D. C. HORWELL & E. ROBERTS. 1993. Selective ligands for cholecystokinin receptor subtypes CCK-A and CCK-B within a single structural class. Biol. Med. Chem. Lett. **3:** 881–884.
20. BODEN, P., M. HIGGINBOTTOM, D. R. HILL, D. C. HORWELL, J. HUGHES, D. C. REES,

E. ROBERTS, L. SINGH, N. SUMAN-CHAUHAN & G. N. WOODRUFF. 1993. Cholecystokinin dipeptoid antagonists: Synthesis and anxiolytic profile of some novel CCK-A and CCK-B selective and "mixed" CCK-A/CCK-B antagonists. J. Med. Chem. **36:** 552–565.
21. PISEGNA, J. R., A. DEWEERTH, K. HUPPI & S. A. WANK. 1992. Molecular cloning of the human brain and gastric cholecystokinin receptor: Structure, function, expression and chromosomal localization. Biochem. Biophys. Res. Commun. **189:** 269–303.
22. WANK, S. A., J. R. PISEGNA & A. DEWEERTH. 1992. Brain and gastrointestinal cholecystokinin receptor family: Structure and functional expression. Proc. Natl. Acad. Sci. USA **89:** 8691–8695.
23. NAKATA, H., T. MATSUI, M. ITO, T. TANIGUCHI, Y. NARIBAYASHI, A. NAKAMURA, K. KINOSHIKAZU, K. CHIHARA, S. HOSODA & T. CHIBA. 1992. Cloning and characterization of gastrin receptor from ECL carcinoid tumor of *Mastomys Natalensis*. Biochem. Biophys. Res. Commun. **187:** 1151–1157.
24. HERGET, T., S. F. BROOKS, S. BROAD & E. ROZENGURT. 1992. Relationship between the major protein kinase C substrates acidic 80-kDa protein-kinase-C substrate (80K) and myristoylated alanine-rich C-kinase substrate (MARCKS). Eur. J. Biochem. **209:** 7–14.
25. PADGETT, R. A., P. J. GRABOWSKI, M. M. KONARSKA, S. SEILER & P. A. SHARP. 1986. Splicing of messenger RNA precursors. Ann. Rev. Biochem. **55:** 1119–1150.
26. KOZAK, M. 1987. An analysis of 5'-noncoding sequences from 699 vertebrate messenger RNAs. Nucleic Acids Res. **15:** 8125–8148.
27. SIMMS, E., A. F. GAZDAR, P. G. ABRAMS & J. D. MINNA. 1980. Growth of human small cell (oat cell) carcinoma of the lung in serum-free growth factor-supplemented medium. Cancer Res. **40:** 4356–4363.
28. RYBERG, B., J. AXELSON, R. HAKANSON, F. SUNDLER & H. MATTSON. 1990. Trophic effects of continuous infusion of [Lys^{15}]-gastrin-17 in the rat. Gastroenterology **98:** 33–40.
29. WATSON, S., L. DURRANT & D. MORRIS. 1989. Gastrin: Growth enhancing effects on human gastric and colonic tumour cells. Br. J. Cancer **59:** 554–558.
30. JOHNSON, L. R. & P. D. GUTHRIE. 1984. Proglumide inhibition of trophic action of pentagastrin. Am. J. Physiol. **246:** G62–G66.
31. DEMBINSKI, A. B. & L. R. JOHNSON. 1979. Growth of pancreas and gastrointestinal mucosa in antrectomized and gastrin-treated rats. Endocrinology **105:** 769–773.
32. SINGH, P., J. P. WALKER, C. M. TOWNSEND & J. THOMPSON. 1986. Role of gastrin and gastrin receptors on the growth of a transplantable mouse colon carcinoma (MC-26) in Balb/c mice. Cancer Res. **46:** 1612–1616.
33. DOUGLAS, B. R., R. A. WOUTERSEN, J. B. JANSEN, L. C. ROVATI & C. B. LAMERS. 1989. Study into the role of cholecystokinin in bombesin-stimulated pancreatic growth in rats and hamsters. Eur. J. Pharmacol. **161:** 209–214.
34. LAMERS, C. B. & J. B. JANSEN. 1988. Role of gastrin and cholecystokinin in tumours of the gastrointestinal tract. Eur. J. Cancer Clin. Oncol. **24:** 267–273.
35. HOOSEIN, N. M., P. A. KIENER, R. C. CURRY, L. C. ROVATI, D. K. MCGILBRA & M. G. BRATTAIN. 1988. Antiproliferative effects of gastrin receptor antagonists and antibodies to gastrin on human colon carcinoma cell lines. Cancer Res. **48:** 7179–7183.
36. HOOSEIN, N. M., P. A. KIENER, R. C. CURRY & M. G. BRATTAIN. 1990. Evidence for autocrine growth stimulation of cultured colon tumor cells by a gastrin/cholecystokinin-like peptide. Exp. Cell Res. **186:** 15–21.
37. THUMWOOD, C. M., J. HONG, & G. S. BALDWIN. 1991. Inhibition of cell proliferation by the cholecystokinin antagonist L-364,718. Exp. Cell Res. **192:** 189–192.
38. CARNEY, D. N., A. F. GAZDAR & J. D. MINNA. 1980. Positive correlation between histological tumor involvement and generation of tumor cell colonies in agarose in specimens taken directly from patients with small cell carcinoma of the lung. Cancer Res. **40:** 1820–1823.
39. ROZENGURT, E. 1986. Early signals in the mitogenic response. Science **234:** 161–166.
40. ROZENGURT, E. 1991. Neuropeptides as cellular growth factors. Eur. J. Clin. Invest. **21:** 123–134.
41. SETHI, T. & E. ROZENGURT. 1991. Galanin stimulates Ca^{2+} mobilization, inositol phosphate accumulation and clonal growth in small cell lung cancer cells. Cancer Res. **51:** 1674–1679.

42. WOLL, P. J. & E. ROZENGURT. 1991. A neuropeptide antagonist that inhibits the growth of human small cell lung cancer cells *in vitro.* Cancer Res. **51:** 1674–1679.
43. LANGDON, S., T. SETHI, A. RITCHIE, M. MUIR, J. SMYTH & E. ROZENGURT. 1992. Broad spectrum neuropeptide antagonists inhibit the growth of small cell lung cancer *in vivo.* Cancer Res. **52:** 4554–4557.
44. SAMBROOK, J., E. F. FRITSCH & T. MANIATIS. 1989. Molecular cloning: A laboratory manual. Cold Spring Harbor Laboratory Press. Cold Spring Harbor, N.Y.
45. SANGER, F., S. NICKLEN & A. R. COULSON. 1977. DNA sequencing with chain terminating inhibitors. Proc. Natl. Acad. Sci. USA **74:** 5463–5467.
46. MURPHY, A. C. & E. ROZENGURT. 1992. *Pasteurella multocida* toxin selectively facilitates phosphatidylinositol 4,5-bisphosphate hydrolisis by bombesin, vasopressin, and endothelin: Requirement for a functional G protein. J. Biol. Chem. **267:** 25296–25303.
47. CHIRGWIN, J. N., A. E. PRZYBYLA, R. J. MACDONALD & W. J. RUTTER. 1979. Isolation of biologically active ribonucleic acid from scources enriched in riboneuclease. Biochemistry **18:** 5294–5299.
48. FEINBERG, A. P. & B. VOGELSTEIN. 1983. A technique for radiolabeling DNA restriction fragments of high specific activity. Anal. Biochem. **132:** 6–13.

Cholecystokinin Hyperresponsiveness in Dysmotility-Type Nonulcer Dyspepsia

A. S. B. CHUA,[a,d] T. G. DINAN,[b] L. C. ROVATI,[c] AND
P. W. N. KEELING[a]

[a]*Department of Gastroenterology*
St. James' Hospital
James' Street
Dublin 8, Ireland

[b]*Department of Psychological Medicine*
St. Bartholomew's Hospital Medical College
West Smithfield, London ECIA 7BE, England

[c]*Rotta Research Laboratorium*
Via Valosa di Sopra 7
20052 Monza (Milan), Italy

The syndrome of nonulcer dyspepsia consists of a variable combination of persistent, recurrent, and occasionally very disabling symptoms including early satiety, postprandial bloating, abdominal pain, excessive belching, nausea, and vomiting. Depending on the symptom clusters, patients may be categorized into different subgroups.[1] Dysmotility-like dyspepsia describes a group that, on symptoms alone, appears to have abnormal gastrointestinal motility.

Nonulcer dyspepsia is a functional bowel disorder of unknown origin. Recent studies, however, confirmed a high proportion of gastrointestinal dysmotility in these patients, particularly gastric hypomotility and delayed gastric emptying.[2,3] Furthermore, dyspeptic symptoms are frequently related to feeding. Cholecystokinin (CCK) is an established brain-gut peptide that plays an important regulatory role in gastrointestinal function. CCK is involved in the control of food intake in both man and animals.[4,5] It inhibits gastric motility and emptying via a capsaicin-sensitive vagal pathway in rats.[6] In human studies, CCK mediates gastric emptying under physiological conditions.[7] An altered response to CCK may possibly be responsible for the dyspeptic symptoms in nonulcer dyspepsia and may be associated with the frequently observed abnormal gastric motility.

We investigated the effect of intravenous CCK-octapeptide infusion in 30 patients with nonulcer dyspepsia (22 female and 8 male; age range 18–56 years) and compared the response to that in 20 normal healthy controls (12 female and 8 male; age range 24–36 years) and 10 patients with duodenal ulcer (5 female and 5 male; age range 20–40 years). All patients gave full written consent. The dyspeptic symptoms were present at least 3 months, and all had normal upper gastrointestinal endoscopy and normal abdominal ultrasonography. Response to CCK was assessed by an intravenous CCK-8 infusion (6 ng/kg/min) over 10 minutes in a double-blind, cross-over fashion using normal saline solution as placebo. The CCK test was deemed positive when the infusion reproduced the patients' symptoms. The severity of the response was evaluated on a simplified visual analog scale. Results of

---

[d]PRESENT ADDRESS: B-38, Riverdale Park, Bukit Atarabangsa, Ulu Klang, 68000, Ampang, Selangor, Malaysia.

solid-phase gastric emptying tests in the NUD patients were determined using scintigraphic assessment of a standard breakfast labeled with Tc-99m tin colloid and compared with those in 12 healthy controls.

Twenty-seven patients (20 female and 7 male; 90%) with nonulcer dyspepsia had a positive response to the CCK-8 challenge. The most common reproducible symptoms included abdominal pain, abdominal bloating and fullness, nausea, and occasional vomiting. In the healthy controls, four reported mild nausea, whereas four had minor abdominal discomfort. Only 1 of the 10 patients with duodenal ulcer reported significant dyspeptic symptoms on CCK infusion. No subject reported any symptoms on saline infusion. In 10 patients with nonulcer dyspepsia intravenous atropine was successful in fully relieving the symptoms in a dose-dependent fashion. Oral loxiglumide (CCK-A antagonist) 800 mg, taken 1 hour before the CCK challenge, was similarly successful in controlling the symptoms. Solid-phase gastric emptying (analyzed in terms of half-emptying times) differed markedly in both groups, patients with nonulcer dyspepsia having a mean (standard deviation) of 91.3 (23.0) minutes in contrast to 54.6 (10.7) minutes in the healthy controls ($p < 0.001$).

Our results indicated that a high proportion of the patients with dysmotility-type nonulcer dyspepsia had an abnormal response to CCK-8 infusion. In most instances, infusion reproduced the patients' symptoms which may be blocked by atropine and attenuated with loxiglumide. This abnormal hyperresponsiveness to CCK may account for the genesis of dyspeptic symptoms in nonulcer dyspepsia. The effect may be mediated via a vagovagal reflex arc, resulting in perturbation of gastric motility. CCK-A receptors play a role on the afferent limb, whereas cholinergic receptors are important on the efferent limb of this reflex arc.

REFERENCES

1. HEADING, R. C. 1991. Definition of dyspepsia. Scand. J. Gastroenterol. **26** (Suppl 182): 1–6.
2. WALDRON, B., P. T. CULLEN, R. KUMAR, D. SMITH, J. JANKOWSKI, D. HOPWOOD, D. SUTTON, N. KENNEDY & F. C. CAMPBELL. 1991. Evidence for hypomotility in non-ulcer dyspepsia: A prospective multifactorial study. Gut **32**: 246–251.
3. CHUA, A., N. P. KENNEDY, D. HAMILTON, J. J. KEATING & P. W. N. KEELING. 1988. Dysmotility-type non-ulcer dyspepsia is negatively associated with campylobacter-like organisms. Gut **29**: A1437.
4. KISSILEFF, H. R., F. X. PI-SUNYER, J. R. THORNTON & G. P. SMITH. 1981. C-terminal octapeptide of cholecystokinin decreases food intake in man. Am. J. Clin. Nutr. **34**: 154–160.
5. LINDEN, A., K. URNAS-MOBERG, G. FORSBERG, I. BEDNAR & P. SODERSTEN. 1990. Involvement of cholecystokinin in food intake. Concentration of cholecystokinin-like immunoreactivity in the cerebrospinal fluid of male rats. J. Neuroendocrinol. **2**: 783–789.
6. RAYBOULD, H. E. & T. YVETTE. 1988. Cholecystokinin inhibits gastric motility and emptying via a capsaicin-sensitive vagal pathway in the rats. Am. J. Physiol. **255**: G242–G246.
7. LIDDLE, R. A., E. T. MORITA, C. K. CONRAD & J. A. WILLIAMS. 1986. Regulation of gastric emptying in humans by cholecystokinin. J. Clin. Invest. **77**: 992–996.

CCK, Schizophrenia, and Anxiety
CCK-B Antagonists Inhibit the Activity of Brain Dopamine Neurons

KURT RASMUSSEN

Lilly Research Laboratories
Eli Lilly & Co.
Lilly Corporate Center
Indianapolis, Indiana 46285

Hyperactivity of the brain's dopamine system is a widely accepted etiologic hypothesis of schizophrenia,[1] although modifications of this hypothesis have been proposed.[2-5] Support for the dopaminergic hyperactivity hypothesis of schizophrenia has come, in part, from electrophysiological studies showing that antipsychotic drugs have strong effects on the activity of dopamine-containing neurons in the substantia nigra (A9) and ventral tegmental area (A10).[6,7] For example, chronic administration (i.e., 2–3 weeks) of classic antipsychotic drugs (e.g., haloperidol) was shown to be necessary to decrease the number of spontaneously active A9 and A10 dopamine cells. This delayed onset for inhibiting dopamine neuronal activity corresponds to the delayed therapeutic onset of the antipsychotic drugs, inasmuch as antipsychotic drugs also require 2 to 3 weeks of administration before therapeutic effects are seen in schizophrenic patients. A major problem with currently available antipsychotic drugs, in addition to the delayed onset, is extensive motor-related side effects (e.g., involuntary movements, tremor, rigidity, and abnormal facial movements). Interestingly, atypical antipsychotics (i.e., those that produce fewer motor side effects) selectively decrease the number of spontaneously active A10 (and not A9) dopamine cells.[8,9] Thus, it has been hypothesized that the effects of typical antipsychotics on A9 cells underlie their deleterious motor side effects, whereas the common effect of classic and atypical antipsychotic drugs on A10 cells underlie their therapeutic action.

Cholecystokinin (CCK) has been shown to exist in a large proportion of A9 and A10 dopamine neurons.[10] Although the interactions between CCK and dopamine are complex,[11] some studies suggest that CCK can enhance dopamine function. For example, CCK has potent excitatory effects on dopamine cells[12] and has been shown to potentiate dopamine-mediated behaviors.[13,14] Therefore, since dopaminergic hyperactivity may play a role in schizophrenia, CCK antagonists could have antipsychotic actions. In addition, it was recently demonstrated that expression of CCK mRNA in the midbrain dopamine cells of schizophrenic patients is increased compared to that in normal controls.[15] In an effort to evaluate CCK antagonists as potential antipsychotic drugs, we examined several diphenylpyrazolidinone CCK antagonists with a wide range of binding affinities for CCK-B and CCK-A receptors (FIG. 1). We also examined the effects on the number of spontaneously active A10 dopamine cells of CCK-B antagonists from two other structural classes: LY247348, LY202769 (quinazolinones),[16] and L-365,260 (a benzodiazepine).[17]

CCK-B ANTAGONISTS AND SCHIZOPHRENIA

Dopamine Unit Activity

Acute administration of the diphenylpyrazolidinone CCK-B antagonists LY262691, LY262684, LY191009, and LY242040 dose-dependently decreased the number of spontaneously active A10 dopamine neurons. However, both an inactive analog (LY206890) and a CCK-A selective analog (LY219057) did not affect the number of spontaneously active A10 dopamine cells (FIG. 2).[19] The benzodiazepine CCK-B antagonist L-365,260 (FIG. 2) and the quinazolinone CCK-B antagonists LY247348 and LY202769 also decreased the number of spontaneously active A10 dopamine cells.[19,20] Acute administration of LY262691, LY262684, LY191009, and LY242040, but not the CCK-A selective antagonist LY219057 or the inactive analog LY206890, also dose-dependently decreased the number of spontaneously active A9

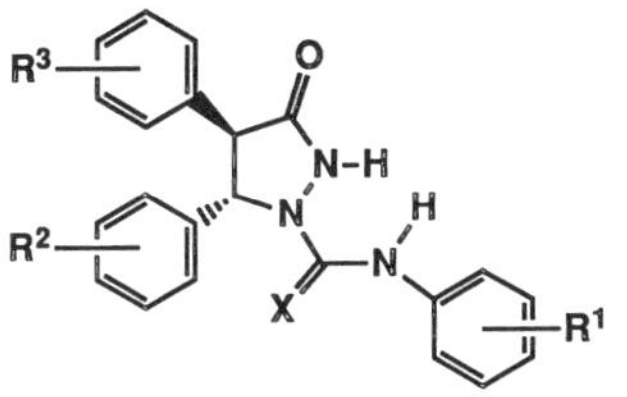

Compound	X	R1	R2	R3	CCK-B IC$_{50}$ (nM)[a]	CCK-A IC$_{50}$ (nM)[a]
LY262684	O	4-Br	2-Cl	2-Cl	6	7,900
LY191009	O	4-CF$_3$	2-Cl	H	10	>10,000
LY262691	O	4-Br	H	H	31	11,600
LY288513[b]	O	4-Br	H	H	16	>30,000
LY242040	O	4-CF$_3$	H	H	44	10,600
LY219057	S	4-Cl, 3-CF$_3$	H	H	510	42
LY206890	O	H	H	H	5200	>>10,000

FIGURE 1. Chemical structure of diphenylpyrazolidinone CCK antagonists and their affinities for CCK-B and CCK-A receptors. [a]From ref. 18. [b](+) optical isomer of LY262691.

dopamine neurons (FIG. 3).[19] Previously, chronic administration (i.e., 2–3 weeks) of antipsychotic drugs was shown to be required to decrease the number of spontaneously active A9 and A10 dopamine cells.[8,9] Therefore, the acute effect of CCK-B antagonists on A9 and A10 dopamine cells may be predictive of an antipsychotic action without a delayed onset. In addition, the effects of LY262691 on A9 and A10 dopamine cells did not abate with chronic administration; administration of LY262691 produced a significant decrease in the number of spontaneously active A9 and A10 dopamine cells in animals pretreated for 21 days with 30 mg/kg per day of LY262691.[21] Therefore, CCK-B antagonists should maintain any antipsychotic activity with chronic administration.

The inhibition of A9 and A10 dopamine neurons produced by chronic administration of antipsychotic drugs has been postulated to arise from a chronic state of strong depolarization (i.e., depolarization inactivation).[22] The depolarization inactivation hypothesis is supported, in part, by studies showing that systemic administration of

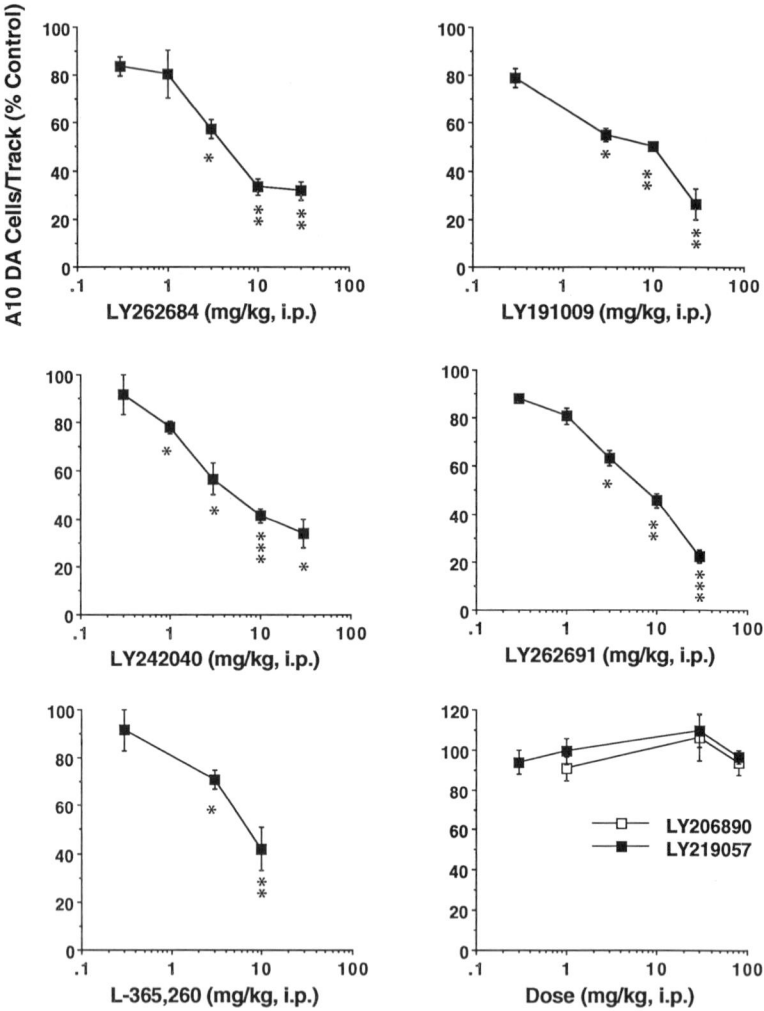

FIGURE 2. Effect of acute administration of CCK antagonists on the number of spontaneously active A10 dopamine (DA) cells; each point represents the mean ± SE of 2–7 animals. Vehicle administration had no significant effect (89 ± 3% of control, $n = 5$). The overall cells/track mean for all control groups was 1.34 ± 0.03 ($n = 82$). *Asterisks* indicate values significantly different from control: $*p < 0.05$; $**p < 0.01$; $***p < 0.001$ (from ref. 19).

apomorphine, a dopamine agonist that hyperpolarizes dopamine cells in control animals, can reverse the effects of chronic administration of antipsychotic drugs and cause previously nonfiring dopamine cells to become active.[22] Findings from our laboratory suggest that the decrease in the number of spontaneously active dopamine cells by LY262691 is not due to depolarization inactivation, because administration of apomorphine did not reverse the effects of acutely or chronically administered LY262691.[21] Further, single-unit recordings revealed that following acute

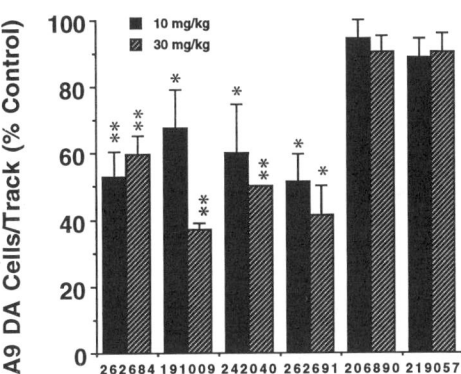

FIGURE 3. Effect of acute administration of CCK antagonists (10 and 30 mg/kg ip) on the number of spontaneously active A9 dopamine (DA) cells; $n = 3$–4 for each group. Vehicle administration had no significant effect (96 ± 4% of control, $n = 3$). The overall cells/track mean for all control groups was 1.16 ± 0.33 ($n = 39$). Asterisks indicate values significantly different from control: *$p < 0.05$; **$p < 0.01$ (from ref. 19).

administration of LY262691, A9 and A10 dopamine cells gradually decrease their activity over time and eventually become completely inactive. This inhibition was reversible by administration of the CCK-B agonist pentagastrin at doses that did not affect baseline activity (FIG. 4).[19] In addition, LY262684 ($n = 3$), LY191009 ($n = 4$), and LY242040 ($n = 4$) were also able to decrease the activity of individual A10 dopamine cells after acute administration (2–4 mg/kg iv). Taken together, these results indicate that CCK-B antagonists decrease the activity of A9 and A10

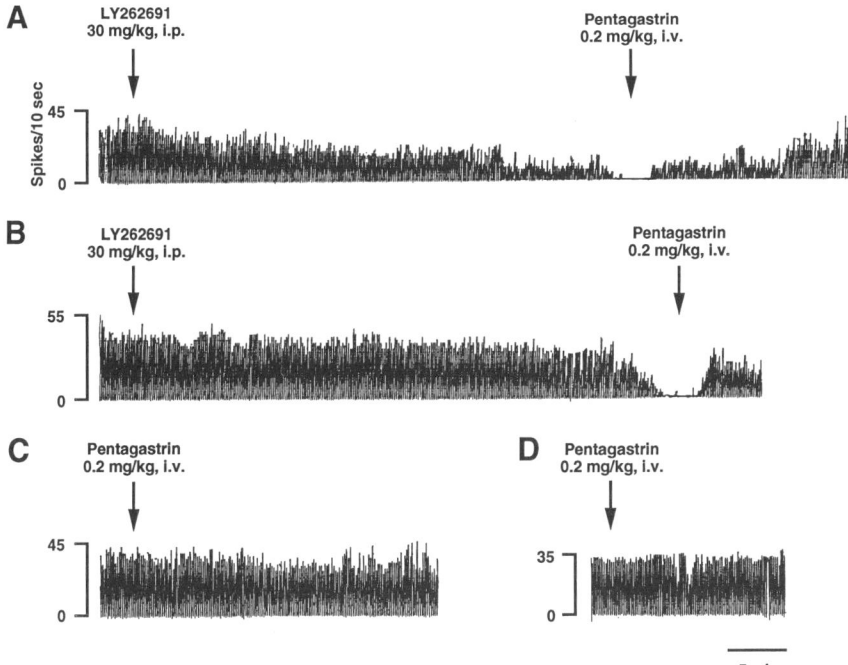

FIGURE 4. Effects of LY262691 and pentagastrin, or pentagastrin alone, on the activity of individual A9 (**A** and **C**) or A10 (**B** and **D**) dopamine neurons (from ref. 19).

dopamine cells through a mechanism different from that of antipsychotic drugs (i.e., not depolarization inactivation).

A recent study reported that administration of the CCK-B antagonist PD 134308 (a peptoid) does not alter the spontaneous activity of A9 or A10 dopamine cells.[23] The apparent discrepancy between the results obtained with a peptoid CCK-B antagonist and those seen with the diphenylpyrazolidinone, benzodiazepine, and quinazolinone CCK-B antagonists could be explained by CCK-B antagonists from different structural classes possessing different pharmacological properties. Inasmuch as PD 13408 has been demonstrated to have poor penetration into the brain following systemic administration,[24] another possible explanation is that PD 13408 was not administered at doses high enough to inhibit the activity of A9 and A10 dopamine cells.

Behavioral Observations

After chronic administration, atypical antipsychotic drugs (e.g., clozapine) selectively decrease the number of spontaneously active dopamine cells in A10 relative to

TABLE 1. Cataleptogenic Effects of Diphenylpyrazolidinone CCK-B Antagonists and Haloperidol

Compound	Dose (mg/kg ip)	Catalepsy Score (sec)			
		Pre	60 Minutes	120 Minutes	180 Minutes
Vehicle		0.9 ± 0.2	1.6 ± 0.4	1.8 ± 0.5	3.7 ± 0.8
LY262684	10	1.9 ± 0.4	1.8 ± 0.7	2.4 ± 1.2	4.8 ± 1.4
	30	1.2 ± 0.3	1.5 ± 0.8	4.3 ± 1.9	6.9 ± 3.6
LY191009	10	1.9 ± 0.5	2.9 ± 1.3	4.6 ± 1.6	4.5 ± 2.1
	30	2.0 ± 0.7	2.4 ± 0.9	3.4 ± 1.5	5.4 ± 2.7
LY262691	10	1.1 ± 0.2	3.8 ± 0.9	3.3 ± 1.2	4.6 ± 2.1
	30	1.5 ± 0.3	2.6 ± 1.1	2.0 ± 0.6	4.9 ± 1.9
LY242040	10	1.5 ± 0.4	1.1 ± 0.1	3.4 ± 1.2	3.2 ± 1.2
	30	3.1 ± 1.2	1.0 ± 0.3	2.9 ± 1.6	2.3 ± 0.6
Haloperidol	0.25	1.8 ± 1.1	2.2 ± 0.3	$9.9^a \pm 2.7$	$23.1^a \pm 4.9$
	0.5	0.9 ± 0.2	3.3 ± 1.7	$17.6^a \pm 2.2$	$33.5^a \pm 8.3$
	1.0	1.2 ± 0.4	$10.6^a \pm 6.3$	$100.0^a \pm 46.2$	$123.9^a \pm 39.7$

^{a}Significantly different from vehicle control group, $p < 0.001$ (from ref. 19).

A9.[8,9] This lack of a decrease of A9 dopamine cells may underlie the reduced propensity of the atypical antipsychotics for producing extrapyramidal side effects. In contrast, diphenylpyrazolidinone CCK-B antagonists, in addition to decreasing the number of spontaneously active A10 cells, also decreased the number of spontaneously active A9 cells (FIG. 3). However, behavioral observations indicate that CCK-B antagonists, unlike classic antipsychotic drugs (e.g., haloperidol), do not produce catalepsy (i.e., maintenance of imposed abnormal postures) (TABLE 1).[19] The occurrence of catalepsy is considered to be a predictor of Parkinsonian-like extrapyramidal side effects. Thus, despite their suppression of A9 dopamine cell firing, CCK-B antagonists compared to classical antipsychotic drugs may also have a reduced propensity for producing extrapyramidal side effects.

As mentioned, a decrease in A10 dopamine unit activity was hypothesized to contribute to the antipsychotic effects of currently available antipsychotic medications.[8,9] However, while CCK-B antagonists inhibit the activity of A10 dopamine cells, they are not active in some behavioral models (i.e., conditioned avoidance responding or reversal of apomorphine- or amphetamine-induced locomotor activity) thought to be predictive of antipsychotic activity (J. D. Leander and H. E. Shannon, unpublished observations). However, rather than being predictive of antipsychotic activity *per se* in man, conditioned avoidance responding and dopamine-agonist-induced locomotor activity tests may simply be sensitive to dopamine antagonist pharmacological activity. Whether CCK-B antagonists have antipsychotic effects in man can only be determined conclusively by clinical trials. The results of these clinical trials will, in turn, help to evaluate the predictive validity of our preclinical models of extrapyramidal side effects and antipsychotic activity.

Dopamine Neurochemistry

It is important to note that the electrophysiological recordings just cited were made in the chloral hydrate anesthetized animal, and chloral hydrate anesthesia has been demonstrated to affect the activity and responsiveness of dopamine cells.[6,25-28] Therefore, in an effort to determine if CCK-B antagonists affect the functional activity of dopamine neurons in the awake, freely moving animal, we examined the effects of LY288513 (the active isomer of LY262691) on dopamine metabolism and release in the olfactory tubercle (a mesolimbic region receiving dopaminergic terminals from the A10 dopamine cells) and the striatum (a region receiving dopaminergic terminals from the A9 dopamine cells). Neurochemical analysis of dopamine and its metabolites (dihydroxyphenylacetic acid [DOPAC], homovanilic acid [HVA], and 3-methoxytyramine [3-MT]) demonstrated that LY288513 dose-dependently decreased the release and metabolism of dopamine in the olfactory tubercle, but not the striatum, after acute treatment, with a time course similar to that of the electrophysiological effects.[29] These neurochemical results corroborate the behavioral observations indicating that CCK-B antagonists are relatively free of locomotor side effects, and they lend further support to the hypothesis that CCK-B antagonists may be efficacious as an antipsychotic medication for schizophrenic patients.

CCK-B ANTAGONISTS AND ANXIETY

Cholecystokinin has been proposed as an etiologic factor in anxiety. The hypothesis that CCK is anxiogenic has been supported by behavioral studies. CCK-B selective agonists (e.g., CCK-4 or pentagastrin) are anxiogenic in mice, rats, and primates.[30,31] CCK-B agonists also induce panic attacks in normal controls and in patients with panic disorder.[32-34] Furthermore, CCK-B antagonists have anxiolytic activity in a variety of animal models of anxiety including the elevated plus-maze, social interaction test, light/dark box, and punished responding.[30,35-37]

In addition to a role in schizophrenia, activation of the A10 dopamine pathway has been hypothesized to play a role in anxiety. The mesoprefrontal dopamine neurons originating in the A10 cell group are activated by a variety of stressors.[38,39] CCK-B antagonists, including LY262691, LY262684, and LY247348, have demonstrated anxiolytic activity in animal models of anxiety.[30,35,37,40] Therefore, a decrease in the number of spontaneously active A10 cells may play a role in the anxiolytic activity that has been observed for CCK-B antagonists. It should be noted that the hypothesized roles of the A10 system in anxiety and schizophrenia may be interrelated inasmuch as stress has been hypothesized to play a role in the etiology of schizophrenic symptoms.[41,42]

FOREBRAIN LOCUS OF ACTION OF CCK-B ANTAGONISTS

The exact locus of action of the CCK-B antagonists on A9 and A10 cells cannot be determined from studies solely employing systemic administration of the compounds. However, the direct effects of CCK on A9 and A10 cell bodies (i.e., both a strong excitation and a potentiation of the inhibitory effects of dopamine agonists) are known to be mediated via CCK-A receptors.[43,44] In addition, binding studies demonstrated that CCK-B receptors have their highest concentrations in the forebrain,[45,46] and efferent projections from some of these forebrain sites were demonstrated to affect A9 and A10 dopamine unit activity (including the number of spontaneously active cells).[22,47] Therefore, one hypothesis is that the effects of CCK-B antagonists on A9 and A10 dopamine cells are mediated through efferents from forebrain sites. To evaluate this forebrain site-of-action hypothesis, we examined the effects of radiofrequency lesions of some of these forebrain projection sites (i.e., caudate-putamen, nucleus accumbens, and medial prefrontal cortex) on the effects of systemic administration of LY262691 on the number of spontaneously active A9 and A10 dopamine cells.

Lesions of the n. accumbens blocked the effects of systemically administered LY262691 on A10, but not A9, dopamine cells. Conversely, lesions of the caudate-putamen blocked the effects of systemically administered LY262691 on the number of spontaneously active A9, but not A10, dopamine cells. Lesions of the medial prefrontal cortex blocked the effects of systemically administered LY262691 on both A9 and A10 dopamine cells.[48] These results indicate that the caudate-putamen plays an important role in mediating the effects of LY262691 on A9, but not A10, dopamine cells; the n. accumbens plays an important role in mediating the effects of LY262691 on A10, but not A9, dopamine cells; and the medial prefrontal cortex plays an important role in mediating the effects of LY262691 on both A9 and A10 dopamine cells.

Since radiofrequency lesions are not selective and destroy both intrinsic cell bodies and any axons projecting through a given nucleus, it is not clear if the effects of lesions on the actions of LY262691 are due to destruction of cell bodies or fibers of passage, or both. Therefore, we also examined the effects of local application of LY262691 directly into the n. accumbens, caudate-putamen, and medial prefrontal cortex. Microinjection of LY262691 into the n. accumbens or medial prefrontal cortex led to a significant decrease in the number of spontaneously active A10, but not A9, dopamine cells (FIGS. 5 and 6).[48] Conversely, microinjection of LY262691 into the caudate-putamen led to a significant decrease in the number of spontaneously active A9, but not A10, dopamine cells (FIG. 7).[48] The specificity of action of any microinjected compound is a concern because the concentration of the compound at the site of action cannot be determined with certainty. The only other receptor for which LY262691 has measurable affinity is the CCK-A receptor, where it displays low, but detectable affinity (FIG. 1). Therefore, we also examined the effects of local application of a structurally related compound (LY219057) with higher affinity for CCK-A receptors than CCK-B receptors (FIG. 1). Microinjection of LY219057 into the n. accumbens or medial prefrontal cortex did not affect the number of spontaneously active A10 dopamine cells, and microinjection of LY219057 into the caudate-putamen did not affect the number of spontaneously active A9

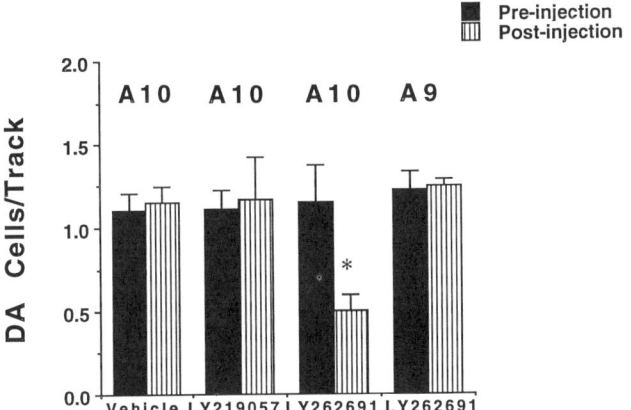

FIGURE 5. Effects of intracerebral microinjection of LY262691, LY219057, or vehicle into the n. accumbens on the number of spontaneously active A10 and A9 dopamine (DA) cells. *Asterisks* indicate values significantly different from control: *$p < 0.05$ (from ref. 48).

dopamine cells (FIGS. 5, 6, and 7).[48] Taken together, these results indicate that the effects of LY262691 on A9 cells are mediated, at least in part, by antagonism of CCK-B receptors in the caudate-putamen, whereas the effects of LY262691 on A10 cells are mediated, at least in part, by antagonism of CCK-B receptors in the n. accumbens and medial prefrontal cortex.

Lesions of the medial prefrontal cortex were able to block the effects of LY262691 on A9 and A10 dopamine cells, yet local injection of LY262691 into the medial prefrontal cortex only affected A10 dopamine cells. These results indicate that CCK-B receptors in the medial prefrontal cortex may not play an important role in the effects of LY262691 on A9 dopamine cells, but the medial prefrontal cortex

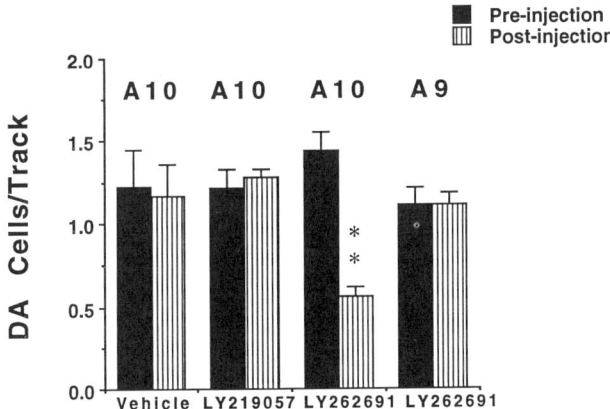

FIGURE 6. Effects of intracerebral microinjection of LY262691, LY219057, or vehicle into the caudate-putamen on the number of spontaneously active A10 and A9 dopamine (DA) cells. *Asterisks* indicate values significantly different from control: **$p < 0.01$ (from ref. 48).

must nevertheless be intact for systemically administered LY262691 to affect A9 unit activity. One possibility is that the excitatory amino acid pathway from the deep layers of the medial prefrontal cortex to medium spiny neurons in the caudate-putamen[49-51] plays a role in the effects of LY262691 on A9 dopamine unit activity.

The results from these radiofrequency lesion and microinjection studies are consistent with known projections from the caudate-putamen to A9,[52] the n. accumbens to A10,[53] and the medial prefrontal cortex to A10.[54] In addition, these results are in accord with previous results indicating that the caudate-putamen plays an important role in mediating the effects of antipsychotic drugs on the number of spontaneously active A9 dopamine cells,[8,22] and with previous results indicating that the n. accumbens plays an important role in mediating the effects of antipsychotic drugs on the number of spontaneously active A10 dopamine cells.[8,47] However, although both antipsychotic drugs and CCK-B antagonists seem to utilize, at least in part, similar anatomical pathways for their effects, these effects are opposite in

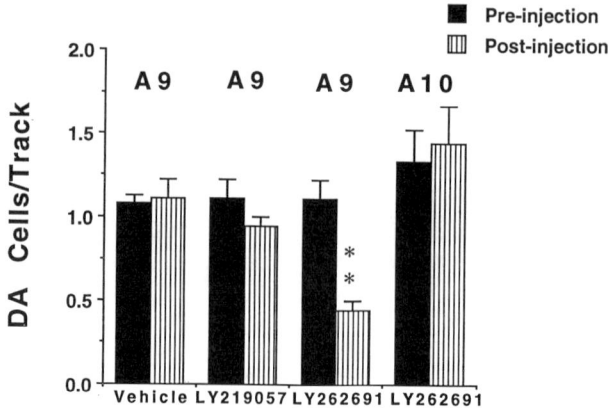

FIGURE 7. Effects of intracerebral microinjection of LY262691, LY219057, or vehicle into the medial prefrontal cortex on the number of spontaneously active A10 and A9 dopamine (DA) cells. *Asterisks* indicate values significantly different from control: $**p < 0.01$ (from ref. 48).

direction. That is, antipsychotic drugs inhibit the activity of dopamine neurons by inducing a chronic state of strong depolarization (i.e., depolarization inactivation).[22] However, CCK-B antagonists inhibit the activity of A9 and A10 dopamine cells without first causing a depolarization.[19] Therefore, the two classes of compounds, albeit via anatomical pathways with at least some overlap, affect A9 and A10 unit activity through very different mechanisms.

CONCLUSIONS

In conclusion, our studies indicate that the firing of A9 and A10 dopamine neurons is suppressed specifically by antagonism of CCK-B, but not CCK-A, receptors. Therefore, an endogenous CCK tone, mediated via CCK-B receptors, affects the spontaneous activity of midbrain dopamine neurons. The effects of CCK-B antagonists on A9 dopamine cells are mediated, at least in part, by antagonism of CCK-B receptors in the caudate-putamen, whereas the effects of CCK-B antagonists on A10 dopamine cells are mediated, at least in part, by antagonism of CCK-B receptors in the n. accumbens and medial prefrontal cortex. These effects on midbrain dopamine neurons suggest that CCK-B antagonists may represent a novel class of antipsychotic drug, with the potential for therapeutic effects in schizophrenic patients, without a delayed onset of action, through a novel mechanism of action. Since CCK-B antagonists have no cataleptogenic effects, their propensity for producing extrapyramidal side effects may also be reduced compared to that of classical antipsychotic drugs. In addition, the effects on midbrain dopamine neurons may play a role in the anxiolytic activity of CCK-B antagonists seen in animals. Confirmation of the predicted antipsychotic and anxiolytic activity of CCK-B antagonists in man awaits clinical trials.

REFERENCES

1. Losonczy, M. F., M. Davidson & K. L. Davis. 1987. The dopamine hypothesis of schizophrenia. In Psychopharmacology: The Third Generation of Progress. H. Y. Meltzer, ed.: 715–726. Raven Press. New York.
2. Weinberger, D. R. 1987. Implications of normal brain development for the pathogenesis of schizophrenia. Arch. Gen. Psychiatry **44**: 660–669.
3. Davis, K. L., R. S. Kahn, G. Ko & M. Davidson. 1991. Dopamine in schizophrenia: A review and reconceptualization. Am. J. Psychiatry **148**: 1474–1486.
4. Deutch, A. Y. 1993. Prefrontal cortical dopamine systems and the elaboration of functional corticostriatal circuits: Implications for schizophrenia and Parkinson's disease. J. Neural. Transm. **91**: 197–221.
5. Grace, A. A. 1993. Cortical regulation of subcortical dopamine systems and its possible relevance to schizophrenia. J. Neural. Transm. **91**: 111–134.
6. Bunney, B. S., J. R. Walters, R. H. Roth & G. K. Aghajanian. 1973. Dopaminergic neurons: Effect of antipsychotic drugs and amphetamine on single cell activity. J. Pharmacol. Exp. Ther. **185**: 560–571.
7. Bunney, B. S. 1992. Clozapine: A hypothesized mechanism for its unique clinical profile. Br. J. Psychiatry **160** (suppl. 17): 17–21.
8. Chiodo, L. A. & B. S. Bunney. 1983. Typical and atypical neuroleptics: Differential effects of chronic administration on the activity of A9 and A10 midbrain dopaminergic neurons. J. Neurosci. **3**: 1607–1619.
9. White, F. J. & R. Y. Wang. 1983. Differential effects of classical and atypical antipsychotic drugs on A9 and A10 dopamine neurons. Science **221**: 1054–1057.
10. Hokfelt, T., L. Skirboll, J. F. Rehfeld, M. Goldstein, K. Markey & O. Dann. 1980. A subpopulation of mesencephalic dopamine neurons projecting to limbic areas contains a cholecystokinin-like peptide: Evidence from immunohistochemistry combined with retrograde tracing. Neuroscience **5**: 2093–2124.
11. Crawley, J. N. 1991. Cholecystokinin-dopamine interactions. Tr. Pharm. Sci. **12**: 232–236.
12. Skirboll, L., A. A. Grace, D. W. Homer, J. Rehfeld, M. Goldstein, T. Hokfelt & B. S. Bunney. 1981. Peptide-monoamine coexistence: Studies of actions of cholecystokinin-like peptide on the electrical activity of midbrain dopamine neurons. Neuroscience **6**: 2111–2127.
13. Crawley, J. N., J. A. Stivers, K. L. Blumstein & S. M. Paul. 1985. Cholecystokinin potentiates dopamine-mediated behaviors: Evidence for modulation specific to a site of coexistence. J. Neurosci. **5**: 1972–1988.
14. Crawley, J. N. 1989. Microinjection of cholecystokinin into the rat ventral tegmental area potentiates dopamine-induced hypolocomotion. Synapse **3**: 346–355.
15. Schalling, M., K. Friberg, K. Seroogy, P. Riederer, E. Bird, S. N. Schiffmann, P. Mailleux, J.-J. Vanderhaeghen, S. Kuga, M. Goldstein, K. Kitahama, P. H. Luppi, M. Jouvet & T. Hokfelt. 1990. Analysis of expression of cholecystokinin in

dopamine cells in the ventral mesencephalon of several species and in humans with schizophrenia. Proc. Natl. Acad. Sci. USA **87:** 8427–8431.
16. YU, M. J., K. J. THRASHER, J. R. MCCOWAN, N. R. MASON & L. G. MENDELSOHN. 1991. Quinazolinone cholecystokinin-B receptor ligands. J. Med. Chem. **34:** 1505–1508.
17. LOTTI, V. J. & R. S. L. CHANG. 1989. A new potent and selective non-peptide gastrin antagonist and brain cholecystokinin receptor (CCK-B) ligand: L-365,260. Eur. J. Pharmacol. **162:** 273–280.
18. HOWBERT, J. J., K. L. LOBB, R. F. BROWN, J. K. REEL, D. A. NEEL, N. R. MASON & L. G. MENDELSOHN. 1992. A novel series of non-peptide CCK and gastrin antagonists: Medicinal chemistry and electrophysiological demonstration of antagonism. *In* Multiple Cholecystokinin Receptors. Progress Toward CNS Therapeutic Targets, C. T. Dourish & S. J. Cooper, eds.: 28–37. Oxford University Press. London.
19. RASMUSSEN, K., J. F. CZACHURA, M. E. STOCKTON & J. J. HOWBERT. 1993. Electrophysiological effects of diphenylpyrazolidinone CCK-B and CCK-A antagonists on midbrain dopamine neurons. J. Pharmacol. Exp. Ther. **264:** 480–488.
20. YU, M. J., J. F. CZACHURA, M. E. STOCKTON, J. R. MCCOWAN & K. RASMUSSEN. 1992. Quinazolilinone CCK-B antagonists decrease the number of spontaneously active dopamine neurons. Soc. Neurosci. Abstr. **18:** 278.
21. RASMUSSEN, K., M. E. STOCKTON, J. F. CZACHURA & J. J. HOWBERT. 1991. Cholecystokinin (CCK) and schizophrenia: The selective CCK-B antagonist LY262691 decreases midbrain dopamine unit activity. Eur. J. Pharmacol. **209:** 135–138.
22. BUNNEY, B. S. & A. A. GRACE. 1978. Acute and chronic haloperidol treatment: Comparison of effects on nigral dopaminergic cell activity. Life Sci. **23:** 1715–1728.
23. MELTZER, L. T., C. L. CHRISTOFFERSEN, K. A. SERPA & A. RAZMPOUR. 1993. Comparison of the effects of the cholecystokinin-B receptor antagonist, PD 134308, and the cholecystokinin-A receptor antagonist, L-364,718, on dopamine neuronal activity in the substantia nigra and ventral tegmental area. Synapse **13:** 117–122.
24. PATEL, S., K. L. CHAPMAN, A. J. SMITH, A. HEALD & S. B. FREEDMAN. 1993. Use of *ex-vivo* binding to estimate brain penetration and central activity of CCK-B antagonists. Ann. N.Y. Acad. Sci., this volume.
25. FREEMAN, A. S., L. T. MELTZER & B. S. BUNNEY. 1985. Firing properties of substantia nigra dopaminergic neurons in freely moving rats. Life Sci. **36:** 1983–1994.
26. KELLAND, M. D., A. S. FREEMAN & L. A. CHIODO. 1989. Chloral hydrate anesthesia alters the responsiveness of identified midbrain dopamine neurons to dopamine agonist administration. Synapse **3:** 30–37.
27. KELLAND, M. D., L. A. CHIODO & A. S. FREEMAN. 1990. Anesthetic influences on the basal activity and pharmacological responsiveness of nigrostriatal dopamine neurons. Synapse **6:** 207–209.
28. DIANA, M., M. GIANPAOLO, A. MURA, F. FADDA, N. PASSINO & G. GESSA. 1991. Low doses of gama-hydroxybutyric acid stimulate the firing rate of dopaminergic neurons in unanesthetized rats. Brain Res. **566:** 208–211.
29. IYENGAR, S., D. LI, R. M. SIMMONS, J. J. HOWBERT & K. RASMUSSEN. 1993. CCK-B receptors tonically modulate A10 dopaminergic neurons selectively: Neurochemical evaluation of LY288513. Soc. Neurosci. Abstr., in press.
30. SINGH, L., M. J. FIELD, J. HUGHES, R. MENZIES, R. J. OLES, C. A. VASS & G. N. WOODRUFF. 1991. The behavioral properties of Cl-988, a selective cholecystokinin-B receptor antagonist. Br. J. Pharmacol. **104:** 239–245.
31. ERVIN, F. R., R. M. PALMOUR & J. BRADWEJN. 1991. A new primate model for panic disorder. Am. Psychiat. Assoc. **144:** (NR216) 100.
32. DE MONTIGNY, C. 1989. Cholecystokinin tetrapeptide induces panic-like attacks in healthy volunteers. Arch. Gen. Psychiatry **46:** 511–517.
33. ABELSON, J. L. & R. M. NESSE. 1990. Cholecystokinin-4 and panic. Arch. Gen. Psychiatry **47:** 395.
34. BRADWEJN, J., D. KOSZYCKI & C. SHRIQUI. 1991. Enhanced sensitivity to cholecystokinin tetrapeptide in panic disorder. Arch. Gen. Psychiatry **48:** 603–610.
35. BARRETT, J. E., M. C. LINDEN, H. C. HOLLOWAY, M. J. YU & J. J. HOWBERT. 1991. Anxiolytic-like effects of the CCK-B antagonists LY262691, LY262684, and LY247348 on punished responding of squirrel monkeys. Soc. Neurosci. Abstr. **17:** 1063.

36. POWELL, K. R. & J. E. BARRETT. 1991. Evaluation of the effects of PD 134308 (Cl-988), a CCK-B antagonist, on the punished responding of squirrel monkeys. Neuropeptides **19:** 75–78.
37. RATAUD, J., F. DARCHE, F, O. PIOT, J. M. STUTZMANN, G. A. BOHME & J. C. BLANCHARD. 1991. Anxiolytic effect of CCK-antagonists on plus-maze behavior in mice. Brain Res. **548:** 315–317.
38. KANEYUKI, H., H. YOKOO, A. TSUDA, M. YOSHIDA, Y. MIZUKI, M. YAMADA & M. TANAKA. 1991. Psychological stress increases dopamine turnover selectively in mesoprefrontal dopamine neurons of rats: Reversal by diazepam. Brain Res. **557:** 154–161.
39. ROTH, R. H., S. Y. TAM, Y. IDA, J. X. YANG & A. Y. DEUTCH. 1988. Stress and the mesocorticolimbic dopamine systems. Ann. N.Y. Acad. Sci. **537:** 138–147.
40. PALMOUR, R., F. R. ERVIN, J. BRADWEJN & J. J. HOWBERT. 1991. Anxiogenic and cardiovascular effects of CCK-4 in monkeys are blocked by the CCK-B antagonist LY262691. Soc. Neurosci. Abstr. **17:** 1602.
41. DOHRENWEND, B. P. & G. EGRI. 1981. Recent stressful life events and episodes of schizophrenia. Schizophrenia Bull. **7:** 12–23.
42. SPRING, B. 1981. Stress and schizophrenia: Some definitional issues. Schizophrenia Bull. **7:** 24–33.
43. HOMMER, D. W., G. STONER, J. N. CRAWLEY, S. M. PAUL & L. R. SKIRBOLL. 1986. Cholecystokinin-dopamine coexistence: Electrophysiological actions corresponding to cholecystokinin receptor subtype. J. Neurosci. **6:** 3039–3043.
44. KELLAND, M. D., J. ZHANG, L. A. CHIODO & A. S. FREEMAN. 1991. Receptor selectivity of cholecystokinin effects on mesoaccumbens dopamine neurons. Synapse **8:** 137–143.
45. HILL, D. R. & G. N. WOODRUFF. 1990. Differentiation of central cholecystokinin receptor binding sites using the non-peptide antagonists MK-329 and L-365,260. Brain Res. **526:** 276–283.
46. WOODRUFF, G. N., D. R. HILL, P. BODEN, R. PINNOCK, L. SINGH & J. HUGHES. 1991. Functional role of brain CCK receptors. Neuropeptides **19:** 45–56.
47. JIANG, L. H., R. J. KASSER & R. X. WANG. 1988. Cholecystokinin antagonist lorglumide reverses chronic haloperidol-induced effects on dopamine neurons. Brain Res. **473:** 165–168.
48. RASMUSSEN, K., J. J. HOWBERT & M. E. STOCKTON. 1993. Inhibition of A9 and A10 dopamine cells by the cholecystokinin-B antagonist LY262691: Mediation through feedback pathways from forebrain sites. Synapse **15:** 95–103.
49. GODUKHIN, O. V., A. D. ZHARIKOVA & V. I. NOVOSELOV. 1980. The release of labeled L-glutamic acid from rat neocaudate-putamen in vivo following stimulation of frontal cortex. Neuroscience **5:** 2151–2154.
50. GERFEN, G. R. 1989. The neostriatal mosaic: Striatal patch-matrix organization is related to cortical lamination. Science **246:** 385–388.
51. GERFEN, C. R. 1992. The neostriatal mosaic: Multiple levels of compartmental organization. Trends Neurosci. **15:** 133–138.
52. BUNNEY, B. S. & G. K. AGHAJANIAN. 1976. The precise localization of nigral afferents in the rat as determined by a retrograde tracing technique. Brain Res. **117:** 423–435.
53. OADES, R. D. & G. M. HALLIDAY. 1987. Ventral tegmental (A10) system: Neurobiology. 1. Anatomy and connectivity. Brain Res. Rev. **12:** 117–165.
54. SESACK, S. R. & V. M. PICKEL. 1992. Prefrontal cortical efferents in the rat synapse on unlabeled neuronal targets of catecholamine terminals in the nucleus accumbens septi and on dopamine neurons in the ventral tegmental area. J. Comp. Neurol. **320:** 145–160.

A Second Generation of Non-Peptide Cholecystokinin Receptor Antagonists and Their Possible Therapeutic Potential

S. B. FREEDMAN,[a,b] S. PATEL,[a] A. J. SMITH,[a]
K. CHAPMAN,[a] A. FLETCHER,[a] J. A. KEMP,[a]
G. R. MARSHALL,[a] R. J. HARGREAVES,[a] K. SCHOLEY,[a]
E. C. MELLIN,[c] R. M. DiPARDO,[c] M. G. BOCK,[c]
AND R. M. FREIDINGER[c]

[a]*Merck Sharp and Dohme Research Laboratories
Departments of Biochemistry and Pharmacology
Neuroscience Research Centre
Terlings Park
Eastwick Road
Harlow, Essex, England*

[c]*Medicinal Chemistry
West Point, Pennsylvania 19486*

The peptide hormone cholecystokinin (CCK) has been demonstrated to act as a neurotransmitter in the central nervous system and to have an important physiological role in peripheral tissues such as the gastrointestinal tract. The peptide is thought to be associated with a number of physiological processes, which include the neural pathways mediating secretion, motility, pain, satiety, anxiety, and neurotransmission. In the 1980s Innis and Snyder[1] and Moran et al.[2] suggested the presence of at least two subtypes of CCK receptors, termed CCK-A and CCK-B/gastrin. In both radioreceptor binding and functional studies, it was shown that these receptors had a distinctive regional distribution and pharmacological specificity. More recently, several developments have led to renewed interest in the cholecystokinin field, including the molecular cloning and characterization of CCK-A and CCK-B/gastrin receptors and the discovery of a more ubiquitous distribution of CCK-A and CCK-B receptors within the CNS and periphery than was previously appreciated. In addition, both animal studies and trials in man have suggested an increasing number of potential therapeutic areas in which CCK has been implicated. All of these developments have led to interest in the identification of selective non-peptide antagonists for both of the CCK receptor subtypes.

FIRST GENERATION NON-PEPTIDE CCK-B ANTAGONISTS

The first available cholecystokinin antagonists were either peptide based or simple derivatives of dibutyryl cGMP.[3] An important breakthrough was the identification of asperlicin as a selective CCK antagonist.[4] This subsequently led to the development of benzodiazepine-based antagonists such as devazepide (MK-329)

[b]Author for correspondence.

and L-365,260 which were the first selective compounds available with high affinity for CCK-A and CCK-B receptors, respectively.[5,6] These compounds enabled the first investigations of the potential therapeutic applications of CCK-A and CCK-B receptors, because they had a number of important advantages over the early antagonists. L-365,260 has high affinity for the human CCK-B receptor and reasonable selectivity compared with the CCK-A receptor (TABLE 1). Furthermore, it has excellent CNS penetration, is orally bioavailable, and has low toxicity. One limiting feature of the compound was its relatively low aqueous solubility and rate of dissolution, which meant that special formulations were required for *in vivo* use. This property prompted a search for a second generation of CCK-B receptor antagonists.

SECOND GENERATION NON-PEPTIDE CCK-B ANTAGONISTS

The remainder of this chapter focuses on the biochemical and pharmacological properties of L-368,935 (*N*-(1,3-dihydro-1-(2-methyl)propyl-2-oxo-5-phenyl-1H-1,4-

TABLE 1. *In vitro* Binding Properties of Acidic Benzodiazepine CCK-B Antagonists Compared to L-365,260[a]

Benzodiazepines	Guinea Pig CCK-B IC_{50} (nM)	Rat CCK-A IC_{50} (nM)	CCK-A/CCK-B Selectivity	Aqueous Solubility (mg/ml)[b]
L-365,260	8.5	680	80	<0.002
L-367,116	4.9	98	20	2.64
L-368,730	1.0	580	580	0.58
L-368,935	0.14	1400	10,000	0.48

[a]Binding results are expressed as the geometric means. All values are a minimum of four independent determinations. CCK-B binding was to guinea pig cerebral cortex; CCK-A binding was to rat pancreas.
[b]Determined at pH 7.4.

benzodiazepin-3-yl)-N-((3-(1H-tetrazol-5-yl)phenyl) urea)), a second generation nonpeptide CCK-B receptor selective antagonist (FIG. 1).

IN VITRO PROPERTIES

The initial strategy to identify more water-soluble antagonists led to the investigation of the effects of modification of the N1 substituent and the meta position of the urea phenyl ring of L-365,260. Of particular interest was the discovery that the acetic acid derivative L-367,116 (FIG. 1) retained high affinity for CCK-B receptors (TABLE 1) and that inclusion of the acidic moiety improved aqueous solubility from <0.002 to 2.64 mg/ml. This compound, however, penetrated relatively poorly into the CNS as seen in an *ex vivo* binding assay with only limited inhibition (<50%) of specific binding at 10 mg/kg intravenously in mouse brain.

To increase the receptor affinity and CNS potency a range of acidic replacements was investigated, and interesting biological activity was observed with a number of tetrazole derivatives. L-368,730, the tetrazole analog of L-365,260 (FIG. 1), showed an eightfold increase in CCK-B receptor affinity and improved the CCK-B/CCK-A

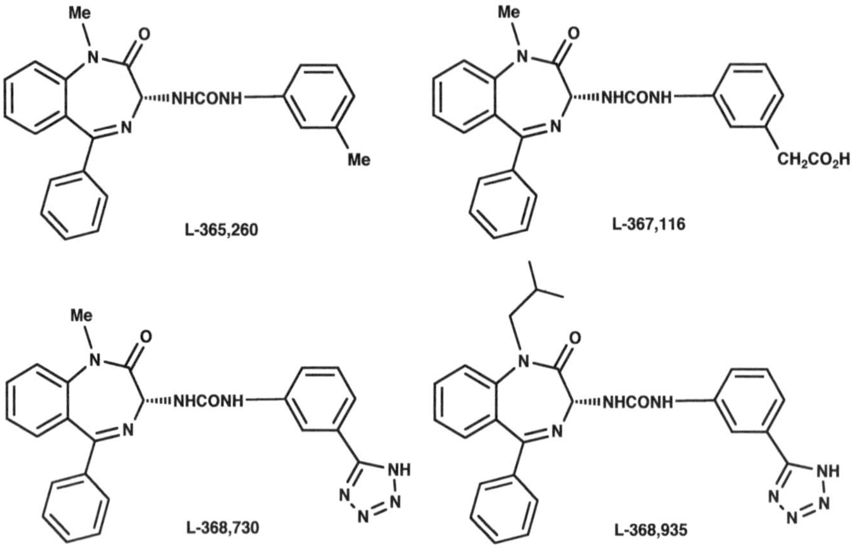

FIGURE 1. Structures of the acidic benzodiazepines L-367,116, L-368,730, and L-368,935 compared with L-365,260.

selectivity from 80 to 580. Replacement of the N1 methyl group by lipophilic alkyl substituents improved both affinity and selectivity. Optimal activity was seen with the isobutyl derivative L-368,935 (CCK-B IC_{50} 0.1 nM) which had a 60-fold increased affinity compared with L-365,260. In comparison with other recently described CCK-B receptor antagonists, such as CI 988[7] and LY 262,691,[8] L-368,935 appeared to be the most potent and selective CCK-B antagonist yet described (10,000-fold CCK-B selective, TABLE 2). The solubility of both tetrazole derivatives was significantly improved compared with L-365,260 (TABLE 1).

L-368,935 retained high affinity for the guinea pig gastrin receptor (IC_{50} 0.30 nM) when measured by the displacement of [^{125}I] gastrin binding to isolated gastric glands, supporting the hypothesis that the CCK-B and gastrin receptor are identical gene products.[9] L-368,730 and L-368,935 also retained high affinity for the human CCK-B receptor from human cerebral cortex (IC_{50} 2.1 and 0.27 nM, respectively),

TABLE 2. *In Vitro* Binding Properties of Second-Generation CCK-B Antagonists Compared to L-365,260[a]

Compound	Class	Guinea Pig CCK-B IC_{50} (nM)	Rat CCK-A IC_{50} (nM)	CCK-A/CCK-B Selectivity
L-365,260	Benzodiazepine	8.5	680	80
LY 262,691	Pyrazolidinone	31[b]	11,500	370
CI988	Dipeptoid	3.3	1500	450
L-368,935	Acidic benzodiazepine	0.14	1400	10,000

[a]Binding results are expressed as the geometric means. All values are a minimum of four independent determinations.
[b]Mouse brain, Howbert *et al.*[8]

but they had no affinity for the benzodiazepine binding site on the GABA-A receptor as measured by [^{3}H] RO 15-1788 binding to rat cortical membranes.

FUNCTIONAL ACTIVITY OF CCK-B ANTAGONISTS

Two models were used to determine the functional activity of the tetrazole derivative L-368,935 *in vitro*. In the rat ventromedial hypothalamic slice preparation, L-368,935 produced a rightward shift of the pentagastrin dose response curve (FIG. 2) with an estimated Kb of 0.6 ± 0.4 nM ($n = 5$). At high concentrations (10 nM) a slight flattening of the dose response curve was observed, probably due to a number of factors. These included the very slow off rate observed with a high affinity compound like L-368,935, and secondly the problems of desensitization associated with CCK, which meant that only very short agonist application times were possible (1 minute). Because of these considerations, it is unlikely that equilibrium would have been reached using this experimental protocol.

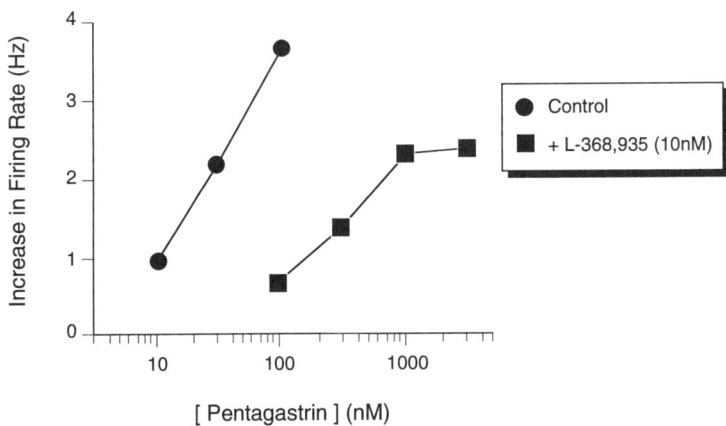

FIGURE 2. Effect of L-368,935 on the rat ventromedial hypothalamic slice preparation.

We recently reported that pentagastrin produces an increase in calcium mobilization in GH3 cells and that this response is mediated by CCK-B receptors.[10] The response curve to pentagastrin (100 nM) was significantly inhibited by both L-365,260 (IC_{50} 220 nM) and L-368,935 (IC_{50} of 9.5 nM), which corresponded to a 23-fold increase in activity for the tetrazole derivative.

These results support the hypothesis that L-368,935 is a selective antagonist with high affinity for CCK-B receptors. There was no evidence for agonist or partial agonist activity in either the VMH slice preparation or the calcium mobilization studies.

IN VIVO PROPERTIES OF CCK-B ANTAGONISTS

The functional activity of the tetrazole antagonist L-368,935 *in vivo* was estimated by its ability to block pentagastrin-induced gastric acid secretion in the anesthetized rat.[11] L-365,260 (ip) blocked the response to pentagastrin dose-dependently with an ED_{50} of 0.83 mg/kg. Following intraperitoneal administration, L-368,935 also dose-dependently blocked this response but was almost an order of magnitude more potent, with an ED_{50} of 0.14 mg/kg (FIG. 3). Since there have been no reports that CCK-B receptor antagonists discriminate between CCK-B and gastrin receptors, these results support the suggestion that L-368,935 is a potent antagonist of CCK-B receptors *in vivo*.

To assess the penetration of these compounds into the central nervous system and estimate their *in vivo* potency, we have examined the activity of L-365,260, L-368,730, and L-368,935 in an *ex vivo* binding model in mouse. In this model mice were administered intravenously with test compound 30 minutes prior to sacrifice. CNS activity of test compound was then quantified by the measurement of residual binding activity in whole brain *ex vivo* using [^{125}I] BHCCK-8S. An important discovery during the development of this assay was the finding that high plasma levels of test compounds could potentially give a false positive in this assay due to the presence of the residual plasma within the blood vessels of the brain. This potential artefact was eliminated by anesthetizing the animals at the end of the experiment and transcardially perfusing with heparinized saline to remove residual blood from brain. The detailed methodology and development are described elsewhere in this volume.[12]

All three compounds dose-dependently inhibited *ex vivo* binding in mouse (TABLE 3), with L-368,935 being most potent with an ED_{50} of 5.6 mg/kg. Interestingly, this corresponded to only a threefold increase compared to that seen with L-365,260 (ED_{50} 13 mg/kg). Although these results suggested that significant amounts of L-368,935 penetrate the CNS, the relative potency compared with that of L-365,260 was less than the comparative differences in *in vitro* affinity between L-365,260 and L-368,935 (60-fold). This suggested that brain penetration of the tetrazole was significantly less than that with L-365,260.

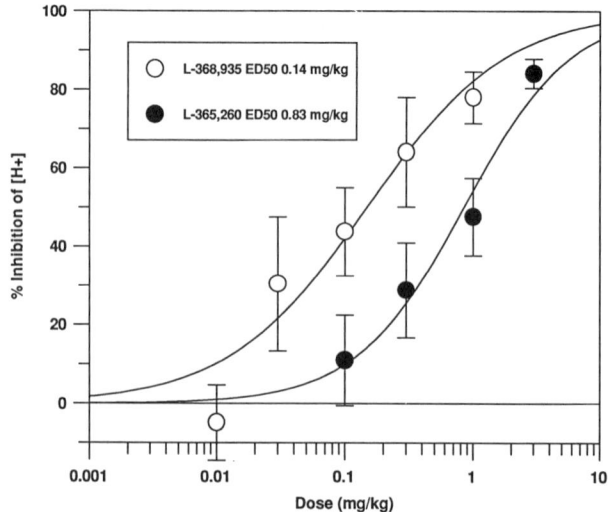

FIGURE 3. Antagonism of pentagastrin-induced gastric acid secretion in the anesthetized rat by L-368,935 and L-365,260.

TABLE 3. Comparison of L-365,260 and L-368,935 *In Vivo*[a]

Benzodiazepine	In Vitro CCK-B affinity IC_{50} (nM)	Ex Vivo Binding ED_{50} (mg/kg iv)	In Vivo Dialysis MED (mg/kg iv)
L-365,260	8.5	13	0.1
L-368,935	0.14	5.6	0.1

[a]*Ex vivo* studies were performed in mouse as described in the text using [^{125}I] BHCCK-8S. Dialysis studies were performed in 200 g male Sprague-Dawley rats.

These results were confirmed in a separate series of experiments using intracerebral dialysis to measure the effects of peripherally administered CCK-B antagonists on CCK-8S–induced aspartic acid release from rat striatum. Barnes and colleagues[13] recently reported that CCK-8S causes an increase in aspartate, glycine, and GABA release from rat striatal slices *in vitro* by a CCK-B receptor mechanism. We recently developed an *in vivo* correlate of this response using anesthetized rats that were previously implanted with microdialysis probes into the striatum (Patel *et al.*, manuscript in preparation). CCK-8S administered through the probe at 1 μM produced a 3- to 4-fold increase in aspartate release, which was blocked dose-dependently by both L-365,260 (MED 0.1 mg/kg) and L-368,935 (MED 0.1 mg/kg) (TABLE 3). These results confirmed previous results in the *ex vivo* binding studies and indicated that significant amounts of L-368,935 penetrated the CNS, albeit to a lesser extent than did L-365,260. These findings were verified by direct measurement using HPLC detection methods of L-368,935 in the CNS of rats following intravenous administration (3 mg/kg). Brain levels of L-368,935 (corrected for drug remaining in residual plasma within the brain) corresponded to 29 ng/g brain tissue 30 minutes after drug administration (M. Graham, personal communication).

CONCLUSIONS

The discovery of benzodiazepines as small molecule, non-peptide antagonists of CCK-B receptors has been important in our understanding of the role of CCK in physiology and disease. The second generation of more selective, higher affinity antagonists, such as L-368,935, which possess improved pharmaceutical properties, will facilitate studies on the therapeutic utility of this class of compound in man.

SUMMARY

The profile of an acidic series of benzodiazepine CCK-B receptor antagonists is described. The tetrazolyl urea derivative L-368,935 had high affinity (CCK-B IC_{50} 0.1 nM) and was one of the most selective (CCK-B/CCK-A 10,000) CCK-B antagonists known. L-368,935 was a CCK-B antagonist with high affinity on the rat ventromedial hypothalamic slice preparation (Kb 0.6 nM) and also blocked pentagastrin-induced calcium mobilization in GH3 cells. L-368,935 had potent *in vivo* activity and antagonized pentagastrin-induced gastric acid secretion in the anesthetized rat and CCK-8S–induced aspartate release using microdialysis in the striatum of conscious rats. Activity within the central nervous system was confirmed by a mouse *ex vivo* binding assay and by direct measurement of the compound within the central nervous system using an HPLC assay. A second generation of CCK-B receptor antagonists such as L-368,935 will be important in determining the therapeutic potential of this class of compound in man.

REFERENCES

1. INNIS, R. B. & S. H. SNYDER. 1980. Distinct cholecystokinin receptors in brain and pancreas. Proc. Natl. Acad. Sci. USA **77:** 6917–6921.
2. MORAN, T. H., P. H. ROBINSON, M. S. GOLDRICH & P. R. MCHUGH. 1986. Two brain cholecystokinin receptors: Implications for behavioural actions. Brain Res. **362:** 175–179.
3. PEIKIN, S. R., C. L. COSTENBADER & J. D. GARDNER. 1979. Actions of derivatives of cyclic nucleotides on dispersed acini from guinea pig pancreas. J. Biol. Chem. **254:** 5321–5327.
4. CHANG, R. S., V. J. LOTTI, J. MONAGHAN, J. BIRNBAUM, E. O. STAPLEY, M. A. GOETZ, G. ALBERS-SCHONBERG, A. A. PATCHETT, J. M. LIESCH, O. D. HENSENS & J. P. SPRINGER. 1985. A potent non-peptide cholecystokinin antagonist selective for peripheral tissues isolated from Aspergillus alliaceus. Science **230:** 177–179.
5. EVANS, B. E., M. G. BOCK, K. E. RITTLE, R. M. DIPARDO, W. L. WHITTER, D. F. VEBER, P. S. ANDERSON & R. M. FREIDINGER. 1986. Design of potent, orally effective, non-peptide antagonists of the peptide hormone cholecystokinin. Proc. Natl. Acad. Sci. USA **83:** 4918–4922.
6. BOCK, M. G., R. M. DIPARDO, B. E. EVANS, K. E. RITTLE, W. L. WHITTER, D. F. VEBER, P. S. ANDERSON & R. M. FREIDINGER. 1989. Benzodiazepine gastrin and brain cholecystokinin receptor ligands-L-365,260. J. Med. Chem. **32:** 13–16.
7. HUGHES, J., P. BODEN, B. COSTALL, A. DOMENEY, E. KELLY, D. C. HORWELL, J. C. HUNTER, R. D. PINNOCK & G. N. WOODRUFF. 1990. Development of a class of selective cholecystokinin type B receptor antagonists having potent anxiolytic activity. Proc. Natl. Acad. Sci. USA **87:** 6728–6732.
8. HOWBERT, J. J., K. L. LOBB, R. F. BROWN, J. K. REEL, D. A. NEEL, N. R. MASON, L. G. MENDEL, J. P. HODGKISS & J. S. KELLY. 1992. A novel series of non-peptide CCK and gastrin antagonists: Medicinal chemistry and electrophysiological demonstration of antagonism. In Multiple Cholecystokinin Receptors in the CNS. C. T. Dourish, S. J. Cooper, S. D. Iversen & L. L. Iversen, eds.: 28–37. Oxford University Press. Oxford, UK.
9. KOPIN, A. S., Y.-M. LEE, E. W. MCBRIDE, L. J. MILLER, M. LU, H. Y. LIN, L. F. KOLAKOWSKI & M. BEINBORN. 1992. Expression cloning and characterisation of the canine parietal cell gastrin receptor. Proc. Natl. Acad. Sci. USA **89:** 3605–3609.
10. SMITH, A. J., S. PATEL & S. B. FREEDMAN. 1993. Characterisation of CCK-B receptors in GH3 cells. Br. J. Pharmacol. **108:** 26P.
11. GHOSH, M. N. & H. O. SCHILD. 1958. Continuous recording of acid gastric secretion in the rat. Br. J. Pharmacol. Chemother. **13:** 54–61.
12. PATEL, S., K. L. CHAPMAN, A. J. SMITH, A. HEALD & S. B. FREEDMAN. 1993. Use of *ex vivo* binding to estimate brain penetration and central activity of CCK-B antagonists. Ann. New York Acad. Sci., this volume.
13. BARNES, S., H. L. WHISTLER, J. HUGHES, G. N. WOODRUFF & J. C. HUNTER. 1991. Effect of cholecystokinin octapeptide on endogenous amino acid release from the rat ventromedial nucleus of the hypothalamus and striatum. J. Neurochem. **56:** 1409–1416.

A Processing-Independent Analysis (PIA) for Human Procholecystokinin and Its Products

LEA I. PALOHEIMO AND JENS F. REHFELD[a]

State University Hospital
Department of Clinical Biochemistry
Rigshospitalet
DK-2100 Copenhagen, Denmark

To study the widespread expression of the human cholecystokinin (CCK) gene and to improve the diagnostic specificity and sensitivity of CCK measurements, we designed an analysis that is independent of the processing of proCCK in both normal CCK-producing cells and neoplastic cells. This principle, named processing-independent analysis (PIA), has been evaluated in detail for progastrin.[1,2]

Using synthetic fragment 62-71 (Asn-Leu-Gln-Asn-Leu-Asp-Pro-Ser-His-Arg) of human proCCK as antigen, antibodies were raised in eight rabbits. Rabbit 89009 produced antibodies of sufficient titer (3.5×10^5), monoclonality (Sips index ~ 1.0), and affinity ($K^o_{eff} \sim 0.88 \times 10^{12}$ l/mol). A radioimmunoassay (using antiserum 89009 and tyrosine-extended 1–10 fragment of human CCK-22 as tracer, that is, specific for the NH_2-terminus of human CCK-22) proved useful for measurement. Thus, after tryptic cleavage at Lys^{61} of proCCK, the assay measures the CCK mRNA translation product irrespective of the degree of processing.

During examination of different tumors, we found an interesting malignant small round cell tumor in the thoracopulmonary region (Askin tumor), in which the processing of proCCK was extraordinary. The tumor contained 10.1 pmol/g of proCCK and its products before and 71.3 pmol/g after tryptic cleavage. By gel filtration (FIG. 1) of the water extract, a large peak eluted at $K_d = 0.03$, which most likely is a mixture of unprocessed proCCK and glycine-extended CCK-83. After tryptic cleavage the proCCK peak increased 20-fold. Normally processed CCK was also present in water extract. Gel filtration of acetic acid extract revealed a mixture of CCK-33/39 ($K_d = 0.53$) and COOH-terminally extended forms of CCK-8 ($K_d = 0.95$), moderate amounts of CCK-83, CCK-58, and CCK-22 ($K_d = 0.21, 0.32,$ and 0.67), and some processing intermediates.

We conclude that monospecific antibodies against NH_2-terminal sequence of CCK-22 are suitable for development of a processing-independent analysis (PIA) for proCCK and its products. Moreover, such a PIA appears useful for quantitation of the CCK gene expression in normal and neoplastic tissue.

---

[a] Address for correspondence: Jens F. Rehfeld, Professor, D.Med & D.Sc., State University Hospital, Department of Clinical Biochemistry, Rigshospitalet, Blegdamsvej 9, DK-2100 Copenhagen, Denmark.

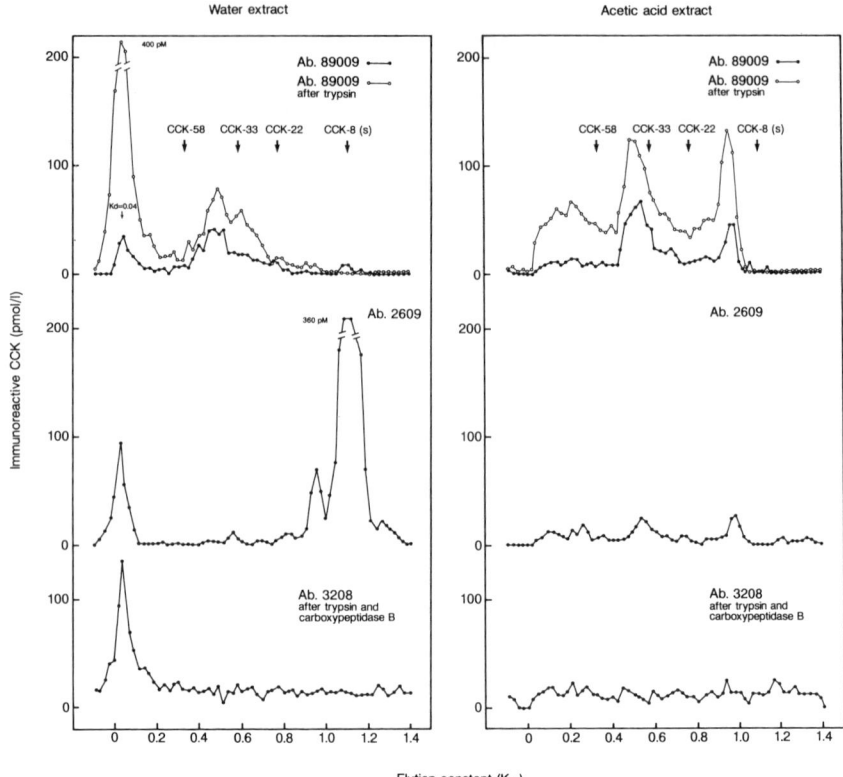

FIGURE 1. Gel chromatography of 1 ml water and acetic acid extracts from an Askin tumor applied to Sephadex G-50 superfine column (10 × 1,000 mm) and eluted at 4°C with 20 mmnol/l barbital buffer, pH 8.4, containing 0.11% bovine serum albumin. Fractions of 1.2–1.3 were collected at a rate of 4 ml/h. Fractions (1:2 diluted) were monitored by radioimmunoassays with Ab 89009 specific for the NH_2-terminal CCK-22, Ab 2609 specific for the common carboxyamidated COOH-terminus of the CCK and gastrin, and Ab 3208 sequence specific for the glycine-extended gastrin and CCK. Expected positions of CCK peptides are indicated by *arrows*. Inasmuch as human CCK-58 was not available for calibration, elution position is marked as reported by others.[3]

REFERENCES

1. BARDRAM, L. & J. F. REHFELD. 1988. Processing-independent radioimmunoanalysis: A general analytical principle applied to progastrin and its products. Anal. Biochem. **175:** 537–543.
2. BARDRAM, L. & J. F. REHFELD. 1989. Production and evaluation of monospecific antibodies for processing-independent sequence of human progastrin. Scand. J. Clin. Lab. Invest. **49:** 173–182.
3. EYSSELEIN, V. E., J. R. REEVE, JR., J. E. SHIVELY, C. MILLER & J. H. WALSH. 1984. Isolation of a large cholecystokinin precursor from canine brain. Proc. Natl. Acad. Sci. USA **81:** 6565–6568.

Regulation of the Human Cholecystokinin Gene

KARIN PEDERSEN, FINN CILIUS NIELSEN, AND
JENS F. REHFELD

Department of Clinical Biochemistry
State University Hospital
Blegdamsvej 9
DK-2100 Copenhagen, Denmark

Expression of the CCK gene is known to be regulated in a tissue-specific and developmentally-specific manner. This study characterizes the *cis*- and *trans*-acting elements in the promoter region that control the transcription of the gene. We cloned ~1,400 base pairs of the promoter region from a size-fractionated λgt10 genomic library. Deletion constructs of the promoter region were performed, and the fragments were fused to the bacterial chloramphenicol acetyl transferase gene (CAT). Relative CAT activity was measured, and the actual binding of proteins to the promoter region was examined by band shifts.

RESULTS AND DISCUSSION

The activity of the promoter region was examined by transient transfections[1] of the deletion constructs into the neuroblastoma cell line SK-N-MC. Relative CAT activity was measured[2] (FIG. 1A). A computer search revealed several motifs of putative binding sites for *trans*-acting factors. Three of the binding sites found in this search were SP-1, AP-1, and USF.[3-5] In FIGURE 1B the position of the three putative binding sites for *trans*-acting factors is indicated.

The binding of *trans*-acting factors to the various regulatory elements was analyzed by band shifts[1] using nuclear extracts[6] from the SK-N-MC cells. A band shift, performed with an SP-1 probe, showed binding of a protein to the probe. The binding was fully displaced with 100 times molar excess of the competitor. Likewise, a band shift was performed with the AP-1 probe and with nuclear extract from SK-N-MC cells. A protein bound to the probe with a low affinity because a 10,000-fold molar excess of competitor was necessary to displace the binding. Results showed that the SP-1 protein bound with a higher affinity to the probe than did the AP-1 protein.

For examination of the USF binding site, two probes were synthesized, one (CCKUSF) with the USF sequence in the CCK promoter region and another (CCKUSFΔ) that exhibits three base substitutions in the putative binding site. The band shift shows a DNA protein complex (FIG. 2), indicated by A, which was displaced by 100 times molar excess of the nonlabeled probe. The mutated probe did not displace the binding, and the protein did not bind to the mutated probe. We conclude that the USF element associates strongly with the *trans*-acting factor.

To confirm that the protein binding to the probe was the USF protein reported,[3] we obtained a USF-specific polyclonal antibody and also some purified recombinant USF protein[3] which was used in a super shift and in band shifts to compare the recombinant USF-DNA complex to the protein-DNA complex formed with nuclear extract from SK-N-MC cells. These two experiments showed that the protein was the USF protein.

CONCLUSION

In this study we identified three positive regulatory elements in the human CCK promoter region. Band shift analyses demonstrated high affinity binding sites for SP-1 and USF proteins. The functional significance of the putative AP-1 site is

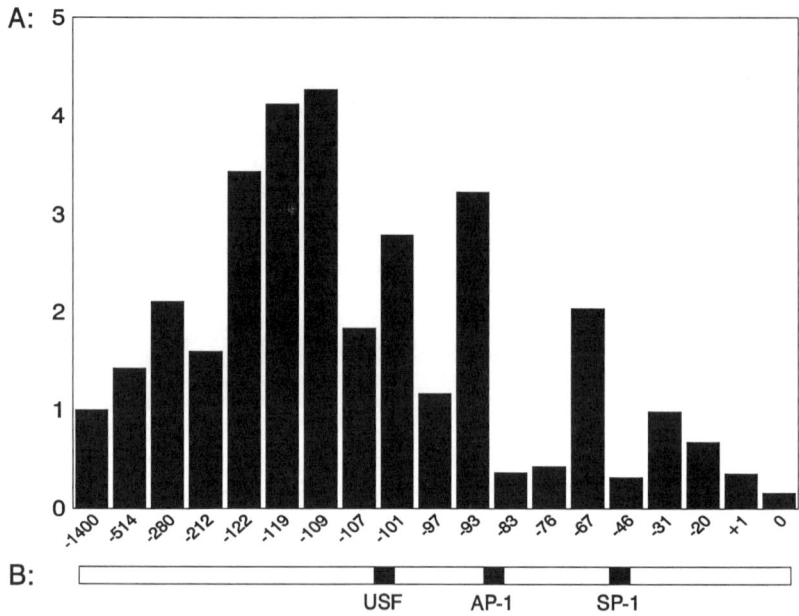

FIGURE 1. Relative CAT activity of the human CCK promoter region. (**A**) Length of the constructs is given on the X axis as the number of bases from the transcriptional start site. The fold induction compared to the longest construct = 1 is shown on the Y axis. (**B**) The position of putative binding sites for *trans*-acting factors.

uncertain because the proteins bound with very low affinity. We conclude that USF and SP-1 may be the major regulatory factors in the human CCK gene.

ACKNOWLEDGMENT

The neuroblastoma cell line SK-N-MC was kindly provided by Dr. Thue W. Schwartz, Laboratory of Molecular Endocrinology, State University Hospital, Copenhagen, Denmark. The recombinant USF protein and antibody was kindly provided by Dr. R. G. Roeder, The Rockefeller University, New York, NY.

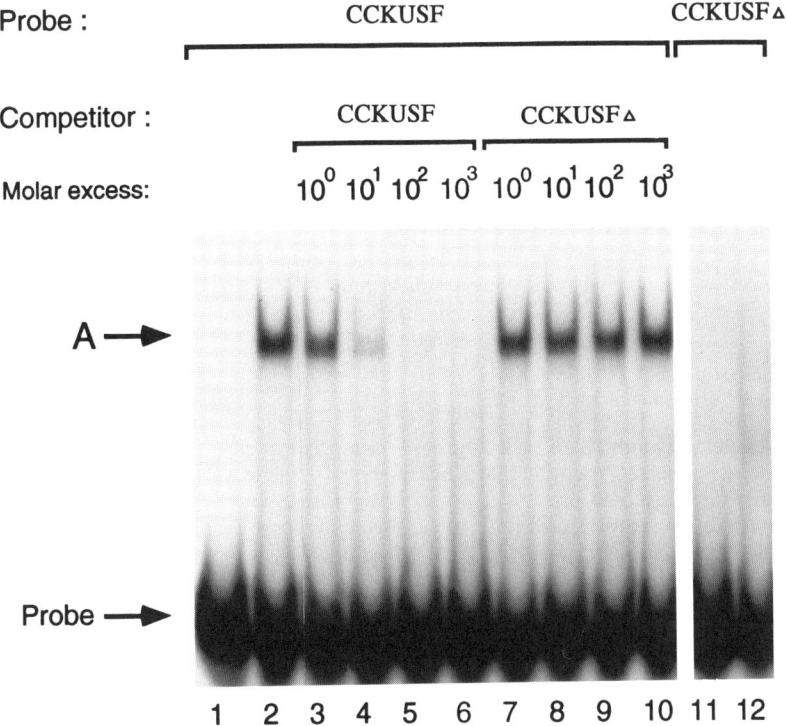

FIGURE 2. CCKUSF and CCKUSFΔ band shift. *Lane 1:* CCKUSF probe; *lane 2:* CCKUSF probe and SK-N-MC extract; *lanes 3–6:* same as lane 2 with CCKUSF competitor as indicated; *lanes 7–10:* same as lane 2 with CCKUSFΔ competitor as indicated; *lane 11:* CCKUSFΔ probe; *lane 12:* CCKUSFΔ probe and SK-N-MC extract.

REFERENCES

1. Current Protocols in Molecular Biology. 1993. John Wiley & Sons. New York.
2. GORMAN, C. 1985. *In* DNA Cloning—A Practical Approach, Vol. II. D. M. Glover, ed.: 143–165. IRL Press. Oxford, UK.
3. SAWADOGO, M., M. W. VAN DYKE, P. D. GREGOR & R. G. ROEDER. 1988. J. Biol. Chem. **263:** 11985–11988.
4. HAUN, R. S. & J. DIXON. 1990. J. Biol. Chem. **265:** 15455–15463.
5. KADONAGA, J. T. 1986. TIBS **11:** 20–23.
6. DIGNAM, J. D., R. M. LEBOVITZ & R. G. ROEDER. 1983. Nucl. Acids Res. **11:** 1475–1489.

cDNA Deduced Procionin

Structure and Expression Pattern in Protochordates Resembles that of Procholecystokinin in Mammals

J. U. THORUP,[a] H.-J. MONSTEIN, A. H. JOHNSEN, AND J. F. REHFELD

*Department of Clinical Biochemistry KB 3014
Rigshospitalet
University of Copenhagen
Blegdamsvej 9
DK-2100 Copenhagen, Denmark*

The cholecystokinin (CCK)-gastrin family comprises peptides sharing an amidated COOH-terminal tetrapeptide that is necessary for biological activity. Cholecystokinin-like peptides are also present in lower vertebrates, but their exact structure and function remain to be elucidated. Recently the octapeptide cionin was identified in the protochordate *Ciona intestinalis*.[1] With sulfated Tyr in the position of both gastrin and CCK, cionin is structurally a hybrid between the two. The present communication describes the structure and function of the cionin gene and its expression pattern in *Ciona intestinalis*.

By the combined use of 3′ RACE[2] and inverse polymerase chain reaction[3] in cloning, we isolated and characterized cDNA clones, which encode cionin. Full-length cDNA is 510 bp long and encodes a 128 amino acid preprocionin molecule (FIG. 1). Furthermore, cionin mRNA is expressed in both the neuronal ganglion and the gastrointestinal tract of *C. intestinalis*. The structure of procionin, having only one copy of cionin per propeptide, does not resemble that of the frog-skin procaeruleins. Procionin shows a greater similarity with proCCK than with progastrin because of both a COOH-terminal position of cionin between a single basic residue and an amidation site and similarity in the COOH-terminal flanking sequence of procionin and proCCK (FIG. 1). The pentapeptide sequence of procionin immediately NH$_2$-terminal to the two O-sulfated tyrosyl residues in the cionin sequence contains two Arg and only one Asp. Hence, the procionin sequence challenges the proposed consensus for tyrosyl O-sulfation[4] and suggests a different substrate specificity of protochordean tyrosyl-protein sulfotransferase. In progastrins and proCCKs, the COOH-terminal amidation site is followed by the tripeptide Ser-Ala-Glu. It has been proposed that phosphorylation of the Ser adjacent to the amidation site is of regulatory significance.[5] Inasmuch as the procionin amidation site is followed by Ala-Ile-Glu rather than Ser-Ala-Glu, phosphorylation is apparently not required for processing at the procionin amidation site.

Radioimmunoassay and chromatography[6-8] showed that the cionin gene is expressed at the peptide level in both the gastrointestinal tract and the neuronal ganglion (FIG. 2). Extracts of the neuronal ganglion contained only the cionin octapeptide amide without traces of precursors or processing intermediates. In contrast, the gastrointestinal extracts also contained significant amounts of glycine-extended cionin. Moreover, antibody G160 did not recognize the gastrointestinal

[a] Corresponding author.

FIGURE 1. (Top) Nucleotide and predicted amino acid sequence of the protochordean procionin peptide. The consensus poly A⁺ addition site AATAAA is underlined. (Bottom) Comparison of sequence homologies between the COOH-terminal parts of procionin, rat proCCK, and rat progastrin. Gaps are introduced to maximize homology between sequences. Dashes denote identity between sequences. Gly is the amide donor for mature peptides.

```
101  GlyHisMetGlnArgMetAspArgAsnTyr ... TyrGlyTrpMetAspPheGlyLysArgAla
     GGTCATATGCAAAGAATGGATCGAAACTAT ... TACGGCTGGATGGATTTTGGTAAAAGAGCA  409

121  IleGluAspValAspTyrGluTyrEnd
     ATCGAAGATGTTGATTATGAATATTAAGAA ... CATATTCATCGTAAAATGAACGTTTTCTTC  469

     GCTCAATGCTTATATTGTTTAAATAAATTT ... CGTGCAACGACAAAAAAAAAAAAA  3'   529
```

Cionin	Met	Asp	Arg	Asn	Tyr	Tyr	Gly	Trp	Met	Asp	Phe	Gly	Lys	Arg
CCK	Ser	–	–	–	Asp	–	–	–	–	–	–	–	Arg	–
Gastrin	Glu	Glu	Glu	Glu	Glu	Ala	–	–	–	–	–	–	Arg	–

Cionin	Ala	Ile	Glu	Asp	Val	Asp	Tyr	Glu	Tyr
CCK	Ser	–	–	–	–	–	–	–	–	Pro	Ser
Gastrin	–	–	–	–	–	–	Glu	Glu	Asp	Gln	Tyr	Asn

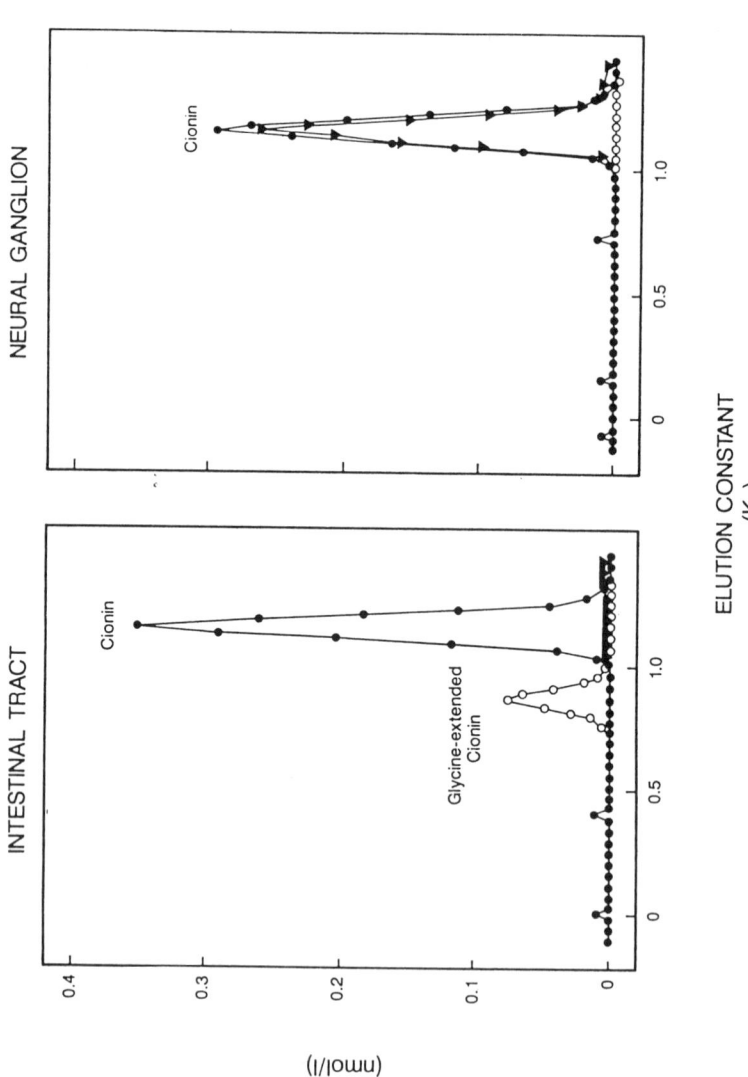

FIGURE 2. Gel chromatography extracts from the gastrointestinal tract (*left*) and neuronal ganglion (*right*) of *Ciona intestinalis*. Fractions were collected and analyzed by specific radioimmunoassays. *Symbols:* (○) antibody 3208; (●) antibody 2609; (▼) antibody G160.

peptide, which accordingly appears to be nonsulfated. Hence, the neuronal processing of procionin is more complete than that of gastrointestinal cells. Thus, the tissue-specific expression and processing of preprocionin resembles that of the mammalian CCK system.

REFERENCES

1. JOHNSEN, A. H. & J. F. REHFELD. 1990. J. Biol. Chem. **269**: 335–338.
2. FROHMANN, M. A., M. K. DUSH & G. R. MARTIN. 1988. Proc. Natl. Acad. Sci. USA **85**: 8998–9002.
3. OCHMAN, H., A. S. GERBER & D. L. HARTL. 1988. Genetics **120**: 621–623.
4. HUTTNER, W. & P. A. BAEURLE. 1988. Modern Cell Biol. **6**: 97–140.
5. DOCKRAY, G. J. et al. 1991. The Stomach as an Endocrine Organ, vol. 15. R. Håkanson & F. Sundler, eds.: 197–210. Fernström Foundation Series.
6. HILSTED, L. & J. F. REHFELD. 1986. Analyt. Biochem. **152**: 119–126.
7. REHFELD, J. F. 1978. J. Biol. Chem. **253**: 4016–4021.
8. CONLON, J. M., T. W. SCHWARTZ & J. F. REHFELD. 1988. Regul. Pept. **20**: 241–250.

Evidence for a Helix-Turn-Helix in the NH$_2$-Terminus of CCK-58

ANDREW K. S. LEE,[a] HUGH B. NICHOLAS, JR.,[b] AND GRACE L. ROSENQUIST[a]

[a]Section of Neurobiology, Physiology and Behavior
University of California
Davis, California 95616

[b]Pittsburgh Supercomputing Center
Pittsburgh, Pennsylvania 15203

Cholecystokinin-58 (CCK-58) is less active than the shorter forms in eliciting amylase release from isolated acinar cells,[1] but when given as a bolus injection, it is more potent in stimulating pancreatic bicarbonate and protein secretion in rats.[2] We present evidence for a stable helix-turn-helix structure that may explain these activity differences.

METHODS

We calculated the hydrophobic moment[3] and Chou-Fasman[4] turn potentials with Genetics Computer Group programs. Test sequences were compared to a reference group of aligned sequences and similarity scores were computed using Profile-SS.[5] Reference sequences were chosen from proteins with packed helices described by Chothia et al.[6] (TABLE 1) and aligned on their contact residues that had relative position numbers of i, i+3, i+4, and i+7 in the sequence. The structure-derived correlation matrix (SCM)[7] was chosen to quantify amino acid similarities. We used the control protein phospholipase A2[8] to evaluate the effectiveness of this method.

RESULTS

Hydrophobic moment analysis of human CCK-58 identified two regions in which an α-helix would have one nonpolar, hydrophobic face and one opposed, polar, hydrophilic face. Chou-Fasman analysis predicted a turn at residues 27–30 between the two α-helices. We hypothesized that the hydrophobic faces of the helices adhere to each other to form a stable helix-turn-helix structure. Profile-SS correctly selected the individual helices in the reference sequences when each was successively omitted from the reference set, and it correctly selected the helices in phospholipase A2 using the complete reference set (TABLE 2). The segment containing the packed helix for a given protein was ranked in the top three scores for 11 of the 16 reference peptides. The top scores for the test sequence, human CCK-58, fell within the range of scores of the known, packed helical segments. The position of the proposed helices in human CCK-58 is based on alignments with the contact residues (vertical

TABLE 1. Alignment of Sequences from 3-4 Packed Helices[a]

Name	+4 Helices Sequence			Name	+3 Helices Sequence		
	i−4	i	i+13		i−6	i	i+13
CPA[b]__124[c]	tIde	IydFmdlL	vaeH..	CPA__186	..qatg	VwfAKkfT	......
LZM[d]__82	..ak	LkpVYdsL	......	LZM__94	....vR	RcaLInmV	fqm...
LZM__94	....	VRrcALiN	mvfQm.	LZM__126	......	WdeAavNL	a.....
LZM__114	....	FtNSlrML	q.....	LZM__143	pnRakr	VitTFrtG	......
SBT[e]__210	...q	YswIIngI	EwaIan	SBT__240	....aA	LkaAvdKA	vas...
TLN[f]__164	inea	IsdIFgtL	vefya.	TLN__260	..rdkl	GkiFYraL	tqyl..
TMV[g]__38	.qqa	RttVQqqF	S.....	TMV__76	..ldpl	ItaLLgtF	d.....
TMV__74	..av	LdpLItaL	lgTFd.	TMV__117	..atvA	IrsAInnL	vnElvr

[a] +4 Helices and +3 Helices refer to helices involved in a 3-4 packing scheme as described by Chothia et al. Contact residues are bold.
[b] Carboxypeptidase A (Swiss-Prot: Cbpa__Bovin).
[c] First residue of sequence from Swiss-Prot database.
[d] Lysozyme (Swiss-Prot: Lycv__Bpt4).
[e] Subtilisin (Swiss-Prot: Subt__Bacam).
[f] Thermolysin (Swiss-Prot: Ther__Bacth).
[g] Tobacco mosaic virus coat protein (Swiss-Prot: Coat__Tmvda).

lines) in the reference set:

```
VSQRTDGESR AHLGALLARY IQQARK AP SG RMS I VKNLQN LDPSHRISDR DYMGWMDF
           |  ||    |              |  ||  |          |
           *HELIX 1*           -TURN- * --HELIX  2-- *
```

DISCUSSION

Our results suggest that a pair of packed α-helices are connected by a turn in human CCK-58. This turn may provide a favorable site for enzymatic cleavage of the peptide to form CCK-33. The proposed helix-turn-helix structure could bring the NH$_2$-terminus, or some other part of the peptide, close to the COOH-terminus and

TABLE 2. Profile-SS Analysis Scores for 3-4 Packed Helices[a]

+4 Helices			+3 Helices		
Name	Rank[b]	Score	Name	Rank	Score
TLN__164	1	445.6	TMV__117	1	347.8
CPA__124	1	441.3	SBT__240	1	339.2
TMV__74	1	401.4	LZM__94	1	328.7
SBT__210	1	397.3	LZM__126	3	307.2
LZM__114	1	395.4	TMV__76	3	303.2
LZM__82	2	390.4	TLN__260	4	285.6
CCKH[c]__31[d]	1	367.3	CCKH__14	1	275.8
TMV__38	8	358.0	CPA__186	21	269.4
LZM__94	12	351.0	LZM__143	28	253.8

[a] Chothia reference sequences: +4 Helices (i to i + 11), +3 Helices (i − 2 to i + 9).
[b] Rank within individual sequence run.
[c] Human cholecystokinin.
[d] First residue of predicted helix.

alter CCK binding and activity. Studies are underway that should conclusively define the structure of CCK-58.

REFERENCES

1. REEVE, J. R., JR., V. EYSSELEIN, G. A. EBERLEIN, P. CHEW, F. J. HO, V. D. HUEBNER, J. E. SHIVELY, T. D. LEE & R. A. LIDDLE. 1991. J. Biol. Chem. **266:** 13770–13776.
2. REEVE, J. R., JR., V. E. EYSSELEIN, H. E. RAYBOULD, R. A. LITTLE & G. EBERLEIN. 1989. The Neuropepetide Cholecystokinin (CCK): Anatomy and Biochemistry, Receptors, Pharmacology and Physiology. J. Hughes, G. Dockray & G. Woodruff, eds.: 47–57. Ellis Forwood Limited. Chichester.
3. EISENBERG, D., R. M. WEISS & T. C. TERWILLIGER. 1984. Proc. Natl. Acad. Sci. USA **81:** 140–144.
4. CHOU, P. Y. & G. D. FASMAN. 1978. Adv. Enzymol. **47:** 45–147.
5. ROPELEWSKI, A., H. NICHOLAS, JR. & M. GRIBSKOV. 1993. In preparation.
6. CHOTHIA, C., M. LEVITT & D. RICHARDSON. 1981. J. Mol. Biol. **145:** 215–250.
7. NIEFIND, K. & D. SCHOMBURG. 1991. J. Mol. Biol. **219:** 481–497.
8. BRUNIE, S., J. BOLIN, D. GEWIRTH & P. B. SIGLER. 1985. J. Biol. Chem. **260:** 9742–9749.

Characterization of Cholecystokinin Receptors in Rat Pancreas

Evidence for Expression of CCK-A Receptors But Not CCK-B (Gastrin) Receptors

WEIGONG ZHOU,[a] STEPHEN P. POVOSKI,[a]
NANCY A. ROSEN,[a] DANIEL S. LONGNECKER,[b] AND
RICHARD H. BELL, JR.[a,c]

[a]*Department of Surgery*
University of Cincinnati College of Medicine and
Veterans Affairs Medical Center
Cincinnati, Ohio 45220

[b]*Department of Pathology*
Dartmouth Medical School
Hanover, New Hampshire 03756

It has previously been demonstrated that guinea pig pancreatic acinar cells, widely used in the study of pancreatic physiology, contain three classes of cholecystokinin (CCK) receptors.[1] First is a high-affinity CCK-A receptor, which has a high affinity for CCK but a low affinity for gastrin. Second is a high-affinity CCK-B (gastrin) receptor which does not discriminate between CCK and gastrin peptides. CCK binds to both receptors with approximately equal affinity, whereas gastrin binds with high affinity only to CCK-B (gastrin) receptors. The third receptor is a low-affinity CCK receptor site which has a low affinity for both CCK and gastrin. In contrast to guinea pig pancreas, it is not known if high-affinity CCK receptors in rat pancreas are CCK-A receptors, CCK-B (gastrin) receptors, or both. Thus, in the present study, we used ^{125}I-Bolton-Hunter-labeled cholecystokinin octapeptide (^{125}I-BH-CCK-8), the specific CCK-A and CCK-B (gastrin) receptor antagonists L364,718 and L365,260, and ^{125}I-gastrin-I to characterize CCK receptors in rat pancreas. Additionally, we used ^{32}P-labeled cDNA probes of the CCK-A receptor and CCK-B (gastrin) receptor coding regions to examine the expression of CCK receptor subtypes in rat pancreas at the messenger RNA level.

MATERIALS AND METHODS

Normal pancreas and liver were obtained from 1- to 2-month-old male Lewis rats. As positive controls for the expression of both the CCK-A and CCK-B (gastrin) receptors, the rat pancreatic carcinoma cell line AR42J and the azaserine-induced rat pancreatic carcinoma DSL-6 were used. Receptor binding assays were performed by the method of von Schrenck *et al.*[2] Pancreatic tissue slices were incubated with: (1) ^{125}I-BH-CCK-8 in the presence of graded concentrations of unlabeled CCK-8; (2)

---

[c]Address for correspondence: Richard H. Bell, Jr., MD, Surgical Service (112), Veterans Affairs Medical Center, 3200 Vine St., Cincinnati, Ohio 45220.

^{125}I-BH-CCK-8 in the presence of graded concentrations of the specific CCK-A receptor antagonist L364,718 or the specific CCK-B (gastrin) receptor antagonist L365,260; (3) ^{125}I-gastrin in the presence or absence of 10 μM unlabeled gastrin-17-I. After 4 hours of incubation, the tissue slices were rinsed, and the radioactivity was counted in a gamma counter. Total RNA was isolated from normal rat pancreas, normal rat liver, AR42J, and DSL-6, electrophoresed in a 1.0% agarose/formaldehyde gel, and transferred to nylon membranes. Blots were hybridized with ^{32}P-labeled probes of the CCK-A receptor and the CCK-B (gastrin) receptor full-length coding regions,[3,4] respectively (kindly provided by Dr. Stephen A. Wank, DDB/NIDDK, NIH, Bethesda, MD).

RESULTS

^{125}I-BH-CCK-8 bound to a single class of high-affinity receptors in normal rat pancreas with K_d of 0.68 ± 0.13 nM and B_{max} of 99.2 ± 15.9 fmol/mg protein. A low-affinity receptor site with K_d of 656 ± 289 nM and B_{max} of 7,768 ± 3,107 fmol/mg protein was also identified. L364,718 was 627 times as potent as L365,260 in inhibiting ^{125}I-BH-CCK-8 binding (K_i 1.0 ± 0.1 vs 627 ± 49 nM, $p < 0.001$). L364,718 bound to normal rat pancreas at a single high-affinity site, whereas no site of high-affinity binding of L365,260 was determined. No saturable binding of ^{125}I-gastrin-I to normal rat pancreas was detected. The ^{32}P-labeled cDNA probe of the CCK-A receptor coding region hybridized with ≈ 2.7-kb mRNA from normal rat pancreas and the positive control pancreatic carcinomas (AR42J and DSL-6); no hybridizing mRNA could be identified at ≈ 2.7 kb from the negative control (normal rat liver) (FIG. 1). The ^{32}P-labeled cDNA probe of the CCK-B (gastrin) receptor coding region hybridized with ≈ 2.7-kb mRNA from the positive control pancreatic

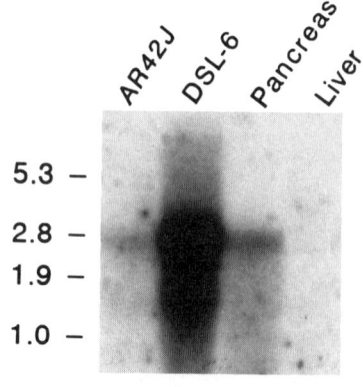
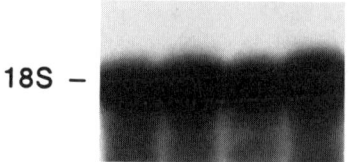

FIGURE 1. Northern blot analysis of CCK-A receptor mRNA from normal rat pancreas and control tissues. Sizes are shown in kilobases (kb). Hybridization of 18S ribosomal RNA was used as a loading control.

FIGURE 2. Northern blot analysis of CCK-B (gastrin) receptor mRNA from normal rat pancreas and control tissues. Sizes are shown in kilobases (kb). Hybridization of 18S ribosomal RNA was used as a loading control.

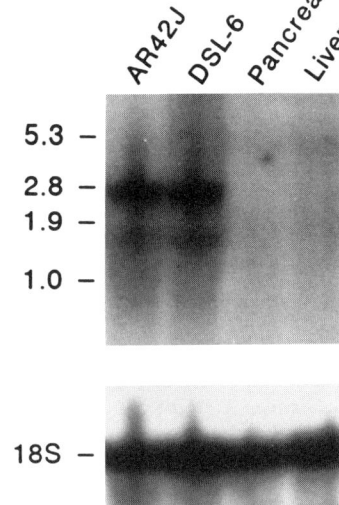

carcinomas (AR42J and DSL-6); no hybridizing mRNA could be identified around 2.7 kb from normal rat pancreas or the negative control (normal rat liver) (FIG. 2).

DISCUSSION

The present study demonstrates that normal rat pancreas expresses only CCK-A receptors. The CCK-A receptor exists in two affinity states, one with high affinity for CCK-8 but low capacity and the other with low affinity for CCK-8 but high capacity. In contrast, CCK-B (gastrin) receptors were absent in normal rat pancreas at both the receptor and messenger RNA level. These results suggest that the rat is a pure *in vivo* model for studying the biological activity of CCK-A receptors in the pancreas.

REFERENCES

1. YU, D.-H., S. C. HUANG, S. A. WANK, S. MANTEY, J. D. GARDNER & R. T. JENSEN. 1990. Pancreatic receptors for cholecystokinin: Evidence for three receptor classes. Am. J. Physiol. **258:** G86–G95.
2. VON SCHRENCK, T., T. H. MORAN, P. HEINZ-ERIAN, J. D. GARDNER & R. T. JENSEN. 1988. Cholecystokinin receptors on gallbladder muscle and pancreatic acinar cells: A comparative study. Am. J. Physiol. **255:** G512–G521.
3. WANK, S. A., R. HARKINS, R. T. JENSEN, H. SHAPIRA, A. DE WEERTH & T. SLATTERY. 1992. Purification, molecular cloning, and functional expression of the cholecystokinin receptor from rat pancreas. Proc. Natl. Acad. Sci. USA **89:** 3125–3129.
4. WANK, S. A., J. R. PISEGNA & A. DE WEERTH. 1992. Brain and gastrointestinal cholecystokinin receptor family: Structure and functional expression. Proc. Natl. Acad. Sci. USA **89:** 8691–8695.

Cholecystokinin Receptors in Cells of the Immune System

MARIE-FRANCOISE LIGNON, NICOLE BERNAD, AND
JEAN MARTINEZ

Chimie et Pharmacologie de Molécules d'Intérêt Biologique
EP CNRS 51
Faculté de Pharmacie
15 Av. C. Flahault
34060 Montpellier, France

Interactions between the central nervous system and the immune system, particularly through neuropeptides, are of growing interest,[1] and the number of reports suggest that brain/gut mediators affect the immune response.[2,3] Identification of immunoreactive forms of cholecystokinin (CCK) in human lymphocytes[4,5] and more recent studies[6,7] suggest a regulatory function of CCK in the immune system. However, initial attemps to characterize CCK receptors on lymphocytes were unsuccessful. Our approach was to use continuous lymphoblastic cell lines to identify CCK receptors in cells of the immune system. This paper summarizes our work on the characterization of CCK receptors in a human leukemia JURKAT T-cell line[8] and the study of their transduction mechanism.[9]

PHARMACOLOGICAL CHARACTERIZATION OF CCK RECEPTORS ON THE HUMAN JURKAT T-LYMPHOCYTE CELL LINE

We used labeled CCK-8 to characterize high-affinity CCK binding sites on a human JURKAT lymphoma cell line. Analysis of the data demonstrated a single class of binding sites with high affinity for the ligand ($K_d = 3.2 \pm 0.5 \cdot 10^{-11}$ M) and a binding capacity of 0.42 fmol/10^6 cells (≈ 500 sites per cell). These CCK binding sites displayed a typical CCK-B pharmacological profile established by the use of several selective agonists and antagonists for the CCK-receptor types, namely, compounds MK-329, the CCK antagonist selective for the peripheral CCK receptor (CCK-A),[10] and compound L-365,260, selective for the central CCK receptor (CCK-B)[11] and the cyclic CCK analog highly selective for the CCK-B receptor developed in our laboratory (e.g., JMV320).[12] The ligand-binding properties of these sites are in good agreement with those found in brain membranes (CCK-B sites) and differ from the predominant type of CCK binding site found in the pancreas (CCK-A type), as shown in TABLE 1.

TRANSDUCTION MECHANISM

Although second messenger systems coupled to CCK-A receptor activation are well documented, intracellular events promoted by CCK-B receptor activation remain largely obscure. Some evidence indicates that CCK-B receptors are coupled

TABLE 1. Abilities of Different CCK Agonists and Antagonists to Inhibit Binding of ^{125}I-BH-CCK-8 to Rat Pancreatic Acini (CCK-A), to Guinea Pig Brain Membranes (CCK-B), and to Human Jurkat T Cells[a]

Compound	Rat Pancreatic Acini	Guinea Pig Brain Membranes	Jurkat T cells
CCK-8	3 ± 0.6	0.20 ± 0.03	0.27 ± 0.04
Boc(Nle28,Nle31)CCK-7	2.3 ± 0.5	0.20 ± 0.02	0.1 ± 0.1
Boc CCK-4	4,000 ± 800	2.6 ± 0.4	1.0 ± 0.1
JMV180	3 ± 0.5	2 ± 0.3	1.5 ± 0.2
JMV320	21,800 ± 2,700	3.2 ± 0.7	0.7 ± 0.1
MK-329	1.5 ± 0.3	280 ± 100	100 ± 6
L-365, 260	370 ± 60	4 ± 1.8	3.3 ± 0.5

[a]Results are expressed as IC$_{50}$(nM) and are means ± SE of at least six separate experiments.

to intracellular calcium mobilization in cerebral tissues[13] or in a small cell lung carcinoma line where CCK-B receptors were located. In JURKAT T cells, changes in intracellular calcium concentration were measured by fura 2 fluorimetry. In these cells, CCK-8 increased the resting intracellular calcium concentration in a dose-dependent manner. The CCK-8–induced increase in (Ca^{2+})$_i$ concentration is rapid, reaching a maximum value in a few seconds, and is followed by a rapid decrease near the basal level. The CCK-8–mediated (Ca^{2+})$_i$ mobilization is not affected in the absence of extracellular calcium, indicating that calcium is mobilized from intracellular stores. The inability of CCK-8 to stimulate (Ca^{2+})$_i$ release in JURKAT T cells after a first stimulation with a maximal dose of CCK-8 indicates that the pool of (Ca^{2+})$_i$ is depleted or the CCK receptor is desensitized to the administration of the second agonist.

To further characterize the pharmacological profile of the response, we investigated the effect of several compounds able to interact with CCK-B receptors. CCK-8, Boc-(Nle^{28,31})-CCK-7, Boc-Trp-Nle-Asp-Phe-NH$_2$, and the cyclic analog JMV320 were found to behave as full agonists in stimulating (Ca^{2+})$_i$ release (TABLE 2). Both compounds Boc-Trp-Nle-Asp-Phe-NH$_2$ and JMV320, which are CCK-B/gastrin selective ligands possessing high binding affinities in JURKAT T cells, stimulated (Ca^{2+})$_i$ release with high potency. Interestingly, compound JMV320 behaved as a gastrin antagonist on gastrin-stimulated growth of human stomach cancer, contain-

TABLE 2. Abilities of Different CCK Analogs to Release Intracellular Calcium or to Inhibit the Response of 10 nM CCK-8 on Calcium Mobilization in Human Jurkat T Cells[a]

Compound	Agonist EC$_{50}$(nM)	Antagonist IC$_{50}$(nM)
CCK-8	2.5 ± 1	
Boc(Nle28,Nle31)CCK-7	8 ± 2	
Boc CCK-4	32 ± 10	
JMV320	25 ± 10	
JMV180		10 ± 2
MK-329		400 ± 100
L-365, 260		20 ± 8

[a]Results are expressed as EC$_{50}$ or IC$_{50}$ values and are means of at least six separate experiments.

ing the gastrin receptor that is linked to $(Ca^{2+})_i$ mobilization.[14] These results suggest that compound JMV320, exhibiting high affinity for the CCK-B/gastrin receptor, is able to discriminate, at least in terms of biological activity, between the central type CCK receptor where it behaves as an agonist and the gastrin receptor where it behaves as a gastrin antagonist.

Compound JMV180 was unable to mobilize $(Ca^{2+})_i$ even at high concentrations (10 mM). Compound JMV180 was a functional antagonist at CCK-B/gastrin binding sites in JURKAT cells, blocking CCK-8–stimulated $(Ca^{2+})_i$ release in a dose-dependent manner. It has partial agonist activity on CCK-A binding sites in rat pancreatic acini where it has been described as an agonist at the high-affinity receptor and as an antagonist at the low-affinity receptor. As expected, both MK329 and L-365,260, the selective CCK-B receptor antagonist, were found to be functional antagonists at the CCK-B/gastrin receptor in JURKAT cells by blocking CCK-8–stimulated $(Ca^{2+})_i$ release in a dose-dependent manner. Accordingly, the selective CCK-B receptor antagonist compound L-365,260 was more potent than MK329, which is in agreement with their relative affinities for the CCK receptor on JURKAT cells.

Further studies are necessary to elucidate the physiological or pathological significance of the presence of these CCK receptors in these malignant lymphoïd cell lines. However, this cell line could provide a useful model for the pharmacological studies of CCK-B receptors and a better understanding of their regulation.

REFERENCES

1. MORLEY, J. E., N. E. KAY, G. F. SOLOMON & N. P. PLOTNIKOFF. 1987. Neuropeptides: Conductors of the immune orchestra. Life Sci. **41:** 527–544.
2. WEIGENT, D. A. & J. E. BLALOCK. 1987. Interactions between the neuroendocrine and immune systems: Common hormones and receptors. Immunol. Rev. **100:** 79–108.
3. O'DORISIO, M. S. & A. PANEIRA. 1990. Neuropeptides and immunopeptides: Messengers in the neuroimmune axis. Ann. N. Y. Acad. Sci. **594:** 1–499.
4. OKAHATA, H., Y. NISHI, K. MURAKI, K. SUMII, Y. MIYACHI & T. USUI. 1985. Gastrin or cholecystokinin like immunoreactivity in human blood cells. Life Sci. **36:** 369–373.
5. DONABEDIAN, R. K., N. ODUM, A. SOLJGANARD, B. K. JACOBSEN & J. REHFELD. 1989. The active neuropeptide cholecystokinin and its inactive precursors are present in human peripheral mononuclear cells. Clin. Res. **37:** 848a.
6. FERRARA, A., M. A. MCMILLEN, H. C. SCHAEFER, K. A. ZUCKER, J. R. GOLDENRING & I. M. MODLIN. 1989. Cholecystokinin mediated calcium signals in human peripheral blood mononuclear cells. FASEB J. **3:** A998.
7. FERRARA, A., M. A. MCMILLEN, H. C. SCHAEFER, K. A. ZUCKER & I. M. MODLIN. 1989. Effect of cholecystokinin receptor blockade on human lymphocyte proliferation. J. Surg. Res. **48:** 354–357.
8. LIGNON, M. F., N. BERNAD & J. MARTINEZ. 1991. Pharmacological characterisation of type B cholecystokinin binding sites on the human T lymphocyte cell line. Mol. Pharmacol. **39:** 615–620.
9. LIGNON, M. F., N. BERNAD & J. MARTINEZ. 1993. CCK increase the intracellular calcium concentration in the human JURKAT T lymphocyte cell line. Eur. J. Pharmacol. **245:** 241–246.
10. CHANG, R. S. L. & V. J. LOTTI. 1986. Biochemical and pharmacological characterization of an extremely potent and selective nonpeptide cholecystokinin antagonist, Proc. Natl. Acad. Sci. USA **83:** 4923–4926.
11. LOTTI, V. J. & R. S. L. CHANG. 1989. A new potent and selective non-peptide gastrin antagonist and brain cholecystokinin receptor (CCK-B) ligand: L-365,260. Eur. J. Pharmacol. **162:** 273–280.

12. RODRIGUEZ, M., M. F. LIGNON, M. C. GALAS, M. AMBLARD & J. MARTINEZ. 1990. Cyclic cholecystokinin analogues that are highly selective for rat and guinea pig central cholecystokinin receptors. Mol. Pharmacol. **38:** 333–341.
13. GALAS, M. C., N. BERNAD & J. MARTINEZ. 1992. Pharmacological studies on CCKB receptors in guinea pig synaptoneurosomes. Eur. J. Pharmacol. **226:** 35–41.
14. ISHIZUKA, J., J. MARTINEZ, C. M. TOWNSEND, JR. & J. C. THOMPSON. 1992. The effects of gastrin on growth of human stomach cancer cells. Ann. Surg. **215:** 5528–5535.

Molecular Cloning, Functional Expression, and Chromosomal Localization of the Human Cholecystokinin Type A Receptor

JOSEPH R. PISEGNA,[a] ANDREAS DE WEERTH,[a]
KONRAD HUPPI,[b] AND STEPHEN A. WANK[a,c]

[a]Digestive Diseases Branch
National Institute of Diabetes and Digestive and Kidney Diseases and the
[b]Laboratory of Genetics
Molecular Genetics Section
National Cancer Institute
National Institutes of Health
Bethesda, Maryland 20892

The cholecystokinin (CCK) family of peptides occurs throughout the gastrointestinal, central (CNS), and peripheral nervous systems.[1,2] Within this family, CCK_A receptors (CCK_A-Rs) have a high affinity for only sulfated CCK. The CCK_A-R is a guanine nucleotide-binding regulatory protein-coupled receptor capable of activating phospholipase C and an increase in intracellular calcium.[2-6]

CCK_A receptors have diverse physiological roles in the gastrointestinal tract and brain. In the gastrointestinal system, CCK_A-Rs mediate gallbladder contraction, pancreatic growth, and enzyme secretion.[2] In the nervous system, CCK_A-Rs are present in mesolimbic neurons, where they regulate dopamine release, and in the hypothalamus and vagus nerve, where they regulate satiety.[7,8] CCK_A-Rs are also expressed on human gastric and pancreatic cancers.[9-11] The growth of some human pancreatic cancer cell lines is stimulated by CCK and inhibited by the CCK_AR-selective antagonist devazepide (L-364,718).[9]

RESULTS AND DISCUSSION

We cloned the human CCK_AR cDNA from a surgical gallbladder specimen using primers obtained from screening a human genomic library under low stringency conditions with a [^{32}P]-labeled probe prepared from the recently cloned rat CCK_A-R cDNA.[12,13] These primers allowed the amplification of a 1686 bp polymerase chain reaction product from a human gallbladder cDNA library. The human CCK_A-R cDNA sequence contained a single long open reading frame encoding a unique 428 amino acid protein having 91% and 92% homology to the rat and guinea pig CCK_A receptors, respectively (FIG. 1).[13,14] The receptor has a calculated molecular mass of 48 kD and is similar in size to the 43 kD deglycosylated core protein previously reported for the human gallbladder CCK_A-R using affinity cross-linking methods.[15]

---

[c]To whom correspondence should be addressed.

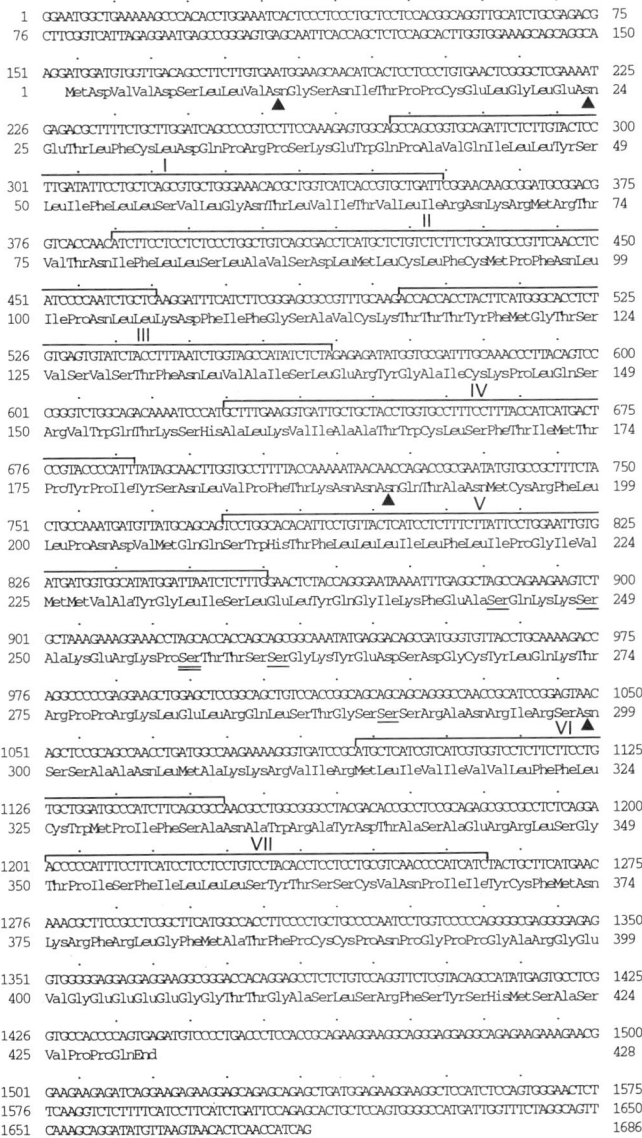

FIGURE 1. Nucleotide and deduced amino acid sequences of the human gallbladder CCK$_A$ receptor cDNA clone. *Solid lines* with Roman numerals I–VII delineate the putative transmembrane domains predicted by the Kyte-Doolittle criteria and homology with the rat and guinea pig CCK$_A$ receptors. *Solid triangles* indicate potential sites for *N*-linked glycosylation. Solid underlines indicate potential protein kinase C (single underline) or protein kinase A (double underline) sites for serine and threonine phosphorylation.[17]

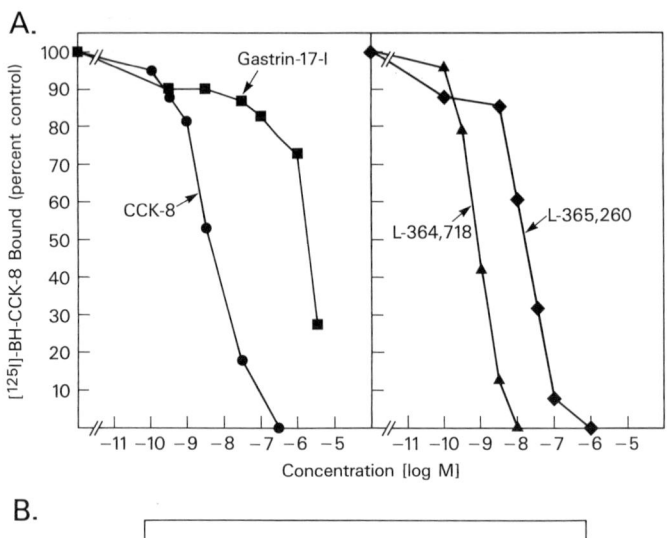

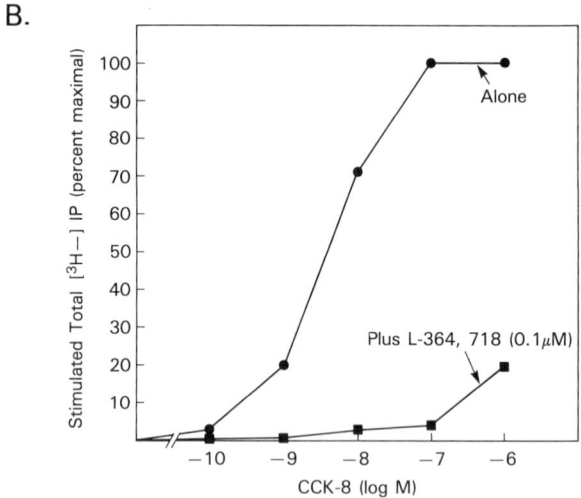

FIGURE 2. (**A**) Ability of CCK receptor agonists and antagonists to inhibit binding of [^{125}I]BH-CCK-8 to COS-7 cells expressing the human CCK$_A$ receptor. COS-7 cells were transfected with the mammalian expression vector pCDL-SRα, containing the human CCK$_A$ receptor cDNA. Transfected COS-7 cells were incubated either with the tracer alone or with increasing concentrations of agonists CCK-8 or gastrin-17-I (*left panel*) or antagonists L-365,260 and L-364,718 (*right panel*). Data are presented as percent saturable binding (total binding in the presence of labeled hormone alone minus binding in the presence of 1 μM CCK-8). (**B**) Ability of CCK-8 alone or CCK-8 plus L-364,718 to stimulate total [^{3}H]inositol phosphate generation in COS-7 cells transfected with the human CCK$_A$ receptor. Data are expressed as the percent of maximal increase obtained using 1 μM CCK-8. CCK-8 (1 μM) increased [^{3}H]inositol phosphates from a basal level of 4,235 ± 808 to 28,676 ± 1,495 dpm.

Hydropathy analysis reveals seven regions of hydrophobic residues that correspond to putative transmembrane-spanning regions expected for members of the G-protein–coupled superfamily of receptors.[16] Similar to the rat and guinea pig CCK_A-Rs, the sequence allows for four potential N-linked glycosylation sites, two in the amino terminus, one in the second extracellular loop, and one in the third intracellular loop (FIG. 1).[13,14] There are five potential sites for protein kinase C phosphorylation and one for protein kinase A phosphorylation, all on serines in the third intracellular loop (FIG. 1).

The human CCK_A-R cDNA clone was subcloned in the mammalian expression vector pCDL-SRα and transfected into COS-7 cells using DEAE/dextran. Transient expression of cell surface receptors was assayed 48 hours posttransfection for binding of ^{125}I-Bolton-Hunter-CCK-8 (^{125}I-BH-CCK). ^{125}I-BH-CCK binding was specific and saturable. CCK-8 inhibited binding with high potency ($IC_{50} \cong 3$ nM) and was almost 1,000-fold more potent than gastrin-17-I. The CCK_A receptor selective antagonist L-364,718 inhibited ^{125}I-BH-CCK binding with high potency ($IC_{50} = 1$ nM) and was greater than 30-fold more potent than the CCK_B receptor selective antagonist L-365,260 (FIG. 2A). To determine if the CCK_A-R clone isolated from human gallbladder encodes a functional CCK_A-R capable of activating phospholipase C, we measured the increase of phosphoinositides stimulated by CCK-8 in COS-7 cells expressing the transfected receptor. CCK-8 caused a dose-dependent increase in total inositol phosphates with a detectable increase at 0.1 nM, a half-maximal increase at 3.0 nM, and a maximal increase at 100 nM. This response was nearly completely inhibited by the CCK_A receptor-specific antagonist L-364,718 at 0.1 μM (FIG. 2B). These results are in close agreement with previous results of studies of CCK_A-R on the human neuroblastoma cell line CHP212.[18] High stringency Northern blot analysis of 2 μg of human organ-specific polyadenylated RNA from brain, stomach, pancreas, kidney, liver, lung, and gallbladder using a [^{32}P]-labeled-human CCK_A-R cDNA full-length coding region probe identified a 6-kb hybridizing transcript only in gallbladder. Chromosomal localization studies map the human CCK_A-R to chromosome 4. Localization of the CCK_A receptor to chromosome 4 and the previous localization of the CCK_B receptor to chromosome 11 suggest that these genes may be regulated independently.[17]

SUMMARY

The results presented here describe for the first time the molecular cloning of the human CCK_A-R. Expression of the recombinant receptor shows the expected subtype pharmacology and coupling to phosphoinositide hydrolysis reported for the native human CCK_A-R.[18] This knowledge will enhance our understanding of its distribution, pharmacology, and structure and will improve our understanding of its physiological role in the gastrointestinal and nervous systems in humans. Ultimately, this should hasten the understanding and therapy of gastrointestinal and neuropsychiatric disorders.

REFERENCES

1. HILL, D. R., N. J. CAMPBELL, T. M. SHAW & G. N. WOODRUFF. 1987. J. Neurosci. **7:** 2967–2976.
2. JENSEN, R. T., S. A. WANK, W. H. ROWLEY, S. SATO & J. D. GARDNER. 1989. Trends Pharmacol. Sci. **10:** 418–423.

3. CHANG, R. S. L. & V. J. LOTTI. 1986. Proc. Natl. Acad. Sci. USA **83:** 4923–4926.
4. MERRIT, J. E., C. W. TAYLOR, R. P. RUBIN & J. W. PUTNEY. 1986. Biochem. J. **236:** 337–343.
5. INNIS, R. B. & S. H. SNYDER. 1980. Proc. Natl. Acad. Sci. USA **77:** 6917–6921.
6. CHEW, C. S. & M. R. BROWN. 1986. Biochim. Biophys. Acta **888:** 116–125.
7. CRAWLEY, J. N. 1991. Trends Pharmacol. Sci. **12:** 232–236.
8. MORAN, T. H., P. H. ROBINSON, M. S. GOLDRICH & P. R. MCHUGH. 1975. Brain Res. **362:** 986–989.
9. SMITH, J. P., T. E. SOLOMON, S. BAGHERI & S. KRAMER. 1990. Dig. Dis. & Sci. **35:** 1377–1384.
10. MILLER, L. J. 1984. Am. J. Physiol. **247:** G402–G410.
11. PEARSON, R. K., M. HADAC & L. J. MILLER. 1989. Am. J. Physiol. **256:** G1005–1010.
12. SCHJOLDAGER, B., X. MOLERO & L. J. MILLER. 1989. Gastroenterology **96:** 1119–1125.
13. WANK, S. A., R. HARKINS, R. T. JENSEN, H. SHAPIRA, A. DE WEERTH & T. SLATTERY. 1992. Proc. Natl. Acad. Sci. USA **89:** 3125–3129.
14. DE WEERTH, A., J. R. PISEGNA & S. A. WANK. 1993. Am. J. Physiol. **265:** G1116–G1121.
15. SCHJOLDAGER, B., X. MOLERO & L. J. MILLER. 1990. Regul. Pept. **28:** 265–272.
16. DOHLMAN, H. G., M. G. CARON & R. J. LEFKOWITZ. 1987. Biochemistry **26:** 2657–2663.
17. PISEGNA, J. R., A. DE WEERTH, K. HUPPI & S. A. WANK. 1992. Biochem. Biophys. Res. Comm. **189:** 296–303.
18. BARRETT, R. W., M. E. STEFFEY & A. W. WOLFRAM. 1989. Mol. Pharmacol. **35:** 394–400.

CCK_8-Evoked Ca^{2+} Mobilization in Pancreatic Acinar Cells

Evidence for a Regulatory Role of Protein Kinase C by Phosphorylation-Dependent Inhibition of Signaling through the High-Affinity CCK Receptor

P. H. G. M. WILLEMS, H. J. M. VAN HOOF,
M. G. H. VAN MACKELENBERGH, J. G. J. HOENDEROP,
S. E. VAN EMST–DE VRIES, AND J. J. H. H. M. DE PONT

Department of Biochemistry
University of Nijmegen
P.O. Box 9101
NL-6500 HB Nijmegen, the Netherlands

Treatment of pancreatic acinar cells with phorbol esters, such as TPA, leads to inhibition of cholecystokinin (CCK)-evoked Ca^{2+} mobilization.[1] The aim of the present study was to investigate the mechanism underlying this negative feedback role of protein kinase C.

MATERIALS AND METHODS

Rabbit pancreatic acinar cells were prepared by enzymatic digestion, using collagenase and hyaluronidase, as previously described.[2] Isolated acinar cells, resuspended in a Krebs-Ringer bicarbonate medium (pH 7.4), were incubated in the presence of 5 μM fura-2-AM for 30 minutes at 37°C. Fura-2–loaded acinar cells were resuspended in a HEPES/Tris medium (pH 7.4), and fluorescence measurements were carried out at 37°C using a dual wavelength spectrofluorophotometer. The fluorescence emission ratio at 490 nm was monitored after excitation at 340 and 380 nm. In each experiment, the maximal increase in fluorescence emission ratio, evoked by the secretagogue studied, was set at 100%, to which all other values were related.

RESULTS AND DISCUSSION

Using a digital-imaging technique, we previously showed that submaximal concentrations of the COOH-terminal octapeptide of cholecystokinin (CCK_8) evoke the dose-dependent recruitment of acinar cells in terms of receptor-mediated Ca^{2+} mobilization.[2] Therefore, the increase in fluorescence emission ratio ($R^{340}/_{380}$) obtained from a suspension of CCK_8-stimulated acinar cells is largely proportional to the number of responding cells and thus reflects an increase in the average free cytosolic Ca^{2+} concentration ($[Ca^{2+}]_{i,av}$).

Effects of TPA on the CCK_8-Evoked Increase of the Average $[Ca^{2+}]_i$ in a Suspension of Pancreatic Acinar Cells

Stimulation of a suspension of fura-2–loaded acinar cells with CCK_8 resulted in a transient increase in $[Ca^{2+}]_{i,av}$ (not shown), the altitude of which was clearly dose-dependent, reaching a maximum at 0.1 nM CCK_8 (FIG. 1). Pretreatment of the cells with TPA for 3 minutes resulted in a rightward shift of the dose-response curve for the effect of CCK_8 on the peak increase in $[Ca^{2+}]_{i,av}$. The effect of TPA was dose-dependent but reached a maximum, that is, a rightward shift of one order of magnitude, at a concentration of 10 nM. The inhibitory effect of TPA was completely overcome by 10 nM CCK_8. By contrast, the rightward shift evoked by the receptor-antagonist D-lorglumide was, in principle, infinite, demonstrating its competitive nature (not shown). Both the observation that the stimulatory effect of submaximal CCK_8 concentrations is inhibited by TPA and the finding that the inhibitory effect of TPA is dose-dependently reversed by maximal CCK_8 concentrations led to the hypothesis that protein kinase C, either directly or indirectly, inhibits signaling through the high-affinity CCK receptor without affecting signaling through the low-affinity CCK receptor.[3]

Effects of TPA on the JMV-180–Evoked Increase of the Average $[Ca^{2+}]_i$ in a Suspension of Pancreatic Acinar Cells

The foregoing hypothesis was tested by investigating the effect of TPA pretreatment on the response evoked by the high-affinity CCK receptor agonist JMV-180. At

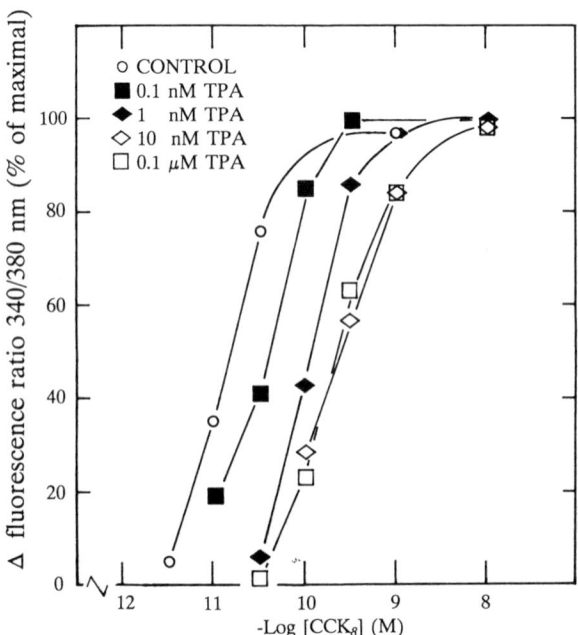

FIGURE 1. Effect of TPA on the dose-response curve for the CCK_8-evoked increase in $[Ca^{2+}]_{i,av}$.

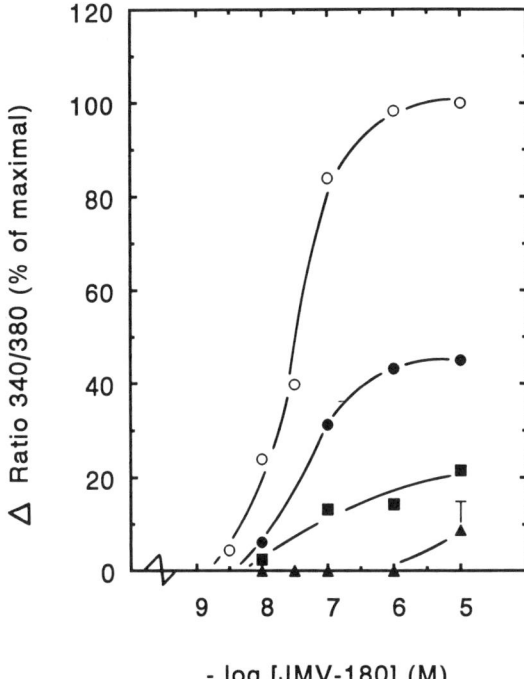

FIGURE 2. Effect of TPA on the dose-response curve for the JMV-180–evoked increase in $[Ca^{2+}]_{i,av}$.

a concentration of 0.1 μM, TPA virtually completely inhibited the stimulatory effect of JMV-180 (FIG. 2). Data presented demonstrate that protein kinase C, either directly or indirectly, inhibits signaling through the high-affinity CCK receptor. The CCK_A receptor was recently cloned and was shown to possess four potential phosphorylation sites for protein kinase C. This opens the possibility that protein kinase C acts directly on the receptor itself, thereby converting it from a high-affinity state to a low-affinity state.

REFERENCES

1. WILLEMS, P. H. G. M., I. G. P. VAN NOOIJ, H. E. M. G. HAENEN & J. J. H. H. M. DE PONT. 1987. Biochim. Biophys. Acta **930**: 230–236.
2. WILLEMS, P. H. G. M., S. E. VAN EMST-DE VRIES, C. H. VAN OS & J. J. H. H. M. DE PONT. 1993. Cell Calcium **14**: 145–159.
3. WILLEMS, P. H. G. M., H. J. M. VAN HOOF, M. G. H. VAN MACKELENBERGH, J. G. J. HOENDEROP, S. E. VAN EMST-DE VRIES & J. J. H. H. M. DE PONT. 1993. Pflügers Arch. **424**: 171–182.

Gastrin$_{13}$ Binds to CCK$_B$ Brain Membrane Receptors Coupled to G Protein in Guinea Pig Brain Membranes

J. C. LALLEMENT, J. C. GALLEYRAND, A. C. LIMA-LEITE,
P. FULCRAND, AND J. MARTINEZ

Chimie et Pharmacologie de Molécules d'Intérêt Biologique
EP CNRS 51
Faculté de Pharmacie
15 Av. Charles Flahault
34060 Montpellier, France

Cholecystokinin (CCK) is one of the most widely distributed brain neuropeptides. It occurs in the whole nervous system in several molecular forms in which CCK-8 predominates.[1] Cholecystokinin and gastrin share the same C-terminal pentapeptide sequence, and proper gastrin-17 immunoreactivity have also been found in the central nervous system and medulla oblongata in small but significant amounts.[2–4] Cholecystokinin binding to brain tissue preparations was the subject of several studies, leading to good knowledge of CCK receptor repartition and pharmacology throughout the nervous system.[5] Binding experiments were performed using ^{125}I-CCK$_8$,[6] [^{3}H]-CCK$_8$,[7] ^{125}I-CCK$_{33}$,[8] as well as [^{3}H]-CCK$_4$[9] and [^{3}H]pentagastrin[10] which represent the common C-terminal sequence of CCK and gastrin and are selective CCK$_B$ radioligands. Binding studies using longer forms of gastrin were performed with various gastrin ligands in which the tyrosine residue located in the C-terminal part of the molecule was labeled by ^{125}I. Iodination of tyrosine-12 in Gastrine-17 or gastrin analogs leads to labeled ligands that might interfere with specific properties of gastrin compared to CCK, because the position of the tyrosine is crucial in gastrin and CCK molecules. Therefore, the use of ^{125}I-BH-[Leu^{15}]-gastrin-(5-17), a newly synthesized probe having the biological activity of gastrin and in which the integrity of tyrosine located in the C-terminal part of the molecule have been respected,[11] led us to the characterization of specific gastrin-binding sites on guinea pig brain membranes. Recent works after the cloning purification of CCK$_B$ receptor (CCK$_B$R) and gastrin receptor (GR) from various mammal tissues[12,13] strongly suggested that CCK-B and gastrin receptors are the same receptors.

Indeed, ^{125}I-BH-[Leu^{15}]-gastrin-(5-17) binds, on guinea pig brain membranes, to a homogeneous population of binding sites (B_{max} is about 17.3 ± 3.3 fmol/mg of protein) with high affinity (K_d = 0.53 ± 0.03 nM) (FIG. 1). The nonpeptide antagonists L-365,260, selective for CCK$_B$R, and MK-329, selective for CCK$_A$R, inhibited ^{125}I-BH-[Leu^{15}]-gastrin-(5-17) binding with IC$_{50}$'s of 6.5 ± 0.9 nM and 96 ± 15 nM, respectively, in accordance with their selectivity. ^{125}I-BH-[Leu^{15}]-gastrin-(5-17) binding is completely inhibited by CCK-8 as well as the unlabeled homologous peptide. [Leu^{15}]-gastrin-(5-17) is able to completely inhibit ^{125}I-BH-CCK$_8$ binding. These inhibition-competition studies showed that ^{125}I-BH-[Leu^{15}]-gastrin-(5-17) bound to the CCK$_B$R. However, ^{125}I-BH-[Leu^{15}]-gastrin-(5-17) and ^{125}I-BH-CCK$_8$ binding were compared, and Scatchard studies indicated that ^{125}I-BH-CCK$_8$ binds to a single class of high-affinity binding sites (Kd = 0.045 ± 0.007 nM; B$_{max}$ is about 50.6 ± 8.4 fmol/mg of protein) (FIG. 1). ^{125}I-BH-CCK$_8$ and ^{125}I-BH-[Leu^{15}]-gastrin-(5-17) bind

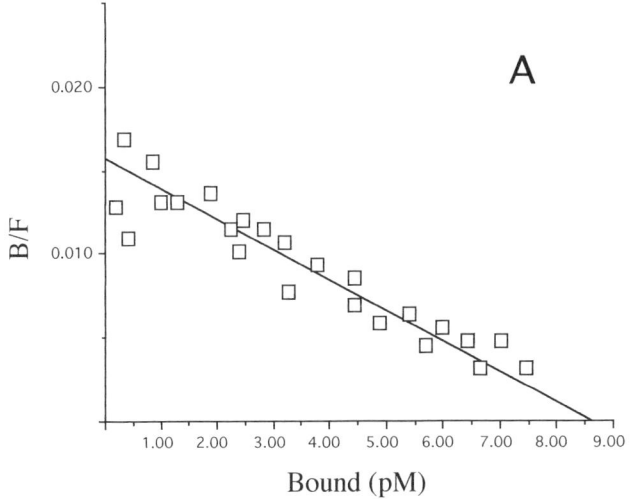

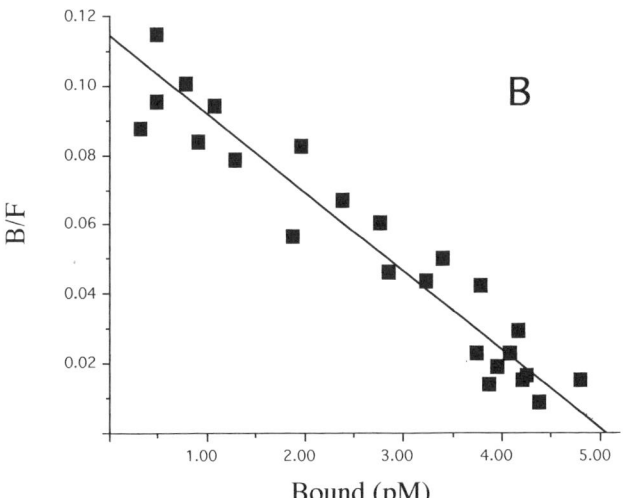

FIGURE 1. Scatchard analysis of ^{125}I-BH-(Leu^{15})-gastrin-(5-17) (**A**) and ^{125}I-BH-CCK-8 (**B**) binding to guinea pig brain membrane preparation as a function of radiolabeled peptide concentration.

to guinea pig brain membranes with almost the same maximal binding capacities, whereas they differ in binding affinity. No evidence was found to suggest that gastrin binds to selective binding sites other than CCK$_B$R.

The influence of monovalent and divalent cations on ^{125}I-BH-[Leu^{15}]-gastrin-(5-17) and ^{125}I-BH-CCK$_8$ binding was tested. In the absence of Mg^{2+}, both labeled ligand binding was significantly decreased, whereas it was strongly increased by removal of Na^+ and K^+. The influence of stable guanyl nucleotides on ^{125}I-BH-[Leu^{15}]-gastrin-(5-17) and ^{125}I-BH-CCK$_8$ binding was also tested (FIG. 2). ^{125}I-BH-[Leu^{15}]-gastrin-(5-17) binding was strongly affected by GTPγS, whereas ^{125}I-BH-CCK$_8$ binding was only slightly reduced. Saturation experiments followed by Scatchard analysis of the ^{125}I-BH-[Leu^{15}]-gastrin-(5-17) binding data suggested that the stable analogs of GTP decreased the affinity of the ligand, whereas the number and homogeneity of binding sites remained unaffected. Scatchard analysis of ^{125}I-BH-CCK$_8$ binding data clearly showed that GTPγS was unable to significantly modify the affinity and maximal binding capacity. Competition studies performed with GTPγS confirmed the results of binding experiments and Scatchard replot, showing a

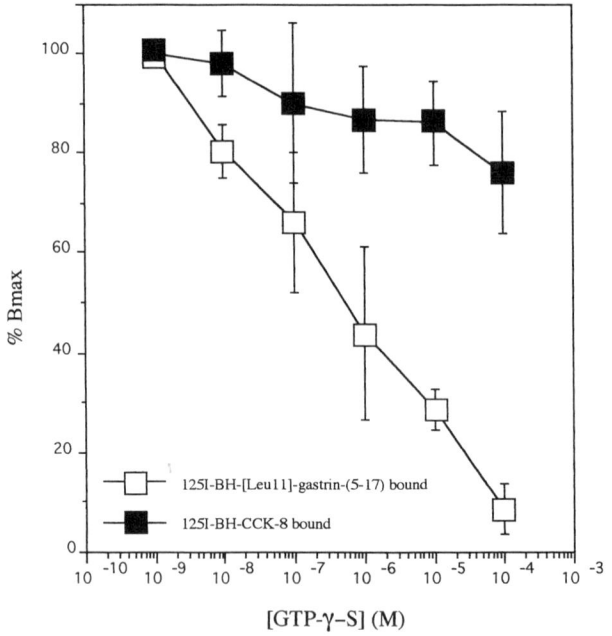

FIGURE 2. Effects of GTPγS on binding of ^{125}I-BH-[Leu^{15}]-gastrin-(5-17) and ^{125}I-BH-CCK$_8$ to guinea pig brain membranes.

decrease in affinity for gastrin but not for CCK$_8$ in displacing ^{125}I-BH-[Leu^{15}]-gastrin-(5-17) or ^{125}I-BH-CCK$_8$ binding.

This study indicated that gastrin$_{13}$ binds to a brain population of CCK$_B$R. The influence of GTPγS on ^{125}I-BH-[Leu^{15}]-gastrin-(5-17) and ^{125}I-BH-CCK$_8$ binding strongly suggested that they are differently coupled to G protein through the same molecular target.

REFERENCES

1. DOCKRAY, G. J. 1976. Immunochemical evidence of cholecystokinin-like peptides in brain. Nature **264:** 568–570.
2. REHFELD, J. F. 1978. Localization of gastrin to neuro- and adeno-hypophysis. Nature **271:** 771–773.

3. REHFELD, J. F., H. F. HANSEN, L. I. LARSSON, K. STENGAARD-PEDERSEN & N. A. THORN. 1984. Gastrin and cholecystokinin in pituitary neurons. Proc. Natl. Acad. Sci. USA **81:** 1902–1905.
4. REHFELD, J. F. & J. M. LUNDBERG. 1983. Cholecystokinin in feline vagal and sciatic nerves: Concentration, molecular forms and transport velocity. Brain Res. **275:** 341–347.
5. WOODRUFF, G. N., D. R. HILL, P. BODEN, R. PINNOCK, L. SINGH & J. HUGHES. 1991. Functional role of brain CCK receptors. Neuropeptides **19** (Suppl.): 45–56.
6. DIETL, M. M., A. PROBST & J. M. PALACIOS. 1987. On the distribution of cholecystokinin binding sites in the human brain: An autoradiographic study. Synapse **1:** 169–183.
7. VAN DJIK, A., J. G. RICHARDS, A. TRZECIAK, D. GILLESSEN & H. MÖHLER. 1984. Cholecystokinin receptors: Biochemical demonstration and autoradiographical localisation in rat brain and pancreas using [^{3}H]cholecystokinin$_8$ as radioligand. J. Neurosci. **4:** 1021–1033.
8. ZARBIN, M. A., R. B. INNIS, K. WALMSLEY, S. H. SNYDER & M. J. JUHAR. 1983. Autoradiographic localization of cholecystokinin receptors in rodent brain. J. Neurosci. **3:** 877–906.
9. DURIEUX, C., D. PELAPRAT, B. CHARPENTIER, J.-L. MORGAT & B. P. ROQUES. 1988. Characterization of [^{3}H]-CCK-4 binding sites in mouse and rat brain. Neuropeptides **12:** 141–148.
10. GAUDREAU, P., R. QUIRION, S. ST. PIERRE & C. B. PERT. 1983. Characterization and visualization of cholecystokinin receptor in rat brain using [^{3}H]pentagastrin. Peptides **4:** 755–762.
11. GALLEYRAND, J.-C., J.-C. LALLEMENT, M.-F. LIGNON, A.-C. LIMA-LEITE, N. BERNAD, P. FULCRAND & J. MARTINEZ. 1993. Characterization of ^{125}I-BH-[Leu15]-gastrin-(5-17) binding on canine fundic mucosal cells and Jurkat cells. Eur. J. Pharmacol., submitted.
12. WANK, S. A., J. R. PISEGNA & A. DE WEERTH. 1992. Brain and gastrointestinal cholecystokinin receptor family: Structure and functional expression. Proc. Natl. Acad. Sci. USA **89:** 8691–8695.
13. LEE, Y. M., M. BEINBORN, E. W. MC BRIDE, M. LU, L. F. KOLAKOWSKI, JR. & A. S. KOPIN. 1993. The human brain cholecystokinin-B/gastrin receptor. J. Biol. Chem. **268:** 8164–8169.

Rat Pancreatic Nucleoside Diphosphate Kinase, a Novel Regulator of Cholecystokinin Receptor Affinity

Cloning and Expression

GEORGE T. BLEVINS, JR.,[a] ELS M. A. VAN DE WESTERLO, PAULETTE M. BLEVINS, AND JOHN A. WILLIAMS

Department of Physiology
University of Michigan Medical School
Ann Arbor, Michigan 48109–0622

We previously demonstrated that the existence of two affinity states of the pancreatic cholecystokinin (CCK) receptor depends on the presence of ATP.[1] Subsequently, we established that the effect of ATP to induce two CCK binding affinity states was biochemically mediated by the enzyme nucleoside diphosphate kinase (NDPK) (manuscript in preparation). Nucleoside diphosphate kinase catalyzes the transfer of high energy gamma-phosphate groups from nucleoside triphosphates to nucleoside diphosphates. In that study the ability of an assortment of nucleoside triphosphates to serve as substrate for NDPK was compared with their ability to induce two binding affinity states of the CCK receptor on rat pancreatic membranes for which previous studies have observed only a single binding affinity state. Nucleoside triphosphates capable of serving as a substrate for NDPK could also induce two CCK binding affinity states on pancreatic membranes, whereas those that could not serve as substrate for NDPK could not induce two CCK binding affinity states. Furthermore, GDP potentiated the effect of ATP on binding (manuscript in preparation). To conclusively identify NDPK we found it necessary to clone and functionally express this enzyme. We report here that the characteristics of the cloned and expressed enzyme are similar to those of pancreatic membrane NDPK and consistent with the ability of this enzyme to induce two CCK binding affinity states.

METHODS

To identify pancreatic NDPK molecularly, it was amplified by the polymerase chain reaction (PCR) from a λgt11 rat pancreatic cDNA library, cloned, expressed, and functionally characterized. Polymerase chain reaction primers were prepared based on the published sequence of rat skeletal muscle NDPK.[2] The 5' primer was a 25-mer (CGGGATCCATGGCCAACAGCGAGCG) which incorporated a *Bam*HI restriction site to facilitate subcloning, and the primer for the complementary strand was a 33-mer (CGGAATTCCTCACTCATACATCCAGTTCTGCGC) incorporating an *Eco*RI restriction site. These primers allowed amplification of a single band of

---

[a] Address for correspondence: George T. Blevins, Jr., Department of Physiology and Biophysics, University of Arkansas for Medical Sciences, 4301 W. Markham Slot 505, Little Rock, AR 72205.

about 465 bp. The cloned PCR product was sequenced using the Sanger dideoxy sequencing protocol. The cloned NDPK was ligated into the expression vector pGEX-KT,[3] which expresses cloned proteins in frame with *Schistosomal* glutathione S-transferase, under the control of the IPTG-inducible *tac* promoter. Transformed bacteria were grown and fusion protein synthesis was initiated by adding IPTG. Cells were lysed by two passes through a French press, and fusion protein was purified by affinity chromatography using glutathione-agarose beads. Fusion protein was used to immunize New Zealand white rabbits, and the rabbits received boosters three times at 5-week intervals, blood was drawn, and immune serum obtained.

RESULTS

The coding sequence of the PCR product was identical to that of rat skeletal muscle NDPK. The apparent molecular weight of the purified fusion protein was 42 kD, consistent with the combined molecular weight of NDPK (18 kD) and GST (26 kD) (FIG. 1). The fusion protein exhibited the activity and kinetic parameters

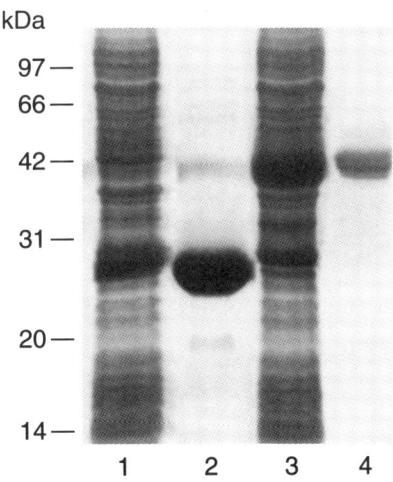

FIGURE 1. Coomassie blue stained 12% SDS-PAGE of recombinant bacterial lysates and purified recombinant proteins. Total bacterial lysate and purified GST (1,2); total lysate from recombinant bacteria and the GST-NDPK fusion protein (3,4). The apparent molecular weight of the purified fusion protein (42 kDa) is consistent with the combined molecular weight of NDPK (18 kDa) and GST (26 kDa). The migration distance and sizes of molecular weight markers are indicated on the *left*.

expected of an NDPK. In typical experiments ATP was utilized with a K_m of 455 μM and GDP with a K_m of 127 μM; the maximal velocity of these reactions averaged 3,400 times that measured in total pancreatic membranes per unit protein. Immunoblots of total pancreatic membranes, performed using the antiserum produced against the recombinant fusion protein, identified a single band with an apparent molecular weight of 18 kD in AR4-2J cell membranes, total, and enriched pancreatic membranes (FIG. 2). The antiserum only weakly recognized NDPK in CHO cells.

DISCUSSION

These findings demonstrate the presence of NDPK in rat pancreas at both the nucleic acid and protein level. The purified recombinant enzyme exhibited kinetic

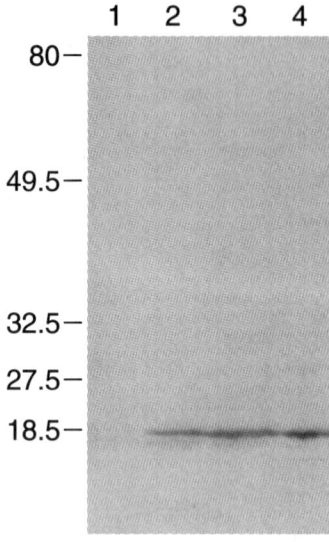

FIGURE 2. Immunoblot of (1) total CHO cell membranes, (2) total AR4-2J cell membranes, (3) total pancreatic membranes, and (4) enriched pancreatic membranes. Membranes (50 μg) were run on a 5–15% gradient SDS-PAGE, transferred to nitrocellulose, and probed with antiserum 553 raised against the GST-NDPK fusion protein.

characteristics consistent with our earlier findings on rat pancreatic membranes. These results provide further support for a role of NDPK in regulating CCK receptor affinity.

REFERENCES

1. BLEVINS, G. T., JR. & J. A. WILLIAMS. 1992. Am. J. Physiol. **263:** G44–G51.
2. KIMURA, N., N. SHIMADA, K. NOMURA & K. WATANABE. 1990. J. Biol. Chem. **265:** 15744–15749.
3. HAKES, D. J. & J. E. DIXON. 1992. Anal. Biochem. **202:** 293–298.

Combined Dose-Ratio Analysis for the CCK-B Antagonist Virginiamycin in Guinea Pig Ileum

M. CORSI, G. DAL FORNO, B. OLIOSI, C. PIETRA,
F. TH. M. van AMSTERDAM, AND D. G. TRIST

Glaxo Research Laboratories
37135 Verona, Italy

Virginiamycin, a macrolide antibiotic produced by fermentation of a strain of *Streptomyces olivaceous*, has been reported to bind selectively to CCK-B receptors.[1] The objective of this study was to determine and to quantify the nature of the interaction of virginiamycin with CCK-B receptors in a functional assay, namely, the guinea pig ileum longitudinal muscle myenteric plexus (LMMP). To verify the selectivity of virginiamycin, binding studies on guinea pig brain and rat pancreas were also included.

METHODS

Binding Studies. The pancreas and brain assays were carried out in male Sprague-Dawley rats (150–200 g) and male Dunkin-Hartley guinea pigs (350 g), respectively. The methods used were described elsewhere.[2] The pKi values for virginiamycin together with CCK-4 and L-365,260 were estimated using [^{3}H]-CCK-8s (60 Ci/mmol) as the radioligand.

Functional Studies. Male Dunkin-Hartley guinea pigs weighing 350–450 g were sacrificed and the LMMP was prepared as described by Dal Forno *et al.*[3] The combined dose-ratio analysis was performed according to the procedure of Shankley *et al.*[4] (L-365, 260 was used as a standard antagonist (A) and its dissociation constant was indicated as K_{BL}.) From the combined dose-ratio analysis the dissociation constant (K_{BV}) for virginiamycin (C) was estimated using the equation: $DR_{AC} = 1 + [A]/(K_{BL}*(1 + [C]/K_{BV}))$[5] where DR_{AC} is the dose-ratio with both antagonists together relative to the curve obtained in the presence of virginiamycin alone.

RESULTS

Virginiamycin Binding to CCK Receptors. The pKi values estimated for CCK-4 ($n = 3$), virginiamycin ($n = 3$), and L-365,260 ($n = 4$) are given in TABLE 1. All three compounds showed marked selectivity for CCK-B receptors (guinea pig brain) in comparison with CCK-A receptors (rat pancreas).

Antagonism of Virginiamycin on CCK-4–Induced LMMP Contraction. The antagonism of virginiamycin was studied using Krebs solution containing the CCK-A selective antagonist L-364,718 at 10 nM. Under these conditions, virginiamycin (1–10 μM) antagonized in a dose-dependent manner the concentration response curve (CRC) to CCK-4. Virginiamycin at 10 μM significantly ($p < 0.05$) depressed the maximal response to CCK-4, and thus only a pA$_2$ could be calculated, which was found to be 6.64 ± 0.06 (SE).

In a combined dose-ratio analysis the standard antagonist L-365,260 (A) competitively antagonized CCK-4–induced contraction with a pK_{BL} value of 8.60 ± 0.16. The Schild plot slope was 1.25 ± 0.15 (95% CL 0.93–1.56). A mixture of L-365,260 (0.1 µM) and 10 µM virginiamycin (C) antagonized the CRC to CCK-4. The dose-ratio analysis predicts that if the two antagonists act on different sites to antagonize CCK-4–induced contraction, the log dose-ratio should be 2.37; however, if the action is on the same site, the log dose-ratio should be 1.49. The log dose-ratio obtained was 1.53. The test statistic (Student's t test) for the multiplicative model was (± SE) 0.810 ± 0.076 ($p < 0.05$), whereas for the additive model the test statistic was 0.027 ± 0.155 ($p > 0.05$). Thus, it is concluded that the two antagonists act on the same site. From the equation described by Trist et al.[5] in the methods section, a pK_{BV} of 6.20 for virginiamycin could be obtained.[1]

TABLE 1. Estimated pKi Values for CCK-4, Virginiamycin, and L-365,260 in Rat Pancreas and Guinea Pig Cortex Binding Assay (pKi ± SE)

	Rat Pancreas	Guinea Pig Cortex
CCK-4	4.27 ± 0.03	7.76 ± 0.12
Virginiamycin	<4.0	6.45 ± 0.05
L-365,260	6.48 ± 0.09	8.53 ± 0.11

CONCLUSIONS

The results suggest that virginiamycin is a competitive antagonist for the CCK-B receptors present in LMMP, and it does not discriminate between CCK-B receptors present in the brain and those present in peripheral tissues (LMMP). The difference between the pA_2 value obtained for virginiamycin and that of its pK_B may be due to the depressive effect on the maximal response of CCK-4.

REFERENCES

1. LAM, Y. K. T., D. BOGEN, R. S. CHANG, K. A. FAUST, O. D. SCHWARTZ, L. ZITANO, G. M. GARRITY, M. M. GAGLIARDI, S. A. CURRIE & H. B. WOODRUFF. 1991. J. Antibiotics **44:** 613–634.
2. VAN DIJK, A., J. G. RICHARDS, D. TRECIAK, D. GILLESSEN & H. MÖHLER. 1984. J. Neurosci. **4:** 1021–1033.
3. DAL FORNO, G., C. PIETRA, M. URCIUOLI, F. T. M. VAN AMSTERDAM, G. TOSON, G. GAVIRAGHI & D. G. TRIST. 1992. J. Pharmacol. Exp. Ther. **261:** 1056–1063.
4. SHANKLEY, N. P., J. W. BLACK, C. R. GANELLIN & R. C. MITCHELL. 1988. Br. J. Pharmacol. **94:** 264–274.
5. TRIST, D. G., P. LEFF, J. W. BLACK, V. P. GERSKOWITCH & N. P. SHANKLEY. 1987. J. Pharmacol. Exp. Ther. **243:** 1043–1047.

CCK-B Antagonists Exhibit Antidepressant-Like Effects and Potentiate Endogenous Enkephalin Analgesia

Correlation with *in Vivo* Binding Affinities and Brain Penetration

C. DURIEUX, M. DERRIEN, R. MALDONADO,
O. VALVERDE, A. BLOMMAERT,
M.-C. FOURNIÉ-ZALUSKI, AND B. P. ROQUES

Laboratoire de Pharmacochimie Moléculaire et Structurale
INSERM U 266-CNRS URA D 1500
4, avenue de l'Observatoire
75006 Paris, France

The existence of a possible physiological antagonism between cholecystokinin (CCK) and enkephalin systems was investigated using an animal model of depression, the conditioned suppression of motility, and the hot plate test in mice. For the latter test, a systemically active inhibitor of enkephalin degrading enzymes, RB 101, was administered to increase the levels of endogenous opioid peptides before injection of selective CCK-B antagonists. The ability of the selective CCK-B agonists and antagonists used in this study to cross the blood-brain barrier was also evaluated using *in vivo* binding techniques.

MATERIAL AND METHODS

In vivo binding techniques were performed as previously reported.[1] Mice were killed 15 minutes after intracerebroventricular administration of 10 pmol [^{3}H]pBC 264. In the conditioned suppression of motility test,[2] the mouse was left in the same cage in which it had received, or not, electric footshocks the day before, and motility changes were observed for 6 minutes. The hot plate test was based on the method of Eddy and Leimbach.[3] The heated surface of the plate was kept at 55 ± 0.5°C. The latency period until the mouse jumped was registered (cut-off time 240 s).

RESULTS

As shown in TABLE 1, CCK-B agonist BC 264 (Boc-Tyr(SO$_3$H)-gNle-mGly-Trp-(NMe)Nle-Asp-Phe-NH$_2$) exhibited a sevenfold higher *in vivo* affinity than did BC 197 after central administration, but a sevenfold lower capacity to cross the blood-brain barrier. *In vivo* affinities and passages to the brain of the two CCK-B antagonists, L-365,260 and RB 211,[4] were similar, whereas the antagonist CI-988 was

TABLE 1. *In Vitro* (K_I) and *in Vivo* (ID_{50}, icv) Apparent Affinities in Mouse Brain of Agonists and Antagonists for CCK-B Receptors[a]

	K_I (nM)	ID_{50} (nmol) after ICV Injection	Inhibition after Peripheral Injection of 20 mg/kg (%)	Estimation of Passage through the BBB (%)
BC 264	0.32 ± 0.02	0.15	48**	0.03
BC 197	33 ± 5	1.0	37**	0.2
L-365,260	5.2 ± 0.6	21% inhibition at 1 nmol	23*	0.1
CI 988	1.2 ± 0.2	3	10	0.02
RB 211	13.6 ± 1.6	10	19*	0.2

[a] Passage across the blood-brain barrier (BBB) was evaluated by establishing the ratio of the doses administered to the brain and at the periphery, producing the same percentage of inhibition of [^{3}H]pBC 264 in the brain. Agonists (iv) and antagonists (ip) were injected 15 and 5 minutes before radioligand administration, respectively. *p < 0.05 and **p > 0.01 compared to control (Student's *t* test).

the most potent in inhibiting [^{3}H]pBC 264 specific binding after intracerebroventricular injection, but it was less efficient in crossing the blood-brain barrier.

The selective CCK-B agonists BC 264 (3 and 30 µg/kg) and BC 197 (3 and 30 µg/kg) intraperitoneally administered 30 minutes before the test to shocked mice induced a decrease in motor activity and had no effect in non-shocked mice. L-365,260 (0.2 mg/kg) administered 15 minutes before BC 264 (30 µg/kg) antagonized the effect of BC 264 in shocked mice (FIG. 1). L-365,260 (0.2 and 2 mg/kg intraperitoneally) and RB 211 (0.02 mg/kg ip) administered 30 minutes before the

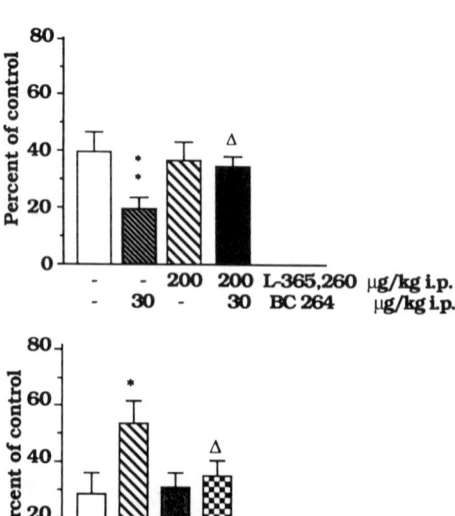

FIGURE 1. Suppression of BC 264-induced decrease in motor immobility measured in shocked mice by L-365,260 and the antidepressant-like effect of L-365,260 antagonized by naltrindole. In the first experiment, L-365,260 was administered 15 minutes before BC 264 (or 45 minutes before the beginning of the test); in the second experiment, the CCK-B antagonist was injected 30 minutes before the test. *$p < 0.05$, **$p < 0.01$ compared to control group, $\Delta p < 0.05$ compared to BC 264 group (first experiment) or compared to L-365,260 group (second experiment).[4]

experiments induced an increase in motor activity only in shocked mice. Moreover, naltrindole (0.3 mg/kg subcutaneously), a selective ∂ opioid antagonist, administered 5 minutes before L-365,260 (0.2 mg/kg) antagonized the effect of L-365,260 in shocked mice (FIG. 1).

RB 101 is a full inhibitor of enkephalin degradation, which induces potent analgesic responses in mice and rats after systemic administration, by increasing the extracellular level of enkephalins.[5] Association of an inactive dose of RB 101 (2.5 mg/kg) with L-365,260 (0.02 and 0.1 mg/kg) or CI-988 (0.3, 1, and 3 mg/kg), but not with the selective CCK-A antagonist L-364,718 (0.02 and 1 mg/kg) produced antinociception in the mouse hot-plate test, whereas the CCK antagonists alone were inactive. This facilitatory effect was reversed by the opioid antagonist naloxone but not by the ∂ opioid antagonist naltrindole, suggesting a selective involvement of μ opioid receptors.

DISCUSSION

The selective agonist BC 197 has a lower affinity, but better brain penetration than does BC 264. Both agonists induced depressant-like effects in mice at similar doses, suggesting that these effects involve brain CCK-B receptors. Moreover, CCK-B antagonists such as L-365,260 induced antidepressant-like effects in mice, which were antagonized by naltrindole, supporting the occurrence of ∂ opioid and CCK-B receptor interactions. Indeed, similar effects also resulted from ∂ opioid receptor activation by endogenous enkephalins.[6] Moreover, the strong potentiation of endogenous enkephalin-related analgesia by CCK-B antagonists supports the existence of an antiopioid effect of CCK_8. Therefore, the possible use of CCK-B antagonists in the treatment of pain or depression warrants further studies.

REFERENCES

1. DURIEUX, C., M. RUIZ-GAYO & B. P. ROQUES. 1991. Eur. J. Pharmacol. **209**: 185–193.
2. KAMEYAMA, T. & M. NAGASAKA. 1982. Pharmacol. Biochem. Behav. **17**: 59–63.
3. EDDY, N. B. & D. LEIMBACH. 1953. J. Pharmacol. Exp. Ther. **107**: 385–389.
4. BLOMMAERT, A. G. S., J. H. WENG, A. DORVILLE, I. MCCORT, B. DUCOS, C. DURIEUX & B. P. ROQUES. 1993. J. Med. Chem., in press.
5. NOBLE, F., J. M. SOLEILHAC, E. SOROCA-LUCAS, S. TURCAUD, M. C. FOURNIÉ-ZALUSKI & B. P. ROQUES. 1992. J. Pharmacol Exp. Ther. **261**: 181–190.
6. BAAMONDE, A., V. DAUGÉ, M. RUIZ-GAYO, I. G. FULGA, S. TURCAUD, M. C. FOURNIÉ-ZALUSKI & B. P. ROQUES. 1992. Eur. J. Pharmacol. **216**: 157–166.

Effect of Hypothalamic Microinjection and Ventricular Perfusion of CCK Receptor Antagonists on Gut Myoelectrical Activity[a]

S. NITECKI, G. J. HARTY, AND J. H. SZURSZEWSKI

Department of Physiology and Biophysics
Mayo Clinic
Rochester, Minnesota 55905

Perfusion of the brain ventricular system with S-CCK-OP replaces the fasting pattern of gut myoelectrical activity with a fed-like pattern by a vagally dependent mechanism.[1,2] The specific brain nuclei that mediate this effect of S-CCK-OP are unknown. Although both CCK-A and CCK-B receptor subtypes are present in the brain,[3] the subtype that mediates the effect of S-CCK-OP on gut myoelectrical activity is not known. Thus, the aims of this study were to determine, in fasting dogs, the brain nuclei that mediate the effect of centrally administered S-CCK-OP and the receptor subtype.

In each of four dogs, myoelectrical activity of the stomach, duodenum, and small intestine was recorded by seromuscularly implanted electrodes. Brain ventricular spaces were perfused through chronically implanted catheters in left and right lateral and fourth ventricles. Hypothalamic nuclei were injected via an array of four microinjectors. Migrating myoelectrical complexes (MMCs) were recorded during: (a) ventricular perfusion with cerebrospinal fluid (CSF) (artificial); (b) ventricular perfusion with CSF-containing either NS-CCK-OP, S-CCK-OP, L-364,718, or L-365,260; (c) single-site hypothalamic microinjections of either CSF, S-CCK-OP, L-364,718, or L-365,260; and (d) ventricular perfusion and hypothalamic injection of S-CCK-OP and one of the antagonists. Each dog ($n = 4$) served as its own control. Ventriculography with omnipaque showed no leakage either to the spinal canal or around brain hemispheres. Ventricular perfusion with either $[I]_{125}$-CCK-OP or S-CCK-OP did not lead to any significant increase in either radioactivity or CCK-like immunoreactivity in the plasma. An active hypothalamic site was identified by a series of experiments in which S-CCK-OP (2 μl, 10^{-3} M) was microinjected at each of the four sites and then at different levels (58–62 mm below dura; 2-mm interval) at each site. Replacement of spontaneously occurring MMCs with a fed-like pattern was considered an active site. A CSF solution containing either S-CCK-OP, L-364,718 (A receptor antagonist), or L-365,260 (B receptor antagonist) was perfused (each, 1.4 pmol/kg/min) from the lateral to the fourth ventricle, while injecting the active hypothalamic site.

All ($n = 12$) perfusions and all ($n = 16$) active site microinjections of S-CCK-OP abolished MMCs and evoked a fed-like pattern. Perfusion or injection with either NS-CCK-OP, L-364,718, or L-365,260 had no effect on spontaneously occurring MMCs. Ventricular perfusion with L-364,718 blocked the conversion from fasted to the fed-like pattern induced by hypothalamic microinjection of S-CCK-OP. How-

[a] This work was supported by NIH DK 17632 and 07198.

ever, perfusion with L-365,260 did not. Microinjection of L-364,718 into an active site before ventricular perfusion with S-CCK-OP blocked its effect. In contrast, microinjection of L-365,260 failed to block the conversion from fasted to the fed-like pattern induced by S-CCK-OP perfusion.

These data show that CCK-A receptors in the hypothalamus mediate the effect of S-CCK-OP on gut myoelectrical activity. Furthermore, the data raise the possibility that conversion of the fasted pattern of myoelectrical activity to the fed pattern after a meal is due to release of S-CCK-OP in a specific hypothalamic nucleus.

REFERENCES

1. BUENO, L. & J.-P. FERRE. 1982. Science **216:** 1427–1429.
2. SCHWARTZ, G. J., P. R. MCHUGH & T. H. MORAN. 1991. Am. J. Physiol. **261:** R64–9.
3. HILL, D. R., T. M. SHAW, W. GRAHAM & G. N. WOODRUFF. 1990. J. Neurosci. **10:** 1070–1081.

Use of *Ex Vivo* Binding to Estimate Brain Penetration and Central Activity of CCK-B Antagonists

SMITA PATEL,[a] KERRY L. CHAPMAN,
ALISON J. SMITH, ANNE HEALD, AND
STEPHEN. B. FREEDMAN

Merck Sharp & Dohme Research Laboratories
Department of Biochemistry
Neuroscience Research Centre
Terlings Park
Eastwick Road
Harlow, Essex, England

Cholecystokinin (CCK) is the most abundant peptide in the central nervous system, found mainly in its octapeptide form, CCK-8S. Cholecystokinin has been implicated in physiological functions including satiety, gallbladder contraction, pancreatic secretion, analgesia, anxiety, and dopamine-mediated behaviors. Of the two subtypes of CCK receptor known to exist, CCK-B receptors predominate in the brain. The recent development of potent and selective CCK-B receptor antagonists has generated interest both in determining the involvement of CCK-B receptors in biological activity and also for the possible therapeutic potential of selective antagonists. To be clinically effective, these compounds need to be orally active and brain penetrable.

In the present study we developed an *ex vivo* binding assay to estimate the central nervous system potency and brain penetration of the systemically administered CCK-B antagonists L-365,260, CI988,[1] and the new benzodiazepine L-368,935.[2] Since the presence of drug within the residual blood in the brain may represent a source of error, this assay incorporates a transcardiac perfusion step to allow clearance of blood from the brain and to avoid overestimation of CNS potency.

METHODS

Radioligand Binding Assays. CCK-B and CCK-A receptor activity of compounds highlighted in this study was determined using binding protocols modified from that described previously.[3]

Estimation of Plasma Content in Mouse Brain. The following protocol was used to determine an appropriate time period for transcardial perfusion in the mouse for effective removal of blood from the brain. Male BKTO mice (25 g) were injected with [^{3}H] inulin (0.25 µCi/mouse intravenously, $n = 4$–8/time point) and anesthetized with isoflurane, blood samples were taken via cardiac puncture, and brains were removed after 0, 5, 10, 20, and 60 seconds of transcardiac perfusion with 0.9% heparinized saline solution at 80–100 mm Hg. Radioactivity was estimated by

---

[a] Author for correspondence.

counting 50 µl of plasma in 10 ml of scintillant and expressed as dpm/µl of plasma. Brains were homogenized in assay buffer (20 mM HEPES, 1 mM EGTA, 5 mM $MgCl_2$, 150 mM NaCl, 0.025% bacitracin, pH 6.5) in a final dilution of 40 mg wet weight per milliliter. Radioactivity in brain was determined by adding 500 µl of brain membrane preparation to 10 ml of scintillant and expressed as dpm/g brain. Brain plasma was determined at each time point by dividing dpm/g (brain samples) by dpm/µl (plasma samples).

Ex Vivo Binding of CCK-B Antagonists. Male BKTO mice (25–30 g) were administered either vehicle or drug (iv). After 30 minutes, animals were anesthetized with isoflurane and transcardially perfused with 0.9% heparinized saline solution for 20 seconds. For intracerebroventricular injections, mice were anesthetized with methoxyflurane, and either L-368,935 (0.1–100 µg/kg), CI988 (1.0–1,000.0 µg/kg), or vehicle (phosphate-buffered saline solution) was injected in 5 µl volume into the ventricles. After 15 minutes, mice were decapitated, brains removed, and membranes prepared as already described. For the binding assay, 100 µl of tissue homogenate was incubated with 50 pM [^{125}I] BH-CCK8S (50 µl), assay buffer (300 µl), and either saline, 1 µM CCK8S (nonspecific), or drug (calibration curve) for 120 minutes at room temperature. Assay was terminated by rapid filtration, and radioactivity was determined by counting filters in an LKB gamma counter. Results were expressed as percentage inhibition of specific binding of [^{125}I] BH-CCK8S for each dose. A plot of percentage inhibition *versus* log dose allowed calculation of ED_{50} values for each drug.

RESULTS

The CCK-B antagonists evaluated in this study, the benzodiazepine L-365,260, the tetrazole L-368,935, and the dipeptoid CI988, exhibit high affinity and selectivity for CCK-B receptors.[2]

Experiments with [^{3}H] inulin showed that the blood content within the CNS was reduced considerably after 20 seconds of perfusion (from 17.3 to 6.3 µl plasma per gram of brain). Increasing perfusion time to 60 seconds did not result in a further reduction in blood content. For subsequent experiments all animals were perfused for 20 seconds before removal of brain.

Results from *ex vivo* binding studies using L-365,260, L-368,935, and CI988 are described in Figures 1 and 2. Both L-365,260 and L-368,935 showed good activity in the assay with dose-dependent inhibition of binding activity (FIG. 1A and B). In contrast, CI988 showed little activity after intravenous administration (FIG. 1C), but it showed potent activity when injected directly into the brain by intracerebroventricular (icv) administration (FIG. 2).

Brain penetration of L-365,260 was estimated by comparing the inhibition of *ex vivo* binding after intravenous administration with a calibration curve generated within each experiment. This involved performing detailed dose response curves to L-365,260 in brain homogenates from vehicle-treated animals. Penetration of L-365,260 into the brain was calculated by dividing the amount present in the brain by the total amount of drug administered x 100 and expressed as mean ± SEM. The values obtained for CNS penetration (0.48 ± 0.07%) confirmed that L-365,260 showed good brain penetration.

DISCUSSION

Biochemical estimation of brain penetration by measurement of the binding activity of compounds in rodent CNS using *ex vivo* methodology has been reported previously.[4,5] In the present study we described an *ex vivo* binding assay in mice which allows simple and rapid measurement of CNS activity of systemically administered CCK-B antagonists. A novel finding is that incorporation of a transcardiac perfusion step allows effective removal of residual blood in the brain, thereby preventing overestimation of CNS activity. This assay showed high CNS activity for the benzodiazepines L-365,260 and L-368,935 but not the dipeptoid CI988. In a recent report, CI988 was claimed to show CNS activity (ED_{50} = 8 mg/kg ip) in an *ex vivo* assay lacking a transcardiac perfusion step.[5] One explanation for the discrepancy between the present study and that of Bertrand and colleagues[5] may possibly be a result of the presence of CI988 in cerebral blood vessels of nonperfused mice. In support of this

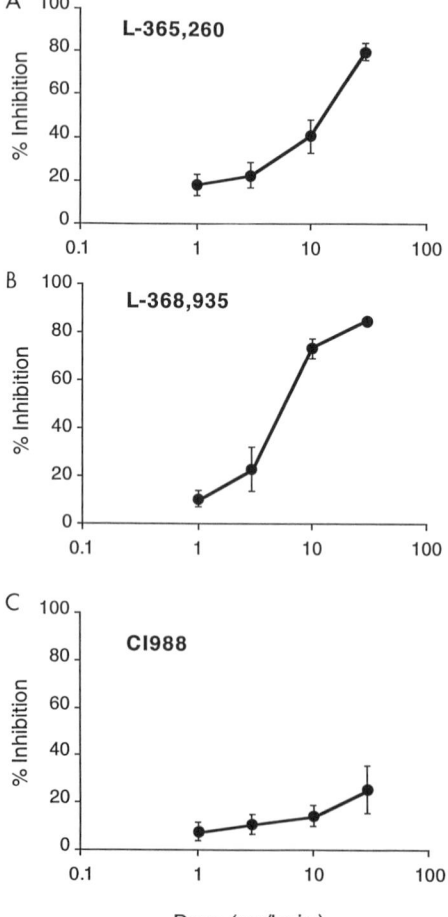

FIGURE 1. (**A**) Intravenous administration of L-365,260 (1.0–30.0 mg/kg, n = 10–12/dose) 30 minutes before sacrifice resulted in a dose-dependent inhibition of *ex vivo* binding of [^{125}I]BH-CCK8S to mouse whole brain compared to vehicle-treated animals (polyethylene glycol: saline:ethanol; 60:30:10). The dose required to inhibit 50% of binding (ED_{50}) was 12.0 mg/kg intravenously. (**B**) Intravenous administration of L-368,935 (1.0–30.0 mg/kg, n = 6/dose) 30 minutes before sacrifice resulted in marked inhibition of *ex vivo* binding of [^{125}I] BH-CCK8S to mouse whole brain compared to vehicle-treated animals (polyethylene glycol:saline:ethanol; 60:30:10) with an ED_{50} of 5.0 mg/kg intravenously. (**C**) Intravenous administration of CI988 (1.0–30.0 mg/kg, n = 7–8/dose) 30 minutes before sacrifice resulted in relatively weak inhibition of *ex vivo* binding of [^{125}I] BH-CCK8S to mouse whole brain compared to vehicle-treated animals (phosphate-buffered saline solution, pH 7.4) with an ED_{50} of > 30.0 mg/kg intravenously. Only limited inhibition of binding was observed at 30.0 mg/kg (26%).

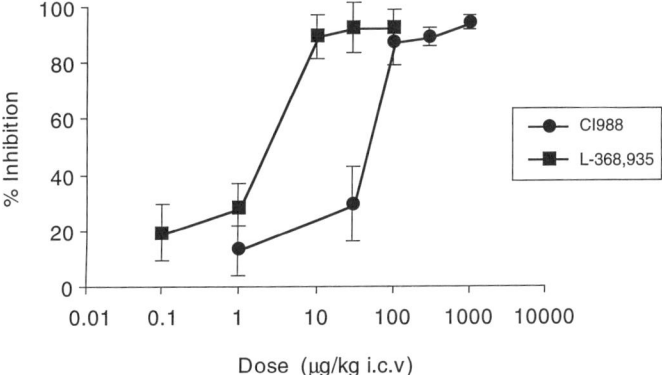

FIGURE 2. CI988 (1.0–1,000 μg/kg, $n = 4$/dose) was administered intracerebroventricularly to lightly anesthetized mice in a volume of 5 μl 15 minutes before *ex vivo* binding studies. Significant dose-dependent inhibition of binding was observed compared to that in vehicle-treated animals (5 μl phosphate-buffered saline solution) with an ED_{50} of 46.0 μg/kg intracerebroventricularly (icv). L-368,935 (0.1–100.0 μg/kg, $n = 4$/dose) was administered icv to lightly anesthetized mice in a volume of 5 μl, 15 minutes before *ex vivo* binding studies. L-368,935 also showed marked inhibition of binding compared to that in vehicle-treated animals (5 μl of phosphate-buffered saline solution) with an ED_{50} of 2.2 μg/kg icv.

hypothesis, when CI988 was given directly into the brain (avoiding penetration across the blood-brain barrier), it showed good CNS activity in agreement with the *in vitro* binding activity of the compound.

The *ex vivo* binding assay described here enables rapid assessment of potentially active compounds in the CNS and is a useful and reliable way of assessing CNS potency and brain penetration of CCK-B antagonists.

REFERENCES

1. HUGHES, J., P. BODEN, B. COSTALL, A. DOMENEY, E. KELLY, D. HORWELL, J. C. HUNTER, R. D. PINNOCK & G. N. WOODRUFF. 1990. Development of a class of selective cholecystokinin type B receptor antagonists having potent anxiolytic activity. Proc. Natl. Acad. Sci. USA **87:** 6728–6732.
2. FREEDMAN, S. B., S. PATEL, A. J. SMITH, K. CHAPMAN, A. FLETCHER, J. A. KEMP, G. R. MARSHALL, R. J. HARGREAVES, K. SCHOLEY, E. C. MELLIN, R. M. DIPARDO, M. G. BOCK & R. M. FREIDINGER. 1993. A second generation of non-peptide cholecystokinin receptor antagonists and their possible therapeutic potential. Ann. N.Y. Acad. Sci., this volume.
3. CHANG, R. S. L. & V. J. LOTTI. 1986. Biochemical and pharmacological characterisation of a new extremely potent and selective nonpeptide cholecystokinin antagonist. Proc. Natl. Acad. Sci. USA **83:** 4923–4926.
4. FREEDMAN, S. B., E. A. HARLEY & S. PATEL. 1989. Direct measurement of muscarinic agents in the central nervous system of mice using *ex vivo* binding. Eur. J. Pharmacol. **174:** 253–260.
5. BERTRAND, P., B. JEANTAUD, S. DREISER, P. LOPEZ, C. GUYNON, M. CAPET, M. C. DUBROEUCQ & A. DOBLE. 1993. Estimation of brain penetration of CCK_B receptor antagonists by an *ex vivo* binding assay. Neuropeptides **24:** 128.

The CCK$_A$ Receptor Antagonist SR 27897 Differentially Influences the Activity of A$_9$ and A$_{10}$ Dopaminergic Neurons in the Rat

V. SANTUCCI,[a] C. GUEUDET,[a] O. THURNEYSSEN,[a]
D. GULLY,[b] P. SOUBRIE,[a] AND G. LE FUR[a]

[a]*Department of Neuropsychiatry*
Sanofi Recherche
34184 Montpellier, France

[b]*Department of Exploratory Biochemistry*
Sanofi Recherche
31036 Toulouse, France

SR 27897 is a potent and selective CCK$_A$ receptor ligand with antagonistic properties in *in vitro* and *in vivo* gastrointestinal models.[1] The compound antagonizes neurobehavioral and biochemical actions of CCK-8S in rodents.[2] CCK$_A$ receptors are probably involved in the facilitation by CCK of the rate-suppressant effect of dopamine D2 agonists such as apomorphine on midbrain dopamine-containing neurons.[3] The present study investigates the effects of SR 27897 in two paradigms involving the electrophysiological properties of dopaminergic neurons submitted to the influence of CCK-8S and apomorphine.

Micropipettes were stereotaxically[4] aimed at the vicinity of A$_9$ or A$_{10}$ neurons in male Sprague-Dawley rats anesthetized with chloral hydrate. The spikes recorded from the micropipette were amplified, filtered, and fed into an intelligent interface via a window discriminator for computer processing. Rate histograms were constructed on line and analyzed off line to determine the number of spikes in given periods.

SR 27897 was first studied for its ability to alter the facilitation by CCK-8S of the apomorphine-induced inhibition of the firing rate of A$_{10}$ cells. SR 27897 was administered intraperitoneally 60 minutes before the experiment. After the firing rate was stabilized, CCK-8S and apomorphine were injected intravenously at an interval of 5 minutes, and the firing rate was monitored for an additional 15–20 minutes. For comparison, devazepide (5 mg/kg) was studied under the same conditions.

The activity of SR 27897 was also investigated against the inhibitory effects of apomorphine alone on A$_9$ and A$_{10}$ cells. The general conditions were the same as in the first study except that apomorphine was injected 5–10 minutes after recording onset.

The weak depression by apomorphine (5 μg/kg iv) of the firing rate of A$_{10}$ cells was potently facilitated by CCK-8S (FIG. 1). This facilitation was dose-dependently prevented by SR 27897 as well as by devazepide (FIG. 1). SR 27897 also dose-dependently attenuated the inhibition by apomorphine (10 μg/kg iv) of the firing rate of A$_{10}$ but not of A$_9$ cells (FIG. 2).

These results show that CCK$_A$ receptor antagonists such as SR 27897 and

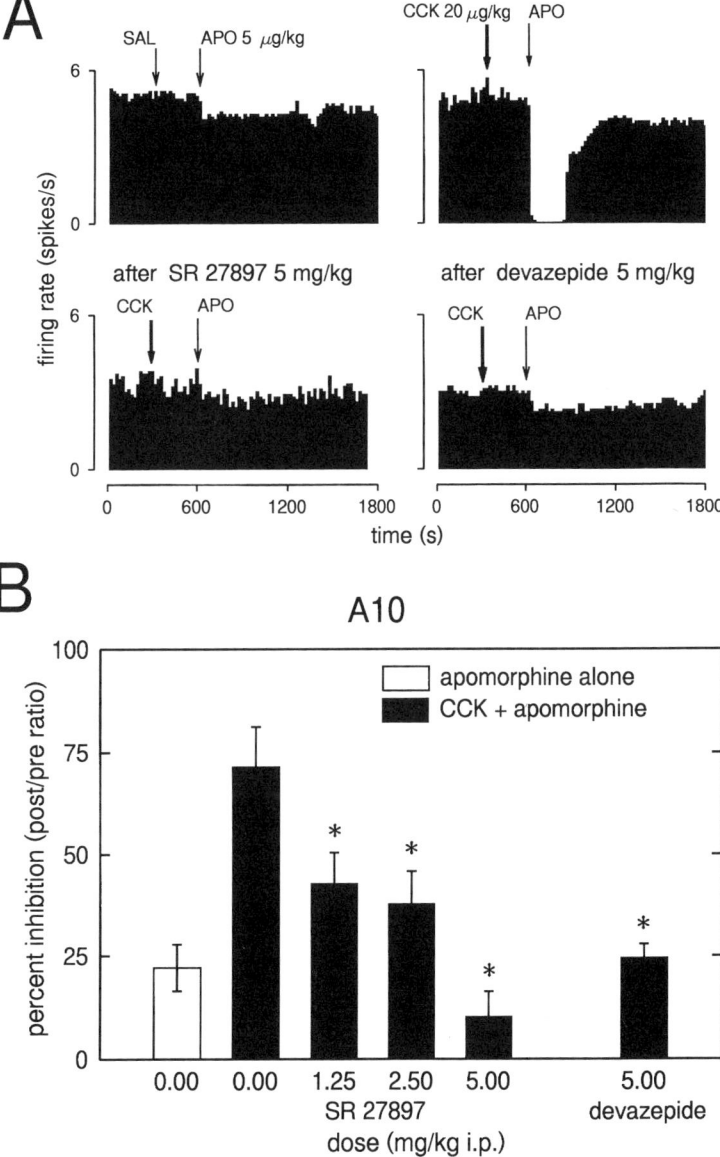

FIGURE 1. Effects of SR 27897 and devazepide on the facilitation by CCK-8S (20 μg/kg iv) of the rate-suppressant effect of apomorphine (APO, 5 μg/kg iv) on A_{10} neurons. (**A**) Typical samples of rate histograms showing the potentiation by CCK-8S of a weak effect of apomorphine and its reversal by the previous (60 min) administration of SR 27897 (5 mg/kg ip) and devazepide (5 mg/kg ip). (**B**) Dose-response relationships of SR 27897 and devazepide. *Bars* indicate the post/pre ratio level of apomorphine-induced inhibition in the absence (0.00) or presence of the compounds.

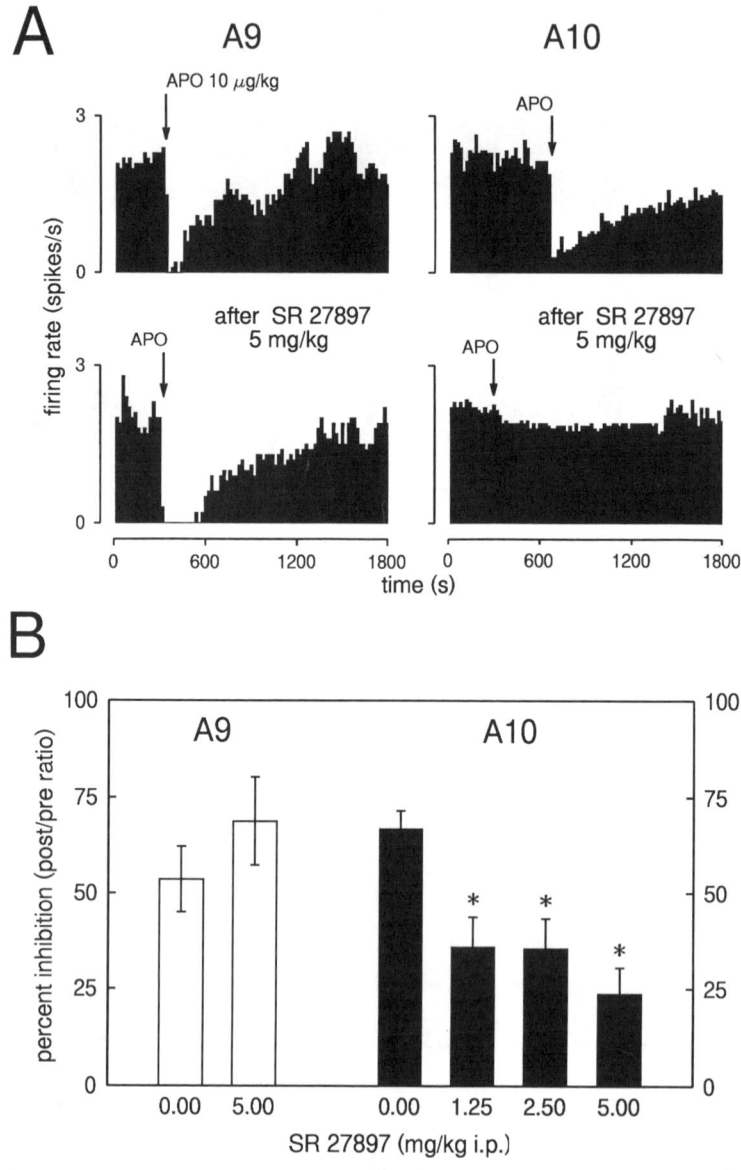

FIGURE 2. Effects of SR 27897 on the inhibition by apomorphine (APO, 10 μg/kg iv) of the spontaneous firing rate of A_9 and A_{10} cells. (**A**) Typical samples of rate histograms showing the antagonistic effect of SR 27897 on the rate-suppressant activity of apomorphine in A_{10} vs A_9 cells. (**B**) Dose-effect relationship of SR 27897. *Bars* indicate the post/pre ratio level of apomorphine-induced inhibition in the absence (0.00) or presence of the compound.

devazepide preferentially affect the changes induced by apomorphine, as well as their potentiation by CCK-8S, in A_{10} vs A_9 dopamine-containing neurons. This selectivity is in line with the reported coexistence of CCK and dopamine in A_{10} cells. The data presented here suggest that CCK_A receptors modulate the activity of dopaminergic neurons of the mesolimbic, but probably not of the nigrostriatal system.

REFERENCES

1. GULLY, D., D. FREHEL, C. MARCY, A. SPINAZZE, L. LESPY, G. NELIAT, J.-P. MAFFRAND & G. LE FUR. 1993. Eur. J. Pharmacol. **232**: 13–19.
2. PONCELET, M., M. ARNONE, M. HEAULME, N. GONALONS, C. GUEUDET, V. SANTUCCI, O. THURNEYSSEN, P. KEANE, D. GULLY, G. LE FUR & P. SOUBRIE. 1993. Naunyn-Schmiedeberg's Arch. Pharmacol. **348**: 102–107.
3. CHIODO, L. A., A. S. FREEMAN & B. S. BUNNEY. 1987. Brain Res. **410**: 205–211.
4. PAXINOS, G. & C. WATSON. 1986. The Rat Brain in Stereotaxic Coordinates. Academic Press. Sydney.

Comparison of the Effects of the CCK-Receptor Antagonist Loxiglumide and the M_1-Receptor Antagonist Telenzepine on the Pancreatic Protein Response to Intraduodenal Tryptophan in Dogs

First Results

STEPHAN TEYSSEN AND MANFRED V. SINGER[a]

Department of Medicine IV (Gastroenterology)
University Hospital of Heidelberg at Mannheim
Theodor-Kutzer Ufer
68135 Mannheim, Germany

Previous studies have shown that atropine[1-4] and truncal vagotomy[2] decrease the pancreatic response to intestinal amino acids such as tryptophan. In conjunction with studies on the latency of the pancreatic enzyme response to intestinal stimuli,[5] we concluded that enteropancreatic cholinergic vagovagal reflexes are quantitatively important mediators of the pancreatic enzyme response to intraduodenal tryptophan. Recently we showed[6] that at least some cholinergic fibers of the enterocholinergic vagovagal reflex which controls the first part of the pancreatic enzyme secretion end on highly selective muscarinic receptors of the subtype M_1.

The present study attempts to determine the relative contribution and possible additive or potentative interaction of the enteropancreatic cholinergic vagovagal reflexes and the hormone cholecystokinin (CCK) as mediators of the pancreatic secretory response to low and high loads of tryptophan.

MATERIALS AND METHODS

In six male and female conscious foxhounds (weighing 24–33 kg) with chronic gastric and pancreatic Thomas fistulas we performed dose response studies of the pancreatic protein response to graded loads of intraduodenal tryptophan (TRP; 0.37–10.0 mmol/h, starting with the lowest dose and tripling the dose every 45 minutes) given against a background of secretin (S; 20.5 pmol/kg/h iv). Studies were repeated in the presence of telenzepine (Tel; 81 nmol/kg/h iv) or loxiglumide (Lox; 10 mg/kg/h iv), or both.

Pancreatic juice was collected continuously and separated into 15-minute samples.

---

[a] Address for correspondence: Manfred V. Singer, MD, Department of Medicine IV (Gastroenterology), University Hospital of Heidelberg at Mannheim, Theodor-Kutzer Ufer, 68135 Mannheim, Germany.

Volume was measured to the nearest 0.1 ml. Concentrations of protein were measured as described previously[7] and outputs calculated.

Synthetic secretin (Secretolin) was bought from Hoechst (Frankfurt, Germany); telenzepine was a gift from Byk Gulden (Konstanz, Germany), loxiglumide was a gift from Rotta Research (Monza, Italy), and L-tryptophan was purchased from Serva Biochemical (Heidelberg, Germany).

All statistical analyses were performed by the statistical analysis system (SAS). p values less than 0.05 were considered significant.

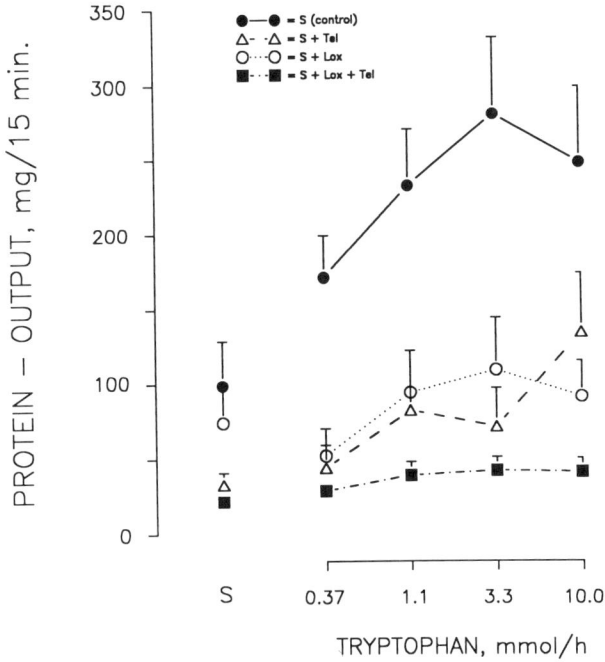

FIGURE 1. Effect of telenzepine (81 nmol/kg/h iv), loxiglumide (10 mg/kg/h iv), and loxiglumide plus telenzepine, respectively, on pancreatic protein output, during secretin (S), and in response to graded loads of intraduodenal tryptophan (0.37–10.0 mmol/h) as compared to control (S without Tel or Lox). Results are means ± SEM of six dogs.

RESULTS

All loads of TRP significantly ($p < 0.05$) increased pancreatic protein output over that seen with S alone. Tel and Tel+Lox but not Lox alone significantly reduced protein output during S by 66% and 78%, respectively. In the presence of Tel only the highest load (10 mmol/h) of TRP significantly increased the protein output over that of S+Tel. Lox and Lox+Tel abolished the response to all loads of TRP (FIG. 1). Tel, Lox, and Lox+Tel significantly inhibited the 3-hour integrated protein response (IPR; g × min) to all loads of TRP by 62%, 86% and 89%, respectively, as compared

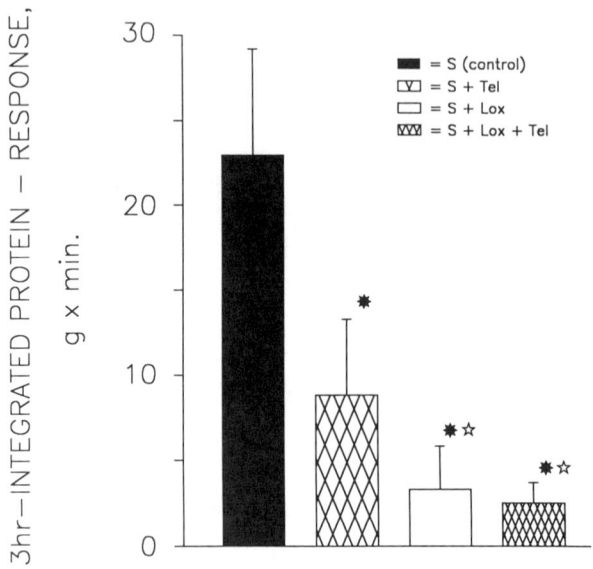

FIGURE 2. Three-hour integrated pancreatic protein responses (g × min) to all loads of intraduodenal tryptophan during intravenous secretin (S), S+Tel, S+Lox, and S+Lox+Tel, respectively. ✱$p < 0.05$ vs control (S); ☆—☆$p < 0.05$ vs S+Tel.

to control (S without Tel or Lox). Inhibition by Lox and Lox+Tel of the 3-hour IPR was significantly higher (24% and 27%, respectively) than that by Tel (FIG. 2).

CONCLUSIONS

These findings indicate that: (1) during secretin, pancreatic protein output is controlled by cholinergic nerves rather than by CCK. (2) The M_1-receptor antagonist Tel and the CCK-antagonist Lox are capable of inhibiting the pancreatic protein response to low and high loads of TRP. Lox preferably inhibits the protein response to high loads of TRP. (3) Both enteropancreatic cholinergic reflexes and the hormone CCK are involved as mediators of the protein response to low and high loads of intraduodenal TRP. (4) Enteropancreatic cholinergic reflexes are probably the dominant mediators of the protein response to low amounts of TRP, whereas CCK is the major mediator of the response to high loads of TRP.

REFERENCES

1. SINGER, M. V., T. E. SOLOMON & M. I. GROSSMAN. 1980. Effect of atropine on secretion from intact and transplanted pancreas in the dog. Am. J. Physiol. **238:** G18–G22.
2. SOLOMON, T. E. & M. I. GROSSMAN. 1979. Effect of atropine and vagotomy on response of transplanted pancreas. Am. J. Physiol. **236:** E186–190.
3. VAZQUEZ-ECHARRI, J., D. BAUMGÄRTNER & M. V. SINGER. 1986. Dose-response effects of atropine on pancreatic secretory response to intestinal tryptophan in dogs. Am. J. Physiol. **251:** G847–851.

4. SINGER, M. V., W. NIEBEL, J. B. M. J. JANSSEN, D. HOFFMEISTER, S. GOTTHOLD, H. GOEBELL & C. B. H. W. LAMERS. 1989. Pancreatic secretory response to intravenous caerulein and intraduodenal tryptophan. Studies before and after stepwise removal of the extrinsic nerves of the pancreas in dogs. Gastroenterology **96:** 925–934.
5. SINGER, M. V., T. E. SOLOMON, J. WOOD & M. I. GROSSMAN. 1980. Latency of pancreatic enzyme response to intraduodenal stimulants. Am. J. Physiol. **238:** G23–29.
6. SINGER, M. V., S. TEYSSEN & U. KÜPPERS. 1991. Influence of the M_1-receptor antagonists telenzepine and pirenzepine on pancreatic secretory response to intraduodenal tryptophan in dogs. Digestion **48:** 34–42.
7. SINGER, M. V. & H. SARLES. 1978. Pancreatic dose-response curves to cholecystokinin determined by two techniques in dogs. Scand. J. Gastroenterol. **13:** 969–974.

Effects of CCK-A Antagonist Devazepide on Inhibition of Feeding by Duodenal Infusion of Oleic Acid in Rats

TODD A. WOLTMAN[a] AND ROGER D. REIDELBERGER

Department of Biomedical Sciences
Creighton University School of Medicine
Omaha, Nebraska 68178
and
Veterans Administration Medical Center
Omaha, Nebraska 68105

Cholecystokinin (CCK) does not appear to produce satiety by an endocrine mechanism. Intravenous CCK doses that inhibit food intake produce plasma CCK levels an order of magnitude larger than those occurring after a meal.[1] Findings showing that suppression of feeding by exogenous CCK is mediated by the low-affinity state of the type A receptor[2] suggest that postprandial plasma levels of CCK are insufficient to produce satiety. Furthermore, immunoneutralization of circulating CCK was recently reported to block the pancreatic secretory response to a maximal dose of CCK and a liquid meal, but to have no effect on food intake.[3] Yox et al.[4] propose that nutrients in the upper intestine stimulate CCK secretion which acts locally in a paracrine fashion to activate vagal neural inhibition of feeding behavior. Duodenal fat releases CCK and decreases food intake. In rats, CCK receptor antagonists reverse the inhibitory effect of duodenal infusion of oleic acid on *sham* feeding.[4,5] However, in pigs[6] and humans,[7] CCK antagonists were shown to have no effect on oleic acid–induced suppression of *real* feeding. Thus, it is controversial whether endogenous CCK is important in mediating the anorectic effect of duodenal fat. Therefore, we used the type A CCK receptor antagonist devazepide to examine the role of endogenous CCK in duodenal oleic acid–induced inhibition of *real* feeding in rats with free access to food.

Male Sprague-Dawley rats ($n = 7$–13) were prepared with duodenal and jugular vein catheters. At the start of the dark period, nonfasted rats received intravenous injection of devazepide (1 or 2 mg/kg) or vehicle (5% DMSO, 5% Tween 80, and 90% saline solution) 15 minutes before a 2-hour duodenal infusion of oleic acid (45, 62.5, or 90 mM; ED_{40}, ED_{50}, and ED_{80} doses, respectively; 0.13 ml/min) or vehicle. Oleic acid was emulsified in phosphate-buffered saline solution (pH 6.4, 300 mOsm/l) with 1.5% Tween 80 or 1% sodium taurocholate and 0.1% lecithin. Food intake was determined from continuous computer recordings of changes in food bowl weight. Data were analyzed by a two-way repeated measures analysis of variance.

Duodenal infusion of oleic acid inhibited 4-hour food intake dose-dependently whether the emulsifier was Tween 80 or sodium taurocholate/lecithin ($p < 0.00001$). Devazepide injection alone stimulated 4-hour intake ($p < 0.01$); however, there was no significant interaction between oleic acid and devazepide on feeding ($p > 0.10$). Thus, oleic acid was equally effective in suppressing food intake whether devazepide

---

[a] Address for correspondence: Todd A. Woltman, Department of Biomedical Sciences, Division of Physiology, Creighton University, 2500 California Plaza, Omaha, NE 68178.

was injected or not, and devazepide was equally effective in stimulating feeding whether oleic acid was infused or not.

It is uncertain why CCK receptor blockade produced different results in real and sham feeding studies. Differences in feeding paradigm may explain the disparate results. Redundant mechanisms may mediate the anorectic effects of intestinal fat in real feeding conditions, rendering gut CCK nonessential for normal satiety to occur. In real feeding subjects, stimulation of CCK-independent gastric and intestinal mechanisms by ingested food and infused fat, respectively, may have been sufficient to produce the inhibitory response to infused fat. In contrast, in sham feeding animals, duodenal fat stimulation of a CCK-dependent mechanism may have been required for the complete anorectic response to occur, as food stimulation of gastric mechanisms is minimal. An alternative explanation is that the results of sham feeding studies were misinterpreted. Opposing effects of CCK receptor blockade and duodenal infusion of fat on food intake could reflect either a causal relationship between infused fat, endogenous CCK, and suppression of sham feeding, or independent, opposing effects of CCK receptor blockade and infused fat on food intake. For an independent effect of CCK receptor blockade to be clearly shown, CCK antagonists must stimulate food intake similarly in the presence and absence of intestinal fat infusion. This was demonstrated in the present study. In contrast, in the sham feeding studies, CCK receptor blockade increased food intake only when fat was infused into the duodenum. However, in sham feeding and fasted real feeding rats, CCK receptor blockade does not usually elevate intake further because the animals are already ingesting a large quantity of food. Thus, it is reasonable to speculate that an independent effect of CCK receptor blockade may have been expressed in the sham feeding studies during intestinal infusion of fat because food intake was reduced but not during intestinal infusion of saline solution because intake was greatly elevated. In conclusion, these results do not support the hypothesis that CCK mediates the satiety effect of duodenal oleic acid.

REFERENCES

1. REIDELBERGER, R. D., T. J. KALOGERIS & T. E. SOLOMON. 1989. Am. J. Physiol. **256:** R1148–R1154.
2. ASIN, K. E. & L. BEDNARZ. 1992. Pharmacol. Biochem. Behav. **42:** 291–295.
3. REIDELBERGER, R. D., G. VARGA, G. L. ROSENQUIST, R. M. LIEHR, H. WONG & J. H. WALSH. 1991. Int. J. Obesity **15(S3):** 12 (abstr.).
4. YOX, D. P., L. BRENNER & R. C. RITTER. 1992. Am. J. Physiol. **262:** R554–R561.
5. GREENBERG, D., N. I. TORRES, G. P. SMITH & J. GIBBS. 1989. Ann. N.Y. Acad. Sci. **575:** 517–520.
6. GREGORY, P. C., M. MCFADEN & D. V. RAYNER. 1989. Physiol. Behav. **45:** 1021–1024.
7. DREWE, J., A. GADIENT, L. C. ROVATI & C. BEGLINGER. 1992. Gastroenterology **102:** 1654–1659.

The CCK-B Antagonist LY288513 Blocks Diazepam-Withdrawal-Induced Increases in Auditory Startle Response

KURT RASMUSSEN,[a] DAVID R. HELTON,[a]
JAMES E. BERGER,[b] AND ELIZABETH SCEARCE[b]

[a] Lilly Research Labs
Eli Lilly & Co.
Indianapolis, Indiana 46285

[b] Butler University
Indianapolis, Indiana 46208

In humans, withdrawal from the chronic use of benzodiazepines can result in a variety of undesirable side effects, including anxiety. In animals, benzodiazepine withdrawal has also had anxiogenic effects as indicated by decreases in body weight and food intake,[1] disruption of an operant behavior,[2] decreased time spent in the light compartment of a light/dark box,[3] decreased time spent in the open arms of an elevated plus-maze,[4] and increased auditory startle responses.[5] CCK-B antagonists have demonstrated anxiolytic actions in several animal models of anxiety[6] and have blocked the anxiogenic effects of benzodiazepine withdrawal in the light/dark box.[7] The effects of CCK-B antagonists on benzodiazepine-withdrawal-induced increases in the auditory startle response have never been measured. We therefore examined the effects of the selective CCK-B antagonist LY288513 on the auditory startle response in rats undergoing withdrawal from the chronic administration of diazepam.

Male Long-Evans rats on a growth curve (150–350 g) were anesthetized with halothane, and Alzet osmotic minipumps (2ML2; Alza Corp.) were implanted subcutaneously. Pumps were filled with either diazepam (20 mg/kg/day) or vehicle. Before implantation, each pump was primed for 4 hours in physiological saline. All treatment groups contained 10 rats. Twelve days after implantation of pumps, rats were anesthetized with halothane and the pumps were removed. The auditory startle response (peak amplitude, V_{max}) of individual rats was recorded using San Diego Instruments startle chambers (San Diego, CA). Startle sessions consisted of a 5-minute adaptation period at a background noise level of 70 ± 2 dBA immediately followed by 25 presentations of auditory stimuli (120 ± 3 dBA noise, 50-ms duration) presented at 8-second intervals. Peak startle amplitudes were then averaged for all 25 presentations of stimuli for each session. All data are presented as overall session means. Auditory startle responding was evaluated daily on days 13–16 at 24-hour intervals following drug withdrawal.

As observed previously,[5] cessation of chronic diazepam administration resulted in significantly increased auditory startle responses (FIGS. 1 and 2). Administration of 30 mg/kg diazepam 15 minutes before testing blocked the withdrawal-induced increases in startle responding. Administration of 30 mg/kg LY288513 (ip) 60 minutes before startle testing significantly reduced the withdrawal-induced increase in startle responding only on withdrawal day 1. Administration of 60 mg/kg LY288513 (ip) 60 minutes before startle testing significantly reduced the withdrawal-induced increase in startle responding on all days examined.

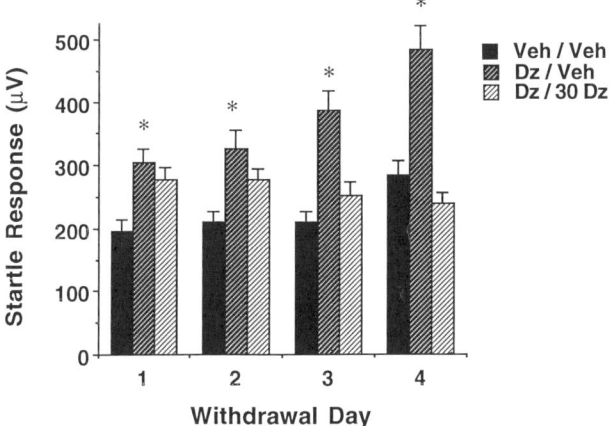

FIGURE 1. Mean (±SE) startle response for rats undergoing withdrawal from chronic administration of diazepam. Startle responses were measured daily for 4 days beginning 24 hours after removal of diazepam- or vehicle-containing minipumps. Rats received either: chronic diazepam and an acute daily pretreatment during withdrawal of vehicle (Dz/Veh) or 30 mg/kg diazepam (Dz/30 mg/kg Dz); or chronic vehicle and an acute daily pretreatment during withdrawal of vehicle (Veh/Veh). $n = 10$ per group; *Significantly different from Veh/Veh, $p < 0.05$.

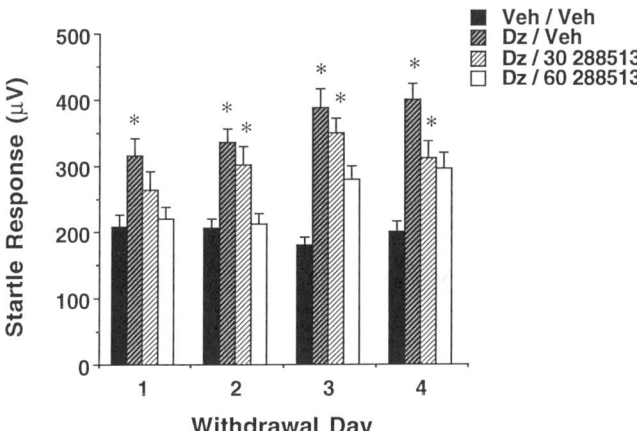

FIGURE 2. Mean (±SE) startle response for rats undergoing withdrawal from chronic administration of diazepam. Startle responses were measured daily for 4 days beginning 24 hours after removal of diazepam- or vehicle-containing minipumps. Rats received either: chronic diazepam and an acute daily pretreatment during withdrawal of vehicle (Dz/Veh), 30 mg/kg LY288513 (Dz/30 LY), or 60 mg/kg LY288513 (Dz/60 LY); or chronic vehicle and an acute daily pretreatment during withdrawal of vehicle (Veh/Veh). $n = 10$ per group; *Significantly different from Veh/Veh, $p < 0.05$.

Acute administration of diazepam or LY288513 blocked the effects of withdrawal of chronic diazepam administration on auditory startle responses. Blockade of the withdrawal-induced increased startle responding with acute diazepam replacement confirms that increased startle responding is due to a lack of diazepam and is not a nonspecific effect of the procedure. The effects of diazepam and LY288513 on diazepam-withdrawal-induced increased startle responding were similar. However, LY288513 has extremely low affinity for both GABA and benzodiazepine receptors (D. O. Calligaro, unpublished observations). Therefore, although the effects of the two types of compounds have a common end-point (reduction of withdrawal symptoms), their mechanisms of action are not identical.

These results indicate that LY288513 and other CCK-B antagonists may be an effective treatment for benzodiazepine withdrawal symptoms in humans.

REFERENCES

1. GOUDIE, A. J. & M. J. LEATHLEY. 1990. Effects of the 5-HT$_3$ antagonist GR38032F (ondansetron) on benzodiazepine withdrawal in rats. Eur. J. Pharmacol. **185:** 179–186.
2. GOUDIE, A. J. & M. J. LEATHLEY. 1992. Effects of the 5HT$_3$ antagonist ondansetron on benzodiazepine-induced operant behavioural dependence in rats. Psychopharmacology **109:** 461–465.
3. COSTALL, B., J. JONES, M. E. KELLY, R. J. NAYLOR, E. S. ONAIVI & M. B. TYERS. 1990. Sites of action of ondansetron to inhibit withdrawal from drugs of abuse. Pharmacol., Biochem. & Behav. **36:** 97–104.
4. ANDREWS, N. & S. E. FILE. 1992. Are there changes in sensitivity to 5-HT$_3$ receptor ligands following chronic diazepam treatment? Psychopharmacology **108:** 333–337.
5. MARTINEZ, J. A., M. J. FARGEAS & L. BUENO. 1992. Physical dependence on diazepam: Precipitation of abstinence syndromes by peripheral and central benzodiazepine receptor antagonists. Pharmacol. Biochem. Behav. **41:** 461–464.
6. RAVARD, S. & C. T. DOURISH. 1990. Cholecystokinin and anxiety. Trends Pharmacol. Sci. **11:** 271–273.
7. SINGH, L., M. J. FIELD, C. A. VASS, J. HUGHES & G. N. WOODRUFF. 1992. The antagonism of benzodiazepine withdrawal effects by the selective cholecystokinin-B antagonist CI-988. Br. J. Pharmacol. **105:** 9–10.

Evaluation of Brain Penetration of CCK-B Antagonists

M. C. DUBROEUCQ,[a] C. GUYON,[a] F. MANFRÉ,[a]
M. CAPET,[a] M. BARREAU,[a] P. BERTRAND,[b]
B. JEANTAUD,[b] A. DOBLE,[b] AND J.-C. BLANCHARD[b]

[a]*Medicinal Chemistry Department and*
[b]*Biology Department of RHÔNE-POULENC RORER*
Centre de recherches de Vitry Alfortville
Vitry sur Seine, France

The development of potent nonpeptide antagonists selective for cholecystokinin (CCK) receptor subtypes offers opportunities to explore the functional role of CCK in the brain and consequently to find therapeutic applications for these compounds. Ureidoacetamides were recently described[1] to present a CCK-B/gastrin antagonist binding profile and an inhibitory effect on CCK responses *in vitro*.[2] To select compounds rationally for subsequent time-consuming behavioral studies, an *ex vivo* binding assay was designed to estimate the brain penetration of these compounds.

EX VIVO BINDING METHOD

Male CD1 mice (20–25 g) were treated either intraperitoneally (ip) or orally (po) with the compound (prepared as a suspension or a solution in 0.025% Tween 80) at doses ranging from 1 to 80 mg/kg. At each time point after administration, the brain was quickly removed and the cerebral tissue (without cerebellum and brainstem) was dispersed (1:4 w/v) in PIPES-HCl buffer.

Aliquots (0.1 ml) of homogenate were incubated with 0.1 ml [^{3}H]p-CCK-8 (0.4 nM final) and 1.1 ml of either CCK-8 (10 μM) or buffer at 25°C for 30 minutes. The samples were then diluted and filtered under vacuum through Whatman GF/B filters, which were rinsed with 2 × 4 ml washes of buffer. Radioactivity was counted in 10 ml of scintillant. Specific binding was defined as that displaceable by 10 μM CCK-8, and all determinations of binding assays were performed in triplicate. The results obtained are a percentage of inhibition of CCK-8 binding.

RESULTS AND DISCUSSION

Easily prepared by a multistep synthesis, compounds belonging to the ureidoacetamide chemical family were evaluated with the technique just described. Introduc-

TABLE 1. CCK-A and CCK-B Receptor Binding Assays and ex Vivo Binding Assays in Guinea Pig Membranes from Pancreas (A) and Cortex (B)

CLogP	R_1	R_2	Binding (IC_{50}, nM) (A)	(B)	Ex Vivo % inhib ip	R_1	R_2	Binding (IC_{50}, nM) (A)	(B)	% inhib ip	Ex Vivo ID_{50} (mg/kg) ip^a	po^a
4.25	H	Me	234	11	0	OMe	±CH(Me)CO$_2$H	2,700	6	90	>40^b	>40
4.25	OMe	Me	143	8	17	"	+CH(Me)CO$_2$H	2,610	5	86	3^b	9
4.16	H	SMe	53	9	12	"	−CH(Me)CO$_2$H	1,255	18	83	>40^b	>40
2.87	"	CH(OH)Me	>1,000	12	10	"	±CH(Me)SO$_3$H	1,350	0.9	90	4	21
3.69	"	CO$_2$H	>1,000	15	65	"	+CH(Me)SO$_3$H	3,295	10	74	9	40
2.87	"	CH$_2$CO$_2$H	>1,000	15	56	"	−CH(Me)SO$_3$H	977	1	89	5	37
1.74	"	SO$_3$H	>1,000	25	35		L-365 260	767	11.5	94	5	9
2.31	"	CH(Me)SO$_3$H	>1,000	1	70		CI-988	646	7.8	82	6	26
3.18	"	CH(Me)CO$_2$H	>1,000	5	56							
3.18	OMe	CH(Me)CO$_2$H	>1,000	6	90							
3.71	OMe	CH(Et)CO$_2$H	>1,000	26	40							

^{a}In each case, the inhibitory effect was well correlated to the logarithm of the dose by linear regression analysis, from which was estimated the half-maximal inhibitory dose.
^{b}Measured 60 minutes after intraperitoneal administration.

tion of hydrophilic and especially acid-type substituent onto the phenyl ring of the ureido moiety in meta position not only increases selectivity for the B-type receptor, but also allows compounds to penetrate the brain. The experimental results obtained with equipotent ligands of the same chemical family indicate optimal brain penetration for compounds whose calculated log P^3 is between 2 and 3.5, which is in agreement with current theories.[4] Extensive studies were performed on two particular racemic compounds and on their corresponding enantiomers. In the carboxylic acid family, the dextrorotatory isomer emerges as the most interesting, giving good results whatever the mode of administration. The sulfonic acid enantiomers are equipotent, but their ID_{50}s are lower than that of the best carboxylic acid derivative. Two other known CCK-B/gastrin antagonists, L-365,260[5] and Cl-988,[6] were evaluated in this model.

In TABLE 1 CCK-A and CCK-B receptor binding assays were carried out with guinea pig membranes from pancreas and cortex, respectively (modification of the method of Saito et al.[7]). The percentage of inhibition of CCK (% inhib ip) binding was measured 30 minutes after ip administration of the compound.

REFERENCES

1. (a) DUBROEUCQ, M. C., C. GUYON, M. BARREAU, C. COTREL, J.-D. BOURZAT, M. CAPET, F. MANFRÉ, P. BERTRAND & G. A. BÖHME. 1992. XIIth International Symposium on Medicinal Chemistry BASEL. poster P-184.A; (b) GUYON, C., M.-C. DUBROEUCQ, M. BARREAU, P. BERTRAND, F. CHENOT, M. FOLKE & A. MADOUX. 1992. XIIth International Symposium on Medicinal Chemistry BASEL. posters P-185.A, P-186.C.
2. BÖHME, G. A., P. BERTRAND, C. PENDLEY, A. DOBLE, C. GUYON, G. MARTIN, J.-M. STUTZMANN, M.-C. DUBROEUCQ, & J.-C. BLANCHARD. 1992. Naunyn-Schmiedeberg's Arch. Pharmacol. **345:** R116.
3. Medchem software (Release 3.52, November 1987). HANSCH, C. Pomona College, Claremont, California.
4. (a) GREIG, N. H. 1989. Implication of the blood-brain barrier and its manipulations. E. A., ed. Plenum Publishing Corp. New York, Vol. 1, 311; (b) HANSCH, C., J. P. BJOKROTH & A. LEO. 1987. J. Pharm. Sci. **76:** 663.
5. LOTTI, V. & R. CHANG. 1989. Eur. J. Pharmacol. **162:** 273–280.
6. SINGH, L., M. J. FIELD, J. HUGHES, R. MENZIES, R. OLES, C. VASS & G. WOODRUFF. 1991. Br. J. Pharmacol. **104:** 239–245.
7. SAITO, A., I. GOLDFINE & J. WILLIAMS. 1981. J. Neurochem. **37:** 483–490.

[³H]SNF 8702 Autoradiography of CCK-B Receptors in Guinea Pig Brain and Studies with a Cloned Rat CCK-B Receptor

RICHARD J. KNAPP,[a] EWA MALATYNSKA,[a]
SHINICHI HASHIMOTO,[b] SUNAN FANG,[c] MARY HUNT,[d]
JAMES K. WAMSLEY,[e] PAM PETERSON,[a]
TERESA ZALEWSKA,[a] VICTOR J. HRUBY,[c]
AND HENRY I. YAMAMURA[a]

The University of Arizona College of Medicine,
[a] Pharmacology and [c] Chemistry Departments
Tucson, Arizona 85724

[b] Biochemical Research Laboratory
Morinaga Milk Industry Co. Ltd.
Kanagawa 228, Japan

[d] Neuropsychiatric Research Institute
Fargo, North Dakota 58107

[e] New York Medical College
Department of Psychiatry
Valhalla, New York 10595

[N-Methyl-Nle^{28,31}]CCK$_{26-33}$ (SNF 8702) interactions with cholecystokinin-B (CCK-B) receptors were characterized with respect to anatomical distribution in guinea pig brain and by measurements of binding affinity and potency at cloned rat CCK-B receptors expressed in COS-7 cells. SNF 8702 is a highly selective CCK-B receptor ligand with over 4,000-fold greater affinity for CCK-B relative to CCK-A receptors.[1] Previous binding studies with membrane homogenates prepared from whole guinea pig brain and selected brain regions suggested the presence of CCK-B receptor heterogeneity.[2] These regional differences led us to examine the anatomical distribution of [³H]SNF 8702 sites to determine if variations from CCK-B distribution seen with Bolton-Hunter ^{125}I-labeled CCK-8 (BH-CCK-8) could be established. COS-7 cells expressing a single cloned CCK-B receptor were used to characterize [³H]SNF 8702 binding to CCK-B receptor affinity states.

MATERIALS AND METHODS

Receptor Autoradiography. Autoradiographic studies were performed using tissue obtained from adult male Hartley guinea pigs (Harlan Sprague-Dawley Inc., Indianapolis, Indiana). Tissue sections were cut to a thickness of 15 μm at −20°C using a cryostat (Bright Instrument company LTD, Huntindon, England) and thaw-mounted on glass slides. Slide-mounted tissue sections were incubated with 2.0 nM [³H]SNF 8702 in the presence or absence of 1.0 μM sulfated CCK-8 for 3 hours. The tissue sections were washed three times for 5 minutes in ice-cold HEPES buffer and rinsed once with distilled water. Autoradiographs were produced by apposing the labeled sections along with brain paste and commercial (^{3}H Microscales) to Hyperfilm ^{3}H (Amersham) for 6 weeks. Films were processed using Kodak D-19 developer and fixer (Kodak, Rochester, New York). Quantitative autoradiographic analyses were performed using a microcomputer imaging densitometric (MCID) system (Imaging Research Inc., Ontario, Canada).

CCK-B Receptor cDNA Cloning and Expression. A cDNA clone including the entire open reading frame of the rat CCK-B receptor described by Wank et al.[3] was produced by the polymerase chain reaction (PCR) method using the flanking primers AGCAGAGCTAAGTGGGACTTCACTGGAGCC (corresponded to positions 106–135 of the 5' untranslated portion of the original CCK-B receptor clone) and TCTTGTCTCTTTCTCCAATCTCCCAACCCC (corresponding to the reversed antisense of positions 1459–1524 of the 3' untranslated region). PCR was performed under standard conditions using rat cDNA (Quick Clone, Clontech, Palo Alto, California) as the template. Nucleotide sequence analysis showed that the cDNA clone produced has complete sequence identity to the corresponding positions of the Wank et al.[3] sequence. The cDNA was subcloned into the pSV-SPORT1 transient expression vector and transfected into COS-7 cells by the DEAE-dextran method. Binding studies were performed 48 hours after transfection. Radioligand binding studies using membranes prepared from the recombinant cells were performed as previously described.[2]

RESULTS AND DISCUSSION

Autoradiography. The distribution of CCK-B receptors labeled by [^{3}H]SNF 8702 shows marked regional differences (FIG. 1). Low receptor densities (10–20 fmol/mg tissue) are observed in the thalamus and substantia nigra (SN). Moderate to high CCK-B receptor densities are seen in the cerebral cortex (21–88 fmol/mg tissue), caudate putamen (CPu), nucleus accumbens (Acb), superior colliculus (SuC), and molecular (MLC) and granular (GLC) layers of the cerebellum. The anterior olfactory nucleus (AONE) shows the highest receptor density (260 fmol/mg tissue). Receptor density values for [^{3}H]SNF 8702 were compared to those of Niehoff[4] obtained for BH-CCK-8 (FIG. 2). The correlation coefficient (r) between the data sets was low (0.693). This difference cannot be attributed to BH-CCK-8 binding to brain CCK-A receptors because these are absent in guinea pig brain.[5] Thus, the low correlation coefficient could be a reflection of differences in CCK-B receptor subtype selectivity between the two radioligands and the presence of such subtypes in the guinea pig brain.

Binding to Recombinant COS-7 Cells. Saturation binding studies ($n = 3$) over a concentration range of 0.1–5.0 nM [^{3}H]SNF 8702 produced data best fit by a one-site model giving a K_d value of 0.8 nM and a B_{max} of 550 fmol/mg protein. The mean Hill slope value was 0.9 which was not significantly different from unity. These data are consistent with previous observations for [^{3}H]SNF 8702 binding to guinea pig cerebral cortical membranes ($K_d = 0.72 \pm 0.08$ nM) but not to guinea pig whole brain or mid-brain thalamus membranes that showed two-site binding. If the two sites observed for guinea pig whole brain (K_d values of 0.29 and 3.3 nM) represented affinity states, we would have expected to see them for the recombinant cells with the concentration range used. Since under the same assay conditions [^{3}H]SNF 8702 shows multiple site binding to some tissue preparations (whole brain and mid-brain thalamus) but not others (cerebral cortex, hippocampus, cerebellum) and since

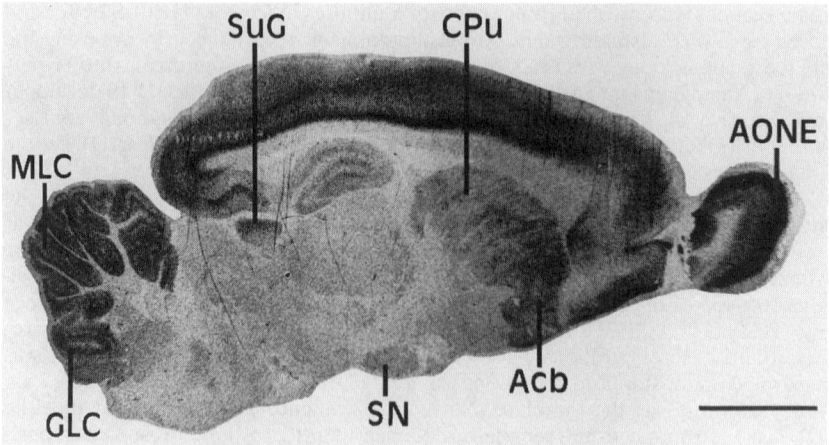

FIGURE 1. CCK-B receptors labeled [³H]SNF 8702 in guinea pig brain. This receptor autoradiograph was prepared from a 15-μm coronal section of guinea pig brain incubated with 2.0 nM [³H]SNF 8702 to label CCK-B receptors. The image represents total binding. Specific binding, determined by subtraction of nonspecific binding observed on an adjacent section incubated with [³H]SNF 8702 in the presence of CCK octapeptide, is not substantially different.

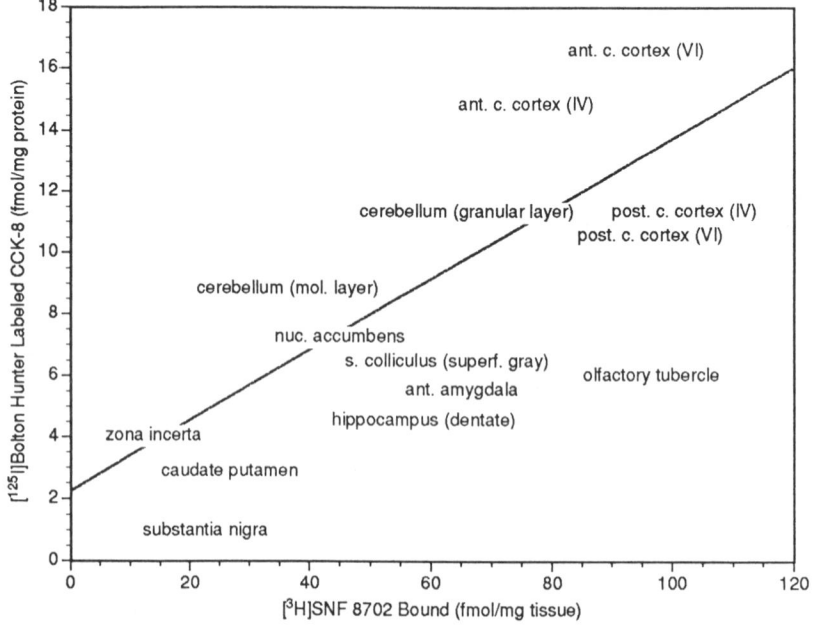

FIGURE 2. Correlation of CCK-B receptor distributions obtained with different radioligands. The figure shows a correlation of CCK-B receptor densities determined by receptor autoradiography using either [³H]SNF 8702 (present study) or [¹²⁵I]Bolton-Hunter–labeled CCK octapeptide.[4] The correlation coefficient is 0.693 for this comparison.

[^{3}H]SNF 8702 shows only single-site binding to a homogeneous population of CCK-B receptors (recombinant rat CCK-B receptor transfected COS-7 cells) without apparent selectivity for affinity states, we conclude that SNF 8702 is a selective ligand for CCK-B receptor subtypes.

REFERENCES

1. HRUBY, V. J., S. FANG, P. KNAPP, W. KAZMIERSKI, G. K. LUI & H. I. YAMAMURA. 1990. Cholecystokinin analogues with high affinity and selectivity for brain membrane receptors. Int. J. Peptide Protein Res. **35:** 566–573.
2. KNAPP, R. J., L. K. VAUGHN, S.-N. FANG, C. L. BOGERT, M. S. YAMAMURA, V. J. HRUBY & H. I. YAMAMURA. 1990. A new, highly selective CCK-B receptor radioligand ([^{3}H][N-methyl-Nle^{28,31}]CCK$_{26-31}$): Evidence for CCK-B receptor heterogeneity. J. Pharmacol. Exp. Ther. **255:** 1278–1286.
3. WANK, S. A., J. R. PISEGNA & A. D. WEERTH. 1992. Brain and gastrointestinal cholecystokinin receptor family: Structure and functional expression. Proc. Natl. Acad. Sci. USA **89:** 8691–8695.
4. NIEHOFF, D. L. 1989. Quantitative autoradiographic localization of cholecystokinin receptors in rat and guinea pig brain using ^{125}I-Bolton-Hunter-CCK8. Peptides **10:** 265–274.
5. HILL, D. R., T. M. SHAW & G. N. WOODRUFF. 1987. Species differences in the localization of "peripheral" type cholecystokinin receptors in rodent brain. Neurosci. Lett. **79:** 286–289.

Effects of Cholecystokinin Octapeptide on Potassium Currents in Cultured Sympathetic Neurons

HU XIAN AND DAVID L. KREULEN

Department of Pharmacology
College of Medicine
The University of Arizona
Tucson, Arizona 85724

Cholecystokinin octapeptide (26–33, CCK_8) is considered to be a neurotransmitter in mammalian prevertebral sympathetic ganglia and is one of the potential mediators of slow excitatory synaptic potential that is evoked with gastrointestinal distention.[1] In intact ganglia and cultured sympathetic neurons, CCK_8 sulfated (CCK_8-S) induces a slow membrane depolarization by acting on CCK_A receptors.[2,3] The present study investigates the ionic mechanisms of the slow membrane depolarizations by CCK_8-S in cultured sympathetic neurons.

The sympathetic neurons from celiac ganglia of guinea pig were enzymatically dissociated and maintained in culture for 3 days to 3 weeks in medium containing guinea pig serum and nerve growth factor (50 ng/ml). The membrane currents were recorded in cultured neurons using whole-cell voltage clamp technique. The pipette solution contained (mM): NaCl 10, KCl 45, K aspartate 100, M_gCl_2 2, EGTA 0.5, ATP 3, GTP 0.3, and HEPES 5 (pH 7.2). The perfusion solution contained (mM): NaCl 145, KCl 5.5, $MgCl_2$ 2, $CaCl_2$ 1.8, TTX 0.0002, and HEPES 10 (pH 7.45).

In 60% of neurons ($n = 160$), application of CCK_8-S (250 nM–1 µM) by the ejection-suction method (duration of exposure: 4 s) evoked a slow inward current at membrane holding potentials of -30 to -60 mV. The peak amplitudes of CCK-induced inward currents were voltage-dependent and varied from 30 to 300 pA. The duration of the inward transients was 2–3 minutes in 49% of cells. However, in 51% of cells, this inward current was sustained more than 3 minutes.

Seventy percent of neurons displayed a voltage-dependent potassium current, which activated at membrane potentials of -30 to -60 mV and showed characteristics of a muscarine-sensitive potassium current (M-current) described in other cell types.[4] The application of CCK_8-S reversibly attenuated the M-current. Thirty percent of celiac neurons did not exhibit the M-current, but rather they exhibited a voltage-independent potassium current. In these neurons, CCK_8-S attenuated this voltage-independent potassium conductance. The reversal potential for the CCK response was -70 to -80 mV, which is close to E_K (-87 mV).

In 18% of neurons tested, CCK_8-S increased a membrane current which was more pronounced at hyperpolarizing potentials (-80 to -110 mV). This response occurred 2–5 minutes after application of CCK_8-S. This current could be a nonselective cation current.

The M-current and the voltage-independent potassium current are involved in the regulation of neuronal membrane potential and firing properties. Inhibition of both of these potassium currents may produce a slow membrane depolarization, resulting in the facilitation of ganglionic transmission. Moreover, the different ionic currents underlying responses to CCK suggests a functional heterogeneity of neurons in sympathetic ganglia.

REFERENCES

1. SCHUMANN, M. A. & D. L. KREULEN. 1986. J. Pharmacol. Exp. Ther. **239:** 618–625.
2. MO, N. & N. J. DUN. 1986. Neurosci. Lett. **64:** 263–268.
3. KNOPER, S. R., A. G. MEEHAN, S. PURNYN, J. S. COGGAN, T. L. ANTHONY & D. L. KREULEN. 1993. Eur. J. Pharmacol. **232:** 65–69.
4. BROWN, D. A. & P. R. ADAMS. 1980. Nature **283:** 673–676.

Cholecystokinin Receptor Subtypes Regulate Dopamine D_2 Receptors in Rat Neostriatal Membranes

Involvement of D_1 Receptors

XI-MING LI, PETER B. HEDLUND, AND KJELL FUXE

Department of Histology and Neurobiology
Karolinska Institutet
Stockholm, Sweden

We previously showed that cholecystokinin octapeptide (CCK-8) *in vitro* increases the affinity of the dopamine (DA) for the D_2 antagonist [^{3}H]spiperone binding sites, but decreases the affinity of the D_2 agonist [^{3}H]NPA (L-(-)-N-propylnorapomorphine) binding sites in rat neostriatal membrane preparations. The current study presents new evidence on the intramembrane regulation by neostriatal CCK receptor subtypes and D_1 receptors on the D_2 receptors.

The homogenate from the Sprague-Dawley rat neostriata in 5 ml of ice-cold 50 mM Tris buffer (pH 7.4) containing 5 mM $MgCl_2$, 1 mM EDTA, and 0.01% L-(+)-ascorbic acid was centrifuged at 45,000 × g for 10 minutes at 4°C. The membranes were preincubated for 30 minutes at 37°C to remove endogenous ligands. Saturation curves with 10 concentrations (0.05–2 nM) of the D_2 agonist [^{3}H]NPA were obtained by incubating the membranes in the Tris buffer also containing 0.05% bovine serum albumen and 1 μM bacitracin for 30 minutes at 25°C using 1 μM of the D_2 antagonist raclopride for the determination of nonspecific binding. Competition experiments with 20 concentrations (1 pM–0.1 mM) of DA or L-(-)-NPA were performed by incubating the neostriatal membranes with 2 nM [^{3}H]raclopride for 30 minutes at 25°C. Kinetic analysis of [^{3}H]NPA binding was performed by incubating the membranes with 1.5 nM [^{3}H]NPA at 25°C for 30 minutes after a 10-minute preincubation with or without CCK-8 (1 nM). Then 10 μM L-(-)-NPA was used to determine the dissociation rate constant. All data were analyzed by iterative nonlinear regression fitting procedures.

TABLE 1 demonstrates that an increase in the K_D value ($p < 0.01$) but not in the B_{max} value of the [^{3}H]NPA binding sites was induced by 0.1 and 1 nM CCK-8. Concentration-response experiments (0.01–100 nM) showed peak action of CCK-8 at 0.1 nM with a 42% increase in the K_D value. Ten nM of the CCK_B antagonist PD134308 blocked this effect. Kinetic analysis demonstrated that the effect of CCK-8 was related to a reduction by 45% in the association rate constant of [^{3}H]NPA. One nM CCK-8 reduced the K_{obs} ($p < 0.01$) and K_1 ($p < 0.01$) values of the radioligand without affecting the K_{-1} value, leading to a 66% increase in the kinetic K_D value ($p < 0.05$).

In contrast, CCK-8 (0.1–100 nM) caused a concentration-dependent decrease in the K_H and K_L values of DA for the D_2 antagonist [^{3}H]raclopride binding sites. This effect was maximal at 1 nM CCK-8 with a similar effect on the K_H (56%, $p < 0.05$) and K_L (50%, $p < 0.01$) values (TABLE 2). Both the CCK_A antagonist L364718 (1 nM) and the CCK_B antagonist PD134308 (100 nM) blocked this effect. The addition of 200 nM SCH23390 (D_1 antagonist) not only fully counteracted the 1 nM CCK-8–

TABLE 1. Effects of CCK-8 on the Binding Characteristics of the Dopamine D_2 Agonist [^{3}H]NPA Binding Sites in Rat Neostriatal Membranes[a]

Treatment	Concentration (nM)	K_D (nM)	B_{max} (fmol/mg protein)
Control		0.327 (0.232–0.436)	406 ± 14
CCK-8	0.01	0.389 (0.360–0.421)	416 ± 15
CCK-8	0.1	0.465 (0.379–0.571)[b]	435 ± 9
CCK-8	1	0.418 (0.337–0.519)[b]	422 ± 18
CCK-8	10	0.386 (0.336–0.445)	426 ± 21
CCK-8	100	0.403 (0.273–0.594)	425 ± 17

[a] K_D values are presented as antilogarithms (geometric means and 95% confidence limits of the geometric mean) of the logarithmically transformed data, and B_{max} values are shown as means ± SEM from nine separate experiments.
[b] $p < 0.01$ vs control group according to the one-factor repeated measure ANOVA followed by the Fisher's protected least square difference (PLSD) test.

induced decreases in the K_H and K_L values of DA for the [^{3}H]raclopride binding sites, but also significantly increased the K_H value. One nM CCK-8 did not change the IC_{50} value of L-(-)-NPA for the [^{3}H]raclopride binding sites. However, in the presence of 200 nM SCH23390, a significant increase in the IC_{50} and a reduction in the B_0 values of L-(-)-NPA was obtained. One nM CCK-8 did not significantly alter the K_H, K_L, and R_H values of DA for the [^{3}H]SCH23390 binding sites. These results indicate that the CCK-8–induced reduction of the affinity of DA for the D_2 antagonist binding sites could not develop until D_1 receptor blockade had been produced. Thus, the activity at D_1 receptors will determine the type of response of D_2 receptors to CCK-8 and can switch it from one of reduced affinity (D_1 blockade) to one of increased affinity (D_1 activation).

In conclusion, the present findings indicate that CCK-8 can reduce or increase the affinity of D_2 receptors in rat neostriatal membrane preparations depending on the activity of the D_1 receptors, the CCK_B receptors being critical for both responses and the CCK_A receptors being critical only for the increase in affinity. Thus, D_1 receptors exert a switching role in the CCK receptor modulation of D_2 receptors.

TABLE 2. Effects of CCK-8 on the Binding Characteristics of the DA D_2 Antagonist [^{3}H]Raclopride Binding Sites in Rat Neostriatal Membranes[a]

Treatment	Concentration (nM)	K_H (nM)	K_L (nM)	R_H (% of total)
Control		3.62 (2.13–6.17)	157 (80–307)	55 ± 4
CCK-8	0.1	3.41 (1.43–8.13)	148 (91–242)	59 ± 6
CCK-8	0.3	1.68 (0.57–5.05)[b]	90 (45–180)[b]	45 ± 8
CCK-8	1	1.61 (0.68–3.85)[b]	78 (44–136)[c]	48 ± 6
CCK-8	3	2.31 (0.77–6.92)	134 (62–286)	56 ± 7
CCK-8	10	2.96 (1.24–7.10)	112 (79–116)	56 ± 7
CCK-8	100	2.87 (1.04–7.89)	105 (70–158)	45 ± 4

[a] K_H and K_L values are presented as antilogarithms (geometric means and 95% confidence limits of the geometric mean) of the logarithmically transformed data, and R_H values are shown as means ± SEM from eight separate experiments.
[b] $p < 0.05$.
[c] $p < 0.01$ vs control group according to the one-factor repeated measure ANOVA followed by the Fisher's protected least square difference (PLSD) test.

Intraduodenal Acid Augments Oleic Acid (C18)-Induced Cholecystokinin Release

R. J. BRODISH,[a,d] B. W. KUVSHINOFF,[a] A. S. FINK,[c]
J. TURKELSON,[d] D. W. McFADDEN,[b]
AND T. E. SOLOMON[d]

Departments of Surgery
[a]*University of Cincinnati and*
Cincinnati and [b]*Sepulveda VAMCs*
Cincinnati, Ohio 45267 and Los Angeles, California 90024
and
Emory University School of Medicine and Atlanta VAMC
Atlanta, Georgia 30033

[d]*Department of Medicine*
Kansas City VAMC
Kansas City, Missouri 64128

Acid-induced pancreatic bicarbonate output is potentiated by oleic acid (C18) and L-phenylalanine. This potentiated response has been attributed to interactions between endogenously released secretin and cholecystokinin (CCK).[1] Potentiation of acid-induced bicarbonate output by L-amino acids, but not by C18, appears to involve neural factors.[2] In this study, we assessed the influence of both acid and extrapancreatic neural elements on C18-induced CCK release in both the innervated and denervated pancreas.

MATERIALS AND METHODS

Pancreatic and CCK responses to intraduodenal perfusion were determined in mongrel dogs with chronic innervated ($n = 6$) or denervated ($n = 5$) pancreatic fistulas. The first set of perfusates consisted of bovine serum albumin (BSA) and C18 (5, 10, and 20 mM), with or without HCl. In acidified solutions, BSA and HCl were adjusted so that each 50 ml contained 2 mEq of acid titratable from initial pH 2.0 to endpoint pH 4.5. Acidified BSA alone (no C18) was perfused in additional studies. All perfusates were adjusted to 300 mOsm and perfused intraduodenally at 200 ml/h. Perfusates were randomly administered for 1 hour followed by a recovery (0.15 M NaCl) hour. Test hours were alternated with recovery hours until all three test doses had been administered. All experiments were replicated in each animal.

Blood samples were collected and separated, and plasma was frozen. Plasma CCK was determined by radioimmunoassay.[3] Pancreatic juice was collected at 15-minute intervals and analyzed for bicarbonate and protein.[4] Each animal's bicarbonate, protein, and CCK responses were averaged and compared using

[c]Address for correspondence: Aaron S. Fink, MD, Department of Surgery, Chief of Surgery, 1670 Clairmont, Decatur, GA 30033.

TABLE 1. Bicarbonate Response to Intraduodenal Oleate

	Mean Incremental HCO_3 Response (mEq/15 min)			
	Innervated		Denervated	
C18 (nM)	C18 (pH 7)	C18 + HCl (pH 2)	C18 (pH 7)	C18 + HCl (pH 2)
5	0.03 ± 0.01	0.71 ± 0.14[a]	0.05 ± 0.01	0.52 ± 0.14
10	0.10 ± 0.03	0.94 ± 0.09[a]	0.18 ± 0.03	0.62 ± 0.09
20	0.15 ± 0.03	1.17 ± 0.13[a]	0.11 ± 0.03	0.86 ± 0.13[a]

NOTE: Values given are the mean ± SEM.
[a] $p < 0.05$ vs C18 (pH 7) by ANOVA.
Bicarbonate response to acidified BSA alone = 0.56 ± 0.16 mEq/15 minutes in innervated and 0.56 ± 0.16 mEq/15 minutes in denervated (NS).

analysis of variance. Statistical significance was assigned at the $p < 0.05$ level. Predicted response was determined by adding the pH 2 BSA + pH 7 oleate responses.

RESULTS

In both groups of animals, oleate-induced pancreatic bicarbonate response was potentiated by acid (TABLE 1). No differences in protein output were noted in either group of animals. In both groups of animals, intraduodenal oleate released CCK in a dose-dependent fashion. Acidification potentiated oleate-induced CCK release in the innervated animals (TABLE 2).

CONCLUSIONS

We conclude that acid augments CCK release evoked by intraduodenal oleate. Inasmuch as CCK release in the denervated animals was not potentiated, this effect may involve extrinsic pancreatic innervation.

TABLE 2. CCK Response to Intraduodenal Oleate

	Mean Incremental CCK Response (pmole)			
	Innervated		Denervated	
C18 (nM)	C18 (pH 7)	C18 + HCl (pH 2)	C18 (pH 7)	C18 + HCl (pH 2)
5	0.25 ± 0.20	0.52 ± 0.10[a]	0.48 ± 0.07	0.68 ± 0.23
10	0.25 ± 0.08	0.93 ± 0.17[a]	0.52 ± 0.16	0.93 ± 0.18
20	0.62 ± 0.07	1.49 ± 0.25[a]	1.49 ± 0.33	1.67 ± 0.36

NOTE. Values given are the mean ± SEM.
[a] $p < 0.05$ vs C18 (pH 7) by ANOVA.
CCK response to acidified BSA alone 0.17 ± 0.09 pmol in innervated and −0.14 ± 0.1 pmol in denervated (NS).

REFERENCES

1. DOTY, J. E., A. S. FINK & J. H. MEYER. 1989. Alterations in digestive function caused by pancreatic disease. Surg. Clin. North Am. **69:** 447–465.
2. FINK, A. S., R. J. BRODISH, B. W. KUVSHINOFF, M. IRVING & A. R. DEMAR. 1993. Potentiation of canine pancreatic bicarbonate output by oleic acid is not neurally dependent. Pancreas, in press.
3. DALE, W. E., C. M. TURKELSON & J. SOLOMON. 1989. Role of cholecystokinin in intestinal phase and meal-induced pancreatic secretion. Am. J. Physiol. **257:** G782–G790.
4. MEYER, J. H. & G. A. KELLY. 1970. Canine pancreatic response to intestinally perfused proteins and protein digests. Am. J. Physiol. **231:** 682–691.

Potentiation of Acid-Induced Pancreatic Bicarbonate Output by Amino Acid Is Mediated by Neural Elements, but Not by Circulating Cholecystokinin

R. J. BRODISH,[a] B. W. KUVSHINOFF,[a] A. S. FINK,[a,c]
D. W. McFADDEN,[b] J. TURKELSON,[d]
AND T. E. SOLOMON[d]

[a]Departments of Surgery
University of Cincinnati and
Cincinnati and [b]Sepulveda VAMCs
Cincinnati, Ohio 45267 and Los Angeles, California 90024
and
Emory University School of Medicine and Atlanta VAMC
Atlanta, Georgia 30033

[d]Department of Medicine
Kansas City VAMC
Kansas City, Missouri 64128

Acid-induced pancreatic bicarbonate output is potentiated by oleic acid and L-phenylalanine (L-P). This potentiated response has been attributed to interactions between endogenously released secretin and cholecystokinin (CCK).[1] We previously showed that neural factors may also regulate potentiation of acid-induced bicarbonate by L-amino acids, but not oleic acid.[2] In this study, we assessed acid's influence on amino acid-induced CCK release in both the innervated and denervated pancreas.

MATERIALS AND METHODS

Pancreatic and CCK responses to intraduodenal perfusion were determined in mongrel dogs with chronic innervated ($n = 6$) or denervated ($n = 5$) pancreatic fistulas. In one set of perfusates, 16, 32, or 64 mM L-(L-P2) or D-phenylalanine (D-P) were acidified with HCl to pH 2. In additional studies, neutral (pH 7) L-phenylalanine (L-P7) was perfused in the same doses. All perfusates were adjusted to 300 mOsm with NaCl and perfused intraduodenally at 200 ml/hr. Perfusates were randomly administered for 1 hour followed by a recovery hour, during which normal saline solution was perfused. All experiments were replicated in each animal.
Blood samples were collected and separated, and plasma was then frozen. Plasma CCK was determined by radioimmunoassay.[3] Pancreatic juice was collected at 15-minute intervals and analyzed for bicarbonate and protein as previously described.[4] Each animal's bicarbonate, protein, and CCK responses were averaged and compared by analysis of variance. Statistical significance was assigned at the $p < 0.05$ level. Predicted response was determined by adding the results of D-P + L-P7.

[c]Address for correspondence: A. S. Fink, MD, Department of Surgery, Chief of Surgery (112), 1670 Clairmont, Decatur, GA 30033.

TABLE 1. Bicarbonate Response to Intraduodenal Phenylalanine

	Mean Incremental HCO$_3$ Response (mEq/15 min)			
	Innervated		Denervated	
L-P (mM)	Predicted	L-P2	Predicted	L-P2
16	0.83 ± 0.07	1.44 ± 0.22[a]	0.76 ± 0.17	1.09 ± 0.42
32	1.13 ± 0.15	1.86 ± 0.31[a]	0.92 ± 0.20	1.26 ± 0.35
64	1.28 ± 0.18	1.95 ± 0.23[a]	0.92 ± 0.19	1.50 ± 0.48

NOTE: Values given are the mean ± SEM.
[a] $p < 0.05$ vs values predicted by ANOVA.

TABLE 2. CCK Response to Intraduodenal Phenylalanine

	Mean Incremental CCK Response (pmol)			
	Innervated		Denervated	
L-P (mM)	Predicted	L-P2	Predicted	L-P2
16	0.45 ± 0.13	0.40 ± 0.09	0.70 ± 0.08	0.83 ± 0.69
32	0.83 ± 0.26	0.80 ± 0.12	1.07 ± 0.23	0.91 ± 0.30
64	1.01 ± 0.39	1.37 ± 0.36	1.11 ± 0.24	1.35 ± 0.70

NOTE: Values given are the mean ± SEM.

RESULTS

In both groups of animals, L-phenylalanine-induced pancreatic bicarbonate response was potentiated by acid (TABLE 1). No differences in protein output were noted in either group of animals. Intraduodenal L-phenylalanine released CCK in a dose-dependent fashion in both groups of animals (TABLE 2). L-phenylalanine–induced CCK release was not augmented by acid (TABLE 2).

CONCLUSIONS

Potentiation of acid-induced bicarbonate output by amino acid appears to be mediated via extrinsic neural elements, but not via circulating CCK.

REFERENCES

1. DOTY, J. E., A. S. FINK & J. H. MEYER. 1989. Alterations in digestive function caused by pancreatic disease. Surg. Clin. North Am. **69:** 447–465.
2. DEMAR, A. R., I. L. TAYLOR, R. R. LAKE & A. S. FINK. 1989. Enteropancreatic reflexes do not mediate potentiation of acid-induced pancreatic bicarbonate output by oleate. Gastroenterology **96:** A118.
3. DALE, W. E., C. M. TURKELSON & T. E. SOLOMON. 1989. Role of cholecystokinin in intestinal phase and meal-induced pancreatic secretion. Am. J. Physiol. **257:** G782–G790.
4. MEYER, J. H. & G. A. KELLY. 1976. Canine pancreatic response to intestinally perfused proteins and protein digests. Am. J. Physiol. **231:** 682–691.

Role of CCK in the Regulation of Dynamic and Tonic Mechanical Response of the Human Gastric Fundus to Lipids

M. A. MESQUITA,[a] D. G. THOMPSON,[a]
N. K. AHLUWALIA,[a] L. E. A. TRONCON,[a] M. D'AMATO,[b]
AND L. C. ROVATI[b]

[a]*University Department of Medicine*
Hope Hospital
Eccles Old Road
Salford M6 8HD, UK

[b]*Rotta Research Laboratorium*
Via Valosa di Sopra 7/9
20052 Monza (MI), Italy

It is well known that cholecystokinin (CCK) is released in response to fatty meals and is involved in the regulation of gastric emptying, CCK retarding,[1] and CCK_A antagonists accelerating meal efflux.[2] It has also been shown that intragastric administration of lipids modifies the mechanical response of the fundus to distention.[3] The present study assesses the role of endogenous CCK in regulating the fat-induced changes in gastric tone and accommodation in humans, using loxiglumide, a potent, selective, and specific CCK_A antagonist.[4-7]

METHODS

Either loxiglumide (5 mg/kg · h) or placebo were intravenously infused in 12 healthy volunteers (7 male, 5 female, mean age 29.6, range 20–43) according to a randomized, cross-over, double-blind design. Fundal pressure-volume relationships were measured before (pre-I) and after (post-I) instillation into the stomach of 250 ml of 10% intralipid by serial recording of pressure in an intrafundal bag connected to a pressure sensor during computer-controlled 50-ml stepwise air inflation (50–600 ml). Compliance, calculated as the slope of the log pressure:volume curves (ml/mm Hg · 10^{-5}), was taken as an index of dynamic properties. Mean pressure, obtained by averaging the recorded values at each inflation step (mm Hg), was taken as an index of the tonic properties of the gastric fundus. Results given are the mean ± SEM, and the differences (pre-I vs post-I) were evaluated by the Wilcoxon signed rank test (two-tailed).

[c]Address for correspondence: Massimo D'Amato, MD, Department of Clinical Pharmacology, Rotta Research Laboratorium, Via Valosa di Sopra 7/9, 20052 Monza (MI), Italy.

RESULTS

Lipid instillation induced a significant increase in fundal compliance which was not affected by loxiglumide (pre-I vs post-I; placebo: 87.6 ± 9.7 vs 47.2 ± 7.0, $p = 0.01$; loxiglumide: 73.5 ± 8.4 vs $52.8 \pm 9.1, p = 0.03$). Loxiglumide prevented the lipid-induced decrease of mean pressure (pre-I vs post-I; placebo: 11.7 ± 0.8 vs $9.7 \pm 0.6, p = 0.004$; loxiglumide 12.1 ± 0.7 vs $11.5 \pm 0.8, p = 0.15$).

DISCUSSION

Loxiglumide, a potent, selective, and specific CCK_A antagonist, prevented the proximal gastric relaxation induced by fat, indicating that CCK plays a major role in the fat-induced changes in gastric tone. Loxiglumide, however, did not affect the gastric relaxation induced by distention, suggesting that this response is not regulated by a CCK_A receptor-mediated mechanism. Moreover, loxiglumide did not prevent the increase in gastric compliance after fat, suggesting that other factors may be involved in the regulation of gastric accommodation. In conclusion, the dynamic and tonic properties of the fundus in response to lipids may be regulated by different mechanisms. Endogenous CCK seems to play a role in the modulation of gastric tone without a major effect on compliance. This increase in the tonic properties of the fundus may thus help explain the prokinetic effect of CCK_A antagonists in man.

REFERENCES

1. LIDDLE, R. A., E. T. MORITA, C. K. CONRAD & J. A. WILLIAMS. 1986. J. Clin. Invest. **77:** 992.
2. FRIED, M., U. ERLACHER, W. SCHWIZER, C. LÖCHNER, J. KOERFER, C. BEGLINGER, J. B. JANSEN, C. B. LAMERS, F. HARDER, A. BISCHOF-DELALOYE, G. A. STALDER & L. ROVATI. 1991. Gastroenterology **101:** 503–511.
3. TRONCON, L. E. A., D. G. THOMPSON, I. FAIRBAIN, N. K. AHLUWALIA, J. BARLOW & L. J. HEGGIE. 1992. Gastroenterology **104:** A528.
4. SETNIKAR, I., M. BANI, R. CEREDA, R. CHISTÈ, F. MAKOVEC, M. A. PACINI & L. REVEL. 1987. Arzneim.-Forsch. **37:** 703.
5. SETNIKAR, I., M. BANI, R. CEREDA, R. CHRISTÈ, F. MAKOVEC, M. A. PACINI & L. REVEL. 1987. Arneim.-Forsch. **37:** 1168.
6. SETNIKAR, I., R. CHRISTÈ, F. MAKOVEC, L. C. ROVATI & S. J. WARRINGTON. 1988. Arzneim.-Forsch. **38:** 716.
7. SETNIKAR, I., R. CHISTÈ, G. GIACOVELLI & L. C. ROVATI. 1989. Arzneim.-Forsch. **39:** 1454.

Selectivity and Potency of New Basic CCK-B Antagonists

L. C. ROVATI, M. D'AMATO, W. PERIS, L. REVEL, AND F. MAKOVEC[a]

Rotta Research Laboratorium S.p.A.
Via Valosa di Sopra 7/9
20052 Monza (MI), Italy

(R)-4-benzamido-5-oxopentanoic acid derivatives (BOPAD) such as CR 1795 and CR 2194 were recently shown to discriminate among the different CCK-receptor subtypes.[1] The present study investigates whether the selectivity and potency of these BOPAD depend on their acidic character.

MATERIAL AND METHODS

CR 1795 and both (R)- and (S)-CR 2194 were condensed with the appropriate amine to obtain the corresponding basic derivatives, CR 2378 and (R)- and (S)-CR 2345, respectively. Both acidic and basic compounds were evaluated for their capacity to inhibit the *in vitro* binding of 25 pM [^{125}I](BH)-CCK-8 to rat pancreatic acini (CCK$_A$)[2] and 25 pM [^{3}H](N-Me,Nlc)-CCK-8 to guinea pig cortex (CCK-$_{B2}$/gastrin)[2,3] and for their ability to inhibit the *in vivo* pentagastrin (30 μg/kg · h)-induced acid secretion in the rat stomach (CCK-$_{B1}$/gastrin).[4] Furthermore, the antisecretory activity *in vivo* in rats[5] and in dogs with a Heidenhain pouch[6] or gastric fistula[7] was evaluated on the most potent compound of the series, (R)-CR 2194 and (R)-CR 2345.

RESULTS

The results of *in vivo* and *in vitro* binding studies are shown in TABLE 1. The antisecretory effect of (R)-CR 2194 and (R)-CR 2345 was evaluated in the perfused rat stomach where the ID$_{50}$ (mg/kg, $p = 0.05$ fiducial limits) were 11.0 (8–15) and 9.0 (6–13), *versus* pentagastrin 30 μg/kg iv, >100 and 15.1 (10–22) *versus* histamine 3 μg/kg iv, and >100 and 22.9 (13–39) *versus* carbachol 30 μg/kg iv, respectively. The *in vivo* antisecretory activity in dogs is shown in TABLE 2.

DISCUSSION

The introduction of a basic moiety in (R)-4-benzamido-5-oxopentanoic acid derivatives did not modify the receptor subtype stereoselectivity, but it decreased the potency of CCK$_A$ antagonists and increased that of the CCK$_B$/gastrin antagonists.

---

[a] Address for correspondence: Francesco Makovec, Department of Pharmacology, Rotta Research Laboratorium S.p.A., Via Valosa di Sopra 7/9, 20052 Monza (MI), Italy.

TABLE 1. *In Vivo* and *In Vitro* Binding Activity of Acidic and Basic 4-Benzamido-5-Oxopentanoic Derivatives in Different Models

Compound	IC_{50} μM[a] (^{125}I) (BH)-CCK-8 Rat Pancreatic Acini	ID_{50} mg/kg[b] Pentagastrin IV (30 μg/kg × h)	IC_{50} μM[c] (^{3}H) Pentagastrin Guinea Pig Gastric Glands	IC_{50} μM[d] (^{125}I) CCK-8 Rat Cortex	IC_{50} μM[e] (^{3}H) (N-Me-Nle) CCK-8 Guinea Pig Cortex
	CCK-A	CCK-B1/Gastrin	CCK-B1/Gastrin	CCK-B2/Gastrin	CCK-B2/Gastrin
(R)-lorglumide	0.05 (0.03–0.1)	IN[f]	28.6 (16–52)	3.0 (2–5)	5.6 (4–8)
(R) CR-2194 (acidic)	13.5 (10–18)	11.0 (8–15)	0.4 (0.2–0.9)	0.6 (0.4–0.8)	1.4 (1–2)
(S) CR-2194 (acidic)	38.4 (25–58)	44.0 (33–59)	24.0 (12.8–45.1)	3.0 (1.9–4.7)	15.8 (7.5–33.2)
CR-1795 (acidic)	0.03 (0.02–0.05)	IN[f]	23.7 (10.1–55.6)	0.5 (0.2–1.5)	3.8 (1.8–7.1)
(R) CR 2345 (basic)	6.6 (4–11)	9.0 (6–13)	0.6 (0.2–2)	4.8 (4–6)	0.7 (0.5–1)
(S) CR 2345 (basic)	35.7 (15–86)	IN[f]	17.5 (11–29)	IN[g]	IN[g]
CR 2378 (basic)	1.5 (1–2)	IN[f]	NT[h]	1.0 (14–67)	16.0 (12–21)

[a]IC_{50}: μM displacing concentration and $p = 0.05$ fiducial limits required to inhibit by 50% the specific binding of 25 pM (^{125}I) (BH)-CCK-8 in rat pancreatic acini (CCK-A).
[b]ID_{50}: compound dose in mg/kg iv (bolus) and $p = 0.05$ fiducial limits required to inhibit by 50% the acid secretion induced by 30 μg/kg per hour of pentagastrin iv infusion.
[c]IC_{50}: μM displacing concentration and $p = 0.05$ fiducial limits required to inhibit by 50% the specific binding of 10 nM (^{3}H) pentagastrin in guinea pig gastric glands.
[d]250 pM [^{3}H](N-Me-Nle) CCK-8 in guinea pig cortex.
[e]25 pM (^{125}I) CCK-8 in rat cortex, respectively.
[f]IN = the antisecretive effect of 30 mg/kg is less than 20%.
[g]IN = ineffective 100 μM.
[h]NT = not tested.

TABLE 2. Effect of (R)-CR 2194 and (R)-CR 2345 on Gastric Acid Secretion in Dogs with Gastric Fistula after Intravenous Bolus Administration and with the Heidenhain Pouch after Oral Administration[a]

	Gastric Fistula		Heidenhain Pouch	
	0–60 min	0–120 min	0–60 min	0–120 min
(R)-CR 2194	5.9 (1–28)	12.5 (4–35)	28.8 (25–31)	34.7 (33–37)
(R)-CR 2345	7.6 (5–9)	10 (8–11)	23.8 (11–30)	23.4 (11–30)

[a] Results are expressed as ID_{50} (mg/kg; mean ± SEM; n = 4–6).

Furthermore, the selectivity of these compounds depends on the steric hindrance for both CCK_A and CCK_B/gastrin antagonists, while that on the acidic character of the molecule only for CCK_A antagonists.

(R)-CR 2345 is the most potent CCK_{-B1}/gastrin antagonist of the new class of basic (R)-4-benzamido-5-oxopentane derivatives. In the binding models of CCK_{-B1}/gastrin and CCK_{-B2}/gastrin antagonism (R)-CR 2345 seems to be equally active as the acidic parent compound (R)-CR 2194. Both the compounds are weak CCK_A antagonists. The antigastrin activity of (R)-CR 2345 is stereospecific, because its (S)-enantiomer is ineffective. In the *in vivo* models of CCK_B/gastrin antagonism, (R)-CR 2194 and (R)-CR 2345 show the same antigastrin potency pattern in all animal species tested, that is, rat and dog. Further studies are in progress to better characterize the antigastrin activity of (R)-CR-2345, which inhibits also both histamine- and carbachol-stimulated gastric acid secretion in the rat.

The nonpeptide structure and the activity after oral administration indicate that both these compounds could be studied for their clinical potential.

REFERENCES

1. MAKOVEC, F., W. PERIS, L. REVEL, R. GIOVANETTI, L. MENNUNI & L. C. ROVATI. 1992. J. Med. Chem. **35:** 28–38.
2. INNIS, R. B. & S. H. SNYDER. 1980. Proc. Natl. Acad. Sci. USA **77:** 6971–6921.
3. MAKOVEC, F., L. MENNUNI, W. PERIS, L. REVEL & L. C. ROVATI. 1993. Biorg. & Med. Chem. Lett. **3:** 861–866.
4. BERGLINDH, T. & K. J. OBRINK. 1976. Acta Physiol. Scand. **96:** 150–159.
5. GHOSH, N. M. & H. O. SCHILD. 1958. Br. J. Pharmacol. **13:** 54–61.
6. ANDERSSON, S. 1960. Acta Physiol. Scand. **50:** 105–112.
7. ANDERSSON, S. & S. OLBE. 1964. Acta Physiol. Scand. **60:** 51–56.

Differential Effects of CCK on Longitudinal and Circular Smooth Muscle of Chicken Ileum

Mechanisms Involved

E. FERNÁNDEZ, M. T. MARTÍN, A. G. FERNÁNDEZ, AND
E. GOÑALONS

Department of Cell Biology and Physiology
Veterinary Faculty
Universitat Autònoma de Barcelona
08193 Barcelona, Spain

This work attempts to determine the effects of cholecystokinin (CCK) on chicken ileum longitudinal and circular smooth muscle and to study the mechanisms involved in the responses.

MATERIAL AND METHODS

L364,718 and L365,260 were kindly donated by Merck Sharp and Dohme. All other chemicals and peptides were commercially obtained. White Leghorn chickens (δ 6–8 weeks old) were killed and bled. Ileal segments were dissected and longitudinal strips (LI) or rings (CI) kept in 11-ml organ bath at 41°C (buffer composition: NaCl 110 mM; KCl 3.4 mM; $CaCl_2$ 2.6 mM; $MgSO_4$ 0.88 mM; $NaHCO_3$ 25.0 mM; NaH_2PO_4 1.6 mM; glucose 15.0 mM; pH 7.4), bubbled with 95% O_2:5% CO_2 and tied to isometric transducers. Resting tension was 1 g for longitudinal strips and 2.5 g for rings.

RESULTS

Cholecystokinin-sulfated COOH-terminal octapeptide (CCK-8s) caused a dose-dependent contraction of the LI (EC_{50} 8.8×10^{-9} M). The maximum response to CCK-8s was about 30% of that to 10^{-6} M acetylcholine. Cholecystokinin-tetrapeptide (CCK-4) was nearly ineffective even at concentrations 200 times higher than the EC_{50} for CCK-8s. L365,260 slightly inhibited the CCK-8s response on the LI, whereas the decrease caused by L364,718 was not significant. TTX (10^{-6} M) decreased the response to CCK-8s by about 90%. Both ketanserin (10^{-5} M) and methiothepine (10^{-6} M) caused significant reductions in the CCK-8s–induced contraction, whereas atropine (10^{-6} M) did not have any effect. Substance P desensitization (SPd) was achieved by successive exposure of the strips to supramaximal concentrations of the peptide. In strips incubated with 10^{-5} M K, CCK-8s response was further reduced after SPd. FIGURE 1 summarizes these results.

CCK-8s induced dose-dependent relaxation (EC_{50} 4.9×10^{-9} M) of the CI. CCK-4 was nearly ineffective even at 2×10^{-6} M. L364,718 had only slight effects on

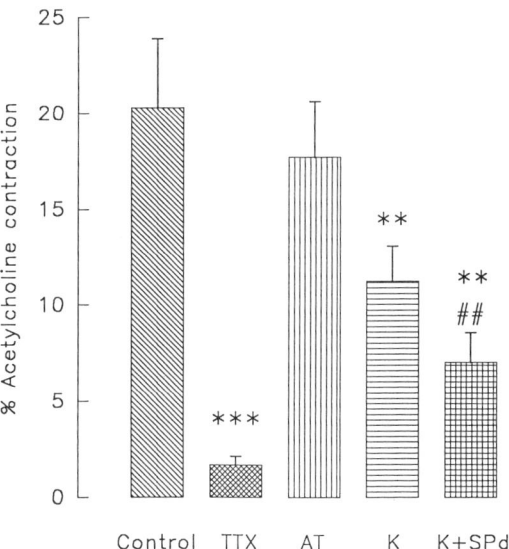

FIGURE 1. Effects of different treatments on the response of chicken longitudinal ileum to 10^{-8} M CCK-8s. Abbreviations and concentrations of the different substances are given in the text. ***$p < 0.001$ vs control; **$p < 0.01$ vs control; ##$p < 0.01$ vs ketanserin. AT = atropine; K = ketanserin; SPd = substance P desensitization.

the inhibitory responses to CCK-8s. L364,260 did not cause significant effects. The presence of TTX (10^{-6} M) completely blocks the CCK-8s–induced relaxation. CI incubated in the presence of L-NO-Arg exhibited a reduced response to CCK-8s. Incubation with L-Arg (10^{-4} M) restored the CCK-8s response. Ileal rings desensitized to ATP (ATPd) by successive exposures to supramaximal concentrations (10^{-4} M) exhibited a reduced response to CCK-8s. FIGURE 2 summarizes these data.

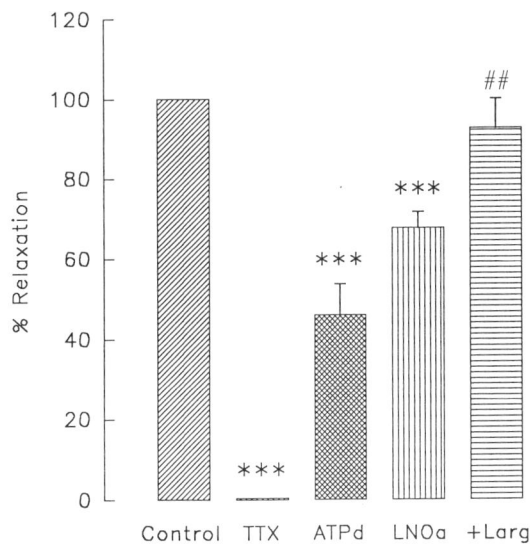

FIGURE 2. Effects of different treatments on the response of circular muscle of chicken ileum to 10^{-8} M CCK-8s. LNOa = response in the presence of L-NO-Arg; +Larg = response after incubation with L-arg. ***$p < 0.001$ vs control; ##$p < 0.01$ vs LNOa. ATPd = ATP desensitization.

DISCUSSION

The potency order of the CCK agonists tested in the LI indicate that the receptors present in this preparation are similar to the mammalian CCK-A receptors. In contrast, L364,718, a CCK-A receptor antagonist,[1] failed to decrease significantly the CCK effects, whereas L365,260, a CCK-B receptor antagonist,[1] caused a significant decrease. In any case, the concentration of L365,260 required to cause inhibition is higher than that which is effective in mammalian preparations.[2] Failure of L364,718 to inhibit CCK-stimulated pancreatic secretion in birds was previously reported.[3] These data suggest that CCK receptors present in chicken ileum differ from both CCK-A and CCK-B receptors described in mammals.

Cholecystokinin receptors present on LI are mainly neurally located, as TTX decreases the response by about 90%. The fact that atropine does not modify the response to CCK indicates that the interaction of CCK with receptors on enteric neurons does not result in acetylcholine release. It was previously shown that 5HT2- and 5HT1D-like receptors are present on chicken LI.[4] The fact that both ketanserin, a 5HT2 receptor antagonist,[5] and methiothepine, a 5HT1-5HT2 receptor antagonist,[5] decrease the CCK-8s response indicates that the interaction of this peptide with neural receptors results in release of serotonin (5HT). However, the blockade of 5HT-receptors does not completely block the contraction induced by CCK-8s, suggesting that additional mediators are involved. The fact that after the addition of ketanserin SPd may still cause a further reduction in the CCK-8s response indicates that both 5HT and substance P mediate the contraction induced by CCK-8s.

Concerning the circular muscle, CCK-8s induces marked relaxation, which is partly antagonized by L364,718. L365,260 did not cause significant effects. The fact that TTX completely blocks the relaxant response to CCK-8s demonstrates a neural location for its receptor. It was also shown that ATPd tissue and the presence of L-NO-Arg, an inhibitor of NO synthesis,[6] decrease CCK-8s–induced relaxation. This suggests that both mediators are involved in the response of circular muscle to CCK-8s.

REFERENCES

1. FREIDINGER, R. M. 1989. Med. Res. Rev. **9:** 271–290.
2. LUCAITES, V. L., L. G. MENDELSOHN, N. R. MASON & M. COHEN. 1991. J. Pharmacol. Exp. Ther. **256:** 695–703.
3. CAMPBELL, B., A. GARNER, R. DIMALINE & G. J. DOCKRAY. 1991. Am. J. Physiol. **261:** G16–G21.
4. MARTIN, M. T., A. G. FERNÁNDEZ, E. FERNÁNDEZ & E. GOÑALONS. 1992. Life Sci. **52:** 1361–1369.
5. HOYER, D. 1989. In The Peripheral Actions of 5-Hydroxytryptamine. J. R. Fozard, ed.: 72–99. Oxford University Press. Oxford, UK.
6. BRIEJER, M. R., L. M. A. AKKERMANS, A. L. MEULEMENS, R. A. LEFEBVRE & J. A. J. SCHUURKES. 1992. Br. J. Pharmacol. **107:** 756–761.

CCK-8 Contracts the Gallbladder and Colon through Different Mechanisms in the Ferret

S. MITAN AND BEVERLEY GREENWOOD[a]

Lilly Research Laboratories
Eli Lilly and Company
Indianapolis, Indiana 46285

Cholecystokinin (CCK) is found in abundance within the alimentary tract and has major effects on gastrointestinal smooth muscle motility such as gallbladder contraction, inhibition of gastric emptying, and stimulation of small intestinal and colonic motility. In the gallbladder the contractile response to CCK-8 is thought to occur via CCK-A receptors located on either smooth muscle cells or neurons.[1,2] Compelling evidence supports a neural mechanism of action by CCK in the colon[3–5]; however, the CCK receptor subtype(s) mediating the contractile response to CCK-8 is unknown. This study (1) measures *in vivo* and *in vitro* motility responses of the gallbladder and colon to CCK-8, (2) determines the CCK receptor subtype(s) mediating the responses, and (3) investigates the mechanisms by which CCK contracts the gallbladder and colon.

METHODS

Studies were conducted using fasted (18-hour) male ferrets (Triple F Supplier, Sayre, Pennsylvania) weighing 0.8–1.5 kg. Anesthesia was induced with urethane (1.5 g/kg, ip, Sigma Chemical Company, St. Louis, Missouri), a tracheal tube was inserted to provide a clear airway for breathing, and body temperature was maintained at 38°C using a homeothermic blanket (Harvard Apparatus, South Natick, Massachusetts). The left jugular vein was cannulated (PE-50, inner diameter 0.58 mm, outer diameter 0.97 mm) for the subsequent administration of drugs, and the left carotid artery was cannulated (PE-90, inner diameter 0.86 mm, outer diameter 1.27 mm) for continual measurement of blood pressure and heart rate. To record gallbladder motility, a saline-filled catheter (PE-50) attached to a pressure transducer was inserted into the gallbladder lumen through the common bile duct. Concurrently, colonic motility was monitored using a strain gauge transducer sewn onto the colonic musculature. Following a 30-minute stabilization period, sulfated CCK-8 was given at doses of 100, 300, and 700 ng/kg intravenously (iv), with a 10-minute stabilization period between CCK-8 doses. Antagonists were administered (iv) after another 30-minute stabilization period, and the CCK-8 dose-response curve was repeated beginning 5 minutes later.

RESULTS AND DISCUSSION

In vivo intravenous administration of CCK-8 (10–700 ng/kg iv) contracts the ferret gallbladder and colon in a dose-dependent manner with an ED_{50} of 458 ng/kg

[a] Address for correspondence: Dr. Beverley Greenwood, GI Research, Lilly Research Laboratories, Eli Lilly & Co., Lilly Corporate Center, 28/1, Indianapolis, IN 46285.

in the gallbladder and 160 ng/kg in the colon. These ED_{50} values suggest sensitivity differences in the gallbladder and colonic motor responses to CCK, possibly due to either variations in the CCK receptor reserve between the gallbladder or colon or a difference in the CCK receptor subtype mediating the contractile responses. As illustrated in FIGURE 1A, the CCK-A receptor antagonist L364,718, given at a dose of 1 mg/kg iv ($n = 3$), inhibited the gallbladder and colonic contractions induced by CCK-8 given at a dose of 300 ng/kg. In contrast, the CCK-B receptor antagonist (L365,260 at 1 mg/kg iv, $n = 6$) had no effect on CCK-8–induced gallbladder contractions, but it significantly ($p < 0.01$) reduced colonic contractions (FIG. 1B). Neither the muscarinic antagonist atropine (1 mg/kg iv) nor the nicotinic ganglionic blocker hexamethonium (20 mg/kg iv), given alone or in combination, had an effect on CCK-8–induced gallbladder contractions. This pattern of response in the gallbladder suggests that CCK-8 has a direct effect on gallbladder smooth muscle in the ferret. In the colon, atropine significantly inhibited the CCK-8–induced colonic motility response ($82 \pm 9.2\%, p < 0.001$), whereas the inhibitory effect of hexamethonium ($11 \pm 18\%, n = 7$) was not statistically different from control experiments. These data suggest that the increase in colonic motility induced by CCK-8 involves muscarinic but not nicotinic neurotransmission.

In isolated segments of ferret gallbladder and colon, CCK-8 stimulates smooth muscle contractility. CCK-8 stimulated smooth muscle activity in the gallbladder

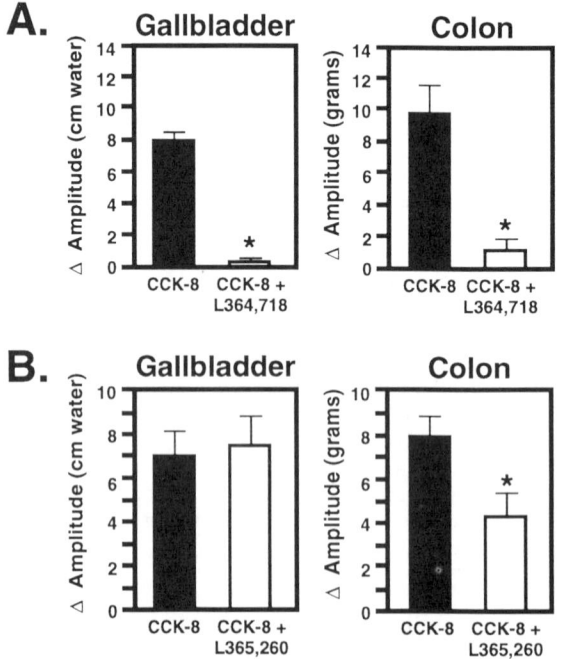

FIGURE 1. In the anesthetized ferret, intravenous administration of the CCK-A antagonist L364,718 at a dose of 1 mg/kg significantly inhibited the CCK-8–induced gallbladder ($p < 0.001$) and colonic contractions ($p < 0.05$). Furthermore, administration of the CCK-B antagonist L365,260 at a dose of 1 mg/kg had no effect on gallbladder motility induced by CCK-8, but it significantly inhibited the CCK-8–induced colonic motility ($p < 0.01$).

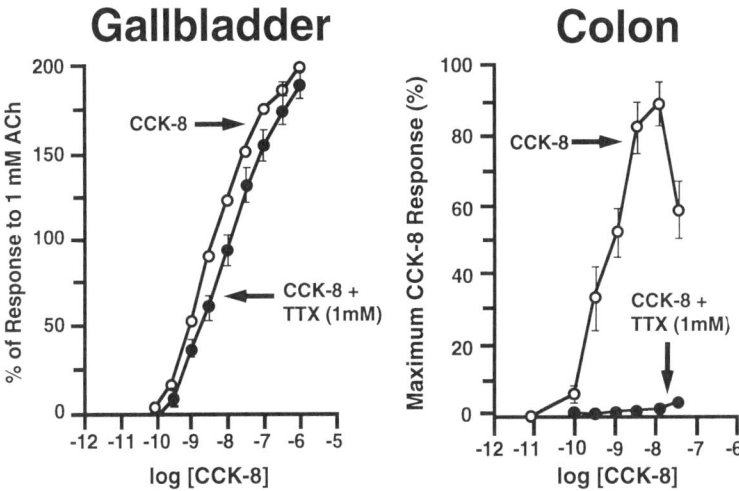

FIGURE 2. *In vitro,* CCK-8 stimulation of gallbladder contractility is not inhibited by the neurotoxin tetrodotoxin which suggests a direct effect of CCK-8 on gallbladder smooth muscle. In the colon, contractility is stimulated by neural mechanisms inasmuch as tetrodotoxin significantly inhibits the effect of CCK-8 ($p < 0.001$).

with an ED_{50} of 4.6×10^{-9} M and in the colon with an ED_{50} of 5.7×10^{-10}M. These data further substantiate the sensitivity difference between the gallbladder and colon. Furthermore, *in vitro* the neural component to the CCK-8–induced colonic motor response was confirmed inasmuch as administration of a neurotoxin, tetrodotoxin (10^{-6}M), abolished the colonic contractions induced by CCK-8 (10^{-10} to 10^{-7} M). In the same series of *in vitro* experiments, tetrodotoxin was without effect on the gallbladder contractions induced by CCK-8 (FIG. 2). In summary, our studies demonstrate that in the anesthetized ferret, CCK-8 stimulates gallbladder contractility via CCK-A receptors located on the smooth muscle. In the colon, CCK-8 stimulates motility through CCK receptors located on neurons; however, the relative importance of CCK-A and CCK-B receptors in mediating the CCK-8–induced colonic motility response remains to be determined.

REFERENCES

1. YAU, W. M., G. M. MAKHLOUF, L. E. EDWARDS & J. T. FARRAR. 1973. Mode of action of cholecystokinin and related peptides on gallbladder muscle. Gastroenterology **65:** 451–456.
2. MAWE, G. M. 1991. The role of cholecystokinin in ganglionic transmission in the guinea-pig gallbladder. Am. J. Physiol. **439:** 89–102.
3. HELLSTROM, P. M. 1985. Atropine and naloxone block the colonic contraction elicited by cholecystokinin and pentagastrin. Acta Physiol. Scand. **124:** 25–33.
4. WILEY, J. & C. OWYANG. 1987. Participation of serotonin and substance P in the action of cholecystokinin on colonic motility. Am. J. Physiol. **252:** G431–435.
5. BARONE, F. C., W. E. BONDINELL, T. J. LABOSH, R. F. WHITE & H. S. ORMSBEE, III. 1989. Cholecystokinin stimulates neuronal receptors to produce contraction of the canine colon. Life Sci. **44:** 533–542.

Stimulation by the Ancestral Member of the CCK/Gastrin Family, Cionin, of Trout Gallbladder Contraction

ANDERS H. JOHNSEN,[a] BIRGIT SCHJOLDAGER,[b] AND
JØRGEN JØRGENSEN[c]

*Departments of [a]Clinical Biochemistry and [b]Gynecology
Rigshospitalet and
[c]Department of Gynecology
Hvidovre Hospital
University of Copenhagen
Copenhagen, Denmark*

Cholecystokinin (CCK) and gastrin constitute a peptide family sharing the amidated COOH-terminal tetrapeptide -Trp-Met-Asp-Phe · NH_2 which is crucial for biological activity of both. In mammals, gallbladder contraction is induced by sulfated CCK (CCK-s), whereas gastrin has a much lower potency. As indicated by specific radioimmunoassays, CCK-like peptides are also present in lower vertebrates, but their exact structures and functions remain to be elucidated. Recently, the ancestral cionin was identified in the protochordate *Ciona intestinalis*.[1] With two sulfated Tyr's, cionin is structurally a hybrid of CCK and gastrin (FIG. 1). The coho salmon gallbladder smooth muscle receptors do not distinguish between CCK and gastrin, but require the peptide to be sulfated.[2] These findings suggest that the endogenous peptide resembles cionin. The present work (1) investigates the effect of cionin on smooth muscle contraction of the rainbow trout (*Oncorhyncus mykiss*) gallbladder and (2) evaluates the potencies of the highly specific (in mammalian systems) receptor antagonists L-364,718 (specific for CCK_A-receptors) and L-365,260 (specific for CCK_B- or gastrin type-receptors).

Experiments were performed essentially as described by Vigna and Gorbman.[2] Our results confirm and extend this previous report. Cionin, CCK-8-s, and gastrin-17-s induced concentration-dependent contractions of muscle strips with equal efficacy and similar potency, ED_{50} being 42 nM, 23 nM, and 74 nM, respectively (FIG. 2). These were significantly different from the potencies of the nonsulfated forms,

Cionin   Asn-Tyr-Tyr-Gly-Trp-Met-Asp-Phe·NH_2
                    SO_3 SO_3

CCK   Asp-Tyr-Met-Gly-Trp-Met-Asp-Phe·NH_2
                    SO_3

Gastrin   -Glu-Ala-Tyr-Gly-Trp-Met-Asp-Phe·NH_2
                    (SO_3)

FIGURE 1. Structure of cionin compared to mammalian CCK-8-s and COOH-terminal part of gastrin.

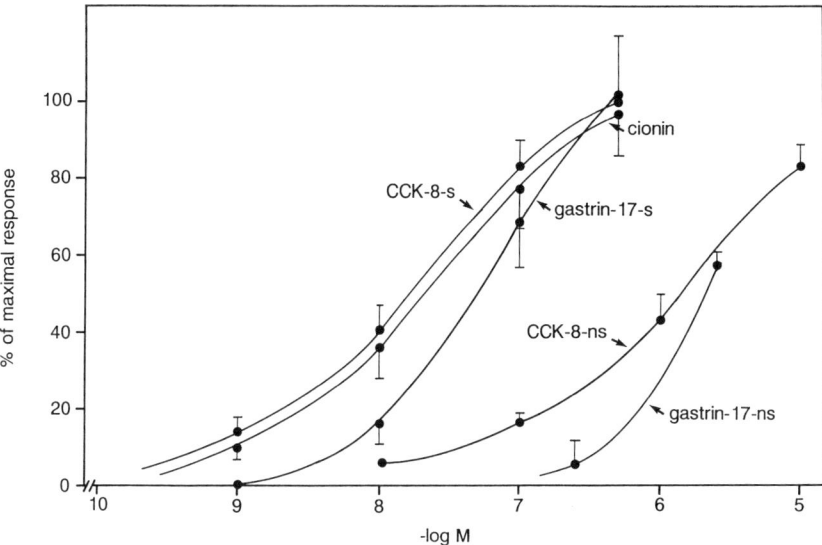

FIGURE 2. Stimulation of gallbladder smooth muscle contraction by cionin and related peptides. For each experiment the preparation was stimulated with increasing concentrations of peptides. Responses are expressed as % of maximal contraction (obtained with $5 \cdot 10^{-7}$ M CCK-s). Values represent means ± SEM of n experiments. $n = 6$ (cionin, CCK-8-s, and gastrin-17-s), 4 (CCK-8-ns), and 3 (gastrin-17-ns).

ED_{50} being 1.7 μM (CCK-8) and 2.0 μM (gastrin-17). The antagonists (from a 10 mM stock solution in DMSO) had no effect when added alone. Ten μM of L-364,718 and L-365,260 both weakly but significantly inhibited CCK-8-s, cionin, and gastrin-17-s induced contractions in a competitive way (data not shown). L-365,260 shifted the dose response curves 1½ log to the right. Surprisingly, L-364,718 was even weaker, shifting the curves ½ log.

The selectivity of the trout gallbladder receptor for sulfated peptides but nonselectivity between CCK and gastrin is not due to the demand of a double sulfated agonist resembling cionin. The results obtained with the antagonists indicated some resemblance with CCK_B receptors. This is in contrast to the dependency on sulfation resembling CCK_A receptors. However, the antagonists have been characterized in mammalian systems, and even between mammals marked differences are seen. Thus, dog CCK_B receptor binds both L-364,718 and L-365,260 radically different than does the human receptor. This discrepancy was due to a single amino acid substitution.[3] Hence, conclusions should be drawn cautiously. Apparently the trout receptor is distinct from the mammalian receptors at least in the region(s) important for binding of agonists and antagonists.

REFERENCES

1. JOHNSEN, A. H. & J. F. REHFELD. 1990. Cionin: A disulfotyrosyl hybrid of cholecystokinin and gastrin from the neural ganglion of the protochordate *Ciona intestinalis.* J. Biol. Chem. **265:** 3054–3058.

2. VIGNA, S. R. & A. GORBMAN. 1977. Effects of cholecystokinin, gastrin, and related peptides on coho salmon gallbladder contraction *in vitro*. Am. J. Physiol. **232:** E485–E491.
3. BEINBORN, M., Y.-M. LEE, E. W. MCBRIDE, S. M. QUINN & A. S. KOPIN. 1993. A single amino acid of the cholecystokinin-B/gastrin receptor determines specificity for non-peptide antagonists. Nature **362:** 348–350.

Inhibitory Action of CCK-OP on Rat Proximal Colon

S. KISHIMOTO,[a] H. MACHINO, H. KOBAYASHI,
K. HARUMA, G. KAJIYAMA, A. MIYOSHI, AND K. FUJII

*Department of Medicine
Hiroshima University and
Physiology Section
Hiroshima College of Women
Hiroshima 734, Japan*

Using a miniature strain gauge force transducer implanted in the serosal site of rat proximal colon, we showed that bolus intraperitoneal injection of cholecystokinin octapeptide (CCK-OP) caused partial inhibition of phasic contractile activity of circular muscle which appeared in the fasting state in conscious rats.[1] This study attempts to ascertain the inhibitory action of CCK-OP and to assess the inhibitory mechanism of this peptide.

MATERIALS AND METHODS

Experiments were performed 3 days after surgery, and recordings were continued for 10 days. Myoelectric activity was recorded with an amplifire system through a bridge box set at a time constant of 0.1 s. Each animal was fasted overnight before the experiment. For this study, we used CCK-OP (Protein Research, Japan) 1.55×10^{-2} μmol/kg, which caused maximal inhibition of fasting phasic contractions of the proximal colon. A specific CCK-A receptor antagonist, loxiglumide (CR1505, Rotta Chemicals, Italy) 1 mg/kg, was injected intraperitoneally in rats before CCK-OP administration. Atropine sulfate (Daiichi Chemical, Japan) 1.0 mg/kg and hexamethonium (C_6, Sigma Chemical, USA) 200 mg/kg were also injected in rats before CCK-OP administration, respectively. Acetylcholine of 0.5 mg/kg was also used for the C_6 study.

RESULTS

Cholecystokinin octapeptide partially inhibited phasic and rhythmical contractions of the circular muscle of the proximal colon in the fasting state of conscious rats (FIG. 1A). Atropine sulfate blocked the contractions that remained after CCK-OP administration (FIG. 1B). Loxiglumide partially blocked the inhibitory action of CCK-OP on fasting contractions (FIG. 2A), whereas C_6 did not cause any changes in the inhibition of CCK-OP on both fasting and acetylcholine-stimulated contractions (FIG. 2B).

[a]Address for correspondence: Dr. Shinya Kishimoto, Department of Internal Medicine, Hiroshima University School of Medicine, 1-2-3 Kasumi, Minami-ku, Hiroshima 734, Japan.

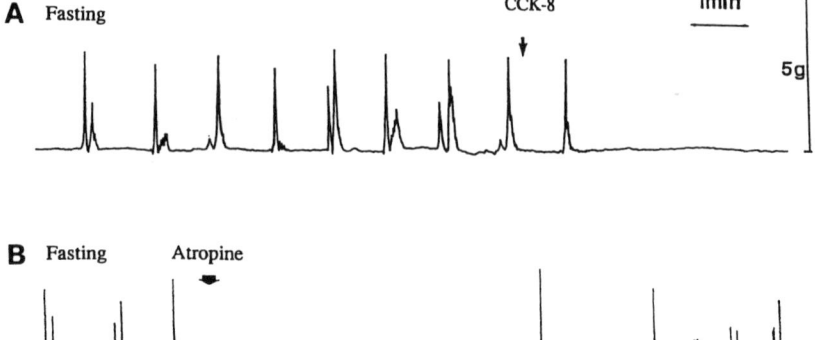

FIGURE 1. (**A**) CCK-OP partly relaxed the phasic contractions of the proximal colon during the fasting state in the unanesthetized rat. (**B**) Atropine sulfate also partly blocked these phasic contractions. Furthermore, atropine also blocked the contractions that remained after CCK-OP, which are not shown in the figure.

DISCUSSION

These data confirm that CCK-OP relaxed the circular muscle of the proximal colon of conscious rats.[1,2] Our results also showed that the inhibitory action of the peptide was mediated, at least in part, by CCK-A receptors on smooth muscle cells directly in one pathway and by stimulation of intramural postganglionic inhibitory neurons in the other. We conclude that the inhibitory action of CCK-OP is at least under the control of two different mechanisms.

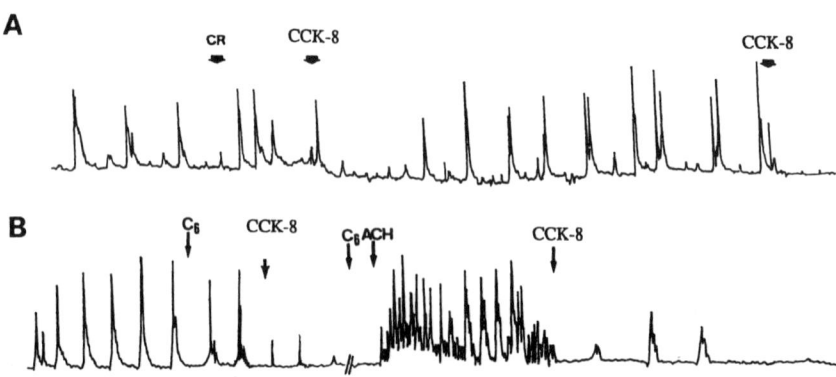

FIGURE 2. (**A**) A specific CCK-A receptor antagonist, loxiglumide (CR1505), blocked the inhibitory action of CCK-OP on phasic contractions of the proximal colon in the fasting rat. (**B**) The inhibitory action of CCK-OP on circular muscle of the proximal colon at the fasting and stimulated state was not blocked by hexamethonium (C_6) when it was administered to rats before CCK-OP.

REFERENCES

1. KISHIMOTO, S., H. KOBAYASHI, A. MIYOSHI & K. FUJII. 1989. Effect of CCK-OP on circular muscle motility of the rat proximal colon. J. Smooth Muscle Res. **25:** 226–228.
2. KISHIMOTO, S., H. KOBAYASHI, A. MIYOSHI & K. FUJII. 1992. Further study of inhibitory effect of CCK-8 in the conscious rat proximal colon. J. Gastrointest. Motil. **4:** 227 (Abstr.).

Gastrin-Releasing Peptide and CCK after Intraduodenal Inhibition of Proteases

H. KÖHLER, R. NUSTEDE, R. STREICH, AND F.-E. LÜDTKE

Department of General Surgery
University of Göttingen
Robert-Koch-Str. 40
37075 Göttingen, Germany

The intraduodenal inhibition of proteases may induce pancreatic secretion and growth. The mediators of the so-called "negative feedback mechanism" are still unknown. We investigated the role of gastrin-releasing peptide (GRP) and CCK after intraduodenal application of the protease inhibitor camostate.

MATERIAL AND METHODS

Six dogs were fitted with a modified Herrera pancreatic fistula. After a recovery period the following studies were performed:

1. GRP was infused intravenously at the rate of 30 pmol $\times$ kg^{-1} $\times$ h^{-1} for 120 minutes. This dose avoids unphysiological plasma concentrations of the peptide. Blood samples for GRP and CCK determinations were drawn at 15-minute intervals. Protein content was determined in simultaneously collected samples of pancreatic secretions.
2. Thirty minutes after the start of the infusion an anti-GRP immunoglobulin (200 µg) solution was given intravenously as a bolus.
3. The same procedure as in 2 was performed but with nonspecific rabbit immunoglobulin.
4. Camostate (600 mg in 10 ml of water) was instilled into the duodenum 30 minutes after specimens were collected for determining basal conditions. Blood samples were drawn, plasma concentrations of GRP and CCK were determined, and the simultaneously collected pancreatic secretions were analyzed.
5. The method described in 4 was repeated with the additional intravenous application of anti-GRP after 30 minutes.

ASSAYS

Protein concentrations were determined by the method of Lowry. CCK and GRP plasma concentrations were determined by radioimmunoassay.

RESULTS

1. The intravenous application of GRP at the rate of 30 pmol $\times$ kg^{-1} $\times$ h^{-1} GRP avoids unphysiological, detectable concentrations of the peptide in peripheral blood.

Although we were unable to detect an increase in circulating CCK concentrations after application of this GRP dose, marked stimulation of pancreatic protein secretion was observed.

2. Secretion was directly affected by the application of specific immunoglobulin solution; an increase in secretion was not observed. Plasma concentrations of GRP and CCK remained in a basal range (FIG. 1).

3. Application of the nonspecific immunoglobulin solution had no effect on pancreatic secretion.

4. Intraduodenal application of the protease inhibitor caused a significant, biphasic secretory increase in pancreatic secretion.

5. The second secretory peak which occurred after administration of the protease inhibitor was not observed after the immunoglobulin infusion (FIG. 2).

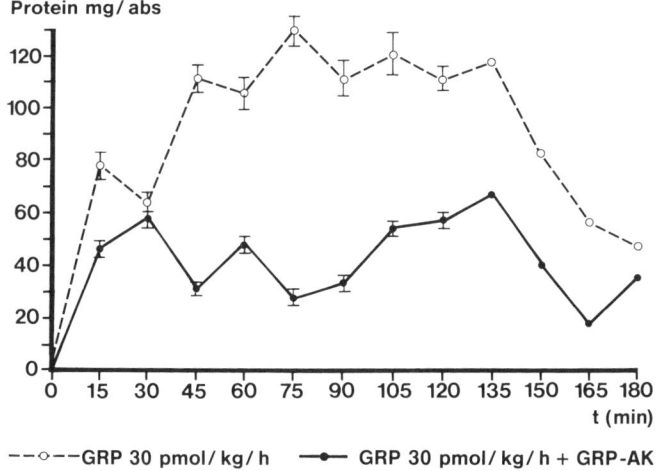

FIGURE 1. Stimulation of pancreatic protein secretion after intravenous application of GRP (30 pmol/kg/h) alone and after application of GRP + GRP-antibody.

DISCUSSION

These data confirm that stimulation of basal pancreatic secretion in the dog occurs after intraduodenal administration of a potent protease inhibitor.[1] They contradict previous data in dogs[2] which were primarily based on draining pancreatic secretions. On the other hand, they confirm the more recent results of Shiratori et al.[3] To our knowledge this study represents the first time that intraduodenal protease activity was modified *in situ* by the administration of camostate.

No evidence was found to support the supposition that circulating CCK concentrations were involved. This means that the mediator of the increase in pancreatic secretion observed after administration of camostate still remains unknown. An analogous situation exists in humans. In 1989 Adler et al.[4] published a study describing a similar secretory profile after camostate. The second peak in secretion observed 45–75 minutes after camostate was markedly diminished by the administration of the CCK-receptor antagonist loxiglumide (CR 1505), while peripheral CCK concentrations remained unchanged.

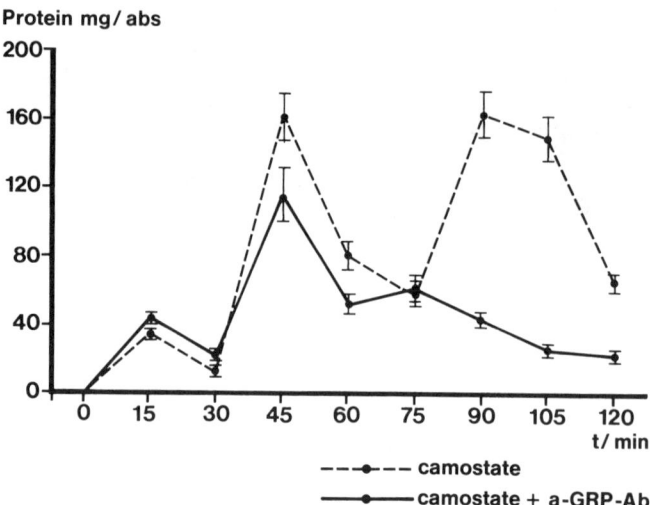

FIGURE 2. Protein output of the exocrine pancreas after intraduodenal application of camostate and after camostate and intravenous application of GRP antibody solution.

Stimulation of peripheral CCK concentrations, which occurs after intravenous application of large doses of GRP, was not observed. The possible role of GRP in regulating the secretion of the exocrine pancreas and the observed negative feedback, which is suggested by our data, may therefore be neurally mediated.[5]

REFERENCES

1. NUSTEDE, R., H. KÖHLER, B. FISCHER, R. STREICH, O. SCHUNK & A. SCHAFMAYER. 1988. Neurotensin and the negative feedback regulation of pancreatic lipase secretion. Pancreas **5:** 612 (Abstr.).
2. KOGIRE, M., K. INOUE, R. HOSOTANI, Y. S. HUANG, J. C. THOMPSON & T. TOBE. 1989. Pancreatic secretion and the release of cholecystokinin after a meal in dogs with and without exclusion of pancreatic juice. Scand. J. Gastroenterol. **24:** 507–512.
3. SHIRATORI, K., Y. JO, K. Y. LEE, T. M. CHANG & W. Y. CHEY. 1988. A hormonal role on negative feedback mechanism in intestinal phase of exocrine pancreatic secretion in dogs. Biomed Res. **1**(Suppl.): 116.
4. ADLER, G., M. REINSHAGEN, I. KOOP, B. GÖKE, A. SCHAFMAYER, L. C. ROVATI & R. ARNOLD. 1989. Differential effects of atropine and a cholecystokinin receptor antagonist on pancreatic secretion. Gastroenterology **96:** 1158–1164.
5. HOLST, J. J., S. KNUHTSEN & O. V. NIELSEN. 1989. Role of gastrin-releasing peptide in neural control of pancreatic exocrine secretion. Pancreas **5:** 581–586.

Role of CCK in the Physiological Control of Gastroduodenal and Intestinal Motility in Chickens

V. MARTINEZ, M. JIMENEZ, E. FERNANDEZ,
E. GOÑALONS, AND P. VERGARA

Department of Cell Biology and Physiology
Veterinary Faculty
Universitat Autònoma de Barcelona
08193-Bellaterra, Barcelona, Spain

In birds, gastroduodenal (GD) coordination is a clear event; each gastric contraction is followed by one or more duodenal spikes.[1] Duodenal refluxes are also part of GD motility. The only study in birds using cholecystokinin (CCK) demonstrates that this peptide could induce GD refluxes.[2] In avian species, small intestinal motility is organized in migrating myoelectric complexes (MMC), which are present in both fed and fasting states.[3] In species that eat large and infrequent meals (i.e., humans or dogs), the MMC pattern is disrupted by postprandially released hormones.[4,5] The MMC in these species has been described as an "all-or-nothing" phenomenon.[6] The finding that in some species, such as chickens, the MMC is not disrupted postprandially suggests a modulatory role for postprandial hormonal output.

The objectives of this work were: (1) to characterize the gastrointestinal motor response to exogenous CCK in chickens, and (2) to correlate these motor actions with those effects observed during CCK endogenous release. The comparative approach of this study permits an understanding of the regulatory mechanisms involved in the control of gastrointestinal motility.

MATERIAL AND METHODS

Electromyographic recordings were undertaken in chickens chronically implanted with either five (stomach [3] and duodenum [2]) or eight (jejunum [1] and ileum [2]) triplets of electrodes. Catheters were also chronically placed in the distal esophagus and the proximal ileum for intraluminal lipid infusion. Total electrical activity was integrated (time intervals of 1 minute),[7] and changes in GD activity and MMC were determined.

RESULTS

Effects of Exogenous CCK in GD Motility. CCK8 ($10^{-10} - 10^{-8}$ mol/kg, $n = 7$ for each dose) were infused for 10 minutes. CCK8 ($3 \times 10^{-10} - 10^{-8}$ mol/kg/min × 10 min) disrupted GD coordination, producing dose-dependent gastric inhibition concurrent with nonmigratory duodenal hyperactivity (FIG. 1). The smaller dose of CCK8 (10^{-10} mol/kg/min × 10 minutes) did not significantly modify total GD electrical activity; however, analysis of the GD cycle showed a significant increase in

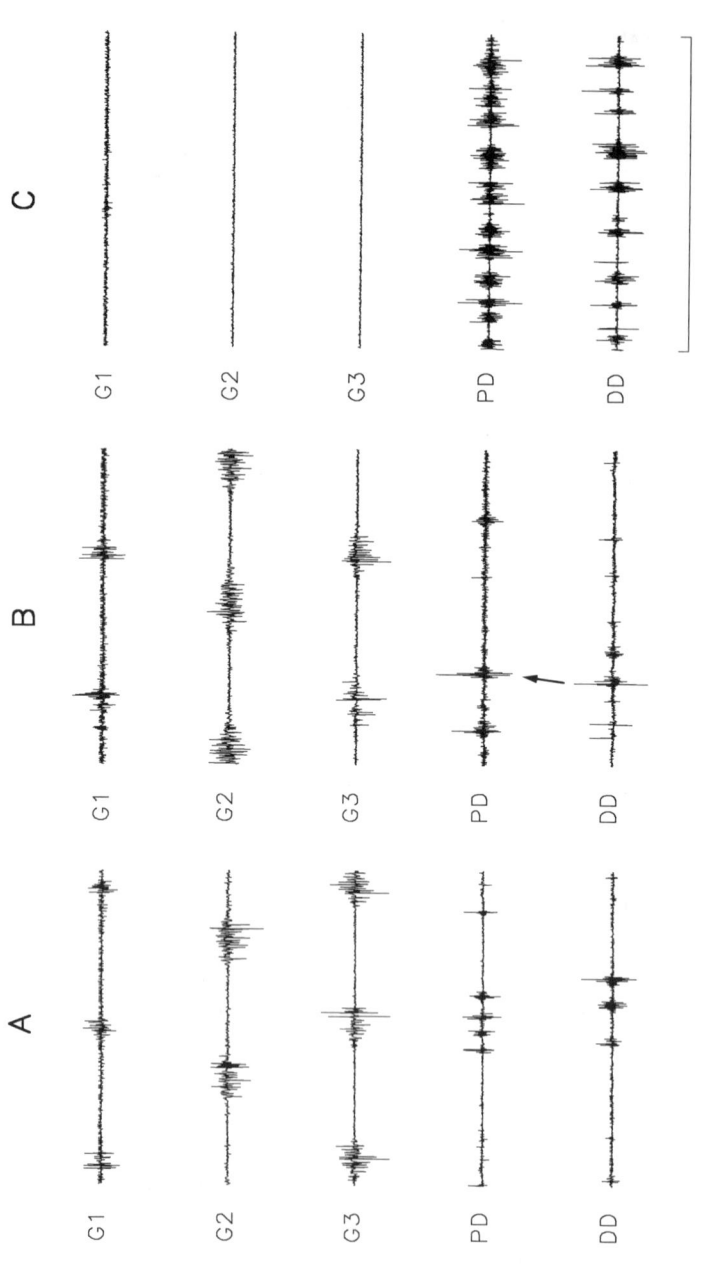

FIGURE 1. Gastroduodenal electrical activity in three different experimental conditions: (**A**) control; (**B**) during infusion of CCK8 10^{-10} mol/kg/min (*arrow* points to duodenal antiperistaltic activity); and (**C**) during infusion of CCK8 10^{-8} mol/kg/min. G1, G2, and G3 = gastric electrodes; PD and DD = proximal and distal duodenum, respectively.

the number of duodenal antiperistaltic spike bursts (0.57 ± 0.32 antiperistaltic spike bursts/10 minutes during the control period vs 2.86 ± 0.79 during the CCK8 infusion, $p < 0.05$, mean ± SEM) (FIG. 1).

Effects of Exogenous CCK on Small Intestinal Motility. CCK8 infusion during the fed state caused dose-dependent effects. Doses of 10^{-11} and 3×10^{-11} mol/kg/min × 2 h ($n = 5$ for each one) induced a dose-related elongation of the MMC and slowed the speed of propagation of phase 3. CCK8 at a dose of 10^{-10} mol/kg/min × 2 h ($n = 5$) disrupted the MMC. When CCK8 (10^{-12} mol/kg/min × 3 h, $n = 6$) was infused in fasting animals, changes in MMC characteristics resembled those observed in fed animals: shortness of the MMC, reduction of the propagation speed of the phase 3, and displacement of the site of origin from the stomach to the duodenum or jejunum (FIG. 2).

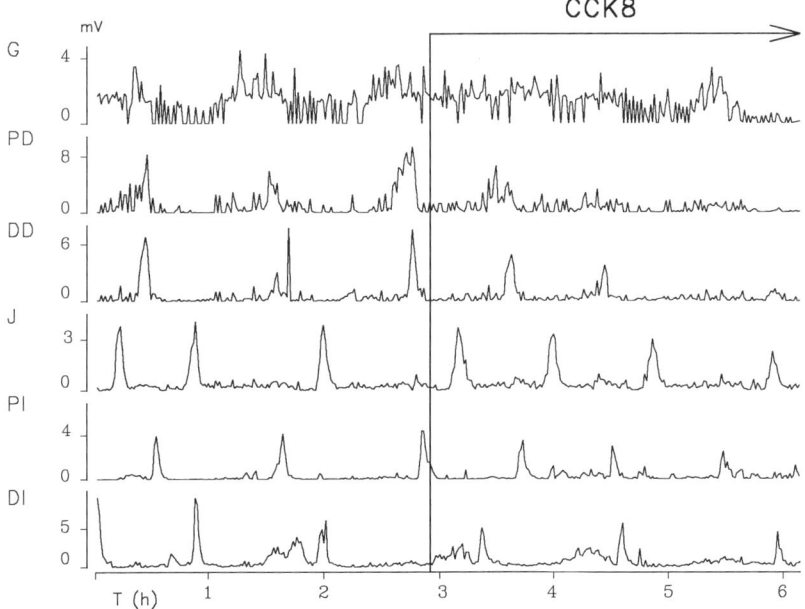

FIGURE 2. Integrated recording of the gastrointestinal electrical activity of a chicken in fasting state. Figure shows the effect of CCK (10^{-12} mol/kg/min) infusion. G = stomach; PD and DD = proximal and distal duodenum, respectively; J = jejunum; PI and DI = proximal and distal ileum, respectively.

Effects of Endogenous CCK Release in Gastrointestinal Motility. To induce endogenous CCK release, either oleic acid or triolein (6.3×10^{-3} mol/30 min) was infused through the esophagus ($n = 8$) or the ileum ($n = 8$). Both esophageal and ileal infusion of oleic acid induced a significant decrease in gastric electrical activity. Analysis of duodenal motility showed a significant increase in antiperistaltic spike bursts (0.87 ± 0.55 antiperistaltic spike bursts/10 minutes during the control period vs 4.25 ± 0.89 10 minutes after starting the ileal infusion of oleic acid; $p < 0.001$; mean ± SEM). Triolein induced similar changes when infused into the esophagus but not when infused into the ileum. Either esophageal or ileal infusion of oleic acid

(6.3×10^{-3} mol/2 h) produced an elongation of the MMC and a reduction in the speed of propagation of phase 3. Disruption of the MMC was not observed in any case.

DISCUSSION

Results show that CCK participates in the physiological regulation of gastrointestinal motility in chickens, as described in mammals. CCK actions in the gastroduodenal area probably induce a delay in gastric emptying by increasing duodenal antiperistaltic activity and inhibiting gastric contractions. Neither endogenous CCK nor low doses of exogenously infused CCK disrupt the MMC pattern. In fasting animals, CCK infusion induces similar changes in this pattern to those observed in fed animals. However, doses of CCK higher than 10^{-10} mol/kg/min totally disrupt the MMC. These results show that in avian species: (1) the MMC should not be described as an "all-or-nothing" phenomenon, as in mammals, and (2) endogenous CCK modulates the MMC characteristics but does not disrupt them. Altogether, these results suggest that the mechanisms involved in the control of gastrointestinal motility are similar throughout the phylogenetical evolution. A search should be made for differences in different sensitivities of these mechanisms in relation to the ingestive behavior of the different species.

REFERENCES

1. ROCHE, M. & Y. RUCKEBUSCH. 1978. Am. J. Physiol. **4:** E670–E677.
2. SAVORY, C. J., G. E. DUKE & R. W. BERTOY. 1981. Comp. Biochem. Physiol. **70A:** 179–189.
3. CLENCH, M. H., V. M. PIÑEIRO-CARRERO & J. R. MATHIAS. 1989. Am. J. Physiol. **256:** G598–G603.
4. THOR, P., J. LASKIEWICK, P. KONTUREK & S. J. KONTUREK. 1988. Am. J. Physiol. **255:** G489–G504.
5. MUKHOPADHYAY, A. K., P. THOR, E. M. COPELAND, L. R. JOHNSON & N. W. WEISBRODT. 1977. Am. J. Physiol. **232:** 44–47.
6. WINGATE, D. L., H. H. THOMPSON, E. A. PEARCE & A. DAND. 1978. In Proceedings of the Sixth International Symposium of GI Motility. J. H. L. Duthi, ed.: 47–58. MTP Press. Lancaster, UK.
7. JIMENEZ, M., V. MARTINEZ, P. VERGARA & E. GOÑALONS. 1992. Poult. Sci. **71:** 1531–1539.

Cholecystokinin in Human Stomach

Immunohistochemical Investigations on the Distribution and the Effects on Gastric Motility *in Vitro*

S. MICHALSKI,[a] H. HERKEN,[b] K. GOLENHOFEN,[c]
G. LEPSIEN,[a] R. NUSTEDE,[a] H. KÖHLER,[a]
AND F. E. LÜDTKE[a]

[a]*Department of General Surgery and*
[b]*Department of Histology*
University of Göttingen
Göttingen, Germany

[c]*Department of Physiology*
University of Marburg
Marburg, Germany

Enteric neuropeptides and gastrointestinal hormones play an important role in modifying gastric motility. Cholecystokinin (CCK) delays gastric emptying *in vivo* and *in vitro*.[1] In a previous study we saw regional differentiation, with maximum excitatory effects in the longitudinal muscle layer of the antrum and in the outer pyloric ring which were not blocked by atropine or tetrodotoxin, and direct effects on smooth muscle are supposed.[2]

Inasmuch as no systematic investigation of the different regions of the human stomach was made, our aim was to reveal the distribution of CCK using immunohistochemistry and to compare these results with the effect on smooth muscle strips from the same regions.

MATERIALS AND METHODS

Surgical samples of the entire stomach wall from human fundus, corpus, antrum, and the prepyloric, pyloric, and postpyloric region were obtained at surgery for gastric cancer ($n = 13$) and ulcer disease ($n = 4$). Sections showed no pathological findings. Muscle strips were transferred to a conventional, thermostatically controlled organ bath at 37°C, and mechanical activity was measured under auxotonic conditions by a mechanoelectrical transducer and a direct recorder.

Polyclonal antibodies to CCK-8 and CCK 10–20 (Milab, Sweden) at a dilution of 1:240 were used. Fresh samples were fixed in Bouin's fluid, Zamboni's fixative, and embedded in paraffin. The PAP method with imidazole enhancement was used to reveal the antigen-antibody reaction.[3]

RESULTS

Measurements of mechanical activity demonstrated regional differentiation of human stomach with strong excitatory effects of CCK on the longitudinal muscle

TABLE 1. Localization of Maximal Excitatory Effects on Smooth Muscle (SM) and of CCK-Immunoreactive Endocrine Cells (EC) in Human Stomach

	Fundus	Corpus	Antrum	Prepyloric	Pylorus	Postpyloric
EC	/	/	/	+	+	/
SM	/	/	+	+	+	/

layer of the antrum and the muscle layer of the outer pyloric ring (TABLE 1), which were not blocked by atropine or tetrodotoxin application. Cholecystokinin was found only in the endocrine mucosa cells of the prepyloric region and the pyloric ring in all human stomachs with no difference between samples with gastric cancer and those with ulcer disease (TABLE 1, FIG. 1).

DISCUSSION

The detection of CCK in endocrine mucosa cells in the distal part of the stomach where maximal excitatory effects on smooth muscle were seen indicates a physiologically important role for CCK in regulating the gastroduodenal region in man. Besides indirect pathways, this peptide also modulates gastric emptying through a local paracrine release with effects on smooth muscle of the pyloric region.

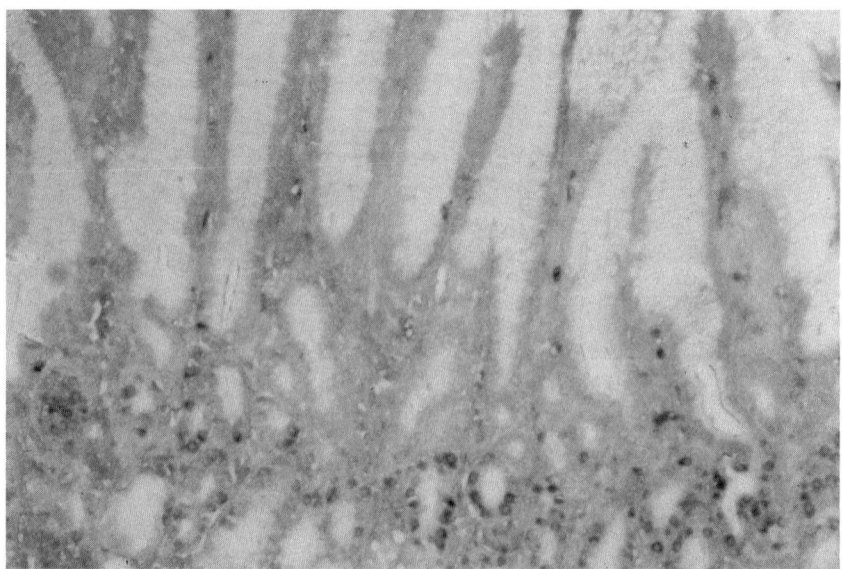

FIGURE 1. Cholecystokinin-immunoreactive endocrine cells in the mucosa of the human pylorus.

REFERENCES

1. ANICA, S. M. 1982. Effects of cholecystokinin and caerulein on gastric emptying. Eur. J. Pharmacol. **85:** 195–199.
2. LÜDTKE, F. E., K. GOLENHOFEN & C. KÖHNE. 1988. Direct effects of cholecystokinin on human gastric motility. Digestion **39:** 210–218.
3. STRAUS, W. 1982. Imidazole increases the sensitivity of the cytochemical reaction for peroxidase with diaminobenzidine at a neutral pH. J. Histochem. Cytochem. **30:** 491–493.

Role of Substance P in the Regulation of Ion Transport by CCK_A and CCK_B Receptors in Mouse Ileum

R. K. RAO,[a] S. LEVENSON,[a] S.-N. FANG,[b] V. J. HRUBY,[b]
H. I. YAMAMURA,[a] AND F. PORRECA[a]

*Departments of [a]Pharmacology and [b]Chemistry
University of Arizona
Tucson, Arizona 85724*

Cholecystokinin (CCK) functions as an enteric neurotransmitter[1] and regulates a variety of gastrointestinal functions including gastric secretion,[2] smooth muscle contraction,[3] and intestinal secretion.[4] Two distinct CCK-specific receptors have been described in various tissues and termed CCK_A and CCK_B receptor subtypes. Although initially it was believed that only CCK_A receptors were functional in peripheral tissues (such as gastrointestinal tract), more recent studies have demonstrated the presence of both CCK_A and CCK_B receptors at peripheral sites such as guinea pig ileum.[3,5] Various forms of CCK show differences in selectivity for CCK receptors. Thus, whereas $CCK_8(s)$ shows high affinity for both CCK_A and CCK_B receptors, CCK_4 and gastrin bind with high affinity only to CCK_B receptors. Application of $CCK_8(s)$ to guinea pig ileum results in contraction of the muscle mediated through the release of substance P and acetylcholine after actions at CCK_A receptors, while application of CCK_4 contracts this tissue through CCK_B receptors through release only of acetylcholine.[3] In our present studies we characterized CCK effects on mouse ileal ion transport with respect to involvement of specific CCK receptor subtypes as well as the potential involvement of release of substance P as a transmitter.

Male ICR mice (35–40 g), allowed free access to food and water, were used in all studies. Small segments of ileal sheets were mounted to standard Ussing flux chambers (surface area 0.65 cm^2). Mucosal and serosal surfaces of the tissue were bathed independently with 10 ml of Krebs-Ringer solution containing 10 mM of either α-D-glucose (serosal) or mannitol (mucosal) and gassed constantly with 95% O_2/5% CO_2 at 37°C. Ion transport was studied by measuring the transmural short circuit current (I_{sc}) and potential difference (PD) across mouse ileal sheets. Agonists and antagonists were added to the medium bathing the serosal surface, and the maximum change in I_{sc} and PD was recorded. We characterized the effects of $CCK_8(s)$, CCK_4, and SNF 9007 (Asp-Tyr-D-Phe-Gly-Trp-Trp-[N-Me]Nle-Asp-Phe-NH_2) on mouse ileal I_{sc} using highly subtype-selective CCK receptor antagonists and [D-Pro^4,D-Trp^{7,9}]substance P 4-11, a substance P antagonist (SPA). SNF 9007 was identified through a synthesis effort[6] aimed at the design of highly selective agonists for subtypes of CCK receptors and was identified as binding selectively to CCK_B (A_{50}, 0.55 nM), rather than CCK_A ($A_{50} > 10,000$ nM), receptors.[7]

Serosal $CCK_8(s)$, CCK_4, and SNF 9007 produced brief, concentration-related increases in I_{sc} without changing tissue conductance, suggesting a net pro-secretory effect of CCK in this tissue, a finding that is consistent with previous studies in guinea pig ileum.[4] The A_{50} (and 95% confidence limit) values for serosal application of peptides were calculated to be 0.56 (0.45–0.70), 63.6 (41.8–96.8), and 10.9 (6.5–18.2) nM for $CCK_8(s)$, CCK_4 and SNF 9007, respectively. L364,718 (100 nM), a selective CCK_A receptor antagonist, blocked the actions of $CCK_8(s)$, but not those of CCK_4 or

SNF 9007. In contrast, L365,260 (100 nM), a selective CCK_B receptor antagonist, blocked the actions of CCK_4 and SNF 9007, but not those of $CCK_8(s)$. Such selective activation of intestinal CCK_A and CCK_B receptors was previously demonstrated using contractile responses of longitudinal smooth muscle from guinea pig ileum.[3] Serosal pretreatment with tetrodotoxin (20 nM), a neural conductance blocker, or chlorisondamine, a ganglionic blocker, almost completely blocked the actions of all peptides studied. Furthermore, these peptides produced no significant response in preparations of ileum physically stripped of the enteric ganglia and muscularis externa; these mucosal preparations did not respond to 1,1-dimethyl-4-phenylpiperazinium (DMPP) and were therefore considered functionally aganglionic. Pretreatment of ileum with SPA (10 μM) produced a transient decrease in I_{sc} and a return to baseline within 5 minutes; SPA pretreatment blocked the actions of $CCK_8(s)$ (3 nM), CCK_4 (1,000 nM), and SNF 9007 (30 nM). At higher concentrations, CCK_4 (3–10 μM) produced an increase in I_{sc} which was not sensitive to SPA pretreatment. In contrast, SNF 9007 (up to 10 μM) remained completely inactive, and a higher concentration of $CCK_8(s)$ (10 μM) produced only a minor response in SPA pretreated tissues.

These data suggest the involvement of substance P in the mediation of CCK effects on mouse ileal I_{sc} through both CCK_A and CCK_B receptors. The present results differ from those of Lucaites et al.[3] in which smooth muscle contraction induced by $CCK_8(s)$, but not CCK_4, was sensitive to substance P antagonists. The actions of $CCK_8(s)$, CCK_4, and SNF 9007 differ in terms of their receptor selectivity in this tissue, with $CCK_8(s)$ showing activity through CCK_A receptors whereas the latter compounds act through CCK_B receptors. Sensitivity to the actions of smaller doses of these agonists to SPA suggests involvement of substance P in effects mediated by both subtypes of CCK receptor. In contrast, higher concentrations of CCK_4, but not SNF 9007, appear able to overcome blockade of substance P receptors. This finding suggests differences in (1) efficacy of CCK_4 and SNF 9007 at CCK_B receptors which may activate a substance P-independent pathway or (2) the presence of different subtypes or affinity states of CCK_B receptors in mouse ileum.

REFERENCES

1. WILLIAMS, J. A. 1982. Cholecystokinin: A hormone and a neurotransmitter. Biomed. Res. **3:** 107–121.
2. PATEL, M. & C. F. SPRAGGS. 1992. Functional comparisons of gastrin/cholecystokinin receptors in isolated preparations of gastric mucosa and ileum. Br. J. Pharmacol. **106:** 275–282.
3. LUCAITES, V. L., L. G. MENDELSOHN, N. R. MASON & M. L. COHEN. 1991. CCK-8, CCK-4 and gastrin-induced contractions in guinea pig ileum: Evidence for differential release of acetylcholine and substance-P by CCK-A and CCK-B receptors. J. Pharmacol. Exp. Ther. **256:** 695–703.
4. KACHUR, J. F., S.-X. WANG, G. W. GULLIKSON & T. S. GAGINELLA. 1991. Cholecystokinin-mediated ileal electrolyte transport in the guinea pig. Characterization of receptor subtypes. Gastroenterology **101:** 1428–1431.
5. GAUDREAU, P., S. ST-PIERRE, C. B. PERT & R. QUIRION. 1987. Structure-activity studies of the C- and N-terminal fragments of cholecystokinin 26–33 in guinea pig isolated tissues. Neuropeptides **10:** 9–18.
6. HRUBY, V. J., S. N. FANG, W. KNAPP, W. KAZMIERSKI, G. K. LUI & H. I. YAMAMURA. 1990. Cholecystokinin analogues with high affinity and selectivity for brain membrane receptors. Int. J. Peptide Prot. Res. **35:** 566–573.
7. SLANINOVA, J., R. J. KNAPP, J. WU, S. N. FANG, T. KRAMER, T. F. BURKS, V. J. HRUBY & H. I. YAMAMURA. 1991. Opioid receptor binding properties of analgesic analogues of cholecystokinin octapeptide. Eur. J. Pharmacol. **200:** 195–198.

Cholecystokinin-Induced Pancreatic Growth Involves the High-Affinity CCK Receptor and Concomitant Activation of Tyrosine Kinase and Phospholipase D

N. RIVARD, G. RYDZEWSKA, AND J. MORISSET

Département de biologie
Université de Sherbrooke
Sherbrooke (Québec), Canada J1K 2R1

Occupation of the high-affinity binding sites by cholecystokinin (CCK) or by the high-affinity CCK receptor agonist JMV-180 caused full stimulation of amylase release from rat pancreatic acini.[1] Although it is well documented that pancreatic enzyme secretion is mediated by the occupation of the CCK receptor through activation of PL-C–associated hydrolysis of phosphatidylinositol 4,5-bisphosphate, the production of IP_3 and DAG, as well as intracellular Ca^{2+} mobilization,[2] the mechanism(s) by which CCK induces growth of the pancreas is still unknown. The aim of the present study was to determine which class of CCK receptor is involved in pancreatic growth and to establish if the CCK-induced growth process involves concomitant tyrosine kinase and phospholipase D activation.

MATERIALS AND METHODS

Male Sprague-Dawley rats were prepared with jugular silastic cannulas for caerulein (0.25 µg $kg^{-1}h^{-1}$) or JMV-180 (50, 100, 150, and 300 µg kg^{-1} h^{-1}) infusions for 4 days or for 30 minutes to 4 hours. After sacrifice, the pancreas was evaluated for weight and contents of protein, RNA, and DNA. Parts of the gland were taken to prepare membrane and cytosol fractions for tyrosine kinase activity or digested with collagenase to prepare acini for phospholipase D activity evaluation.

RESULTS

After 4 days of JMV-180 and caerulein infusion, pancreatic growth occurred. JMV-180 induced a dose-dependent growth response with a maximal effect at 300 µg kg^{-1} h^{-1} comparable to the caerulein response. Maximal increases in pancreatic weight (152.6%), total protein (133.7%), total DNA (53.2%), and total RNA (174%) were obtained with the 300-µg dose of JMV-180. With regard to the transduction signals, JMV-180 (300 µg kg^{-1} h^{-1}) significantly increased membrane tyrosine kinase activity after 1 hour of treatment with a maximal increment of 74% after 3 hours. Parallel increases of less magnitude were also observed in cytosolic tyrosine kinase activity with a maximal increase of 35% observed after 2 hours of infusion. Under the same conditions, JMV-180 was associated with significant increases of 127% and 262% above control values in phospholipase D activity at 30 minutes and 1-hour stimulation, respectively. The phosphatidic acid production represents 4.26% and 6.8% of total radioactivity present in total phospholipids after 30 minutes and 1 hour of JMV-180 compared to 1.88% in the control. From *in vitro* studies performed on dispersed pancreatic acini, JMV-180 caused a dose-dependent phospholipase D activation with significant increases observed from 10 nM up to 10 μM and a maximal response at 1 μM in the presence of 200 μM of propranolol. A final confirmation of this phospholipase D activation by JMV-180 came from the production of phosphatidylethanol through the phospholipase D-catalyzed transphosphatidylation reaction specific to phospholipase D.

DISCUSSION

These data clearly show that occupation of the high-affinity CCK receptors by JMV-180 can induce pancreatic growth as evidenced by significant increases in pancreatic mass and contents of protein, RNA, and DNA. These data also suggest that initiation of pancreatic growth may involve concomitant early activation of tyrosine kinase and phospholipase D. Indeed, tyrosine phosphorylation of proteins catalyzed by tyrosine kinase has been shown to play an important role in the regulation of cellular growth and differentiation.[3] Although we cannot yet associate increased phosphatidic acid production with pancreatic cell proliferation, phosphatidic acid has been described as a potential mitogenic signal in different cell systems.[4] Our current data demonstrate for the first time that CCK stimulates pancreatic growth through the occupation of the high-affinity receptor and that concomitant early tyrosine kinase and phospholipase D activation may be among the early biochemical reactions involved in the initiation and regulation of this growth process.

REFERENCES

1. GALAS, M. C., M. F. LIGNON, M. RODRIGUEZ, C. MENDRE, P. FULCRAND, J. LAUR & J. MARTINEZ. 1988. Am. J. Physiol. **254:** G176–G182.
2. MATOZAKI, T., B. GÖKE, Y. TSUNODA, M. RODRIGUEZ, J. MARTINEZ & J. A. WILLIAMS. 1990. J. Biol. Chem. **265:** 6247–6254.
3. DANGOTT, L. J., D. PUETT & N. H. MELNER. 1986. Biochim. Biophys. Acta **886:** 187–194.
4. FUKAMI, K. & T. TAKENAWA. 1992. J. Biol. Chem. **267:** 10988–10993.

Role of Intraluminal Nutrients in Feedback Regulation of Pancreatic Enzyme Secretion

ALAN W. SPANNAGEL AND GARY M. GREEN

Department of Physiology
University of Texas Health Science Center
San Antonio, Texas 78284

The importance of intraluminal nutrients in stimulating cholecystokinin (CCK) secretion and pancreatic enzyme secretion when pancreatic proteases are not present in the lumen is unclear. In the rat, previous reports showed either a requirement for mixed nutrients, a need for peptone only, or no requirement for nutrients.[1-3] To clarify this issue, we studied the effect of different nutrients on the pancreatic protein secretory response (an indicator of CCK release) to bile-pancreatic juice diversion in a new conscious rat model, the jejunal bypass rat.[4]

MATERIALS AND METHODS

Rats were prepared with biliary, pancreatic, intestinal, and intravenous cannulas. Jejunal bypass surgery was performed, creating a 25-cm self-emptying jejunal blind loop. During recovery (4 days), the jejunal blind loop was nourished by a continuous infusion of a liquid diet (Vital, Ross Laboratories). (A) The effect of pancreatic juice diversion from the jejunal blind loop on pancreatic protein secretion, during the infusion of either saline solution or Vital into the jejunal blind loop, was examined ($n = 5$). (B) During infusion of different nutrients into the jejunal blind loop, pancreatic protein secretion was monitored for 2 hours in the presence of bile-pancreatic juice and for 4 hours after acute bile-pancreatic juice diversion from the jejunal blind loop ($n = 5$). (C) With bile-pancreatic juice chronically diverted from the jejunal blind loop, saline solution was infused into the jejunal blind loop for 3 hours to established a baseline pancreatic secretory rate followed by each nutrient at 1 ml/h for 4 hours or at 5 ml/h for 2 hours ($n = 5-7$). The nutrients used were Vital (1 Kcal/h), 5% protein (lactalbumin), 5% peptone (lactalbumin hydrolysate), 5% mixed L-amino acids (derived from lactalbumin), 5% D-glucose, 200 mM L-glutamine, and 2.5% oleic acid. In some instances, atropine was administered (100 μg/kg/h iv) or MK329 (Merck Sharp and Dohme) was given as an iv bolus (0.5 mg/kg).

RESULTS

(A) The pancreatic hypersecretory response to pancreatic juice diversion requires the presence of intraluminal nutrients (FIG. 1). (B) The incremental protein outputs (mg/kg/30 min) during acute bile-pancreatic juice diversion were 0.56 ± 1.04 (L-amino acids), 1.47 ± 1.45 (D-glucose), 5.45 ± 1.23 (L-glutamine), 11.50 ± 1.85

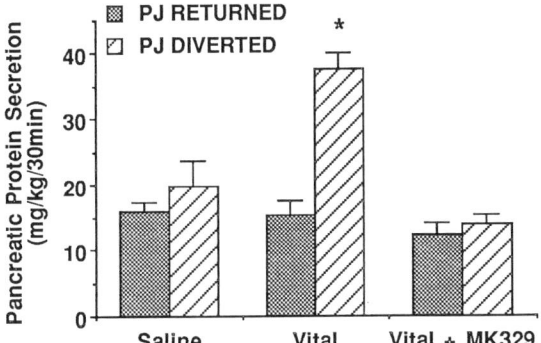

FIGURE 1. Effect of pancreatic juice (PJ) diversion from a jejunal blind loop on pancreatic protein secretion during infusion of either saline solution or a mixed diet (Vital) into the jejunal blind loop. Vital is a nutritionally complete, partially hydrolyzed diet containing 16% peptone, 4% fat, 70% carbohydrates, and 10% vitamins and minerals. *Asterisk* denotes significantly different from all other groups ($n = 5, p < 0.05$, paired and unpaired t tests).

(Vital), and 12.78 ± 1.81 (peptone). (C) The incremental protein outputs (mg/kg/30 min) during the infusion of each nutrient at 1 ml/h were 0.67 ± 2.74 (L-glutamine), 1.82 ± 1.95 (protein), 2.24 ± 1.71 (L-amino acids), 3.09 ± 0.84 (D-glucose), 5.14 ± 1.42 (oleic acid), 13.36 ± 2.23 (peptone), and 18.65 ± 2.30 (Vital). Cholecystokinin receptor blockade and cholinergic receptor blockade eliminated the response to peptone (FIG. 2). Oleic acid stimulated a significant increase in pancreatic protein secretion, but the response was not maintained.

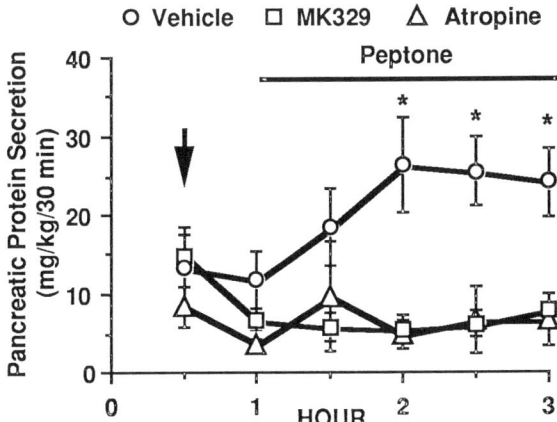

FIGURE 2. Effect of CCK receptor blockade or cholinergic receptor blockade on peptone-stimulated pancreatic protein secretion. Peptone was infused at a rate of 5 ml/h into the jejunal blind loop in rats with chronic bile-pancreatic juice diversion from the jejunal blind loop. At the *arrow*, rats were treated with MK329 or with atropine. *Asterisk* denotes significantly different from basal output ($n = 5, p < 0.05$, paired t test).

In summary, peptone is the major stimulant of pancreatic enzyme secretion in the absence of pancreatic proteases, and this stimulation may depend on a cholinergic pathway. Cholecystokinin appears to be the major humoral mediator of this nutrient effect, as CCK-receptor blockade with MK329 eliminated the response to Vital (FIG. 1) and peptone (FIG. 2).

DISCUSSION

In the rat, peptone can stimulate CCK secretion when the pancreatic proteases are prevented from inhibiting CCK secretion (bile-pancreatic juice diversion); therefore, the peptides released during protein digestion could be stimulating CCK secretion and pancreatic enzyme secretion, inasmuch as intraluminal protein, like bile-pancreatic juice diversion, removes this inhibition of CCK secretion (protein-protease binding). Peptides appear to mediate the effect of peptone because the mixed L-amino acids failed to significantly stimulate pancreatic enzyme secretion. In conclusion, bile-pancreatic juice diversion-stimulated CCK release and bile-pancreatic juice diversion-stimulated pancreatic enzyme secretion require the presence of intraluminal nutrients, and the results obtained in this study indicate that the peptides in peptone are the specific nutrients needed.

REFERENCES

1. LEVAN, V. H., R. A. LIDDLE & G. M. GREEN. 1987. Gut **28** (S1): 25–29.
2. CUBER, J. C., G. BERNARD, T. FUSHIKI, C. BERNARD, R. YAMAMISHI, E. SUGIMOTO & J. A. CHAYVIALLE. 1990. Am. J. Physiol. **259:** G191–G197.
3. MIYASAKA, K., D. GUAN, R. A. LIDDLE & G. M. GREEN. 1989. Am. J. Physiol. **257:** G175–G181.
4. SPANNAGEL, A. W. & G. M. GREEN. 1992. Pancreas **7:** 759.

On the Influence of CCK Receptor Blockade on GRP-Mediated Pancreatic Secretion

F. STÖCKMANN,[a] R. NUSTEDE,[b] R. SCHLEMMINGER,[b]
H. KÖHLER,[b] G. RAMADORI,[a] AND H.-J. PEIPER[b]

[a]Department of Medicine and
[b]Department of Surgery
University of Göttingen
Göttingen, Germany

Gastrin-releasing peptide (GRP) is thought to play a role in the stimulation of exocrine pancreatic secretion. This study investigates the contribution of CCK-dependent mechanisms on the stimulatory influence of GRP on the pancreas.

MATERIALS AND METHODS

Six mongrel dogs under general anesthesia were fitted with a modified Herrera fistula[1] for collection of pancreatic juice. On separate days 30, 100, and 200 pmol $\times$ kg^{-1} $\times$ h^{-1} GRP intravenously were administered over a period of 120 minutes. Plasma concentrations of CCK (antibody 160) and GRP (COOH-terminal antibody) as well as pancreatic juice (protein and enzymes) were analyzed over 180 minutes. In a second experimental series the highly potent CCK receptor antagonist L-364,718 (MK-329 in a dosage of 0.1 mg/kg b.wt.) was applied intraduodenally 30 minutes before the intravenous infusion of 30 pmol $\times$ kg^{-1} $\times$ h^{-1} GRP. Plasma CCK and GRP levels as well as pancreatic juice were again analyzed as in the first experimental series.

RESULTS

The intravenous application of 100 and 200 pmol $\times$ kg^{-1} $\times$ h^{-1} respectively induced marked stimulation of exocrine pancreatic secretion and an increase in plasma concentrations of GRP and CCK. Plasma GRP levels were far above physiological values, which only could be achieved by infusion of 30 pmol $\times$ kg^{-1} $\times$ h^{-1} of GRP. Under these conditions exocrine pancreatic secretion was still significantly increased.

Although the intravenous application of small amounts of GRP (30 pmol $\times$ kg^{-1} $\times$ h^{-1}) alone did not stimulate plasma CCK concentrations, a distinct increase in peripheral CCK plasma levels up to 6.6 pmol/L was observed after the intraduodenal administration of L-364,718. Coincidentally, pancreatic exocrine secretion was diminished after CCK-receptor blockade.

DISCUSSION

Only the small dose of 30 pmol × kg^{-1} × h^{-1} GRP intravenously avoided high plasma concentrations, which have no physiological relevance.[1] Simultaneously no increase in plasma CCK levels was observed. Thus, the GRP-mediated stimulation of exocrine pancreatic secretion does not seem to depend on increased plasma CCK levels.

Until now, the role of CCK in the mediation of GRP- or bombesin-stimulated exocrine pancreatic secretion has been discussed controversially. Wisner et al.,[2] using a rat model, administered large doses of bombesin intravenously (0.2 and 1.0 nmol × h^{-1} × g^{-1}). The subsequent administration of the CCK receptor antagonist L-364,718 (1 mg/kg b.wt.) had no influence on the stimulation of exocrine pancreatic secretion. Plasma concentrations of CCK were not measured.

Similar observations were reported by Terashima et al.[3] and Herzig et al.[4] in rats using 5 μg of bombesin and the specific CCK receptor antagonist L-364,718 (1 mg × kg^{-1} × h^{-1}). However, we demonstrated a marked reduction in exocrine pancreatic secretion with a lower dosage of the CCK receptor antagonist MK-329 (similar to L-364,718). Although we were unable to detect any correlation between peripheral CCK concentrations and the stimulation of exocrine pancreatic secretion, there might be additional CCK-mediated mechanisms that could be of relevance for the increased secretion after intravenous GRP infusion.

The increase in plasma CCK concentrations to postprandial levels after administration of the CCK receptor antagonist might be explained by a different gallbladder function as described by Cantor et al.[5] However, a final explanation is still lacking.

Exocrine pancreatic secretion in conscious dogs is significantly stimulated by the intravenous infusion of small amounts of GRP. Plasma GRP levels are not increased during infusion, as this is physiological in postprandial conditions. No increase in plasma CCK levels was observed in these experimental conditions which is in contrast to previous reports.[3,4] Nevertheless, whether hitherto unknown CCK-mediated mechanisms play an important role in the regulation of exocrine pancreatic secretion (i.e., neuronal release of CCK from intrapancreatic nerves with paracrine action) has to be investigated in further experiments.

REFERENCES

1. DOCKRAY, G. J. 1987. Physiology of enteric neuropeptides. In L. R. Johnson, ed. Physiology of the Gastrointestinal Tract, 2nd Ed.: 41–66. Raven Press. New York.
2. WISNER, J. R., S. OZAWA & I. G. RENNER. 1988. Evidence against cholecystokinin mediation of basal and bombesin-stimulated pancreatic secretion in the rat. Gastroenterology 95: 151–155.
3. TERASHIMA, H., H. T. DEBAS & N. W. BUNNETT. 1992. Effects of cholecystokinin and gastrin antagonists on pancreatic exocrine secretion stimulated by gastrin-releasing peptide. Pancreas 6: 212–219.
4. HERZIG, K. H., D. S. LOUIE & C. OWYANG. 1988. In vivo action of bombesin on exocrine pancreatic secretion in the rat: Independence of cholecystokinin and cholinergic mediation. Pancreas 3: 292–296.
5. CANTOR, P., S. OLSEN, B. J. GERTZ, J. GJORUP & H. WORNING. 1991. Inhibition of cholecystokinin stimulated pancreaticobiliary output in man by the cholecystokinin receptor antagonist MK-329. Scand. J. Gastroenterol. 26: 627–637.

Diurnal Variation in the Effects of Type A CCK Receptor Antagonist Devazepide on Meal Patterns in Rats

DANIEL A. CASTELLANOS[a] AND
ROGER D. REIDELBERGER

*Department of Biomedical Sciences
Creighton University School of Medicine
Omaha, Nebraska 68178
and
Veterans Administration Medical Center
Omaha, Nebraska 68105*

Cholecystokinin (CCK) has been shown to play a role in satiety in a variety of species. Several studies used specific CCK receptor antagonists to block the effects of endogenous CCK and showed a stimulation of feeding in rats,[1,2] pigs,[3] and monkeys.[4] However, it remains to be determined if CCK is equally important in producing satiety at different times in an animal's diurnal cycle. To examine this question, we administered devazepide, a specific CCK-A receptor antagonist, intravenously throughout a 24-hour period and measured its effects on food intake, mean meal size, meal frequency, meal duration, and latency to first meal.

Male Sprague-Dawley rats ($n = 12-16$) surgically prepared with chronic jugular vein catheters had free access to ground chow and water while on a 12:12 light/dark cycle. After postoperative recovery, animals were tethered to single-channel infusion swivels. When acclimated, devazepide (1 mg/kg) or vehicle (5% DMSO, 5% Tween 80, and 90% saline solution) was injected intravenously during separate experiments at 0, 4, 8, 12, 16, and 20 hours after lights out. Feeding patterns were determined from continuous computer recordings of changes in food bowl weights. Effects of CCK receptor blockade on various feeding parameters during the 4-hour period after devazepide injection were evaluated by ANOVA (SYSTAT program).

Devazepide significantly increased 4-hour cumulative food intake at 0 ($n = 13$, $p < 0.01$), 4 ($n = 16$, $p < 0.05$), 16 ($n = 14$, $p < 0.01$), and 20 hours ($n = 15$, $p < 0.05$). Devazepide had no significant effect at either 8 or 12 hours after lights out; this was the transitional period from the dark to light cycle. The increases in cumulative food intake during the dark cycle (0 and 4 hours after lights out) were qualitatively different from the increases in food intake during the animal's light cycle (16 and 20 hours after lights out). Stimulation in 4-hour intake occurred through an increase in mean meal size at 0 hour ($n = 13, p < 0.05$). The stimulation in 4-hour intake at 16 hours after lights out occurred through an increase in meal frequency ($n = 14$, $p < 0.05$) and a decrease in latency to first meal ($n = 14$, $p < 0.01$). The increase in 4-hour intake at 20 hours after lights out was due to an increase in meal frequency ($n = 16, p < 0.05$).

Our results suggest that endogenous CCK acts to suppress feeding behavior

---

[a]Address for correspondence: Daniel A. Castellanos, Creighton University School of Medicine, Department of Biomedical Sciences, Division of Physiology, 2500 California Street, Omaha, NE 68178.

throughout most of the diurnal cycle, with it having no effect during the transition from dark to light. Also, during the early dark period, endogenous CCK acts both within and between meals to decrease meal size and increase intermeal interval. During the latter part of the light period, CCK appears to act primarily by increasing the intermeal interval.

REFERENCES

1. REIDELBERGER, R. D. & M. F. O'ROURKE. 1989. Am. J. Physiol. **257:** R1512–R1518.
2. HEWSON, G., R. G. LEIGHTON & J. HUGHES. 1988. Br. J. Pharmacol. **93:** 79–84.
3. EBENEZER, I. S., C. DE LA RIVA & B. A. BALDWIN. 1990. Physiol. Behav. **47:** 145–148.
4. MORAN, T. H., P. J. AMEGLIO, H. J. PAYTON, G. J. SCHWARTZ & P. R. MCHUGH. Am. J. Physiol., in press.

Cholecystokinin Inhibits Food Intake at a Peripheral Extragastric Site

T. T. ZITTEL,[a,b,c] B. V. ELM,[b] R. K. TEICHMANN,[b]
H. D. BECKER,[b] AND H. E. RAYBOULD[a]

[a]CURE/UCLA Digestive Diseases Center
Department of Medicine
University of California
Los Angeles, California 90073

[b]University Hospital
Department of Abdominal and Transplantation Surgery
Tübingen, Germany

Peripheral cholecystokinin (CCK) is thought to inhibit food intake by activating CCK-A receptors at a gastric and/or vagal afferent site.[1] If this effect persists after gastrectomy, then peripheral extragastric CCK receptor sites that regulate food intake might exist. The aims of our study were to determine: (1) if exogenous CCK inhibits food intake after gastrectomy in rats; (2) if blockade of endogenous CCK increases food intake and body weight after total gastrectomy in rats; and (3) which CCK receptor subtypes (CCK-A or CCK-B) are involved.

MATERIALS AND METHODS

One-hour solid food intake was measured after a 4-hour fasting period in gastrectomized (total gastrectomy, reconstruction by Roux-en-Y, $n = 4$) and unoperated littermates ($n = 4$) and intraperitoneal injection with either vehicle, CCK8 (7 nmol/kg), MK329 (CCK-A receptor antagonist) (0.1 mg/kg) + CCK8, or L365,260 (CCK-B receptor antagonist) (0.1 mg/kg) + CCK8. In a separate study, gastrectomized rats were restricted to a 12-hour feeding period after surgery (20–100 postoperative days) during which they received twice daily either vehicle, MK329 (0.01 or 0.1 mg/kg) or L365,260 (0.01 or 0.01 mg/kg) subcutaneously. Food intake and body weight were measured daily. Data are presented as mean ± standard error of mean (SEM). Differences between treated groups were determined by analysis of variance followed by Fisher's LSD Test. A probability of $p < 0.05$ was significant.

RESULTS

One-hour food intake after a 4-hour fasting period was reduced in gastrectomized rats compared to control rats (0.49 ± 0.01 vs 1.36 ± 0.07 g/100 g body weight [BW], $p < 0.001$). Exogenous CCK reduced 1-hour food intake after a 4-hour fast in gastrectomized and control rats by 53 ± 9% and 54 ± 9%, respectively (ns). This response was abolished by MK329 (0.1 mg/kg) in gastrectomized rats and was

[c]Address for correspondence: Tilman T. Zittel, MD, CURE/UCLA Digestive Diseases Center, VA Wadsworth, Bldg 115, Rm 115, Wilshire & Sawtelle Blvd, Los Angeles, CA 90073.

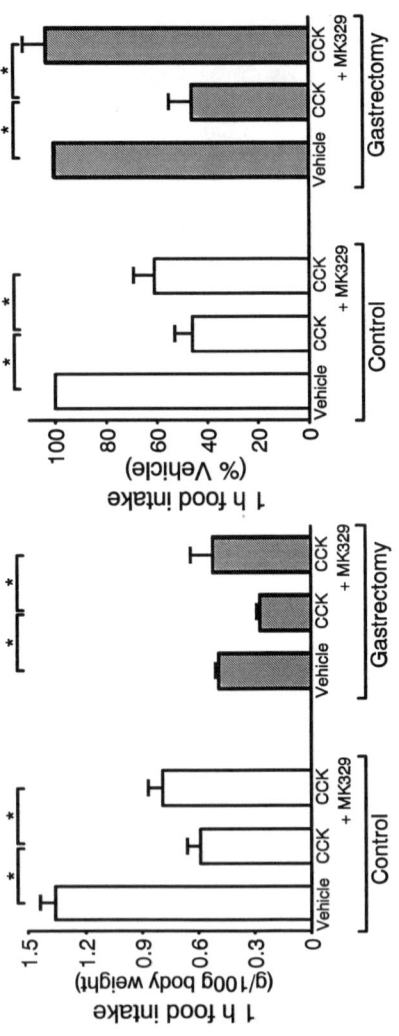

FIGURE 1. One-hour food intake was reduced in gastrectomized (▨) compared to control (□) rats. Exogenous CCK was equipotent in inhibiting food intake in control and gastrectomized rats. *$p < 0.05$.

reversed by 26 ± 8% in control rats (FIG. 1). L365,260 had no effect on exogenous CCK-induced inhibition of 1-hour food intake in both groups.

Blockade of endogenous CCK by chronic MK329 treatment as well as chronic L365,260 treatment after gastrectomy increased postoperative food intake (TABLE 1) and reduced postoperative weight loss (vehicle treatment: 15 ± 2 g/100 g BW; MK329 [0.1 mg/kg]: 5 ± 2 g/100 g BW, $p < 0.01$ vs vehicle; L365,260 [0.01 mg/kg or 0.1 mg/kg]: 8 ± 2 g/100 g BW, $p < 0.05$ vs vehicle).

DISCUSSION

In the present study, CCK was equipotent in inhibiting food intake in control and gastrectomized rats, indicating that CCK can inhibit food intake at a peripheral extragastric site. It has been reported that abdominal vagotomy blocks the satiety effects of CCK.[2] This is somewhat contrary to our results, because total gastrectomy should include abdominal vagotomy. However, it is possible that extragastric vagal

TABLE 1. Effect of CCK Receptor Antagonist Treatment on Food Intake after Total Gastrectomy in Rats[a]

		Treatment			
		MK329		L365,260	
Postoperative Day	Vehicle ($n = 12$)	0.01 ($n = 5$)	0.1 ($n = 5$)	0.01 ($n = 6$)	0.1 mg/kg ($n = 6$)
20–39	108 ± 5 g	107 ± 8 g	123 ± 8 g[b]	129 ± 7 g[b]	114 ± 7 g
40–59	104 ± 3 g	111 ± 4 g	120 ± 4 g[c]	118 ± 4 g[c]	115 ± 4 g[b]
60–79	99 ± 4 g	104 ± 6 g	108 ± 6 g	104 ± 5 g	115 ± 3 g[b]
80–99	93 ± 4 g	103 ± 6 g	106 ± 6 g	104 ± 5 g	104 ± 5 g
20–99	404 ± 10 g	426 ± 16 g	457 ± 16 g[c]	457 ± 14 g[c]	449 ± 14 g[b]

[a]Food intake is expressed as g/100 g preoperative body weight.
[b]$p < 0.05$ vs vehicle treatment.
[c]$p < 0.01$ vs vehicle treatment.

branches such as the hepatic or celiac branch might have been preserved.[3] Therefore, CCK could activate CCK receptors on extragastric branches of the vagus nerve.[4] However, there are other reports that the inhibitory effect of exogenous CCK on food intake is not completely abolished after vagotomy.[1,5] This indicates that extravagal peripheral CCK receptor sites regulating food intake might exist. Inasmuch as CCK receptor binding sites have been shown on dorsal root ganglia,[6] spinal afferents are a possible candidate. The peripheral receptor sites activated by exogenous CCK are CCK-A receptors, because the inhibitory effect of exogenous CCK on food intake was abolished by CCK-A, but not by CCK-B receptor blockade in gastrectomized rats. This is in accordance with a previous report.[7]

Chronic blockade of endogenous CCK by both CCK-A and CCK-B receptor antagonists increased food intake and body weight after gastrectomy in rats, indicating that endogenous CCK is able to inhibit food intake at an extragastric site. The CCK-A receptor antagonist possibly blocks peripheral CCK-A receptors, as we could block exogenous CCK-induced inhibition of food intake with a CCK-A receptor antagonist in gastrectomized rats. In contrast, the CCK-B receptor antagonist possibly blocks central CCK-B receptors, because we could not block exogenous CCK-induced inhibition of food intake by a CCK-B receptor antagonist, and peripheral CCK does not cross the blood-brain barrier.[8]

In conclusion, we found evidence that exogenous and endogenous CCK inhibits food intake at a peripheral, extragastric, possibly extravagal CCK-A receptor site after gastrectomy in rats. Additionally, endogenous CCK released and acting at CCK-B receptors inside the central nervous system seems to be involved in the regulation of food intake after gastrectomy in rats.

REFERENCES

1. MURPHY, R. B., L. H. SCHNEIDER & G. P. SMITH. 1988. Peripheral loci for the mediation of cholecystokinin-induced satiety. *In* Cholecystokinin Antagonists. R. Y. Wang & R. Schoenfeld, eds.: 73–91. Alan R. Liss Inc. New York.
2. SMITH, G. P., C. JEROME, B. J. CUSHIN, R. ETERNO & K. J. SIMANSKY. 1981. Abdominal vagotomy blocks the satiety effect of cholecystokinin in the rat. Science **213**: 1036–1037.
3. POWLEY, H. L., J. C. PRECHTL, E. A. FOX & H.-R. BERTHOUD. 1983. Abdominal considerations for surgery of the rat abdominal vagus: Distribution, paraganglia and regeneration. J. Auton. Nerv. Syst. **9**: 79–97.
4. MORAN, T. H., G. P. SMITH, A. M. HOSTETLER & P. R. MCHUGH. 1987. Transport of cholecystokinin binding sites in subdiaphragmatic vagal branches. Brain Res. **415**: 149–152.
5. GARLICKI, J., P. K. KONTUREK, J. MAJKA, N. KWIECIEN & S. J. KONTUREK. 1990. Cholecystokinin receptors and vagal nerves in control of food intake in rats. Am. J. Physiol. **258**: E40–E45.
6. GHILARDI, J. R., C. J. ALLEN, S. R. VIGNA, D. C. VCVEY & P. W. MANTYH. 1992. Trigeminal and dorsal root ganglion neurons express CCK receptor binding sites in the rat, rabbit, and monkey: Possible site of opiate-CCK analgesic interactions. J. Neurosci. **12**: 4854–4866.
7. DOURISH, C. T., A. C. RUCKERT, F. D. TATTERSALL & S. D. IVERSEN. 1989. Evidence that decreased feeding induced by systemic injection of cholecystokinin is mediated by CCK-A receptors. Eur. J. Pharmacol. **173**: 233–234.
8. PASSARO, E., H. DEBAS, W. OLDENDORF & T. YAMADA. 1982. Rapid appearance of intraventricularly administered neuropeptides in the peripheral circulation. Brain Res. **241**: 338–340.

Expression of CCK-A and CCK-B/Gastrin Receptors in Enterochromaffin-Like Cell Carcinoids of *Mastomys natalensis*

OLA NILSSON,[a,d] LARS KÖLBY,[b] BO WÄNGBERG,[b] STEPHEN A. WANK,[c] AND HÅKAN AHLMAN[b]

Departments of [a]Pathology and [b]Surgery
Sahlgrenska Hospital
Göteborg, Sweden

[c]*NIH/NIDDK/Digestive Diseases Branch*
Bethesda, Maryland 20892

Gastric carcinoids in man are rare, but they occur more frequently in patients with chronic atrophic gastritis or Zollinger-Ellison syndrome as part of an MEN-I syndrome. Both of these conditions are associated with long-standing hypergastrinemia, and gastrin has therefore been suggested as important in the development of these tumors. Experimental studies in rats appear to support the gastrin hypothesis, because gastric carcinoids can be induced by life-long acid inhibition with concomitant hypergastrinemia. Recently, we demonstrated rapid induction of enterochromaffin-like (ECL) cell carcinoids in *Mastomys natalensis* subjected to histamine$_2$-receptor blockade.[1] To evaluate the role of gastrin in this tumor model, we investigated the expression of CCK-A and CCK-B/gastrin receptors in the stomach of normal and tumor-bearing *Mastomys*.

MATERIALS AND METHODS

Animals. The African rodent *Praomys (Mastomys) natalensis* was used in the present study.[1] Animals were given histamine$_2$-receptor blocker (loxtidine, kindly supplied by Glaxo, UK) in the drinking water for 2–12 months. At the end of the treatment period animals were killed by decapitation, blood was collected for determination of plasma gastrin, and the stomachs were taken for morphologic examination and Northern analysis.

Morphology. Specimens of the gastric corpus were fixed in buffered paraformaldehyde and embedded in paraffin wax. Endocrine cell proliferation and carcinoid formation were studied by indirect immunoperoxidase techniques using antibodies to chromogranin A and histamine.

Northern Analysis. Total RNA was prepared by acid guanidine isothiocyanate-phenol-chloroform extraction. Purified mRNA was obtained using the PolyATtract system (Promega). Samples of total RNA and purified mRNA were electrophoresed, blotted onto nylon membranes, and hybridized with ^{32}P-labeled riboprobes under

---

[d]Address for correspondence: Ola Nilsson, MD, Department of Pathology, Sahlgrenska Hospital, S-413 45 Göteborg, Sweden.

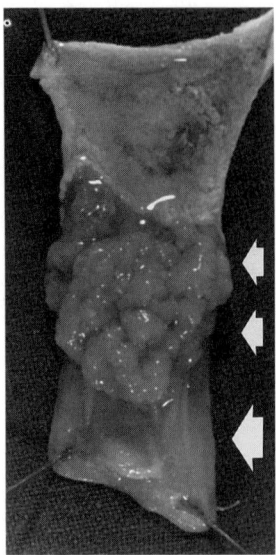

FIGURE 1. Gross appearance of stomach from loxtidine-treated *Mastomys*. The oxyntic mucosa is occupied by a tumor *(small arrows)*, whereas the antral mucosa is unaffected *(large arrow)*.

FIGURE 2. Micrograph showing enterochromaffin-like cell carcinoid in the oxyntic mucosa of loxtidine-treated *Mastomys*. Immunoperoxidase technique using chromogranin antibodies.

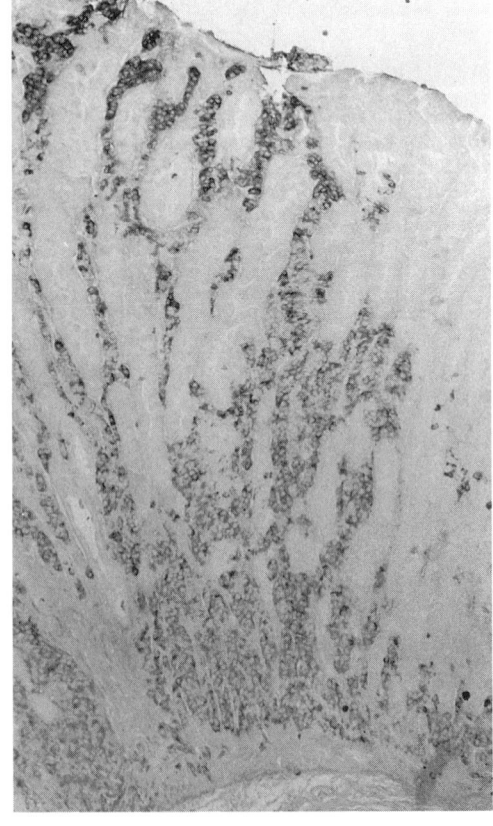

FIGURE 3. Northern blot showing CCK-A receptor expression in normal oxyntic mucosa (C) and in gastric carcinoids of *Mastomys* treated with loxtidine for 5 (L1) or 12 (L2) months.

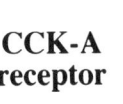
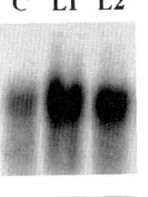

high stringency conditions. ^{32}P-labeled antisense RNA probes were generated with SP6 or T7 RNA polymerases from linearized plasmids carrying one of the following inserts: 1.5-kb rat CCK-A receptor cDNA,[2] 2.4-kb rat CCK-B/gastrin receptor cDNA,[3] and 0.25-kb mouse β-actin cDNA. Specific labeling of membranes was detected using a Phosphorimager (Molecular Dynamics).

RESULTS

Loxtidine treatment of *Mastomys* induced sustained hypergastrinemia with plasma gastrin values 3–4 times those of control animals. Gross tumors were present in the gastric corpus (oxyntic mucosa) in one third of animals treated for 6 months and in more than two thirds of animals treated for 12 months or longer (FIG. 1). Immunocytochemical analysis of the gastric corpus revealed rapid proliferation of ECL cells with the successive appearance of hyperplastic (2 months), dysplastic (4–6 months), and neoplastic (6 months or longer) ECL cell lesions (FIG. 2). Northern analysis demonstrated high expression of CCK-A receptor mRNA (3.5-kb transcript) in normal oxyntic mucosa and in carcinoid tumors (FIG. 3). CCK-B/gastrin receptor mRNA (2.7-kb transcript) was also abundant in normal oxyntic mucosa as well as in tumor tissues (FIG. 4).

DISCUSSION

Praomys (Mastomys) natalensis is a unique animal model in which the development of ECL cell carcinoids can be studied. Histamine$_2$-receptor blockade (induced

FIGURE 4. Northern blot showing CCK-B/gastrin receptor expression in normal oxyntic mucosa (C) and in gastric carcinoids of *Mastomys* treated with loxtidine for 5 (L1) or 12 (L2) months.

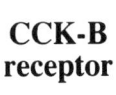
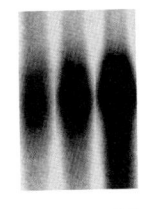
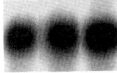

by loxtidine treatment) causes sustained hypergastrinemia and promotes ECL cell proliferation and carcinoid tumor growth in the gastric mucosa. The abundance of CCK-A and CCK-B/gastrin receptor mRNA in normal oxyntic mucosa suggests that this tissue is very sensitive to stimulation by CCK/gastrin. Furthermore, carcinoid tumors also expressed high levels of CCK-A and CCK-B/gastrin receptors, indicating that both of these receptors may be of importance in the control of tumor growth following histamine$_2$-receptor blockade. However, further studies using this experimental model and selective CCK-A and CCK-B receptor antagonists are necessary to elucidate the exact role of these receptors in ECL cell carcinoid formation.

REFERENCES

1. NILSSON, O., B. WÄNGBERG, L. JOHANSSON, E. THEODORSSON, A. DAHLSTRÖM, I. M. MODLIN & H. AHLMAN. 1993. Rapid induction of enterochromaffinlike cell tumors by histamine$_2$-receptor blockade. Am. J. Pathol. **142:** 1173–1185.
2. WANK, S. A., R. HARKINS, R. T. JENSEN, H. SHAPIRA, A. DE WEERTH & T. SLATTERY. 1992. Purification, molecular cloning and functional expression of the cholecystokinin receptor from rat pancreas. Proc. Natl. Acad. Sci. USA **89:** 3125–3129.
3. WANK, S. A., J. R. PISEGNA & A. DE WEERTH. 1992. Brain and gastrointestinal cholecystokinin receptor family: Structure and functional expression. Proc. Natl. Acad. Sci. USA **89:** 8691–8695.

Growth of Azaserine-Induced Putative Preneoplastic Nodules in the Rat Pancreas Is Mediated Specifically by Way of Cholecystokinin-A Receptors

STEPHEN P. POVOSKI,[a] WEIGONG ZHOU,[a]
DANIEL S. LONGNECKER,[b] BILL D. ROEBUCK,[c]
AND RICHARD H. BELL, JR.[a,d]

[a]*Department of Surgery*
University of Cincinnati College of Medicine and
Veterans Affairs Medical Center
Cincinnati, Ohio 45220

Departments of [b]*Pathology and* [c]*Pharmacology and Toxicology*
Dartmouth Medical School
Hanover, New Hampshire 03756

The peptide hormone cholecystokinin (CCK) has been shown to stimulate the growth of azaserine-induced putative preneoplastic acinar cell nodules in the rat pancreas.[1,2] However, it is not known if this growth-stimulating effect is mediated specifically by way of CCK-A receptors, CCK-B receptors, or both. Thus, the present study assesses the effect of highly selective, high-affinity CCK agonists on azaserine-induced putative preneoplastic nodules to determine which CCK receptor subtype(s) mediates growth of these lesions during the early stages of azaserine-induced pancreatic carcinogenesis.

MATERIALS AND METHODS

Sixteen-day-old male Lewis rats received a single intraperitoneal injection of azaserine at 30 mg/kg body weight (BW). Starting on day 21, rats were injected subcutaneously once daily, 5 days per week for 16 consecutive weeks with either (1) CCK-8 (nonselective CCK agonist; cholecystokinin octapeptide; 2.50 µg/kg BW); (2) A-71623[3] (selective CCK-A agonist; *tert*-butyloxycarbonyl-Trp-Lys(ϵ-N-2-methyl-phenylaminocarbonyl)-Asp-(N-methyl)-Phe-NH$_2$; 1.84 µg/mg/kg BW); (3) SNF-8815[4] (selective CCK-B agonist; [(2R,3S)-β-MePhe^{28}, N-MeNle^{31}]CCK$_{26-33}$; 2.40 µg/kg BW); or (4) normal saline solution (control). Rats were subsequently sacrificed, and body weights and pancreatic weights were determined. Quantitative morphometric analysis of acidophilic atypical acinar cell foci and nodules (AACN) was performed according to the criteria of Roebuck *et al.*[5] Statistical analysis was performed by one-way analysis of variance (ANOVA) followed by a Bonferroni multiple-comparison test. Statistical significance was assumed when $p < 0.05$.

---

[d]Address for correspondence: Richard H. Bell, Jr., MD, Surgical Service (112), Veterans Affairs Medical Center, 3200 Vine Street, Cincinnati, Ohio 45220.

TABLE 1. Body and Pancreatic Weights

Treatment	No. of Rats	Body Weight (g)	Pancreatic Weight (g)
CCK-8	17	421 ± 18	1.578 ± 0.136[a,b]
A-71623 (A-agonist)	18	423 ± 19	1.978 ± 0.138[a,b,c]
SNF-8815 (B-agonist)	18	422 ± 21	1.283 ± 0.180
Control	17	424 ± 20	1.299 ± 0.128

NOTE: Values are means ± SD.
[a] $p < 0.001$ vs control by ANOVA/Bonferroni.
[b] $p < 0.001$ vs SNF-8815 (B-agonist) by ANOVA/Bonferroni.
[c] $p < 0.001$ vs CCK-8 by ANOVA/Bonferroni.

RESULTS

The effects of the cholecystokinin agonists on body weight and pancreatic weight are shown in TABLE 1. No significant difference in mean body weight was observed between the treatment groups. Pancreatic weight was significantly increased in the CCK-8 treatment group ($p < 0.001$) and the A-71623 treatment group ($p < 0.001$) as compared to the control group and the SNF-8815 treatment group. Furthermore, the increase in pancreatic weight seen in the A-71623 treatment group was significantly greater ($p < 0.001$) than that seen in the CCK-8 treatment group. No significant difference in pancreatic weight was seen between the SNF-8815 treatment group and the control group.

The results of quantitative morphometric analysis for acidophilic AACN are shown in TABLE 2. The number of AACN per cubic centimeter, the number of AACN per pancreas, the mean diameter per AACN, and the AACN volume as percentage of pancreas were significantly increased in the CCK-8 treatment group ($p < 0.001$) as compared to the control group and the SNF-8815 treatment group. Likewise, the number of AACN per pancreas, the mean diameter per AACN, and the AACN volume as a percentage of pancreas were significantly increased in the A-71623 treatment group ($p < 0.001$) as compared to the control group and the SNF-8815 treatment group. Furthermore, the increase in mean diameter per AACN and AACN volume as the percentage of pancreas seen in the A-71623 treatment group was significantly greater ($p < 0.001$) than that seen in the CCK-8 treatment group. No significant difference in volumetric data was seen between the SNF-8815 treatment group and the control group.

TABLE 2. Quantitative Morphometric Analysis of Acidophilic AACN in Azaserine-Treated Rats

Treatment	Total No./cm^3	Total No./Pancreas	Mean Diameter (μm)	Volume as % of Pancreas
CCK-8	436 ± 97[a,b]	690 ± 174[a,b]	510 ± 89[a,b]	4.027 ± 1.556[a,b]
A-71623 (A-agonist)	373 ± 77	742 ± 186[a,b]	643 ± 83[a,b,c]	6.535 ± 2.035[a,b,c]
SNF-8815 (B-agonist)	305 ± 109	401 ± 196	376 ± 53	1.068 ± 0.577
Control	324 ± 76	420 ± 107	381 ± 31	1.114 ± 0.352

NOTE: Values are means ± SD.
[a] $p < 0.001$ vs control by ANOVA/Bonferroni.
[b] $p < 0.001$ vs SNF-8815 (B-agonist) by ANOVA/Bonferroni.
[c] $p < 0.001$ vs CCK-8 by ANOVA/Bonferroni.

DISCUSSION

In the present study, CCK-8 (nonselective CCK agonist) and A-71623 (selective CCK-A agonist) stimulated pancreatic growth and the development of acidophilic AACN, whereas SNF-8815 (selective CCK-B agonist) had no effect. Additionally, the growth-promoting effect induced by A-71623 (selective CCK-A agonist) was significantly greater than that produced by CCK-8 (nonselective CCK agonist). These findings demonstrate that the growth of azaserine-induced putative preneoplastic lesions in the rat pancreas is mediated specifically by CCK-A receptors.

REFERENCES

1. LHOSTE, E. F., B. D. ROEBUCK & D. S. LONGNECKER. 1988. Stimulation of the growth of azaserine-induced nodules in the rat pancreas by dietary camostate (FOY-305). Carcinogenesis **9:** 901–909.
2. DOUGLAS, B. R., R. A. WOUTERSEN, J. B. M. J. JANSEN, A. J. L. DEJONG, L. C. ROVATI & C. B. H. W. LAMERS. 1989. Influence of cholecystokinin antagonist on the effects of cholecystokinin and bombesin on azaserine-induced lesions in rat pancreas. Gastroenterology **96:** 462–469.
3. LIN, C. W., K. SHIOSAKI, T. R. MILLER, D. G. WITTE, B. R. BIANCHI, C. A. W. WOLFRAM, H. KOPECKA, R. CRAIG, F. WAGENAAR & A. M. NADZAN. 1990. Characterization of two novel cholecystokinin tetrapeptide (30–33) analogues, A-71623 and A-70874, that exhibit high potency and selectivity for cholecystokinin-A receptors. Mol. Pharmacol. **39:** 346–351.
4. HRUBY, V. J., S. FANG, G. TOTH, D. JIAO, T. O. MATSUNAGA, N. COLLINS, R. KNAPP & H. I. YAMAMURA. 1991. Highly potent and selective cholecystokinin analogues for the CCK-B receptor. In Peptides 1990. E. Giralt & D. Andreu, eds.: 707–709. ESCOM Science Publishers B.V. Leiden.
5. ROEBUCK, B. D., K. J. BAUMGARTNER & C. D. THRON. 1984. Characterization of two populations of pancreatic atypical acinar cell foci induced by azaserine in the rat. Lab. Invest. **50:** 141–146.

Endogenous CCK in the Control of Gastric Secretory Response to Meal in Normal Subjects and Duodenal Ulcer Patients

J. W. KONTUREK, R. STOLL, W. DOMSCHKE,
AND S. J. KONTUREK

Department of Medicine B
University of Münster
Münster, Germany
and
Institute of Physiology
University of Krakow
Krakow, Poland

Patients with duodenal ulcer, as a group, tend to secrete more acid than do normal subjects both at rest and in response to secretory stimulation. Several pathophysiological defects in the regulation of gastric acid secretion have been suggested. As the major stimulant of acid secretion after ingestion of a meal is increased plasma gastrin, the duodenal ulcer patients have impaired inhibition of both acid secretion and gastrin release by a fat-containing or acidified meal.[1] The mechanisms by which fat or acid inhibits gastric acid secretion are not fully defined, but recent studies in healthy humans with highly selective cholecystokinin (CCK) receptor antagonists such as loxiglumide suggest that CCK may play an important role in this inhibition.[2,3]

This study examines the influence of endogenous CCK on the gastric pH profile after feeding of a standard meal with and without the addition of fat in normal subjects and duodenal ulcer patients using a highly selective antagonist of type A CCK receptors, loxiglumide.

MATERIAL AND METHODS

Studies were carried out in 10 healthy volunteers (aged 21–24 years) and 10 duodenal ulcer patients. Gastric secretion was stimulated by oral administration of a 500-ml standard liquid meal (Fresubin, Fresenius, Germany), with or without the addition of 15% soybean oil and with or without pretreatment with 1,200 mg of loxiglumide orally. After the meal all subjects underwent 3-hour intragastric pH recording using antimony pH electrodes (Digitrapper, Synectics, Sweden). Plasma samples were drawn for gastrin, CCK, pancreatic polypeptide (PP), and somatostatin determination by specific radioimmunoassay.

RESULTS

A standard meal in healthy controls raised the median 3-hour intragastric pH to about 4.8 (FIG. 1) and increased plasma gastrin levels by 57%, CCK by 177%, PP by 100%, and somatostatin by 39% (FIG. 2). The addition of fat in these normal subjects significantly increased the median 3-hour intragastric pH and prolonged the pH

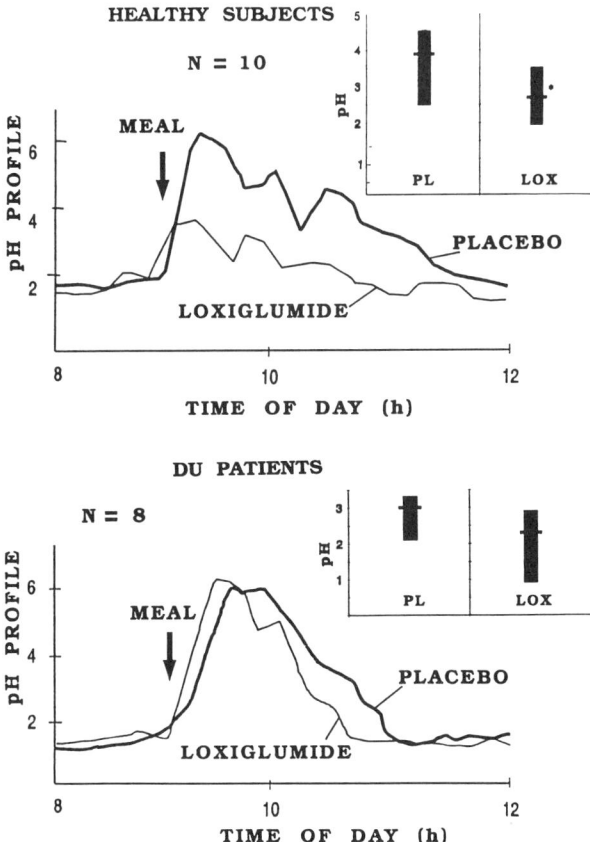

FIGURE 1. Median intragastric pH (with interquartile distance) in healthy subjects ($n = 10$) and duodenal ulcer (DU) patients ($n = 10$) treated with placebo (PL) or loxiglumide (LOX) 1.2 g orally. Columns are Box-Whisker plots for 3-hour postprandial measurement periods with median values. *Asterisk* indicates significant decrease from the value obtained with placebo treatment; $p < 0.05$.

decline after the meal while reducing the increment in plasma gastrin and enhancing plasma CCK. Loxiglumide significantly reduced the median 3-hour postprandial pH (to about 2.5) and reversed the changes in the pH profile caused by the addition of fat. Plasma gastrin and CCK almost doubled, whereas plasma PP and somatostatin

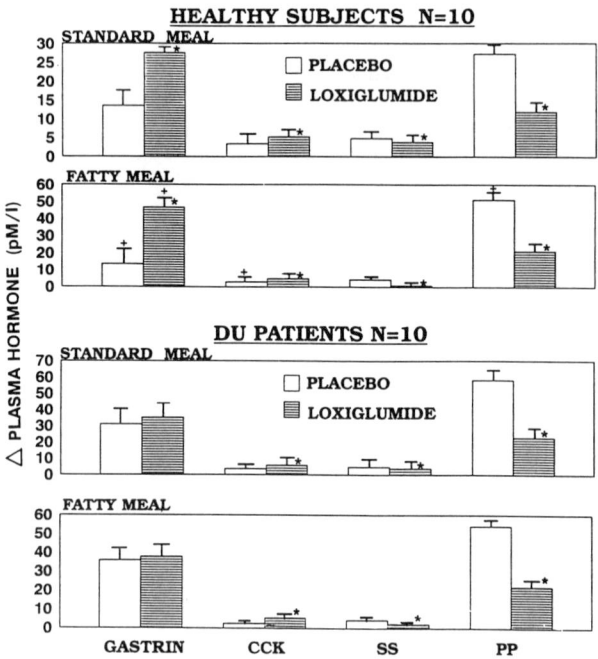

FIGURE 2. Increments in plasma levels of gastrin, cholecystokinin (CCK), somatostatin (SS), and pancreatic polypeptide (PP) in response to a standard meal with and without the addition of 15% soybean oil in tests with and without pretreatment with loxiglumide in healthy subjects ($n = 10$) and duodenal ulcer (DU) patients ($n = 10$). *Asterisk* indicates a significant ($p < 0.05$) change from the values obtained in control tests without loxiglumide. *Cross* indicates a significant ($p < 0.05$) change from the corresponding values obtained with a standard meal without fat.

were significantly reduced. Duodenal ulcer patients showed lower postprandial pH (about 3.0) and higher increments in plasma gastrin, but CCK antagonism failed to significantly affect the pH profile (FIG. 1) or the increments in plasma gastrin and somatostatin, respectively (FIG. 2).

DISCUSSION

This study presents evidence that endogenous CCK released by a caloric liquid meal with or without the addition of fat exerts an inhibitory effect on gastric acid secretion as well as gastrin release. The tonic inhibitory effect of CCK on gastric acid secretion might be mediated, at least in part, by the release of somatostatin, which is liberated by CCK *in vitro*.[4] In duodenal ulcer patients, the gastric acid and plasma gastrin inhibitory response to endogenous CCK is less marked than that in healthy subjects, suggesting a defect in the action of this hormone on gastric secretion and gastrin release, possibly due to a deficiency of somatostatin.

REFERENCES

1. EYSSELEIN, V. E., T. O. G. KOVACS, J. H. KLEIBEUKER, V. MAXWELL, T. REEDY & J. H. WALSH. 1992. Regulation of gastric acid secretion by gastrin in duodenal ulcer patients and healthy subjects. Gastroenterology **102:** 1142–1148.
2. KONTUREK, J. W., R. STOLL, S. J. KONTUREK & W. DOMSCHKE. 1993. Cholecystokinin in the control of gastric acid secretion in humans. GUT **34:** 321–328.
3. BEGLINGER, C., P. HILDEBRAND, R. MEIER, P. BAUERFEIND, H. HASSLOCHER et al. 1992. A physiological role for cholecystokinin as a regulator of gastrin secretion. Gastroenterology **103:** 490–495.
4. SOLL, A. H., D. A. AMIRIAN, J. PARK, J. D. ELASHOFF & T. YAMADA. 1985. Cholecystokinin potently releases somatostatin from canine fundic mucosal cells in short-term culture. Am. J. Physiol **248:** G569–573.

Second Messenger Activators Regulate CCK mRNA in the Human Neuroepithelioma Cell Line SK-N-MCIXC[a]

B. L. MANIA-FARNELL, B. J. MERRILL,
H. I. YAMAMURA, AND T. P. DAVIS

Department of Pharmacology
College of Medicine
University of Arizona
Tucson, Arizona 85724

The biologically active brain-gut peptide cholecystokinin (CCK) is synthesized in a cell-specific manner in the intestinal tract, central nervous system (CNS),[1,2] pituitary,[3] and male germ cells.[4] A large number of studies indicate that brain CCK, predominantly present as the octapeptide CCK-8, functions as a neurotransmitter or neuromodulator.[5] Several biological functions associated with central CCK include effects that are directly related to the gastrointestinal tract, for instance, effects on gastric acid secretion, satiety, and feeding behaviors.[6]

The role that CCK plays is linked to the mechanisms that regulate its biosynthesis and metabolism. Inasmuch as processing and metabolic enzymes are distributed similarly throughout the brain, biosynthetic rates of peptide precursors are generally determined by cellular contents of their encoding mRNAs.[7]

In this study, regulation of cholecystokinin mRNA expression was examined in the human neuroepithelioma cell line SK-N-MCIXC. This cell line expresses the human CCK gene at high levels and performs posttranslational processing of CCK.[8,9] Therefore, SK-N-MCIXC cells should provide a good *in vitro* model in which to study both the tissue-specific control of the induction of the CCK gene and the mechanisms responsible for the differential protein processing of the CCK precursor in neuronal systems.

To examine the effect of the cyclic AMP (cAMP) second messenger pathway on CCK mRNA in SK-N-MCIXC cells, the cells were treated with either the phosphodiesterase inhibitor isobutyl-methylxanthine (IBMX) or 8-bromo cAMP, a nonhydrolyzable analog of cAMP. Phorbol-12-myristate-13 acetate (PMA), a tumor-promoting phorbol ester and potential activator of phospholipase-dependent protein kinase C, and the inactive phorbol ester, 4α phorbol, were used to determine if the protein kinase C second messenger pathway influenced CCK mRNA levels. Additionally PMA and IBMX were added to the cells in combination, to reveal possible synergistic interactions between the two second messenger pathways. Cells were also treated with the DMSO vehicle; this treatment showed no effect ($n = 4$, $df = 6$, $t = .271$, NS). CCK mRNA was quantitated, after 12-hour drug treatments, with Northern blot analysis. The CCK probe was a 550 bp *Alu*I-*Alu*I fragment of exon 2 of the human CCK gene.[10] The β-actin probe was a 1-kb chicken cDNA fragment. cDNA probes were labeled using a random primed DNA labeling kit (Boehringer Mannheim Biochemica, Indianapolis, Indiana). [α-^{32}P]dCTP 3000 Ci/mmol (NEN, Boston, Massachusetts) was used to label the probe. Autoradiograms were analyzed with a Bio-Rad model 620 densitometer (Richmond, California). Cholecystokinin

---

[a] This work was supported by NIDDK grant DK 36289 and MH 42600 to T. P. Davis.

levels were standardized against β-actin levels. Statistical analysis was performed with the Student's t test for grouped data.

Activation of both cAMP and protein kinase C second messenger pathways increased CCK mRNA levels in SK-N-MCIXC cells. IBMX at a 5.0 μM concentration had no effect on CCK mRNA levels ($n = 3$, $df = 4$, $t = .271$, NS); however, 0.5 mM IBMX raised CCK mRNA levels 1.8-fold ($n = 3$, $df = 4$, $t = 2.785$, $p < 0.05$) (FIG. 1). Eight-bromo cAMP (0.5 mM) produced a 1.4-fold increase in CCK mRNA levels ($n = 3$, $df = 4$, $t = 3.053$, $p < 0.05$) (FIG. 1).

PMA (0.5 μM) increased CCK mRNA levels in SK-N-MCIXC cells approximately 2.5-fold ($n = 4$, $df = 6$, $t = 5.949$, $p < 0.01$) (FIG. 2). As expected, 4α phorbol

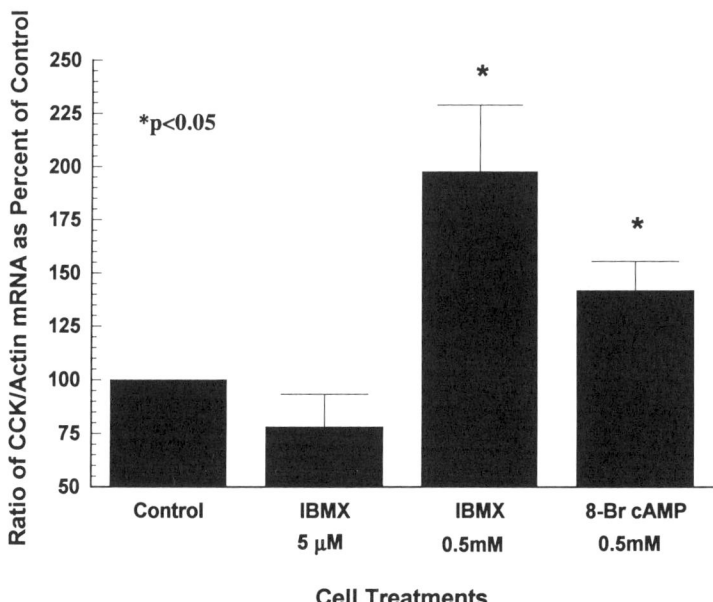

FIGURE 1. Levels of CCK mRNA after 12-hour treatments were determined by Northern blot analysis with a human CCK cDNA hybridization probe. IBMX at a 5.0 μM concentration did not affect CCK mRNA levels; 0.5 mM IBMX raised CCK mRNA levels 1.8-fold. Eight-bromo cAMP (0.5 mM) produced a 1.4-fold increase in CCK mRNA levels (*$p < 0.05$).

(0.5 μM) had no effect on CCK mRNA levels ($n = 3$, $df = 4$, $t = 0.562$, NS) (FIG. 2). PMA in combination with 5.0 μM and 0.5 mM IBMX increased CCK mRNA levels threefold ($n = 3$, $df = 4$, $t = 5.105$, $p < 0.01$) and 2.7-fold ($n = 3$, $df = 4$, $t = 4.615$, $p < 0.01$), respectively (FIG. 2). These values were not significantly different from the levels produced by PMA alone, suggesting that the two systems are not acting synergistically in SK-N-MCIXC cells or that under these experimental conditions the maximal increase in these cells is threefold.

Our results indicate that the levels of CCK mRNA in SK-N-MCIXC cells are regulated by both cAMP and protein kinase C-dependent mechanisms. These results in combination with previous data from this laboratory, which demonstrated: (1) the

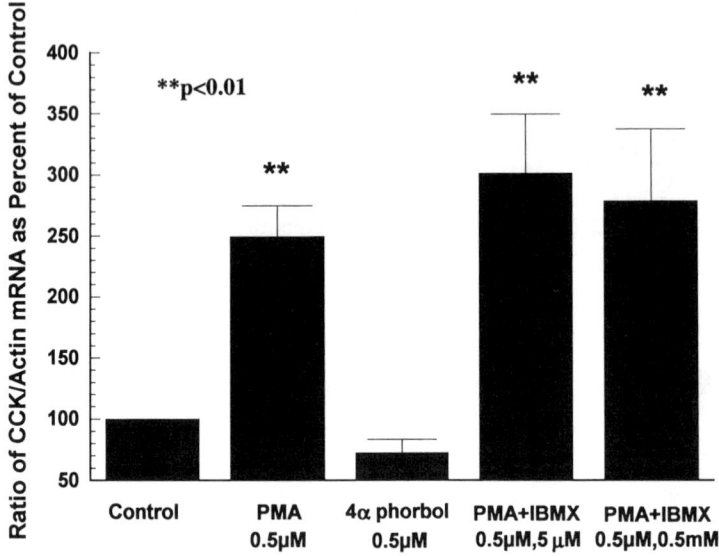

FIGURE 2. After 12-hour treatments, PMA (0.5 μM) increased CCK mRNA levels in SK-N-MCIXC cells approximately 2.5-fold. Four α phorbol (0.5 μM) had no effect on CCK mRNA levels. PMA in combination with 5.0 μM and 0.5 mM IBMX increased CCK mRNA levels 3- and 2.7-fold, respectively. These values were not significantly different from the levels produced by PMA alone (**$p < 0.01$).

presence of storage granules containing glycine extended CCK; (2) regulated and constitutive release of proCCK and its cleaved products; (3) mRNA for the intracellular processing enzymes prohormone convertase 1 and 2 and furin; and (4) the extracellularly localized, membrane-associated CCK-metabolizing enzyme neutral endopeptidase 24.11,[9] suggest that the SK-N-MCIXC cell line can be used as a model system to study drug, neurotransmitter, and steroid effects on CCK processing and metabolism.

REFERENCES

1. DOCKRAY, G. J. 1983. *In* Brain Peptides. D. T. Krieger, M. J. Brownstein & J. B. Martin, eds.: 851–869. Wiley. New York, NY.
2. REHFELD, J. F. 1988. J. Mol. Endocrinol. **1**: 87–94.
3. REHFELD, J. F. 1987. Proc. Natl. Acad. Sci. USA **84**: 3019–3023.
4. PERSSON, H., J. F. REHFELD, A. ERICSSON, M. SCHALLING, M. PELTO-HUIKKO & T. HÖKFELT. 1989. Proc. Natl. Acad. Sci. USA **86**: 6166–6170.
5. VANDERHAEGHEN, J. J., C. DESCHEPPER, F. LOTSTRA, G. VIERENDEELS & J. SCHOENEN. 1982. Cell Tissue Res. **223**: 463–467.
6. BEINFELD, M. C. 1983. Neuropeptides **3**: 411–427.
7. DAVIS, T. P. 1991. *In* Stress, Neuropeptides, and Systemic Disease. J. A. McCubbin, P. G. Kaufman & C. B. Nemeroff, eds. :149–177. Academic Press, Inc. Orlando, FL.
8. VERBEECK, M. A. E. & J. P. H. BURBACH. 1990. FEBS **268**: 88–90.
9. KONINGS, P. N. M., B. MANIA-FARNELL, M. C. BEINFELD, B. OAKES, R. DAY, N. G. SEIDAH & T. P. DAVIS. 1993. Neuropeptides **25**: 19–30.
10. TAKAHASHI, Y., K. KATO, Y. HAYASHIZAKI, T. WAKABAYASHI, E. OHTSUKA, S. MATSUKI & M. IKEHARA. 1985. Proc. Natl. Acad. Sci. USA **82**: 1931–1935.

Loxiglumide, a CCK-A Antagonist, in Irritable Bowel Syndrome

A Pilot Multicenter Clinical Study

P. A. CANN,[a] L. C. ROVATI,[b,f] H. L. SMART,[c]
R. C. SPILLER,[d] AND P. J. WHORWELL[e]

[a] *Middlesbrough General Hospital*
Middlesbrough, UK

[b] *Department of Clinical Pharmacology*
Rotta Research Laboratorium
20052 Monza, Italy

[c] *Royal Hallamshire Hospital*
University of Sheffield
Sheffield, UK

[d] *Queen's Medical Centre*
University of Nottingham
Nottingham, UK

[e] *University Hospital of South Manchester*
Manchester, UK

Cholecystokinin (CCK) is a neurohormonal peptide that is involved in the regulation of several digestive functions, contributing to the control of motility and secretions at different organ levels. Evidence indicates that CCK might be involved in the pathogenesis of irritable bowel syndrome (IBS).[1] Loxiglumide (CR 1505, that is, D,L-4-[3,5-dichlorobenzoylamino]-5-[N-3-methoxy-propil-pentylamino]-5-oxo-pentanoic acid) is a potent, selective, competitive, and orally bioavailable CCK_A receptor antagonist,[2,3] and it is the most widely used in physiological and therapeutic human studies.[4,5] Interestingly, loxiglumide appeared to accelerate colonic transit in healthy volunteers and chronic constipated elderly subjects[6,7] and to regulate regional colonic transit in IBS patients with different bowel habit patterns.[8] CCK_A antagonists have been proposed as potential candidates for drug treatment of IBS,[9] and we were therefore interested in testing the efficacy of loxiglumide on IBS symptoms in a pilot dose-response study, using doses only minimally affecting other gastrointestinal physiological functions such as gallbladder contraction.[10]

PATIENTS AND METHODS

Patients who, in the absence of organic digestive diseases, complained of abdominal pain and a disturbance of bowel habit for at least 6 months and on at least 3 days a week (to be confirmed by diary cards during a 2-week baseline period) were assigned to oral treatment with either placebo or loxiglumide 200 or 400 mg three

---

[f] Address for correspondence: Lucio C. Rovati, MD, Department of Clinical Pharmacology, Rotta Research Laboratorium S.p.A., Via Valosa di Sopra 7/9, 20052 Monza (MI), Italy.

times daily for 8 weeks, according to a randomized, double-blind, parallel-group design. Seventy-two patients satisfied the criteria for evaluation. Fourteen symptoms, mainly related to abdominal pain/discomfort and bowel habits, were each rated on a 100-mm VAS and on a 0–4 scale. Overall efficacy assessment by either patients or physicians were also recorded. Based on a forecasted placebo response rate of 40% and at least on a 15–20% superiority in one of the loxiglumide groups, ~100 patients per group would be necessary to show statistical significance (with alfa = 0.05 and beta = 0.2). This pilot study was designed to confirm this hypothesis and to be tested in larger trials. "Therapeutic responders" were patients with a positive overall efficacy assessment by patients themselves or physician and a decrease $\geq 25\%$ (compared to baseline) in an overall symptom score defined by the sum of VAS of the considered symptoms.

RESULTS AND CONCLUSIONS

Oral loxiglumide 400 mg three times daily for 8 weeks induced a significant improvement in IBS symptoms (including abdominal pain, distention, and change in bowel habit) compared to placebo and to a lower dose of 200 mg three times daily. This effect was more evident in constipation-predominant patients (C-IBS), and indeed abdominal pain and distention and constipation showed a ~50% improvement rate. The effects of loxiglumide on diarrhea-predominant IBS patients (D-IBS) were of similar magnitude (including diarrhea itself), but the sample size was small and placebo induced a similarly high response. Overall (sum of all symptoms in all patient subgroups), loxiglumide 400 induced a 63% ($n = 24$) responder rate, loxiglumide 200 57% ($n = 23$), and placebo 48% ($n = 25$). Loxiglumide superiority was confirmed, to a similar extent, by both the patients' and physicians' overall assessment, but the patients gave both doses of loxiglumide an equal score. Both patient and physician differentiated the active drug from placebo in the C-IBS subgroup, whereas the D-IBS subgroup was very sensitive also to the placebo effect. The three treatments were equally well tolerated. In conclusion, the CCK_A antagonist loxiglumide is a promising drug in the treatment of IBS according to the results of this first pilot study. Further larger trials are necessary to confirm these results and the possible role of CCK in the pathophysiology of IBS.

REFERENCES

1. HARVEY, R. F. & A. E. READ. 1973. The Lancet i: 1.
2. SETNIKAR, I., M. BANI, R. CEREDA, R. CHISTÈ, F. MAKOVEC, M. A. PACINI, L. REVEL, L. C. ROVATI & L. A. ROVATI. 1987. Arzneim.-Forsch. 37: 703.
3. SETNIKAR, I., M. BANI, R. CEREDA, R. CHISTÈ, F. MAKOVEC, M. A. PACINI & L. REVEL. 1987. Arzneim.-Forsch. 37: 1168.
4. ROVATI, L. C. 1991. Int. J. Pancreatol. 8: 215.
5. ADLER, G. & C. BEGLINGER, eds. 1991. Springer-Verlag. Berlin-Heidelberg.
6. MEYER, B. M., B. A. WERTH, C. BEGLINGER, P. HILDEBRAND, J. M. B. J. JANSEN, D. ZACH, L. C. ROVATI & G. A. STALDER. 1989. Lancet II: 12.
7. MEIER, R., C. BEGLINGER, M. THUMSHIRN, B. MEYER, L. C. ROVATI, G. GIACOVELLI, M. D'AMATO & K. GYR. 1993. J. Gastrointest. Mot. 5: 129.
8. BARROW, L., P. E. BLACKSHAW, C. G. WILSON, L. C. ROVATI & R. C. SPILLER. 1992. J. Gastrointest. Mot. 4: 207.
9. READ, N. W. 1991. In Cholecystokinin Antagonists in Gastroenterology: Basic and Clinical Status. :214. Springer-Verlag. Berlin-Heidelberg.
10. MALESCI, A., C. DEFAZIO, S. FESTORAZZI, C. BONATO, A. VALENTINI, M. TACCONI, M. BEKKERING, G. GIACOVELLI, M. D'AMATO & L. C. ROVATI. 1992. Arzneim.-Forsch. 42: 1359.

Clinical Efficacy and Prokinetic Effect of the CCK-A Antagonist Loxiglumide in Nonulcer Dyspepsia

A. S. B. CHUA,[a] M. BEKKERING,[b] L. C. ROVATI,[b,c]
AND P. W. N. KEELING[a]

[a]*Department of Gastroenterology*
St. James' Hospital
James Street
Dublin 8, Ireland

[b]*Rotta Research Laboratorium S.p.A.*
Via Valosa di Sopra 7/9
20052 Monza (MI), Italy

Although the etiology and pathophysiology of nonulcer dyspepsia remain unknown, abnormalities in gastrointestinal motility, more particularly delayed gastric emptying, are found in a substantial proportion of patients.[1] Cholecystokinin (CCK) significantly delays gastric emptying in humans,[2] whereas loxiglumide (CR 1505, i.e., D,L-4[3,5 dichlorobenzoylamino]-5-[N-3-methoxy-propilpentylamino]-5-oxo-pentanoic acid), a potent, selective, competitive, orally bioavailable CCK-A receptor antagonist,[3,4] is known to accelerate gastric emptying in healthy volunteers[5] as well as in patients with nonulcer dyspepsia.[6] Therefore, it was interesting to study the clinical efficacy and gastrokinetic effect of loxiglumide in patients with nonulcer dyspepsia with delayed gastric emptying using a dosage schedule to partially impair gallbladder contraction.[7]

PATIENTS AND METHODS

A randomized, double-blind, parallel group, placebo-controlled trial was carried out in 28 symptomatic outpatients with nonulcer dyspepsia (8 male, 20 female, aged 19–59 years, mean age 33). All patients complained of early satiety, postprandial bloating, and abdominal pain for at least 6 months and at least 3 days a week. The other inclusion criteria included normal upper gastrointestinal endoscopy, normal abdominal ultrasonography, a positive CCK provocation test (symptom appearance after CCK-8 6 ng/kg·min iv infusion), and delayed (half-emptying time [$t_{1/2}$] > 60 minutes for the solid phase) gastric emptying of a radiolabeled, mixed solid-liquid meal of about 400 Kcal. Patients were randomly assigned to placebo or loxiglumide 400 mg three times daily for 8 weeks if after a 2-week baseline period their symptoms were still present. Up to 15 symptoms of nonulcer dyspepsia were each evaluated on a 100-mm Visual Analogue Scale to generate a Cumulative Symptom Score (CSS).

---

[c]Address for correspondence: Lucio C. Rovati, MD, Department of Clinical Pharmacology, Rotta Research Laboratorium S.p.A., Via Valosa di Sopra 7/9, 20052 Monza (MI), Italy.

The effect of treatments was evaluated as the percentage of improvement in the CSS at 2, 4, and 8 weeks compared to baseline.

RESULTS

Despite a high rate of placebo response, a quicker, more pronounced, and sustained symptomatic relief was observed during treatment with loxiglumide (FIG. 1). "Responders" were defined as patients with symptomatic improvement, that is, a decrease of ≥ 15% in the CCS after 8 weeks. There were 11 of 12 responders (91.7%)

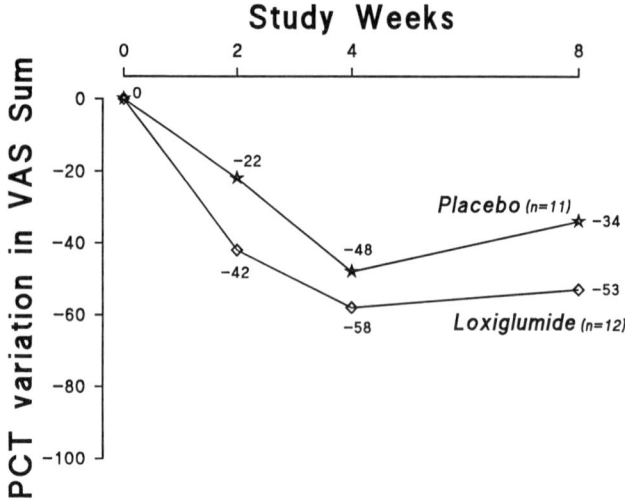

FIGURE 1. Average percent (PCT) variation in the overall symptom score (VAS sum) at each clinic visit in comparison with that of baseline in patients who completed the 8-week treatment period ($n = 23$). Patients in the loxiglumide group had earlier onset of efficacy than did those receiving placebo, and this was maintained up to the end of the study. Indeed, considerable improvement was reached already after 2 weeks, with a peak after 4 weeks that was maintained at the end of treatment. In the placebo group maximum effect is reached after 4 weeks of treatment, but then a clear trend is noted for the total score to return to baseline levels. The two AUCs are significantly different ($p < 0.05$) by ANOVA.

on loxiglumide compared to only 6 of 11 (54.5%) on placebo ($p = 0.04$, chi-square test). Similar results were obtained according to the patients' overall efficacy judgment. An intention-to-treat analysis, including also those patients who prematurely dropped out of the study, showed a response rate of 12 of 14 (85.7%) on loxiglumide vs 7 of 14 (50%) on placebo ($p = 0.04$, chi-square test). Gastric emptying (measured as $t_{1/2}$) could only be evaluated at the end of the treatment period in 12 patients. Loxiglumide induced a significant (paired Student's t test) acceleration only of solid phase gastric emptying ($t_{1/2}$ (mean ± SEM): baseline, 8 weeks: 85.9 ± 9.1, 60.7 ± 5.5; $n = 7$, $p = 0.02$), whereas placebo did not show any effect (71.6 ± 7.1,

66.0 ± 6.2; $n = 5$, $p > 0.5$). No correlation was observed between acceleration in gastric emptying and clinical improvement.

DISCUSSION AND CONCLUSION

Oral loxiglumide 400 mg three times daily for 8 week was significantly superior to placebo in controlling symptoms of nonulcer dyspepsia. Loxiglumide appears to act quicker and provide more sustained symptomatic relief. It showed a significant trend for a prokinetic effect of gastric emptying of solids, thus confirming previous observations, but no definite correlation was noted between symptomatic improvement and acceleration of gastric emptying. In conclusion, the CCK-A antagonist loxiglumide is effective in the treatment of symptoms of nonulcer dyspepsia and has a prokinetic effect. Further studies in a larger patient population are necessary to confirm these results as well as to determine the mechanism of action of the drug and the role of CCK in the pathogenesis of the disease.

REFERENCES

1. MALAGELADA, J. R. 1991. Scand. J. Gastroenterol. **26** (suppl. 182): 29.
2. LIDDLE, R. A., E. T. MORITA, C. K. CONRAD & J. A. WILLIAMS. 1986. J. Clin. Invest. **77**: 992.
3. SETNIKAR, I., M. BANI, R. CEREDA, R. CHISTÈ, F. MAKOVEC, M. A. PACINI, L. REVEL, L. C. ROVATI & L. A. ROVATI. 1987. Arzneim.-Forsch. **37**: 703.
4. SETNIKAR, I., M. BANI, R. CEREDA, R. CHISTÈ, F. MAKOVEC, M. A. PACINI & L. REVEL. 1987. Arzneim.-Forsch. **37**: 1168.
5. MEYER, B. M., B. A. WERTH, C. BEGLINGER, P. HILDEBRAND, J. B. M. J. JANSEN, D. ZACH, L. C. ROVATI & G. A. STALDER. 1989. Lancet **II**: 12.
6. LI BASSI, S., L. C. ROVATI, G. GIACOVELLI, L. BOLONDI & L. BARBARA. 1990. Gastroenterology **98**: A77.
7. MALESCI, A., C. DEFAZIO, S. FESTORAZZI, C. BONATO, A. VALENTINI, M. TACCONI, M. BEKKERING, G. GIACOVELLI, M. D'AMATO & L. C. ROVATI. 1992. Arzneim.-Forsch. **42**: 1359.

Cholecystokinin in the Hormonal Stimulation of Amino Acid Uptake and Pancreatic Enzyme Secretion

J. W. KONTUREK, A. GABRYELEWICZ,
R. STOLL, AND W. DOMSCHKE

Department of Medicine B
University of Münster
Münster, Germany
and
Department of Medicine
Medical School of Białystok
Białystok, Poland

Physiologic stimulation of exocrine pancreatic secretion as occurs after ingestion of a meal has been ascribed to activation of cholinergic reflexes and to the interaction of various gut hormones on pancreatic acinar cells. Cholecystokinin (CCK) and secretin are considered the major physiologic stimulants of pancreatic secretion. On pancreatic stimulation with CCK and secretin, enzymatic protein synthesis is increased 8- to 10-fold[1] and is accompanied by a significant reduction in plasma amino acids[2] presumably utilized in enzyme synthesis. This study evaluates the role of CCK in the control of exocrine pancreatic secretion and amino acid uptake during hormonal stimulation with caerulein and secretin using the highly selective antagonist of type A CCK receptors, loxiglumide.

MATERIAL AND METHODS

Seven healthy male volunteers (aged 21–27 years) were intubated with a double-lumen duodenal tube on two separate occasions. In the first series of tests, duodenal aspirates were collected during a 30-minute basal period and after stimulation with intravenous infusion of caerulein (50 pmol/kg-h) plus secretin (80 pmol/kg-h) during three consecutive 15-minute periods for determination of volume and output of HCO_3 and amylase.

During all tests, blood samples were drawn at 15-minute intervals for total plasma amino acid assay by a ninhydrin method described previously[2] to assess the activity of pancreatic enzyme synthesis. Additionally, changes of gallbladder volume and plasma pancreatic polypeptide concentrations were determined by ultrasound and specific radioimmunoassay, respectively.

On separate occasions, the same subjects underwent the same tests as just described, but the caerulein-secretin infusion was combined with a constant dose of loxiglumide (20 μmol/kg-h iv).

TABLE 1. Volume of Duodenal Aspirate, Bicarbonate, and Protein Output, Pancreatic Polypeptide (PP) Concentration, and Gallbladder (GB) Volume after Infusion of Caerulein (50 pmol/kg-h iv) and Secretin (80 pmol/kg-h iv) in Tests without (C + S) and with the Addition of Loxiglumide 20 μmol/kg-h iv) (C + S + LOX)[a]

	Aspirate Volume (ml/15 min)	HCO_3 (mmol/15 min)	Protein (mg/15 min)	PP (pM/L)	GB Volume (ml)
Basal	27 ± 9	0.3 ± 0.1	26 ± 4.6	18.6 ± 4.3	26 ± 8
C + S	68 ± 19[a]	9.4 ± 1.8[a]	93 ± 14[a]	134 ± 16[a]	2 ± 0.4[a]
C + S + LOX	81 ± 17[a]	11.4 ± 2.1[a]	51 ± 8.3[a,b]	68 ± 11.6[a,b]	22 ± 7[b]

[a] Significant change compared to basal values ($p < 0.01$).
[b] Significant change over control values.

RESULTS

Infusion of caerulein plus secretin significantly increased the volume of aspirate from basal 27 ± 9 to 68 ± 19 ml/15 minutes and the output of HCO_3 from 0.3 ± 0.1 to 9.4 ± 1.8 mM/15 minutes. The level of pancreatic polypeptide significantly increased from 18.6 ± 4.3 to 134 ± 16 pM/L, and the gallbladder volume was reduced from an initial 26 ± 8 ml to 2 ± 0.4 ml. After the addition of loxiglumide to the secretin-caerulein infusion, volume and HCO_3 in duodenal aspirates were unchanged, but pancreatic polypeptide release was decreased about 50% and gallbladder contractions were almost completely abolished (TABLE 1).

With secretin plus caerulein, amylase output rose from basal 5.8 ± 0.7 to 11.6 ± 1.2 KU/15 minutes, whereas plasma amino acid level decreased from an initial

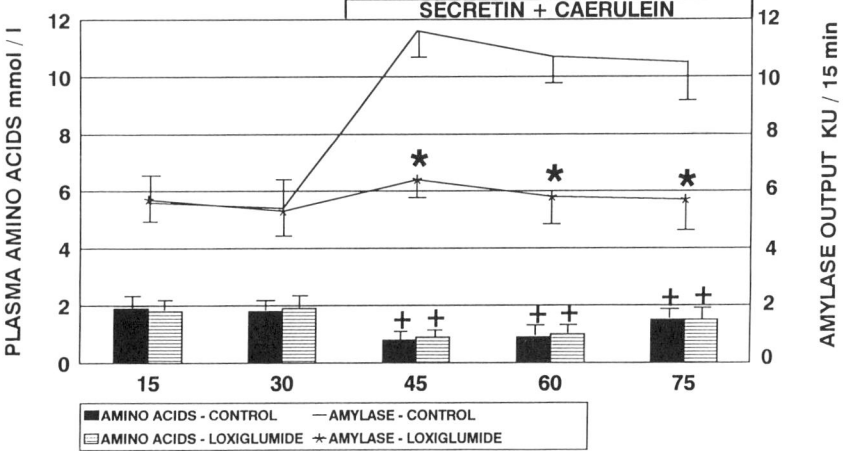

FIGURE 1. Plasma amino acid concentration and amylase output after pancreatic stimulation with caerulein (50 pmol/kg-h iv) and secretin (80 pmol/kg-h iv) in tests with and without the addition of loxiglumide (20 μmol/kg-h iv). *Asterisk* indicates significant change in amylase output compared to control values. *Cross* indicates significant change in plasma amino acids level compared to initial values ($p < 0.01$).

1.96 ± 0.3 to 1.09 ± 0.3 mmol/L ($p < 0.01$). After the addition of loxiglumide, amylase output decreased about 40%, but the total plasma amino acid level was unchanged (FIG. 1).

DISCUSSION

These results show that activation of type A CCK receptors is involved in caerulein-secretin–stimulated pancreatic enzyme secretion and gallbladder contraction, in agreement with previous observations.[3,4] Furthermore, we demonstrated that the increase in pancreatic enzyme secretion after hormonal stimulation is accompanied by a significant decrease in total plasma amino acids presumably utilized for enzyme synthesis.[2] CCK receptor antagonism did not affect plasma amino acids, suggesting that via activation of type A receptors CCK may not be involved in pancreatic protein synthesis.

REFERENCES

1. SOLOMON, T. E. 1987. Control of exocrine pancreatic secretion. *In* Physiology of the Gastrointestinal Tract. 2nd ed. L. R. Johnson, ed. 7:1173–1207. Raven. New York.
2. DOMSCHKE, S., G. HEPTNER, S. KOLB, D. SAILER, M. U. SCHNEIDER & W. DOMSCHKE. 1986. Decrease in plasma amino acid level after secretin and pancreozymin as an indicator of exocrine pancreatic function. Gastroenterology **90:** 1031–1038.
3. FRIED, M., U. ERLACHER, W. SCHWIZER, C. LOCHNER, *et al.* 1991. Role of cholecystokinin in the regulation of gastric emptying and pancreatic enzyme secretion in humans. Gastroenterology **101:** 503–511.
4. HILDEBRAND, P., C. BEGLINGER, K. GYR, J. B. JANSEN, L. C. ROVATI *et al.* 1990. Effects of a cholecystokinin receptor antagonist on intestinal phase of pancreatic and biliary responses in man. J. Clin. Invest. **85:** 640–646.

Summary and Conclusions

VAY LIANG W. GO

*The Brain Research Institute
University of California, Los Angeles
Los Angeles, California 90024–1761*

To all of you who came from Asia, Australia, Europe, and from throughout the Americas, many thanks for your active participation in our international meeting of May 1993. You were all magnanimous in your willingness to share information and knowledge in a very collegial and stimulating way. Your contributions to this conference served to advance, to a very great degree, our understanding of this particular neuropeptide, cholecystokinin.

I would also like to thank our sponsors, particularly the National Institute of Diabetes, Digestive, and Kidney Diseases; the National Science Foundation; the American Gastroenterological Association, and all the other industrial supporters listed in the table of contents. They made it possible for us to meet at Chatham, on beautiful Cape Cod, Massachusetts. This was a truly superb site for discussing where we have been, where we are now, and what the future may hold for research and clinical applications of cholecystokinin in health and disease. The ambiance of our meeting site did much, I think, to stimulate our thinking and our desire to learn more.

Quite frankly, the success of this conference truly exceeded the already high expectations of my fellow organizers, and much of this can be attributed to the conference coordinator, Joyce M. Fried, who worked wonders to turn the conference organizers' ideas and wishes into reality. I extend my warmest gratitude to her. My thanks also go to Mr. Bill Boland and his staff at the New York Academy of Sciences for allowing us to publish the proceedings in this volume. Finally, I want to acknowledge Dr. Martin W. Dodge, my assistant editor on the journal *Pancreas,* for coordinating the publication of these proceedings.

Although there were simply too many outstanding presentations at the symposium to say that any one or two stood above the rest, I would like, if I may, to highlight some of the findings that attracted my personal interest:

- Larger molecular forms of cholecystokinin, CCK_{58}, do exist, but the biosynthesis of cholecystokinin and its processing enzymes still needs to be defined, both in the gut endocrine I cell and in cerebral and spinal CCK neurons.
- The chemical structure of the common amidated COOH-terminus pentapeptide of CCK and gastrin has now been identified in several mammalian and nonmammalian vertebrates as part of a larger molecular form of peptide. This indicates that genes with different evolutionary histories encode the CCK-like peptides in various species.
- Cholecystokinin gene expression is regulated at multiple levels by dietary as well as neurohormonal factors.
- Since the physiology, biochemistry, and molecular biology of cholecystokinin receptors have undergone intense study, we have achieved the molecular cloning of cholecystokinin receptor families.
- Development of novel CCK analogs and first and second generation antagonists has contributed significance and, on some occasions, has even made us

revise our concepts of the neurophysiology and neuropharmacology of cholecystokinin.
* We have begun to appreciate the role cholecystokinin plays in its effect on human behavior (e.g., satiety, anxiety, panic disorders, and schizophrenia), in addition to its regulatory role in gastrointestinal functions.

Truly, we have obtained a great deal of new, important knowledge, not just from the symposium's oral lectures, but also through the contributions of the many people who presented their work in the poster sessions. Through these and our informal exchanges, we have begun to comprehend to a greater degree the roles that cholecystokinin plays in the sensory pathways and in the interactions of the brain-gut axis. We have also begun to understand the role of CCK as it interrelates with other neurotransmitters, both amine and amino acids and classical neurotransmitters, in the regulation of higher cerebral functions in health and disease, and to see the future role CCK will play in the neuroimmune axis.

The knowledge we are building in the mechanism and actions of cholecystokinin and its receptors is forming the basis for developing new agonists and antagonist agents. That development will open a new era for the role of cholecystokinin and its integrative functions in human health and diseases.

In addition, CCK has become a noble peptide, presenting us a road map to follow in investigating the form, pathways, and functions of other neuropeptides.

This volume truly reflects the extent of our current knowledge of cholecystokinin, as it stood by the end of this May 1993 symposium. I wish for all of us great vigor in pursuing our common academic interest in this peptide, and I hope we may meet again in 2 or 3 years to review our accomplishments over the intervening period.

Subject Index

Acetylcholine, 41
Acid-base interactions amd exocrine pancreatic secretion, 199–205
Agonists
　CCK-8s and pentagastrin as, pharmacology of, 129–130
　selective CCK receptor, 93–99, 101
Agoraphobia, 273
Amino acid analysis, 16–17
Amino acids and nonpeptide antagonist affinity, 67–78
Amylase release from pancreatic acini, CCK-58 and CCK-8 in, 15–16
Analogs
　of JMV180, biological evaluation of, 79–86
　synthetic, of CCK-7 and CCK-8, 107–116
Anorexia, CCK-induced, 232–233
Antagonist affinity, nonpeptide, 67–78
Antagonist pharmacology, 130–133
Antagonists
　gastrin and CCK-B, 118–119
　selective CCK receptor, 93–99, 101
　SR 27897 as, 364–367
　virginiamycin as, 353–354
Antroduodenal motility and CCK-A blockade, 222
Anxiety
　CCK in, 273–280
　and schizophrenia, 300–309
Apomorphine-induced inhibition of dopamine neuron firing, 364–367
Askin tumor, processing of proCCK in, 319–320
Asp-Phe amides, 39–40
Auditory startle reflex and LY288513, 374–376
Autoradiography of CCK-B receptors in brain, 380–383
Azaserine-induced pancreatic carcinogenesis, 439–441

Benzodiazepines, 312–318
　and CCK interactions, 132–133
　in panic disorder, 274
　withdrawal of, 374–376
Bicarbonate, ductal, and acinar lumen function, 199–205
Bile acids and pancreatic proteases inhibit CCK release, 174–177
Bile and bile acids, inhibition of CCK release by, 167–174
Bombesin, 41
Brain
　CCK action in, ionic mechanisms in, 129–135

CCK_B receptors
　autoradiography of, 380–383
　gastrin 13, and G protein binding, 346–348
　dopamine system of, and CCK-B antagonists, 306–399
　penetration of, and CCK-B antagonists, 360–363, 377–379
Brain-gut axis, 358–359
Brain regions, CCK, and satiety, 242–251
Brain stem, distention-induced c-fos immunoreactivity in, 164–166

C-fos in rat brain stem, gastric distention and, 164–166
Ca^{2+} mobilization, CCK8-evoked, in pancreas, 335–336, 343–345
Caerulein and cholecystokinin-pancreozymin, 4
Calcium influx in pancreatic acinar cell, 41–45
cAMP second messenger pathway and CCK mRNA, 446–448
Cancer, small cell lung, CCK in, 283–294
Capsaicin, 262–264
　and gastric motility and emptying, 143, 152
Carboxyl-terminal alpha amide structure, 4
Carcinogenesis, pancreatic, and CCK, 180–194, 439–441
Carcinoids, gastric, and CCK receptors, 435–438
CCK. See also Cholecystokinin
CCK "A" receptors, 15, 19
CCK "B" receptors, 19
CCK analogs, 457–458
CCK antagonists, 457–458
　and food intake, 431–434
　and meal size, 237
CCK/gastrin receptor antagonists CR 2345 and CR 2194, 395–397
CCK receptor affinity and nucleoside diphosphate kinase, 350–352
CCK receptor agonists and pancreatic growth, 422–423
CCK receptor antagonists
　and exocrine pancreas, 368–370
　and gut myoelectrical activity, 358–359
CCK receptor blockade
　and pancreatic enzyme secretion, 424–426
　in GRP-mediated pancreatic secretion, 427
CCK-4 as panicogenic agent, 275–280
CCK-7, synthetic analogs of, 111–112
CCK-8
　and dopamine D2 receptors, 386–387

459

and feeding after microinjection into brain, 249–251
and gastrin, 118–119
-evoked Ca^{2+} mobilization in pancreatic acini, 343–345
in gallbladder and colon in ferret, 401–403
in nonulcer dyspepsia, 298–299
inhibitory action of, on rat colon, 407–408
receptor binding of, 14–15
synthetic analogs of, 111–112
CCK-58, 457–458
and physiology of cholecystokinin, 18–19
as released form of cholecystokinin, 13
as stored form of cholecystokinin, 11–13
helix-turn-helix in NH$_2$ terminus of, 328–330
in several species, 14
natural and synthetic, 11–20
receptor binding of, 14–15
synthesis of, 17–18
bioactivity of, 18
CCK$_A$ and CCK$_B$/gastrin receptors in gastric carcinoids, 435–438
CCK$_A$ antagonist
and gastric response to fat, 393–394
devazepide and satiety, 372–373
in irritable bowel syndrome, 449–450
in nonulcer dyspepsia, 451–453
CCK$_A$ receptor antagonists, 261, 407–408
and gastric secretion, 442–444
and gastrointestinal motility, 226–227
and pancreatic enzyme secretion, 454–456
and satiety, 429–430
SR 27897, 364–367
CCK$_A$ receptors, 88–103
and pancreatic carcinogenesis, 439–441
and substance P, 420–421
expression of, 53
identical, in gallbladder and pancreas, 50–53
in gallbladder, effect of CCK-8 on, 401–403
in gastrointestinal system and brain, 338–341
in pancreatic acinar cells, 81–82
in rat pancreas, 331–333
in small cell lung cancer, 290–294
molecular cloning of, 338–341
selective antagonist for, 133–135
site of, 237–238
CCK$_B$ antagonist LY288513 and auditory startle response, 374–376
CCK$_B$ antagonists
and anxiety, 305–306
and enkephalin analgesia, 355–357
and schizophrenia, 301–305
brain penetration of, 360–363, 377–379

inhibit brain dopamine neurons, 300–309
new, 395–397
nonpeptide
first generation, 312–313
second generation, 313
CCK$_B$/gastrin antagonists, nonpeptide, 118–119
CCK$_B$/gastrin receptor, 67–78
in small cell lung cancer, 284–294
CCK$_B$ receptors, 88–103
and gastrin 13 binding, in brain, 346–348
and substance P, 420–421
and virginiamycin, 353–354
antagonists in panic disorder, 276
autoradiography of, 380–383
expression of, 58
by gallbladder, 56
in brain membrane, 81–83
in Jurkat T cells, 81–83, 84, 86
selective antagonist for, 133–135
cDNA deduced procionin, 324–327
cDNAs encoding precursors of gastrin, CCK, and caerulein, 36–37
Cells of immune system, CCK receptors in, 334–336
Cellular growth factors, neuropeptides as, 292–293
Cerebral cortex, CCK in, 158
Cholecystokinin, 358–359, 360–363
analogs, biological evaluation of, 79–86
for studying CCK$_B$ receptor, 107–116
and dopamine-mediated behaviors, 138–141
and enkephalin, antagonism between, 355–357
and exocytosis in pancreatic acini, 203–204
and gallbladder function, 207–213
and gastric motility, 219–223
and gastrointestinal function, 143–155
and gastrointestinal smooth muscle, 398–400
and nonulcer dyspepsia, 298–299
and pancreatic carcinogenesis, 439–441
and pancreatic function and morphology, 180–194
and satiety, 232–234, 236–240, 242–251
and vagal afferent activity, 121–127
bioactivity of, 14
biosynthesis of, 457–458
discovery of, 2
endogenous, and food intake, 255–264
and gastric secretion after food, 442
family of peptides and receptors, 207–213
gastric fundus, and lipids, 393–394
gastrin-releasing peptide, and proteases, 410–412
gene expression, 457–458

SUBJECT INDEX

in rat intestine, 22–29
gene, regulation of, 321–323
historical perspectives on, 1–7
in anxiety and panic disorder, 273–280
in cerebral cortex and at spinal level, 157
in gastroduodenal and intestinal motility, 413–416
in human stomach, 417–418
in nonmammalian vertebrates, 32–37
in pancreatic enzyme synthesis and secretion, 454
in rat brain, 129–135
in satiation and satiety, 268–270
in small cell lung cancer, 283–294
mode of action of, 133–135
mRNA in neuroepithelioma cell line SK-N-MCIXC, 446
octapeptide and potassium currents, 384–385
pancreatic growth induced by, 422–423
peripheral, and food intake, 431–434
physiology of, 11–20
processing-independent analysis for, 319
receptor antagonists, nonpeptide, 312–317
receptor family, 49–64
receptor subtypes
  and dopamine, 386–387
  multiple, 88–103
receptors
  high- vs low-affinity, 343–345
  in cells of immune system, 334–336
  in rat pancreas, 331–333
release, acid-induced, 388–389, 391–392
research on, 1–7
schizophrenia, and anxiety, 300–309
secretion
  and bile and bile acids, 167–170
  intraluminal nutrients in, 424–426
type A receptors, molecular cloning of, 338–341
Cholinergic system and CCK, interaction between, 183
Chou-Fasman analysis of CCK-58, 328
CI988, brain penetration of, 360–363
Cionin, 33–36, 207
  stimulation of trout gallbladder muscle by, 404–405
Cloning, molecular, 457–458
  of CCK_A receptors, 338–341
  of nucleoside diphosphate kinase, 350–352
  of rat CCK-B receptor, 380–383
Colon
  effect of CCK-8 on, in ferret, 401–403
  proximal, inhibitory action of CCK-8 on, 407–408
Cortex, cerebral, CCK in, 158
Corticostriatal pathway, CCK in, 158–159

Cyclic AMP, 41
Cyclic GMP mediating calcium entry, 43–44

D-amino acids, 7
D-tryptophan in CCK analogs in rat pancreatic acini, 83
Depression and CCK-B antagonists, 355–357
Dermorphin, 7
Devazepide, 237
  and dopaminergic neurons, 364–367
  and satiety, 372–373, 429–430
  as CCK_A receptor antagonist, 124–125
Diazepam and auditory startle response, 374–376
Diet and CCK gene expression, 22–25
Dietary fat and gastrointestinal motility, 226–230
Diphenylpyrazolidinone, 301
Dopamine, behavior mediated by, CCK modulation of, 138–141
Dopamine D2 receptors and CCK-8, 386–387
Dopamine neurons of brain, CCK-B antagonists inhibit, 300–309
Dopaminergic neurons and SR 27897, 364–367
Duodenal ulcer, CCK, and gastric secretion, 442–444
Duodenal vagal afferent responses to CCK, 125–127
Dyspepsia
  nonulcer, CCK-8 in, 298–299
  loxiglumide in, 451–453

Electrophysiology of CCK responses in rat brain, 131
Enkephalin analgesia and CCK-B antagonists, 355–357
Enterokinase and cholecystokinin, 5
Estrogen and CCK, 239
Exocrine pancreas
  secretion of, 203–204
  and CCK, 454–456

Fat, dietary, and gastrointestinal motility, 226–230
Feedback inhibition of CCK by pancreatic proteases, 167–177
Feedback regulation, CCK and neural pathways in, 153–155
Food intake
  and CCK, 255–264
  and peripheral cholecystokinin, 431–434
  release of hypothalamic CCK during, 244–251
  suppression of, by CCK, 121–127, 243–244

Fundus, gastric, response of, to fat and CCK, 393–394

G protein in gastrin 13 and CCK_B receptor binding, 346–349
Gallbladder
 and CCK-8 in ferret, 404–403
 and loxiglumide, 183–184, 185
 and secretin, 2
 of trout, cionin stimulation of, 404–405
Gallbladder CCK_A receptor
 expression of, 50–53
 in vitro studies of, 209–213
 in vivo studies of, 208–209
Gastrectomy, CCK, and food intake, 431–434
Gastric chief cells, 93
Gastric distention and c-fos in rat brain stem, 164–166
Gastric emptying and CCK receptor antagonists, 220–221
Gastric function, postprandial, CCK and, 143–145, 146
Gastric motility
 and CCK, 143, 417–418
 and CCK-8 analogs, 112–113
Gastric secretion, endogenous CCK, and food intake, 442–444
Gastric vagal afferent responses to CCK, 125–127
Gastrin, 207–208
 isolation of, 3
Gastrin 13, binding of, to CCK_B brain membrane receptors, 346–348
Gastrin [Ca^{2+}] mobilization in small cell lung cancer, 290–291
Gastrin receptors
 and CCK-B, 67–78
 and parietal cells, 63
Gastrin-like peptides from different species, 32
Gastrin-releasing peptide
 and CCK, 410–412
 in exocrine pancreatic secretion, 427
Gastrocolonic reflex and CCK, 222
Gastroduodenal motility
 and CCK-8 analogs, 112–113
 cholecystokinin in, 413–416
Gastrointestinal motility and CCK-A receptor antagonist, 226–230
Gastrointestinal tract, CCK in regulating function in, 143–155
Gene expression, CCK, 27
Genome project, 6
Glucagon and CCK, 239
GP2/PG matrix in zymogen granule membranes, 201–202

GP2/THP family of GPI-anchored proteins, 201–202
Growth factors, CCK and gastrin as, 292–293

H elix-turn-helix in NH_2-terminus of CCK-58, 328–330
Hormones, intestinal, and CCK gene expression, 25–26
Hybridization in identifying CCK receptor family members, 58–63
Hydrophobic moment analysis of CCK-58, 328
Hypothalamus
 microinjection of, with CCK, 358–359
 release of CCK from, and satiety, 249–251

I leum
 contraction and CCK-8 analogs, 113–115
 smooth muscle in, and CCK, 398–400
 substance P and CCK in, 420–421
 virginiamycin and CCK-B receptor binding in, 353–354
Imipramine and panic disorder, 276
Immune system, CCK receptors in cells of, 334–336
Immunoreactivity, invertebrate CCK-like, 39–40
Intestinal extracts, satiating effect of, 236–240
Intestinal motility, cholecystokinin in, 413–416
Intestinal satiety and endogenous CCK, 255–264
Intestine, rat, cholecystokinin gene expression in, 22–29
Intraluminal nutrients in pancreatic enzyme secretion, 424–426
Invertebrate CCK-like immunoreactivity, 39–40
Irritable bowel syndrome, loxiglumide in, 449–450

J MV180, 335–336, 344–345
 and pancreatic growth, 422–423
JMV180 cholecystokinin analogs, biological evaluation of, 79–86
JMV320, 334
Jurkat T-cells, CCK receptors in, 334–336

L -364,718 and CCK_A receptors, 93–99
L-365,260, 313–318, 334–336
 as CCK_B antagonist, 124–125
 brain penetration of, 360–363
 in CCK-B receptor binding, 353–354
L-368,935, 313–318

L-tryptophan in CCK analogs in rat pancreatic acini, 83
Loxiglumide, 222, 226–230, 237, 407–408
and exocrine pancreatic secretion, 368–370
and gastric secretion after food intake, 442–444
and satiety, 268
in gallbladder and pancreas, and CCK, 183–184
in irritable bowel syndrome, 449–450
in nonulcer dyspepsia, 298–299, 451–453
Loxtidine and gastric carcinoids, 435–438
LymnaDFamides, molluscs, 39
Lymphocytes, CCK in, 334–336

M

ethionine oxidation, 3
Migrating myoelectric complexes, 4
MK329, 221, 261, 263, 334–336
mRNA and diet, 22–29
Muscle, gastrointestinal, and cholecystokinin, 398–400
Myoelectrical activity of stomach, fasting, 358–359

N

eural elements, extrapancreatic, and CCK release, 388–389
Neurobiology of panic disorder, 273
Neuroepithelioma cell line SK-N-MCIXC and CCK mRNA, 446–448
Neuronal cholecystokinin, 5
Neurons
 chemoreceptive, and CCK, 255
 gastric mechanoreceptive, and CCK, 147
 sympathetic, and CCK8, 384–385
Neuropeptides
 as cellular growth factors, 292–293
 molluscan, a new family of, 39–40
Nonpeptidal receptor agonists and antagonists, 6
Nonpeptide antagonist affinity, 67–78
Nonulcer dyspepsia
 dysmotility-type, and CCK, 298–299
 loxiglumide in, 451–453
Nucleoside diphosphate kinase and CCK receptor affinity, 350–352
Nucleus accumbens, medial posterior *versus* anterior, 138–141
Nutrients, intraluminal, in pancreatic enzyme secretion, 424–426

O

leate and cholecystokinin release, 388–389

P

ancreas
 acinar cells of, Ca^{2+} mobilization in, 343–345

and CCK_A receptor expression, 50
and nucleoside diphosphate kinase, 350–352
carcinogenesis of, azaserine-induced, and CCK, 439–441
CCK release in, induced by acid, 388–389
endocrine, and cholecystokinin, 184–187
exocrine, and cholecystokinin, 181–184
rat, cholecystokinin receptors in, 331–333
secretion of, and loxiglumide, 368–370
Pancreatic acinar and duct cell secretion, coordinated, 203–205
Pancreatic acinar cells
 and CCK, 187
 calcium influx in, 41–45
 CCK-8 related analogs in, and binding, 108–111
 express CCK_A receptors, 50
 JMV180 and JMV179 analogs in, 79–86
Pancreatic enzymes
 secretion of, and cholecystokinin, 454–456
 intraluminal nutrients in, 424–426
Pancreatic proteases, inhibition of CCK release by, 174–177
Pancreatic secretion, 424–426, 454–456
 exocrine, and acid-base interaction, 199–205
 GRP-mediated, CCK receptor blockade in, 427
 induced, 410–412
Pancreozymin, discovery of, 2
Panic disorder, CCK in, 273–280
Pepsinogen release, 90–91, 94
Peptide analogs in differentiating receptor subtypes, 112–115
Peptides
 and cholecystokinin in nonmammalian vertebrates, 32–37
 cholecystokinin family of, 207–208
Peptone and CCK secretion, 424–426
Pharmacology of CCK responses in rat brain, 131
Phorbol ester (TPA) in treatment of pancreatic acini, 343–345
Phospholipase D in CCK-induced pancreatic growth, 422–423
Phospholipid effect, 6
Physiology of cholecystokinin, 11–20
PIA. *See* Processing-independent analysis
Potassium currents, CCK8, and sympathetic neurons, 384–385
Processing-independent analysis (PIA) for procholecystokinin, 319
Procholecystokinin
 mammalian, and cDNA deduced procionin, 324–327
 processing-independent analysis for, 319

Procionin, cDNA deduced, and mammalian CCK system, 324–327
Protein kinase C
  and CCK mRNA, 446–448
  in CCK8-evoked Ca^{2+} mobilization, 343–345
Pylorus, CCK receptors in, 238

R adioligand binding of CCK in gallbladder, 210–213
Reagents for studying cholecystokinin physiology, 11–20
Receptor binding of CCK-8 and CCK-58, 15
Receptor, gastrin, and CCK-B, 67–78
Receptor subtypes for cholecystokinin, 88–103
Receptors
  CCK, in cells of immune system, 334–336
  CCK_A and CCK_B (gastrin), in rat pancreas, 331–333
  structure of, 50
  selective antagonists for, 133–135
  cholecystokinin family of, 207–208
  for CCK on vagal and spinal afferents, 152–153
  pancreatic, and CCK-8 related peptides, 108–111

S atiation and satiety, regulation of, by CCK, 268–270
Satiety
  and cholecystokinin, 232–234, 236–240, 268–270
  and devazepide, 372–373
  and effect of CCK on brain regions, 242–251
  intestinal, and endogenous CCK, 255–264
Schizophrenia, cholecystokinin, and anxiety, 300–309
Scintigraphy, 221
Secretin, discovery of, 1
Sensory neurons, CCK in, 159–160
SK-N-MCIXC and cholecystokinin mRNA, 446–448
Small cell lung cancer and CCK, 283–294
[^{3}H]SNF 8702 autoradiography of CCK-B receptors in brain, 380

Somatostatin and CCK gene expression, 25, 27, 29
SP-1 protein binding, 321–322
Spinal cord, CCK in, 159–160
SR 27897 and dopaminergic neurons in rat, 364–367
Stomach and cholecystokinin, 417–418
Substance P and CCK in mouse ileum, 420–421
Sympathetic neurons, potassium currents, and CCK8, 384–385
Synaptosomal endoproteases, 5

T aste aversion conditioning, 232–234
Telenzepine and exocrine pancreatic secretion, 368–370
Trypsin inhibitor and plasma CCK levels, 22–25
Tyrosine kinase in CCK-induced pancreatic growth, 422–423

U lcer, duodenal, CCK, and gastric secretion, 442–444
Ureidoacetamides
  and CCK response, 377–379
  antagonist activity of, 118–119
USF protein binding, 321–323

V agal afferent fibers and CCK receptors, 238
Vagal sensory neurons and CCK in food intake, 255–264
Vagus nerve
  and CCK-induced suppression of food intake, 121–127
  and gastric emptying, effect of capsaicin on, 152–153
Vasoactive intestinal peptide (VIP), 3
Ventromedial hypothalamic slice, 315
Vertebrates, nonmammalian, cholecystokinin in, 32–37
Virginiamycin and CCK-B receptor binding in ileum, 353–354

Z ymogen granule membranes and acid-base interactions, 201

Index of Contributors

Ahlman, H., 435–438
Ahluwalia, N. K., 393–394
Amblard, M., 79–87

Bahnson, T. D., 41–48
Barbara, G., 226–232
Barbara, L., 226–232
Barreau, M., 377–379
Becker, H. D., 431–434
Beglinger, C., 219–225
Beinborn, M., 67–78
Bekkering, M., 451–453
Bell, R. H., Jr., 331–333, 439–441
Berger, J. E., 374–376
Bernad, N., 79–87, 334–337
Bertrand, P., 118–120, 377–379
Blanchard, J. C., 118–120, 377–379
Blevins, G. T., Jr., 350–352
Blevins, P. M., 350–352
Blommaert, A., 355–357
Bock, M. G., 312–318
Boden, P., 129–137
Böhme, G. A., 118–120
Bradwejn, J., 273–282
Brenner, L. A., 255–267
Broberger, C., 157–164
Brodish, R. J., 388–390, 391–392

Cann, P. A., 449–450
Capet, M., 118–120, 377–379
Castel, M.-N., 157–164
Castellanos, D. A., 429–430
Chapman, K., 312–318, 360–363
Chew, P., 11–21
Chua, A. S. B., 298–299, 451–453
Corinaldesi, R., 226–232
Corsi, M., 353–354
Crawley, J. N., 138–142

D'Amato, M., 393–394, 395–397
Dal Forno, G., 353–354
Davis, T. P., 446–448
Davison, J. S., 164–166
De Giorgio, R., 226–232
De Pont, J. J. H. H. M., 343–345
De Weerth, A., 49–66, 338–342
Derrien, M., 355–357
Dinan, T. G., 298–299
Dionne, V. E., 41–48
DiPardo, R. M., 312–318
Doble, A., 118–120, 377–379
Dockray, G., 157–164
Domschke, W., 442–445, 454–456
Dubroeucq, M. C., 118–120, 377–379
Durieux, C., 355–357

Elm, B. V., 431–434
Ervin, G. N., 232–235
Evans, C., 11–21
Eysselein, V. E., 11–21

Fang, S., 380–383
Fang, S.-N., 420–421
Fernández, A. G., 398–400
Fernández, E., 398–400, 413–417
Fink, A. S., 388–390, 391–392
Fletcher, A., 312–318
Fourmy, D., 79–87
Fournie-Zaluski, M.-C., 355–357
Franzoso, L., 226–232
Fraser, K., 164–166
Freedman, S. B., 312–318, 360–363
Freedman, S. D., 199–206
Freidinger, R. M., 312–318
Fujii, K., 407–409
Fulcrand, P., 346–349
Fuxe, K., 386–387

Gabryelewicz, A., 454–456
Galas, M. C., 79–87
Galleyrand, J. C., 346–349
Gibbs, J., 236–241
Go, V. L. W., 226–232, 242–254, 457–458
Golenhofen, K., 417–419
Goñalons, E., 398–400, 413–416
Green, G. M., 167–179, 424–426
Greenwood, B., 401–403
Gueudet, C., 364–367
Gukovskaya, A., 41–48
Gully, D., 364–367
Guyon, C., 118–120, 377–379

Hao, J.-X., 157–164
Hargreaves, R. J., 312–318
Harty, G. J., 358–359
Haruma, K., 407–409
Hashimoto, S., 380–383
Hauad, L., 79–87
Heald, A., 360–363
Hedlund, P. B., 386–387
Heintges, T., 180–198
Helton, D. R., 374–376
Herget, T., 283–297
Herken, H., 417–419
Herrera-Marschitz, M., 157–164
Ho, F. J., 11–21
Hoenderop, J. G. J., 343–345
Hökfelt, T., 157–164
Hoshino, M., 107–117
Hruby, V. J., 380–383, 420–421

Hughes, J., 157–164
Hunt, M., 380–383
Huppi, K., 338–342

Iguchi, K., 107–117

Jansen, J. B. M. J., 268–272
Jeantaud, B., 377–379
Jensen, R. T., 88–106
Jimenez, M., 413–416
Johnsen, A. H., 39–40, 324–327, 404–406
Jørgensen, J., 404–406

Kajiyama, G., 407–409
Kashimoto, K., 107–117
Keeling, P. W. N., 298–299, 451–453
Kemp, J. A., 312–318
Kishimoto, S., 407–409
Knapp, R. J., 380–383
Kobayashi, H., 407–409
Köhler, H., 410–412, 417–419, 427–428
Kölby, L., 435–438
Konturek, J. W., 442–445, 454–456
Konturek, S. J., 442–445
Kopin, A. S., 67–78
Koszycki, D., 273–282
Kreil, G., 32–38
Kreulen, D. L., 384–385
Kuvshinoff, B. W., 388–390, 391–392
Kuwahara, A., 107–117

Lallement, J. C., 346–349
Lamers, C. B. H. W., 268–272
Laur, J., 79–87
Le Fur, G., 364–367
Lee, A. K. S., 328–330
Lee, Y.-M., 67–78
Lepsien, G., 417–419
Levenson, S., 420–421
Li, M., 107–117
Li, X.-M., 386–387
Liddle, R. A., 11–21, 22–31
Lieverse, R. J., 268–272
Lignon, M.-F., 79–87, 334–337
Lima-Leite, A. C., 346–349
Lin, J.-T., 88–106
Lloyd, K. C. K., 143–156
Longnecker, D. S., 331–333, 439–441
Lüdtke, F.-E., 410–412, 417–419
Luthen, R., 180–198

Maccarini, M. R., 226–232
Machino, H., 407–409
Makovec, F., 395–397
Malatynska, E., 380–383
Maldonado, R., 355–357

Manfré, F., 377–379
Mania-Farnell, B. L., 446–448
Mantey, S. A., 88–106
Marshall, G. R., 312–318
Martin, G., 118–120
Martín, M. T., 398–400
Martinez, J., 79–87, 334–337, 346–349
Martinez, V., 413–416
Masclee, A. A. M., 268–272
McBride, E. W., 67–78
McFadden, D. W., 388–390, 391–392
Meana, J. J., 157–164
Mellin, E. C., 312–318
Merrill, B. J., 446–448
Mesquita, M. A., 393–394
Michalski, S., 417–419
Mitan, S., 401–403
Miyoshi, A., 407–409
Mochizuki, T., 107–117
Monstein, H.-J., 324–327
Moran, T. H., 121–128
Morino, P., 157–164
Morisset, J., 422–423
Morselli-Labate, A. M., 226–232
Mutt, V., 1–10

Nicholas, H. B., Jr., 328–330
Niederau, C., 180–198
Nielsen, F. C., 321–323
Nilsson, O., 435–438
Nitecki, S., 358–359
Noel-Artis, A. M., 79–87
Nustede, R., 410–412, 417–419, 427–428

Oliosi, B., 353–354

Paloheimo, L. I., 319–320
Pandol, S. J., 41–48
Patel, S., 312–318, 360–363
Pedersen, K., 321–323
Peiper, H.-J., 427–428
Pendley, C., 118–120
Peris, W., 395–397
Peterson, P., 380–383
Pietra, C., 353–354
Pisegna, J. R., 49–66, 88–106, 338–342
Porreca, F., 420–421
Povoski, S. P., 331–333, 439–441
Puke, M. J. C., 157–164

Qian, J.-M., 88–106
Quinn, S. M., 67–78

Ramadori, G., 427–428
Rao, R. K., 420–421
Rasmussen, K., 300–311, 374–376

INDEX OF CONTRIBUTORS

Raybould, H. E., 143–156, 431–434
Reeve, J. R., Jr., 11–21
Rehfeld, J. F., 39–40, 319–320, 321–323, 324–327
Reidelberger, R. D., 372–373, 429–430
Revel, L., 395–397
Ritter, R. C., 255–267
Rivard, N., 422–423
Rodriguez, M., 79–87
Roebuck, B. D., 439–441
Roques, B. P., 355–357
Rosen, N. A., 331–333
Rosenquist, G. L., 328–330
Rovati, L. C., 226–232, 298–299, 393–394, 395–397, 449–450, 451–453
Rozengurt, E., 283–297
Rydzewska, G., 422–423

Santucci, V., 364–367
Scearce, E., 374–376
Scheele, G. A., 199–206
Schick, R. R., 242–254
Schjoldager, B., 207–218, 404–406
Schlemminger, R., 427–428
Scholey, K., 312–318
Schusdziarra, V., 242–254
Schwartz, G. J., 121–128
Seiger, A., 157–164
Sethi, T., 283–297
Singer, M. V., 368–371
Smart, H. L., 449–450
Smith, A. J., 312–318, 360–363
Smith, G. P., 236–241
Solomon, T. E., 388–390, 391–392
Soubrie, P., 364–367
Spannagel, A. W., 424–426
Spiller, R. C., 449–450
Stanghellini, V., 226–232
Stöckmann, F., 427–428
Stoll, R., 442–445, 454–456
Streich, R., 410–412
Stutzmann, J. M., 118–120
Suzuki, M., 107–117
Szurszewski, J. H., 358–359

Takeda, Y., 107–117
Tamura, C. S., 255–267
Teichmann, R. K., 431–434
Teyssen, S., 368–371

Thompson, D. G., 393–394
Thorup, J. U., 324–327
Thurneyssen, O., 364–367
Trist, D. G., 353–354
Troncon, L. E. A., 393–394
Turkelson, J., 388–390, 391–392

Ungerstedt, U., 157–164

Valverde, O., 355–357
van Amsterdam, F. Th. M., 353–354
van de Westerlo, E. M. A., 350–352
van Emst-de Vries, S. E., 343–345
van Hoof, H. J. M., 343–345
van Mackelenbergh, M. G. H., 343–345
Varro, A., 157–164
Vergara, P., 413–416
Verge, V., 157–164
Vigna, S. R., 11–21

Walsh, J. H., 283–297
Wamsley, J. K., 380–383
Wängberg, B., 435–438
Wank, S. A., 49–66, 88–106, 338–342, 435–438
Wechselberger, C., 32–38
Whorwell, P. J., 449–450
Wiesenfeld-Hallin, Zs., 157–164
Willems, P. H. G. M., 343–345
Williams, J. A., 350–352
Woltman, T. A., 372–373
Woodruff, G. N., 129–137
Wu, S. V., 283–297

Xian, H., 384–385
Xu, X.-J., 157–164

Yaksh, T. L., 242–254
Yamamura, H. I., 380–383, 420–421, 446–448
Yanaihara, C., 107–117
Yanaihara, N., 107–117

Zalewska, T., 380–383
Zhang, X., 157–164
Zheng, L. Q., 107–117
Zhou, W., 331–333, 439–441
Zittel, T. T., 431–434

OHIO UNIVERSITY LIBRARY